NURSING DIAGNOSIS

PROCESS AND APPLICATION

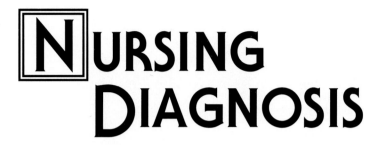

NURSING DIAGNOSIS

PROCESS AND APPLICATION

MARJORY GORDON, PhD, RN, FAAN

Professor of Nursing,
Boston College,
Chestnut Hill, Massachusetts

THIRD EDITION

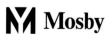 Mosby

St. Louis Baltimore Boston Chicago London Madrid Philadelphia Sydney Toronto

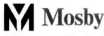

Publisher: Alison Miller
Editor: Timothy M. Griswold
Developmental Editor: Janet Livingston
Project Manager: Gayle May Morris
Editing and Production: University Graphics, Inc.
Manufacturing Supervisor: Betty Richmond

THIRD EDITION

Printed in the United States of America
Composition by Clarinda Company
Printing/binding by R. R. Donnelley & Sons Company

Mosby–Year Book, Inc.
11830 Westline Industrial Drive
St. Louis, Missouri 63146

Library of Congress Cataloging in Publication Data

Gordon, Marjory.
    Nursing diagnosis : process and application / Marjory Gordon.—
3rd ed.
        p.   cm.
    Includes bibliographical references and index.
    ISBN 0-8016-6053-X
    1. Nursing diagnosis. I. Title.
    [DNLM: 1. Nursing Diagnosis.   WY 100 G664n 1993]
RT48.6.G67 1993
616.07′5—dc20
DNLM/DLC   93-31601
for Library of Congress   CIP

    94   95   96   97   /   9   8   7   6   5   4   3   2

Like hues and harmonies of evening—
Like clouds in starlight widely spread—
Like memory of music fled—
Like aught that for its grace may be
Dear, and yet dearer for its mystery.

Thy light alone—like mist o'er mountain driven,
or music by the night—wind sent
through strings of some still instrument,
or moonlight on a midnight stream,
Gives grace and truth to life's unquiet dream.

P. B. Shelley
Hymn to Intellectual Beauty

PREFACE

This third edition of *Nursing Diagnosis: Process and Application* is published approximately 20 years after the first national conference on diagnostic classification was called by Kristine Gebbie and Mary Ann Lavin at St. Louis University. Since 1973 nursing diagnosis has become an integral part of professional nursing practice and has served to make nursing more visible in its contribution to health care. Today, work on classifications for nursing practice has extended to an international effort that involves many countries and cultures around the world.

The relevance of nursing diagnosis to practice, education, and research will sustain enthusiasm for continued development in the years ahead. Since the first edition of this book in 1982, use of nursing diagnosis has grown considerably. Clinical textbooks include nursing diagnoses, and professional nursing associations and health care accrediting agencies view diagnosis as a national standard of professional practice. The American Association of Colleges of Nursing and the National League for Nursing emphasize critical thinking and clinical judgment as essential content in nursing education. The clinical applicability of critical thinking is seen in clinicians' diagnostic and therapeutic judgment.

The purpose of *Nursing Diagnosis: Process and Application* is to integrate nursing diagnosis as a category and as a critical thinking activity. A career in professional nursing requires competence in clinical reasoning, as well as the use of diagnostic categories. Knowledge of terms from a manual is necessary, yet terminology without diagnostic process skills leads to inaccurate clinical judgments. Similarly, diagnostic skill without terminology is akin to speaking ability without language. The success of the first two editions can be attributed to the clear, in-depth treatment of the subject and its application to nursing process, practice, and health care delivery. The chapters in this book provide the beginning professional nursing student with a solid foundation on which to build clinical knowledge and experience.

This edition was written with the expectation that the student will begin to use this book in the first course dealing with nursing process. As clinical experience with clients increases, the reader will find it useful to refer again to the sections on process and application. In fact, development of diagnostic expertise requires a lifelong commitment to learning, and the reader will "see" new things after graduation when this book is reread and clinical knowledge accumulates.

In this edition of *Nursing Diagnosis: Process and Application,* one chapter has been added, all have been updated, most have been revised or extended, and further examples have been added to clarify ideas. Rather than placing questions and exercises at the end of chapters, they are incorporated into the text as a learning tool. Questions that students may raise, or should raise, are included. In some chapters the questions exemplify actual problems informally solicited from undergraduate students learning nursing diagnosis. Raising questions, as a teaching style, encourages students to raise their own questions as they study and use nursing diagnoses.

Exercises followed by a discussion of right and wrong answers are also incorporated into the text. This provides immediate feedback and permits learning to be applied before moving to the next topic. Within the text, salient points are italicized or listed for easier identification by the student. Summaries at the end of each chapter provide a succinct review of major points. Appendixes include current information on diagnoses and their development, simple to complex exercises in aspects of the diagnostic process, and additional content and examples in two areas.

In this edition the major themes from previous editions have been retained: *What is a nursing diagnosis? How are diagnoses made? How are they used in nursing process and in care delivery?*

Nursing diagnosis: concept and category

In *Chapters 1 and 2,* the following important aspects of diagnostic categories are discussed: the evolution of diagnostic categories, the context in which they are used, and nursing diagnosis defined as a concept and a process. Diagnoses are stressed as being important to treatment planning and in articulating the unique perspective of nursing. They are concepts used in clinical reasoning to describe the health status of a person, family, or community. Currently most textbooks and clinical agencies use the North American Nursing Diagnosis Association Diagnostic Classification System. Some are not sufficiently precise, conceptually consistent, or fully descriptive of the unique aspects of nursing. Despite this, clinicians find the available categories useful in thinking about nursing care. Students need to recognize that in any profession, concepts evolve as knowledge evolves from clinical research.

In *Chapter 3,* nursing diagnosis is considered with diagnosis in medicine and in social work. Content on the focus, frameworks, ideas about causality, classification systems, and process is presented. It is important for the student to gain an appreciation that diagnoses in nursing are evolving in a manner similar to that of other professions' diagnoses. In this chapter the student will gain a broad perspective on the major health professions and an appreciation of the similarities and differences between medical and nursing diagnoses. Many professions interact in care delivery, and each has to appreciate the other's focus of practice.

Further information on the major aspects of diagnostic category development and classification is contained in Chapter 12. Issues in development, critiques, and progress in classification are discussed. The student will encounter clinical situations for which a problem has not been described and labeled. This chapter provides information on

how to create a nursing diagnosis. It also provides some hints on helping others move to diagnosis-based practice.

Nursing diagnosis as critical thinking

Many aspects of critical thinking are required in diagnostic reasoning and judgment. New research in this area has resulted in major changes and additions in most of the five chapters dealing with this topic. There is no one diagnostic process that everyone should use all the time. Clinical reasoning situations differ. It may be most useful for students to study the *components* of reasoning and how these apply to the types of tasks they will encounter in clinical practice rather than searching for one reasoning mode. Being aware of the cognitive operations involved will allow flexibility and broad applicability of thinking skills. In Chapters 4 through 8 the reader will find discussions of nursing perspectives, useful information on functional assessment, strategies for collecting and processing information, and the formulation and statement of nursing diagnoses.

The content of *Chapter 4* is based on the assumption that diagnosis in nursing requires taking a nursing perspective on a situation, just as medical diagnosis requires a medical perspective. Grand theories or frameworks, such as self-care agency, adaptation, and others, provide a perspective and a framework for diagnosis, intervention, and outcome projection. *Chapter 5* focuses on functional health patterns. This is a basic framework at a concrete level that can be used as a structure for assessment with any model, including a simple functional model. The reader is helped to see how assessment of health patterns can provide a basic data base for health status assessment and nursing diagnosis. A detailed examination of issues related to the use of functional health patterns in practice is provided. Following this, in *Chapter 6* dysfunctional and potentially dysfunctional health patterns (nursing diagnoses) are discussed. Guidelines for investigating changes from functional to dysfunctional patterns are provided.

Assessment is the information-collection component of the diagnostic process. All elements that combine to make an assessment efficient and accurate are contained in the discussions of *Chapter*

7. Two factors that influence clinical reasoning are described: the type of assessment and the nature of clinical information. The diagnostician's "basic tools" are introduced in this chapter. These include perception, intuition, and inference. Recent work on these abilities and their role in novice and expert thinking is included. *Chapter 8* focuses on the interpretation and clustering of assessment information and the generation of possible diagnoses. Interpretation and clustering of data has been a source of difficulty experienced by learners. In consideration of this, multiple case examples, clear explanations, and a description of sources of possible interpretations are provided. *Chapter 9* deals with another area of difficulty in diagnostic judgment, the formulation of a diagnostic statement. This is the component of judgment wherein ideas about the client's health status are described by diagnostic categories in words that can be communicated. Clear descriptions of useful diagnostic statements are presented. The chapter includes dilemmas identified by undergraduate students and possible solutions; they will be familiar to all novices.

Application of nursing diagnosis

Chapter 10 describes the use of nursing diagnosis in direct care activities, primarily in planning interventions and evaluating outcomes. New work on national practice guidelines is related to nursing diagnosis and treatment. It is stressed that whereas clients may manifest the same diagnosis, care is individualized in the intervention phase. A discussion of who should diagnose, as well as nursing diagnosis and the law, is also included in this chapter.

Chapter 11 is based on the assumption that professional nursing students will eventually assume professional responsibilities. An appreciation must be gained of the issues in nursing practice to which nursing diagnosis applies. Therefore, the relevance of nursing diagnosis to case management, quality assurance, prospective payment and reimbursement, staffing, and other care delivery issues is discussed. *Chapter 12* focuses on issues related to classification and implementation. It ends with a section on future directions of nursing diagnosis and its application.

Many individuals contributed to the development of this book. Early interest in the diagnostic process was stimulated by debates and deliberation with colleagues, especially Carol Soares-O'Hearn and Florence Milliot. Further work in cognitive theory and nursing diagnosis was made possible by a National Institutes of Health Fellowship for doctoral study and by two encouraging advisors, John Dacey and John Travers, and at a later date by a grant from the USDHHS, Division of Nursing, on teaching diagnostic and ethical reasoning with Catherine Murphy. My association with the North American Nursing Diagnosis Association as President and as a member of the Massachusetts Conference Group on Classification of Nursing Diagnosis prompted consideration of specialties other than my own and broader issues of development and implementation. Many lively discussions about diagnosis with colleagues, Ann McCourt in particular, have contributed to this revision. For raising questions that needed answers, I thank graduate students at Boston College. I am also indebted to Beth Porter and undergraduate students who commented on parts of this edition. Finally, gratitude is extended to Terry Van Schaik, Janet Livingston, and Gayle Morris, of Mosby, and to Les Kaplan and Donna Coggshall at University Graphics, who deserve special thanks.

Marjory Gordon

CONTENTS

7 Clinical Information Collection, 121

9 Diagnostic Statements and Diagnostic Errors, 196

APPENDIXES

CHAPTER 1

NURSING DIAGNOSIS: EVOLUTION AND CONTEXT

D uring the twentieth century clinical judgment in nursing evolved into a visible component of practice and an essential concept in education. Nurses have always collected information through the process of assessment and used this information to make judgments about a client's[1] need for care. About three decades ago this process began to be called *nursing diagnosis*. The identification of a diagnostic language permitted labeling of clinical judgments and recognition of health problems that are the unique focus of nursing. The implementation of nursing diagnosis in practice required that nurses sharpen their diagnostic judgment skills and assume responsibility and accountability for their nursing diagnoses.

As nursing diagnosis was implemented in practice settings it became the basis for the assessment of quality nursing care delivery and a measure of accountability to the consumer. Directors of nursing departments in health care agencies began to appreciate that nursing diagnoses combined with medical diagnoses offered a means of determining the number and competency of staff required to deliver care and the cost component of nursing care delivery. Professional practice could now be differentiated from other levels. As clients' records in hospital and community agencies became computerized, statistics on nursing diagnoses, treatments, and outcomes of care became available for practice, research, educational, and health planning purposes. The demand for knowledge about the treatment of health problems described by nursing diagnoses stimulated researchers to focus on these problems. Their research, described in a uniform, common language, could now be found in the literature more easily than before. These developments led to greater use of nursing research and improved care. Are all these developments in place in every health care agency? Not yet, but there is strong evidence that nursing is moving in these directions. For this reason it is important to grasp the concept and definition of nursing diagnosis, as well as its evolution in the profession.

An understanding of nursing diagnosis begins with a knowledge of its development. This chapter traces the concept from its first appearance in the nursing literature to its present role in nursing process, nursing practice, and health care delivery. Chapter 2 discusses the similarities and differences in nursing and medical diagnoses, as well as the conceptual and structural characteristics of diagnostic categories. A broader view of the concept will be attained after studying Chapter 3, which contrasts and compares nursing diagnosis with other health professionals' use of diagnosis in their practice.

The next chapters focus on learning how to make a nursing diagnosis that will direct nursing treatment. The first requirement is a good comprehension of the nursing perspective, which can be gained by examining practice models that guide assessment and diagnosis. These models provide direction for developing nursing treatment plans as well. Chapter 4 considers diagnosis from the perspective of various nursing models. Chapter 5 presents a functional health pattern assessment format compatible with these models. This format for assessment is currently used in a variety of health care settings and permits the nurse to move from data to diagnosis with the least cognitive strain. Chapter 6 contains an overview of nursing diagnoses (i.e., dysfunctional patterns). Having studied what to assess and common diagnoses, the reader will be guided through the diagnostic process, starting with information collection as described in Chapter 7. How to arrive at a diagnostic judgment and problem formulation are the foci of Chapters 8 and 9.

A grasp of nursing diagnosis and the diagnostic process will prepare the reader for Chapter 10, which covers use of diagnosis in direct care. This chapter also includes a discussion of legal and moral accountability, standards of care, and communication through written and computerized records. Chapter 11 contains new views of older practice issues. These issues include the relevance of nursing diagnosis to evaluation of care for purposes of quality assurance, staff allocation, prospective payment, and cost containment. The broader issues of the scope of nursing practice and the development of nursing theory are also related to nursing diagnosis. The development of a classification system for nursing diagnoses is discussed in Chapter 12. A brief review of nursing diagnosis research and of methods for the clinical study of nursing diagnoses is also included in Chapter 12. It is assumed that the reader will be enthusiastic about the concept of diagnosis and wish to influence its development and direction. Chapter 12 reviews methods for identifying and clinically testing diagnostic categories. In summary, this book focuses on the area of practice described by nursing diagnoses. It deals with what a diagnosis is, the diagnostic process, and the application of these concepts to nursing practice.

HISTORICAL TRACES

The term *nursing diagnosis* has had a relatively short history; as an actual practice, it goes back to the founding of modern nursing. Florence Nightingale and her colleagues diagnosed nutritional deficits and other health problems exhibited by Crimean War casualties. On the basis of those nursing diagnoses, interventions were undertaken to improve the system of care in military hospitals. It was nearly a century later before nurses began to recapture the image Nightingale had projected as diagnostician, epidemiologist, and researcher.

In this section an overview of nursing diagnosis will prepare the reader for the more in-depth studies in later chapters. Salient issues related to diagnostic category development[2] and classification will be stressed from the perspective of history-in-context. After 20 years of development, it is interesting to reflect on how diagnosis has influenced nursing and how other developments in nursing have influenced nursing diagnosis.

Evolution of nursing diagnosis

About the middle of the twentieth century the scientific method of problem solving was applied to nursing, which in turn led to the idea of a nursing process. This process involved identifying nursing (therapeutic) problems and deciding on a course of action, marking a change in the role of the nurse. Nursing-prescribed intervention was added to the physician-prescribed intervention that had previously been the essence of practice.

It is interesting, in light of the predicted increase in chronic illnesses, that the first major clinical use of nursing diagnosis was in the care of clients with chronic illness and disability, an area in which physician-prescribed intervention is low. In the early 1960s Bonney and Rothberg[3] employed nursing diagnosis as a client-evaluation instrument to predict needs for nursing care. The objective was to use the clients' nursing diagnoses as predictors of staffing needs in long-term care facilities and as a focus for nursing intervention. As one of the authors commented in a separate paper:

We were determined to show that nursing was a cognitive process, that it wasn't just a simplistic laying on of hands, that it had a process that was logical and consistent, one that could predict outcomes. . . . The crucial point underlying the entire movement (use of nursing diagnosis) is that nursing is a cognitive process (in addition to its intuitive and empathetic aspects) and good nursing care is the result of thoughtful analysis.[4]

Conceptual models of the nursing process appeared in the literature in the late 1960s, and nurses began to identify which treatments and goals were within the province of nursing. In the context of these developments the evolution from nurses' problems (therapeutic problems and goals) to nursing diagnoses (patient problems) occurred. Most influential in this transition were the publication of standards of practice and the first conference on nursing diagnosis.

In 1973 a national invitational conference was called by two faculty members of St. Louis University, Kristine Gebbie and Mary Ann Lavin. The reasons for calling the First Conference on Classification of Nursing Diagnoses were twofold. First, administrators wished to know what nursing data would be included in the computerized documentation systems that were to replace patients' charts. At that time there were no names for the problems within nursing's domain of practice. Nurses used standard medical terminology and extended that terminology to encompass what they saw from a nursing perspective. Second, hospitals, beginning cost containment efforts, wanted to know why two care providers were seeing each patient in an outpatient clinic. Why should a patient see both a nurse and a physician? Did they not do the same thing?[5]

The stated purpose of the first conference was to identify and classify conditions diagnosed and treated by nurses. *Classification,* or *categorization,* involves identifying, naming, and systematically grouping entities based on their relationships. A *diagnostic taxonomy* refers to both the classification system and the rules for classifying conditions. Here the terms *classification system* and *taxonomy* will be used interchangeably. The importance of having categories or classes of diagnoses is that *by placing assessment data in a diagnostic category, one can "explain" the data and draw on all the clinical knowledge about the category stored in memory.*

A number of early writers on nursing diagnosis[6-9] had already used the term *nursing diagnosis* and recognized the importance of clinical judgment, but this first conference represented the initial effort in developing a language to describe diagnostic judgments. Until terminology began to be developed, no clear and consistent language was available for use in clinical settings. Nurses were taught not to make judgments; it was proper to say "appears to be bleeding." Nurses at the first diagnosis conference in 1973 clearly indicated that they made diagnostic and therapeutic judgments and needed a language to communicate these judgments. As classification activities progressed the need for a diagnostic language was challenged by some nurses and physicians. Why did nurses need a different language, and why use the term *diagnosis?*

Well into the 1970s, it was maintained by many that diagnosis was the province of the physician. Levine[10] suggested the word *trophicognosis* to more clearly express the idea of diagnosis in nursing. Others believed that the term *nursing diagnosis* was more easily understood within the healthcare professions. King,[11] a physician, dispelled the notion that only physicians use the cognitive process of diagnosis. A cognitive, or intellectual, process does not belong to any one group. Traditionally, diagnosis was associated with the field of medicine, but times and language change. The word *diagnosis* is now used to refer to a judgment process; for example, you can take your car to a diagnostic clinic. *Nursing diagnosis* is used widely in journals, textbooks, and manuals, indicating its acceptance as a way of describing conditions amenable to nursing intervention. It is interesting that the same concerns about the word *diagnosis* are arising in other countries as they begin implementing nursing diagnosis.

At the First National Conference a list of diagnoses was developed by the clinicians, educators, researchers, and theorists who attended.[5] Some have criticized the fact that the first conference work groups used a biomedical systems approach to identify the conditions nurses diagnose and treat. In 1973 the biomedical approach was the prevailing framework for thinking in clinical situations; thus it was a useful starting point for the participants. The list of diagnoses reflected a scope and focus well beyond biomedical systems. Since 1973 the proceedings of nine additional conferences have been published.[12] During each conference, participants approved diagnostic terms to describe actual and potential health problems or held forums on the diagnoses submitted, which were later voted on by the membership. At present 119 specific diagnoses have been accepted for clinical testing by the North American Nursing Diagnosis Association (NANDA).[13] These diagnoses are listed alphabetically in Appendix A.

Grouping diagnoses under a functional health patterns typology in 1975 enhanced the learning of the diagnostic process and tied assessment categories to diagnosis. The functional health patterns typology, using the NANDA and a few other diagnoses, was later published in the first edition of this book.[14] The grouping of diagnoses is contained in Appendix B and was proposed for clinical use.

For classification purposes (as more diagnoses were accepted nationally), NANDA viewed the alphabetical listing as inadequate. In 1986 diagnoses were placed by NANDA in a framework of human response patterns originally developed by nurse theorists between 1978 and 1982.[15] Currently, diagnoses are arranged according to an adaptation of the theorists' framework (Appendix C). Every two years, following a process of diagnosis review, sets of diagnoses are added to the classification system called *Taxonomy I.*[13]

Most would agree that the list of health problems diagnosed and treated by nurses is incomplete. Work continues on the identification, refinement, and classification of diagnoses. All scientific knowledge is tentative, and this is particularly true of a classification containing health problems, most of which have not been formally tested in clinical practice or subjected to conceptual analysis. It is important to remember this caveat when using diagnostic categories. Although limitations exist, clinicians find that using a diagnostic language greatly facilitates their practice and clarifies what they have to offer clients.

Responsibility for classification system development

The participants in the First National Conference for Classification of Nursing Diagnoses in 1973 established a coordinating body called the Task Force of the National Group for Classification of Nursing Diagnoses. This task force was independent of any professional organization, and its members managed to finance their attendance at meetings creatively. The task force set the direction for the classification work, examined issues, planned conferences, encouraged implementation, and established an office and clearing house at St. Louis University. In 1982 the organization was incorporated as North American Nursing Diagnosis Association, reflecting the collaborative work of nurses in the United States and Canada. A president and

board of directors were elected, and a committee structure was designed, including a working group to review diagnoses submitted, to develop a taxonomy, and to classify the diagnoses that were approved.

Historically a fundamental principle set by Gebbie and Lavin[5] at the First National Conference was that all nurses should feel they could be involved in diagnosis development and classification. Classification belongs to all nurses, not just to an elite group of developers. Thousands of nurses have participated in classification work so far. As will be seen, much work has yet to be done; nurses need to join in the generation, refinement, and classification of nursing diagnoses.[16] As will be explained in Chapter 12 the submission and review process has undergone many changes since 1973.

Other classification systems that contain all or a portion of the diagnoses in the NANDA Taxonomy are the American Nurses Association (ANA) Council of Psychiatric and Mental Health Nursing Classification, the Omaha Visiting Nurses Association Classification of Nursing Problems, and the Georgetown University Home Health Care Classification Project. These systems are discussed in Chapter 12. The majority of health care agencies using professional practice models employ NANDA Taxonomy diagnoses.

In 1988, in its continuing effort to support classification systems for nursing practice and to encourage a unified nursing language system, the ANA recognized NANDA as the organization responsible for development, review, and approval of nursing diagnoses. A collaborative model was established that would use the specialty groups within ANA as reviewers of diagnoses.[17] This action and others discussed in the next section influenced the development of a diagnostic language for clinical practice.

Influences on classification system development

It is interesting to reflect on how nursing diagnosis has influenced (and has been influenced by) dramatic changes in professional nursing in this century. The history of the development of nursing diagnosis is intertwined with the development of nursing. This relationship is not unexpected, since the focus of nursing diagnosis and treatment is the same as the clinical focus of professional nursing.

The recognition by the professional association of the concept of nursing diagnosis as a useful, cognitive tool for practice influenced its implementation. Accountability in practice was a concern in the early 1970s, and the ANA developed standards to guide nurses in evaluating their practice and their accountability to the consumer. The standards were published in 1974; Standard II stated: "Nursing diagnoses are derived from health status data."[18] Consumers could now expect nurses to carry out health assessments and nursing diagnoses to be derived from these data. This supported and encouraged the efforts of the National Task Force on Diagnosis. In turn, people working on the classification of nursing diagnoses were in a position to assist the professional association in implementing national standards at the state level; if diagnoses were to be professionally standardized, a professional language had to be developed and nurses had to be taught that language within the context of the nursing process. When the national standards of practice were published, only one nurse practice act in the United States, that of New York State, mandated diagnosis, and, if asked, most nurses in that state would have been hardpressed to point to a list of nursing diagnoses. None existed.

A second factor that influenced diagnosis was the ANA's 1980 publication *Nursing: A Social Policy Statement,*[19] in which diagnosis was incorporated into the definition of nursing: "Nursing is the diagnosis and treatment of human responses to actual or potential health problems." This definition is similar to that of the New York State Practice Act, which was the first to contain the terms *diagnosis* and *treatment:* "Nursing is the diagnosis and treatment of human responses to actual or potential health problems through such services as. . . ."[20] This act was passed into law in 1972, one year before any listing of diagnoses existed and before the First National Conference on Nursing Diagnosis took place.

At the time the ANA policy statement was published in 1980 the task force and First National Conference participants had guided the development of an alphabetical listing of nearly 50 diagnoses, their definitions, and their defining characteristics. Both the standards of practice and the policy statement made nurses' responsibility to con-

sumers explicit. For professional and legal reasons, the policy statement influenced nurses and many health care agencies across the United States to implement nursing diagnosis. Even more important in the area of accountability were the gradual changes in licensing laws during the 1970s and 1980s. Many state practice acts have been updated to reflect accountability for nursing diagnosis (problem identification) in nursing practice.

Following the social policy statement, a paper was published by Feild and Winslow[21] on the transition to a nursing model of practice. The transition was from disease-focused care to the more holistic diagnosis-based nursing care that represented professional nursing practice. This paper was influential in the implementation of nursing diagnosis in clinical practice. Another major influence on the implementation of nursing diagnosis-based care was the 1992 set of standards published by the Joint Commission on Accreditation of Healthcare Organizations. Their accreditation is highly valued by hospitals and other health care organizations. One standard states that a plan of care, including the identification of nursing diagnoses or other clinical problems, is to be developed for each patient.

It was difficult to find clinical judgment or nursing diagnosis taught in undergraduate curricula in the 1970s and even the early 1980s. In some areas of the country, clinicians, rather than educators, exhibited the greatest interest in implementing diagnosis-based professional practice. In 1986 the American Association of Colleges of Nursing[22] published a report on the essential nursing content of a baccalaureate nursing education. Clearly, the area of clinical judgment was considered to be of critical importance.

Research also lagged behind diagnostic-category identification, causing some to criticize the clinicians' premature implementation of diagnosis. On the other hand clinical research could not be done if diagnosis was not a component of practice.

Diagnostic category development and classification efforts were encouraged during the 1980s by a number of other developments. For example, *Index Medicus* listed *nursing diagnosis* (although only assessment tools could thus be accessed) and *Taber's Dictionary* began to include the current set of nursing diagnoses. By the middle of the decade textbook editors and authors had decided that diagnosis was not a passing trend, and textbooks began carrying the current listing and organizing content using nursing diagnoses. Early in the 1980s the publication of a manual of diagnosis that could be placed in the pocket of a uniform brought diagnoses into daily practice and encouraged implementation. In 1990, when the *Cumulative Index to Nursing and Allied Health Literature* began to index nursing diagnoses, clinicians and researchers could easily access the literature on each diagnosis. Also in 1990 a new journal, *Nursing Diagnosis*, began publication. Literature, textbooks, and manuals on nursing diagnosis increased considerably during the 1980s and 1990s. A few negative journal articles[23-25] and a lack of support from a number of theorists[26] (pp. 81-82) provided food for thought amid the ever-increasing literature on diagnosis and diagnostic judgment.

Clinical application of nursing diagnosis

In the last decade cost containment, quality assurance, and the desire of many consumers to obtain reimbursement for care by nonphysician providers have become important health care issues. It has been suggested that nursing diagnoses may be the basis for third-party (government and private insurers) reimbursement to consumers for nursing services in the community, in addition to reimbursement for delegated medical activities.[27] Quality assurance through peer review would be a mechanism for assuring accountability in reimbursement. Development of home health care reimbursement models based on nursing diagnosis was a resolution adopted by state delegates to the ANA convention in 1984. In addition, at a national conference in 1985, a consensus was reached on a data set for reporting nursing statistics by health care agencies. It was agreed that the Nursing Minimum Data Set to be proposed to the U.S. Department of Health and Human Services include nursing diagnosis.[28] If accepted, this Data Set eventually may influence government reimbursement of the cost of nursing care. National standards, policy statements, practice acts, reimbursement focus, and statistical reporting of nursing diagnosis all emphasize the importance of this concept in practice.

Comments on the usefulness of diagnosis in practice have appeared in the nursing literature since the early 1970s. As may be seen in the bibliography at the end of this book, in recent years the implementation of nursing diagnosis has been considered in such areas as acute care, intensive care, long-term care, community care, and ambulatory care. Its use in all specialty areas of practice has also been described, and frequently occurring diagnoses have been identified in many specialty areas. In addition to direct-care activities, nursing diagnosis has been recognized as useful in quality assurance, staffing distribution, computerized information systems, continuing-care planning, teaching and curriculum, and as a basis for theory development. The wealth of literature currently being published on nursing diagnosis should not suggest that there are no controversial issues. One will be explored in the next section; others will be discussed in later chapters.

Focus of nursing diagnosis

A difficult issue in the development of diagnostic categories has been the definition of nursing diagnosis. What is a nursing diagnosis? What are nurses classifying? Look at Appendix A or C. What broad category would encompass all the diagnoses?

This question is important in the development of diagnoses within a uniform nursing language system for clinical practice. It is also important from a legal perspective. Conditions labeled as nursing diagnoses should be within the legal scope of nursing practice. In the United States practice is controlled by state practice acts; violation of a practice act exposes a nurse to the risk of being accused of malpractice. Since 1973 nursing diagnosis has sometimes been defined as a product of assessment. Yet nurses assess many entities that other professionals claim as their domain: for example, diseases. In the past, the NANDA committee that reviews diagnoses included in their guidelines the definitions shown in the box on p. 7. In 1988 NANDA members voted to replace these with the following definition to guide diagnosis review and classification:

Nursing diagnosis is a clinical judgment about individual, family, or community responses to actual or potential health problems/life processes. Nursing diagnoses provide the basis for selection of nursing interventions to achieve outcomes for which the nurse is accountable.[29,30]

SELECTED DEFINITIONS OF NURSING DIAGNOSIS

Nursing diagnosis is a clinical judgment about an individual, family, or community that is derived through a deliberate, systematic process of data collection and analysis. It provides the basis for prescriptions for definitive therapy for which the nurse is accountable. It is expressed concisely and includes the etiology of the condition when known.[31]

Nursing diagnoses, or clinical diagnoses made by professional nurses, describe actual or potential health problems which nurses by virtue of their education and experience are capable and licensed to treat.[32]

Nursing diagnosis is a concise phrase or term summarizing a cluster of empirical indicators representing patterns of unitary man.[33]

A nursing diagnosis is a concise phrase or term summarizing a cluster or set of empirical indicators, representing normal variations and altered patterns (actual or potential) of human functioning which nurses by virtue of education and experience are capable and licensed to treat.[34]

Note the similarities between the above definition and those in the box above.

What are nurses identifying and classifying? In the previous definition, the answer is actual or potential problems/life processes based on client's manifested human responses. In the box, patterns of unitary humans, actual or potential problems, and altered patterns of human functioning are suggested as foci of diagnosis. Rather than stating the focus of diagnosis, some definitions describe the process of diagnosis and its relationship to intervention and outcome. The difficulty in defining the kinds of conditions described by nursing diagnosis lies in the prevailing theoretical pluralism.

Theoretical or conceptual pluralism describes a situation in which many perspectives and theories of nursing coexist in the one profession. It stems from a belief that at this time multiple perspectives are needed to describe a complex reality, accommodate differing viewpoints, or capture the essence of a social institution, such as nursing. This philosophy also influences consensus on the definition of nursing. National concensus is easier to achieve when diagnosis is defined in *process terms* rather than from one theoretical perspective, such as the self care agency theory, wherein diagnoses describe self care agency deficits. Nurses agree on diagnostic judgment and its place in the nursing process but not necessarily on the focus of judgment. A good example is the definition of nursing diagnosis in the New York State Education Department *Nursing Handbook,*[20] which avoids a conceptual focus entirely:

Nursing diagnosis in the context of nursing practice is the identification and discrimination between physical and psychosocial signs and symptoms essential to the effective execution and management of the nursing regimen. Such diagnostic privilege is distinct from medical diagnosis.

This definition assures the public and members of other professions that nurses do not diagnose and treat medical conditions. Diagnosis is a discrimination task, yet "discrimination between physical and psychosocial signs and symptoms" is not a particularly good description of the diagnostic judgment process.

The ANA was sensitive to the theoretical pluralism that exists in nursing when their Social Policy Task Force defined the focus of diagnosis as "human responses to actual or potential health problems."[19] While this definition was general enough for many perspectives to be included, it is *too* general. It does not provide sufficient discrimination between what are and are not nursing diagnoses within the conceptual focus of nursing. To come full circle: What *is* the conceptual focus of nursing on which all nurses can agree? It may be necessary to live with ambiguity for another century or so; in the meantime, each nurse will have to decide what conceptual focus is most useful in practice and research or is most consistent with personal beliefs about nursing.

Care, cure, and nursing diagnosis

Care and cure are frequently discussed in health care circles. Historically, nursing has been associated with care and medicine with cure; nurses have stressed the art and physicians, the science. Kritek,[35] (p. 583) in a paper suggesting a balance between the art and the science and a need to give words to the elusive, invisible parts, has captured the tradition and the current situation:

While there have always been humans committed to visual, literary, or performing arts, few "service" oriented groups have so persistently labeled their activities "art" as has nursing. Yet nurses seem dumbfounded when attempting to describe that art so dearly prized. Further, this is an era where the dominance of science has persistently defined art as a less powerful, more dispensable force. There seems to be a belief that the centrality of science relegated art to the status of optional . . . that which is most cherished in nursing, those experiences shared with humans during their most vulnerable moments, seem to elude the best efforts at naming. They are often the "stuff" of the most mysterious aspects of the human spirit, and go unnamed for the entire species. Yet they have an overpowering centrality in nursing.

It may seem at first glance that current concepts of caring in nursing are not compatible with the development of nursing diagnosis and nursing science. Kritek goes on to suggest that nursing diagnosis forces confrontation with these issues. On the one hand, the effort to capture what nurses do and to expand the knowledge base for practice are important social responsibilities in a profession created by society. On the other hand, caring has a cognitive component, and the merging of a caring philosophy and nursing diagnosis can only benefit health care delivery.

Nurses have not associated their caring with cure. Cure has been commonly discussed in reference to medicine and disease, but health care is not just the curing of disease. Nurses, particularly in public health, have a tradition of curing social ills. Similarly, should not helping a family regain a feeling of self-competency and worth be classified and valued as curing? We may prefer the word *resolve* rather than *cure* and the sometimes invisible practice of "doing with" rather than "doing for" while helping persons, families, and communities. Yet nursing's "cures" are as valuable as others and in some cases have more impact. Nursing diagnosis involves both care and cure but in a different domain.

International collaboration in diagnosis development

As diagnoses were developed they were translated into many languages. One of the first was French, reflecting the early involvement of nurses from Quebec. Nurses from countries outside North America began to be involved in the biennial classification conferences in the late 1980s, and their attendance has increased progressively. This interest suggested that nursing diagnoses should be entered in the tenth revision of the World Health Organization's (WHO) International Classification of Diseases (ICD). (Yes, the name needs changing!) Listing diagnoses in a section of this classification would facilitate gathering international statistics on nursing; in each country's health care agencies, patients' records could be coded at discharge. Data on health problems would be available for local, state, and national health planning.

In 1989 *Taxonomy I* was modified to conform to international coding, and the ANA submitted it for inclusion in the ICD-10 (Appendix D). The diagnostic categories were called "conditions that necessitate nursing care," a phrase that generates less controversy, internationally, than does "nursing diagnosis." Previously the ANA Council on Computer Applications in Nursing was invited to be involved in the tenth revision of the ICD. The submission of the NANDA taxonomy is awaiting international endorsement before further action will be taken by the WHO; the International Council of Nurses in Geneva plans to seek consensus from member countries.[36]

Nursing diagnoses have been translated into most European and Asian, and some African, languages. There have been national conferences in Australia, the Netherlands, and France, for example. French-speaking nurses have formed an official committee to oversee translation of new diagnoses into the French language. In addition, a European regional group on classification of nursing diagnoses, AFEDI, has been formed and is an affiliate of NANDA. Nurses are in the process of examining whether the diagnoses already identified have cultural relevance in their countries. It is likely that some diagnostic categories in Appendix A will be useful and that some will need clinical study to identify different ways in which a condition is manifested (defining characteristics and different probable causes). Some diagnoses in the NANDA taxonomy will not be applicable to particular cultures. Also, the applicability of diagnoses from other countries (not currently classified in the North American taxonomy) will have to be evaluated by North American colleagues.

As will be discussed in Chapter 12, cultural factors influence the development and use of diagnostic categories. It is predicted that this decade will be marked by increased discussion of nursing diagnosis across countries and cultures. An international nursing diagnosis association will be needed to work toward an international classification of nursing diagnoses. Then nurses around the world will have culturally appropriate diagnostic categories to use in practice. Terms that are not culturally relevant will not be used. This is common practice with other international classifications; countries expand or contract international classifications, adapting them to their own clinical situations.

The question in many nurses' minds in the early 1970s was: Should nurses diagnose? Today the question in most countries is: What are the health problems nurses can competently diagnose and treat? Yet many of the same questions prevalent in the 1980s still exist, as is evident in this excerpt of an address at the Seventh Conference on the Classification of Nursing Diagnoses:

The question for debate can be framed as: Should nursing diagnoses be created to describe all of nursing practice or only that segment of practice that is the unique, independent area of nursing expertise? The answer does not lie in what nurses *do* in practice. All would agree on the realities: some problems are totally within the area of nursing expertise; others require medical diagnosis and treatment carried out/monitored by nurses until patients can manage on their own. The underlying issue is twofold: *What class of health-related problems should nursing diagnoses describe? And when a health-related condition is referred to as a nursing diagnosis, what consequent responsibility and accountability for practice and research does this imply?*[37]

The above questions have many professional, social, and political dimensions that will be discussed in a later chapter. At this point let us consider other ways of defining nursing diagnosis. It has been defined as a concept, or idea, outside the context in which diagnoses are used. The first consideration will be nursing diagnosis in the context of nursing process. It will become clear that nursing diagnosis is just a step in a process that results in care delivery. Attention will be given to how nursing diagnosis relates to assessment, intervention, and evaluation of care. Then nursing diagnosis will be examined in relation to the broader idea of nursing practice. The use of nursing diagnosis in health care delivery will complete the discussion of the contextual aspects of nursing diagnosis.

CONTEXTUAL DEFINITION OF DIAGNOSIS

Sometimes a concept becomes clearer if it is viewed in the context of related ideas rather than in isolation. In this section nursing diagnosis will be examined in its rightful place, within nursing process. *The important understanding to be gained is that nursing diagnosis provides a focus for nursing care planning and evaluation.*

Nursing process will be examined in its own right, then in the context of nursing practice that consists of more than just treating conditions described by nursing diagnoses. Next, a look at the broader context of health care delivery will provide an understanding of the need for collaboration among health professionals, particularly in the treatment of the client's diagnosed conditions. *The major insight to be gained is that nursing diagnoses are not made in isolation.*

Nursing diagnosis in nursing process

Client care is the central focus of nursing. Caring for, about, and with clients are the scientific and humanistic elements. These elements of clinical practice describe a helping, caring relationship actualized through nursing process.

Nursing process is a method of problem identification and problem solving.[38] Although derived from the supposedly objective scientific method, nursing process is not applied in an objective, value-free way. *Human values influence both problem identification and problem solving.* The components of nursing process discussed in textbooks vary but generally include assessment and diagnosis. These are the problem-identification components. Outcome projection, intervention, and outcome evaluation are the problem-solving components. These key components are:

Problem identification
    Assessment
    Diagnosis
Problem solving
    Outcome projection
    Intervention
    Outcome evaluation

Having the key components spelled out encourages deliberation, organization, and thought as opposed to haphazard care planning. This is important when human beings are the recipients of care.

Another way of looking at nursing process is from the perspective of *clinical judgment.* Nursing process involves three interrelated areas of cognition. These are:

Diagnostic reasoning and judgment
Therapeutic reasoning and judgment
Ethical reasoning and judgment

Moral sensitivity and ethical judgment in nurse-client interaction permeates the entire nursing process. This way of defining nursing process stresses the professional dimension characterized by clinical judgment skills.

The components named above only specify a process. The content of nursing process requires a conceptual framework. A *conceptual framework* is a set of concepts that guide general decisions about what to assess and diagnose, what interventions to use, and what to evaluate. In a later chapter a few selected frameworks will be discussed. The objective at this point is to define diagnosis in the context of nursing process. The discussion here will be brief and introductory.

Nursing process begins with the *problem identification phase.* In the first contact with a client a nursing history is taken and an examination is done. This information collection process is referred to as *assessment.* During assessment, actual or potential health problems may be revealed and strengths are identified. Nursing diagnoses are used to describe problems. It is important to understand that problem identification contains elements of uncertainty. One is rarely 100% certain that a diagnosis is valid. This is not peculiar to nursing; all health care providers are faced with the

same situation. In a later chapter methods for dealing with this lack of certainty will be discussed.

When a cluster of signs and symptoms is categorized using a nursing diagnosis, clinical knowledge stored in memory can be retrieved. This knowledge facilitates problem solving or risk factor reduction in the case of a potential problem. In the intervention phase of nursing process diagnosis proves its worth. Once the problem is identified, it provides a focus for problem-solving activities. These include outcome projection, care planning, intervention, and outcome evaluation. The first step in helping a client solve or prevent a problem is to identify clearly the outcome desired. *An outcome is measurable behavior indicating problem resolution or progress toward resolution.* For example, if the diagnosis is High Risk for Skin Breakdown, the desired outcome is intact skin. Did you notice what occurred? *The diagnosis was used as a focus for projecting the outcome.*

When the desired health outcome of a diagnosis is determined (in collaboration with the patient, if possible), the nurse next thinks about what nursing interventions are needed to reach the outcome. Many factors in the client's situation have to be taken into account to individualize care planning. During intervention there is continual assessment and evaluation of the problem, the effectiveness of care, and the progress toward outcome attainment.

This brief overview indicates how nursing diagnoses are used in nursing process. Diagnoses provide a distinct focus for establishing desired outcomes and for making decisions about what interventions are needed. A diagnosis also provides a focus for daily evaluation of a client's progress and for any necessary revision of the care plan. For all these reasons, nursing diagnoses make nursing care delivery easier. Further appreciation of this point will be gained when more specific guidelines and examples are provided in a later chapter.

Nursing diagnosis in nursing practice

A broader view is necessary before nursing diagnosis can be thought of in the context of nursing practice. In this section we will see that nursing practice may include more than the treatment of conditions described by nursing diagnoses. If clients have medical problems, nurses help them carry out medical treatments (i.e., to follow their doctor's orders). It is important to grasp the difference. *With nursing diagnoses, the nurse is responsible for the treatment plan whether determined by the nurse, the patient, or both. In the case of a medical diagnosis the physician is responsible for treatment decisions. The nurse is responsible for helping the patient carry out treatment plans by doing for, doing with, or teaching how.* Aside from the issue of responsibility, in practice the separation of medical diagnoses and nursing diagnoses is artificial. Clients' health problems are interrelated when the whole person is considered. Physicians and nurses work together to help them overcome these problems. The issue that concerns many nurses is, What is the essence of nursing in practice, and is sufficient emphasis given to it? Nursing diagnosis helps clarify these issues.

Nursing diagnoses do not describe the whole of nursing practice. As stated above, clients have other health problems, which are described by medical diagnoses, that are also of concern to nurses. For a moment think of the whole of your practice activities as contained in a circle, such as that illustrated in Fig. 1-1. Think of this circle as 100% of the time you spend in direct client-care activities (ignore administrative tasks for the moment). Move the line to section off the circle in a 90:10 ratio of nursing diagnosis–related care to medically delegated care. This may describe time allocation in long-term care or rehabilitation where nursing diagnosis–related care predominates. For ambulatory or clinic settings, move the line to a 75:25 ratio of nursing diagnosis–related care to delegated care activities.

In home health care or extended care facilities the distribution may be 60:40; with decreased length of stay in hospitals the acuity level of the disease is greater in the home or community than previously seen. The increased acuity of hospitalized clients suggests a 30:70 ratio. Intensive care for problems of physiological instability may result in a 10:90 ratio for activities related to nursing diagnoses and medical diagnoses, respectively.

The line is movable, as is the emphasis nurses place on various aspects of practice. The diagram is a clear visual representation of the principle that nursing diagnosis is used in that aspect of practice

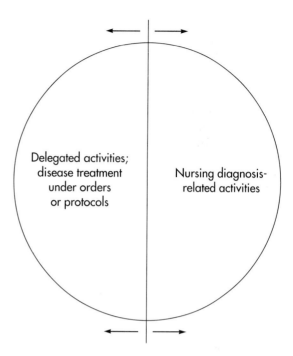

Fig. 1-1   Time spent in direct-care activities of nursing practice.

unique to nursing. No one else is educated to perform this aspect of care. The diagram also makes it clear that nurses do not ignore medical treatment orders or the client's disease; to do so would not be compatible with a holistic approach. It is important to notice also that disease-related nursing care is not considered "nonnursing" activity. The current emphasis on nursing diagnoses has come about because this aspect of practice (diagnosis) has not been described before; the others have.

With a holistic approach to care all health problems are considered simultaneously and in the context of the patient's life. *Treatment priorities are decided by the severity of a health problem and its significance in the client's recovery and future health potential, irrespective of whether they are medical or nursing diagnoses.* In some instances, treating clients' anxiety is more important than a routine dressing change if clients are seen as integrated human beings (as opposed to just physiological or psychosocial beings). At other times, carrying out a medical treatment may be more important to the overall health of the client than treating anxiety. Nursing judgment about priorities is required in these instances. This type of judgment develops with experience.

It is important to point out that clinical judgments in nursing practice are not confined to nursing diagnoses. Judgment is required in reporting changes in the client's medical condition, the response to therapy, administration of drugs, carrying out medical treatments, and seeking consultation with nurse specialists or other health care personnel. Development of clinical judgment continues throughout every nurse's professional career.

Nursing diagnosis in health care delivery

In this section we will use a broader view to encompass nursing process and nursing practice. Health care delivery is the combined objective of many groups: physicians, nurses, administrators, agencies of the federal government, and others. Basic health services are delivered by two professions, nursing and medicine. These basic services to the consumer are supplemented as necessary by a number of other health care providers. For example, when clients' health problems warrant it, referrals can be made to social workers, physical therapists, or psychologists.

Research has demonstrated that collaboration among nurses and physicians is critical to the welfare of patients. An evaluation of mortality was done in the intensive care units of 13 hospitals by comparing actual and predicted death rates for 5030 intensive care patients. Nurse-physician communication was the most important factor contributing to differences in mortality across settings.[39]

Fig. 1-2 symbolizes the components of collaborative care when only a nurse, a physician, and a consultant are involved in providing services. Although the interactions and outcome shown by the arrows do not always take place, coordination represented by arrows toward a central focus is a realistic goal. Clients' contributions to the coordination of their health care management include (1) their personal perceptions of their state of health, (2) their plans, and (3) their health practices. They have expectations that the "specialists" in health care will offer information, recommendations, and care they cannot do themselves. Health professionals formalize clients' health concerns with diagnoses and treatment plans, as the diagram indicates. Thus the major elements are present for joint planning by the client, nurse, and physician.

Coordinated care as illustrated in Fig. 1-2 is not a new idea; it can be found in textbooks dating back 30 years or more. Yet the challenge to implement this coordination still faces the next generation of clinicians in the health care professions. Fig. 1-3 illustrates the current situation in many institutions devoted to health care: "part-and-parcel care delivery." The professions operate more or less separately, and each offers its own "parcel" to the consumer. Nursing has not yet clearly understood what its own contribution is and consequently has not been able to clarify this matter for consumers. The language used in health care circles is not just one of tasks and doing. It deals with what the problem is and what treatment can be offered, a logical approach. If health care is to progress from the situation represented in Fig. 1-3 to that in Fig. 1-2, the first step is for nurses to share, in some clear and concise way, their conceptions of clients' current functional health status and nursing care needs. Nursing diagnoses provide a method for synthesizing and communicating nurses' observations and judgments. As later chapters will show, the ability to communicate the health needs of clients can influence funding of preventive and comprehensive health care services.

It is predicted that chronic diseases will be the major medical problem as the twentieth century ends and the twenty-first century begins. Consistent with this view, the main population using health services will be the "frail elderly." The need currently exists to delay the onset of chronic disease and disability. Underlying early onset are conditions such as obesity, stress management, accidental injuries, and drug abuse (nicotine, alcohol, and others). If the functional health patterns of the population were surveyed, it would probably be found that the nursing diagnosis Health Management Deficit probably outranks all other currently identified medical or nursing problems. Consumers are beginning to realize that they have considerable control of their health through personal health management. Guidance in health management and early detection of dysfunctional health patterns by nurses will contribute to delaying the onset of chronic disease and disability.

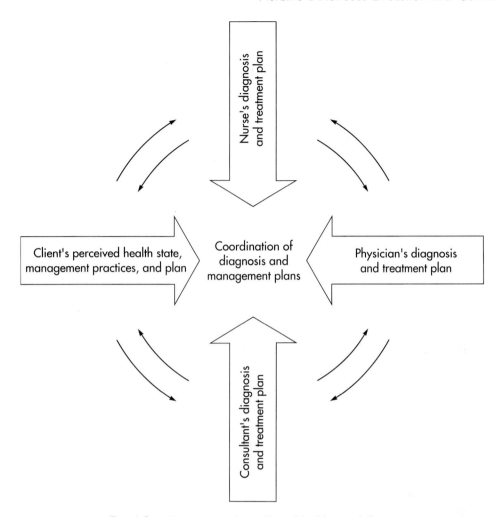

Fig. 1-2   Components of coordinated health care delivery.

SUMMARY

Interest in and enthusiasm about nursing diagnosis are widespread. Nurses in a number of countries recognize the implications for nursing practice, education, and research. In particular, those providing direct care to clients view nursing diagnosis as a way to improve care. As one nurse said, "It helps me to define what I do and to feel good about how I do it." In this chapter, nursing diagnosis was introduced; most of the emphasis was on diagnostic categories rather than diagnostic process. The evolution of nursing diagnosis, responsibility for development, and factors influencing development were reviewed as a basis for discussing clinical application and the issue of what a diagnosis describes. Leaving other conceptual distinctions for a later chapter, consensus exists that a nursing diagnosis is an actual or potential health problem/life process amenable to nursing intervention. The international interest in nursing diagnosis was described, and it was concluded that much could be gained by international collaboration in the development of a unified nursing language system that is useful in clinical practice.

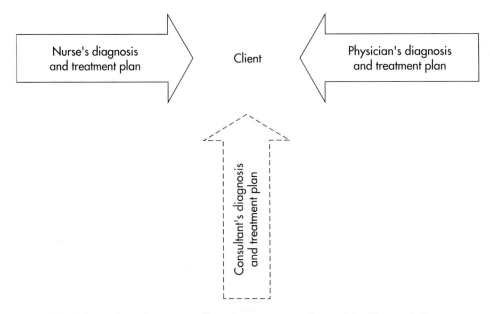

Fig. 1-3 Independent (uncoordinated) components of current health care delivery.

Nursing diagnosis was examined in the context of nursing process in order to establish its essential and practical meaning. Below are the important points in that discussion:

1. A diagnosis provides the focus for the caring relationship established with clients.
2. Nursing diagnosis is used in nursing process as a basis for projecting health outcomes and determining nursing interventions to reach the projected outcomes.

When the broader scope of nursing practice was considered, it was recognized that nurses make many types of clinical judgments. Nursing diagnostic judgments have a particular characteristic that distinguishes them from nursing judgments related to diagnosis and treatment of disease. The major points in this section were:

1. When nursing diagnoses are made, nurses have the responsibility and accountability for determining the treatment plan, as opposed to implementing the plans of other care providers.
2. Nursing practice requires competency in three types of clinical judgment: diagnostic, therapeutic, and ethical. Moral reasoning and ethical judgment are involved in most diagnostic and therapeutic activities.

An examination of health care delivery demonstrated that a variety of professionals make diagnoses and develop treatment plans. Not to be overlooked are clients' perceptions of their health or their health management plans. Ideally, coordinated health care takes all these factors into account. Two important implications for nursing were discussed:

1. Nursing diagnoses represent a clear focus for nursing participation in coordinated planning.
2. Nurses, physicians, consultants, and clients (insofar as their conditions permit) should pool their conceptions of the pertinent health problems and treatment plans in order to coordinate activities.

It has been suggested that the incidence of chronic disease and disability in the population will rise unless there is early diagnosis and treatment of potential problems, such as health management deficits. This is an area in which nurses have much to contribute to improving the health of the population.

NOTES AND REFERENCES

1. The term *client* will be used to refer to individuals, families, and communities.

2. A number of terms will be used synonomously: *diagnostic category, diagnostic concept,* and *nursing diagnosis. Diagnostic category* refers to the name of an actual or potential health problem or condition. It is used when referring to a division in a classification system such as those listed in Appendixes A through D. *Diagnostic concept* is used when referring to the conceptual knowledge base or theoretical underpinnings of the problem and the application of this knowledge to the clinical data. *Nursing diagnosis* is the common term for any of the actual or potential health problems or conditions listed in Appendix A. A *nursing diagnostic statement* refers to the diagnostic judgment labels for a problem and its etiological or related factors; it is usually used to summarize a set of specific signs and symptoms.

3. Bonney V, Rothberg J: *Nursing diagnosis and therapy,* New York, 1983, National League for Nursing.

4. Rothberg JS: *History of nursing diagnosis (audiotape transcript).* Paper presented at the Conference on Nursing Diagnosis, Adelphi University, New York, April 10, 1982.

5. Gebbie KM, Lavin MA: *Classification of nursing diagnoses: proceedings of the first national conference,* St Louis, 1975, Mosby.

6. Abdellah FG, et al: *Patient-centered approaches to nursing,* New York 1961, Macmillan.

7. Fry V: The creative approach to nursing, *Am J Nurs* 53:301, 1953.

8. Komorita NL: Nursing diagnosis, *Am J Nurs* 63:83, 1963.

9. Rothberg JS: Why nursing diagnosis? *Am J Nurs* 67:1000, 1967.

10. Levine M: Trophocognosis: an alternative to nursing diagnosis. In: *Exploring progress in medical-surgical nursing practice,* Proceedings of the ANA Regional Clinical Conference, 2:55-70, San Antonio, Texas, 1965, American Nurses' Association.

11. King LS: What is a diagnosis? *JAMA* 202:714, 1967.

12. Carroll-Johnson R, editor: *Classification of nursing diagnoses: proceedings of the tenth conference,* Philadelphia, 1993, Lippincott, p 306; Carroll-Johnson R, editor: *Classification of nursing diagnoses: proceedings of the ninth conference,* Philadelphia, 1992, Lippincott, p 306; Carroll-Johnson R, editor: *Classification of nursing diagnoses: proceedings of the eighth conference,* Philadelphia, 1989, Lippincott, p 560; McLane A, editor: *Classification of nursing diagnoses: proceedings of the seventh conference,* St Louis, 1987, Mosby, p 478; Hurley M, editor: *Classification of nursing diagnoses: proceedings of the sixth conference,* St Louis, 1986, Mosby, p 513; Kim MJ, Moritz DA, editors: *Classification of nursing diagnoses: proceedings of the third and fourth conferences,* New York, 1982, McGraw-Hill, p 281; Gebbie K, editor: *Classification of nursing diagnoses: proceedings of the second conference,* St Louis, 1976, Clearinghouse for Nursing Diagnoses, St Louis University School of Nursing; Gebbie KM, Lavin MA, editors: *Classification of nursing diagnoses: proceedings of the first national conference,* St Louis, 1975, Mosby.

13. Taxonomy I, revised June, 1992, Philadelphia, 1992, North American Nursing Diagnosis Association.

14. Gordon M: *Nursing diagnosis: process and application,* New York, 1982, McGraw-Hill.

15. The framework containing nine patterns developed by the theorists' group was originally called "Patterns of Unitary Man." See Kim MJ, Mortiz DA, editors: *Classification of nursing diagnoses: proceedings of the third and fourth national conferences,* New York, 1981, McGraw-Hill. Although some have interpreted this work as an outgrowth of Martha Rogers' conceptual framework, it was the creation of the group of theorists listed in Appendix E. Evolution of the Taxonomy as Human Response Patterns was guided by Dr. Phyllis Kritek (Chairperson, 1982-1987) and Dr. Joyce Fitzpatrick (Chairperson, 1987-1992) and the NANDA Taxonomy Committee. Appendix F contains the original and current definitions of the nine patterns.

16. Contact NANDA, 1211 Locust St., Philadelphia, PA 19107. NANDA is composed of nurses actively involved in the identification and classification of nursing diagnoses. Until 1982 it was called the National Group for Classification of Nursing Diagnoses.

17. *Classification systems for describing nursing practice,* Washington, DC, 1989, American Nurses Association; and *Am Nurse,* February 1988, p 5.

18. *Standards of nursing practice,* Washington, DC, 1974, American Nurses Association.

19. *Nursing: a social policy statement,* Washington, DC, 1980, American Nurses Association.

20. New York State Education Department, *Nursing handbook,* Albany, NY, 1992, Author, p 24.

21. Feild L, Winslow EH: Moving to a nursing model, *Am J Nurs* 85:1100, 1985.

22. *Essentials of college and university education for professional nursing: final report,* Washington DC, 1986, American Association of Colleges of Nursing.

23. Mitchell G: Nursing diagnosis: an ethical analysis, *Image* 23:99, 1991.

24. Hagey RS, McDonough P: The problem of professional labeling, *Nurs Outlook* 32:151, 1984.

25. Leininger M: Issues, questions, and concerns related to the nursing diagnosis cultural movement from a transcultural nursing perspective, *J Transcult Nurs* 2:23, 1990; Feild L: Response to published article: nursing diagnosis, *J Transcult Nurs* 3:25, 1991.

26. Randell B: Nursing theory: the 21st century, *Nurs Sci Q* 5:176, 1992.

27. Joel L: DRGs and nursing diagnosis. In Hurley M, editor: *Classification of nursing diagnoses: proceedings of the sixth conference,* St Louis, 1986, Mosby.

28. Werley HH, Lang N, editors: *Identification of nursing minimum data set,* New York, 1987, Springer.

29. Carroll-Johnson R, editor: *Classification of nursing diagnoses: proceedings of the tenth conference,* Philadelphia, 1993, Lippincott, p 306.

30. The definition builds on suggestions from the literature that have become accepted practice, such as the definition derived from a national research study by Shoemaker,[31] comments on outcomes and accountability by Feild and Winslow,[21] and the early definitions by Gordon[32] and McLane.[34]

31. Shoemaker J: Essential features of a nursing diagnosis. In Kim MJ, McFarland G, McLane A, editors: *Classification of nursing diagnoses: proceedings of the fifth conference,* St Louis, 1984, Mosby, p 104.

32. Gordon M: Nursing diagnosis and the diagnostic process, *Am J Nurs* 76:1298, 1976.
33. Roy C: Theoretical framework for classification of nursing diagnosis. In Kim MJ, Moritz DA, editors: *Classification of nursing diagnoses: proceedings of the third and fourth conference,* New York, 1982, McGraw-Hill, pp 215-221.
34. McLane A: A taxonomy of using diagnoses: toward a science of nursing, *Milwaukee Prof Nurse* 20:33, 1979.
35. Kritek P: Risks and realities. In Hannah K et al, editors: *Clinical judgment and decision making: the future with nursing diagnosis.* Proceedings of the International Conference, Calgary, Alberta, Canada New York, 1987, Wiley. See also Loomis ME, Wood DJ: Cure: potential outcome of nursing care, *Image* 15:4-7, 1983.
36. Saba V: ICN to review nursing diagnoses, *Am Nurse,* September 1992. The International Council of Nurses in Geneva, Switzerland, is composed of the national nursing associations of member countries. Most countries belong to this council, which represents nursing in international circles. Congresses are held every four years; in 1993 an International Congress was held in Madrid, Spain.
37. Gordon M: Issues in nursing diagnosis. In McLane A, editor: *Classification of nursing diagnoses: proceedings of the seventh conference,* St Louis, 1987, Mosby, p 17.
38. Many authors use the term *problem solving* to encompass both identification of a problem and its solution. To emphasize the two components, in this text each will be stated explicitly.
39. Knaus WA et al: An evaluation of outcome from intensive care in major medical centers, *Ann Intern Med* 104:410, 1986.

CHAPTER 2

NURSING DIAGNOSIS:
CATEGORY AND PROCESS

S ome words people use to communicate their ideas have two or more definitions. The way in which the word is used clarifies its meaning. So it is with the term *nursing diagnosis*. It refers not only to the process of diagnosing but also to the diagnostic judgment reached and expressed via a category name. The separation of the process and the content of diagnostic judgment is artificial; the two are actually interdependent. Yet it makes learning easier if initially they are considered separately. In this chapter the reader can obtain an in-depth understanding of the conceptual and structural aspects of diagnostic categories. An overview of nursing diagnosis as process will introduce the subject of diagnostic reasoning and judgment. This overview will place the reader in a position to consider who should have the responsibility for diagnostic judgments in clinical practice.

When a nurse describes a client's condition as Impaired Mobility (Level II) Related to Activity Intolerance, two diagnostic category labels are being used. To help the reader understand the meaning of nursing diagnosis as a category for naming a health problem, it will be defined from two perspectives. Its *conceptual* definition and basis will deal with the focus and meaning of nursing diagnosis, and its *structural* definition will describe what it "looks like." Combined with the contextual definition discussed in Chapter 1, this approach should provide a good understanding of

nursing diagnosis as a category for labeling nurses' diagnostic judgments.

CONCEPTUAL DEFINITION OF NURSING DIAGNOSIS

A conceptual definition communicates the meaning of an idea, such as nursing diagnosis. For example, the words "fruit" or "dog" have standardized meanings that can be found in dictionary definitions. There are two purposes in defining the term *nursing diagnosis:*

1. To discriminate among problems that primarily require nursing intervention, referral, or treatment under protocols.
2. To accept or reject diagnoses submitted to NANDA for placement in the taxonomy.

Let us analyze some definitions of nursing diagnosis. The discussion will acquaint the reader with the difficulty in finding a uniformly acceptable definition to guide usage and diagnosis development. This difficulty exists because of theoretical pluralism (where there is not just *one* unified idea about nursing and nursing science). The reader can also appreciate the difficulty encountered by "purists" and scholars who want diagnosis development to proceed along some ideal path. Yet pluralism is not unique to nursing; there are multiple theories of learning in the field of education. In the box on p. 7 see if the definitions provide a specific conceptual focus that would serve the two purposes above. The question is, What is to be classified and called a nursing diagnosis?

An early definition addressed the concerns of the mid-1970s. It stressed a way of differentiating between health problems that required medical treatment and those that required nursing intervention:

Nursing diagnoses, or clinical diagnoses made by professional nurses, describe actual or potential health problems which nurses by virtue of their education and experience are capable and licensed to treat. This definition thereby excludes health problems for which the accepted mode of therapy is prescription drugs, surgery, radiation, and other treatments that are defined legally as the practice of medicine.[1]

To treat, or to provide treatment, refers to the *initiation* of accepted modes of therapy. Some may argue that clarifying domains of practice by using the qualifier "competency to treat" is inadequate; nurses do participate in the treatment of diseases. Nurses do indeed report observations and judgments, carry out physicians' orders that clients cannot carry out for themselves, and diagnose and treat diseases under physician supervision or protocols.[2] These activities of disease-related care are in a sense under the cognitive control of the physician. The nurse must anticipate what the physician would think and do.[3] This is not the case with nursing diagnoses.

The other definitions presented in Chapter 1 did not offer a *specific* conceptual focus. Patterns of human functioning, unitary persons, health problems, responses, life processes, or clinical judgment are general and cannot be used to discriminate between nursing diagnoses and other clinical conditions. Yet general terms may be necessary because nursing has many different schools of thought with different models to describe its focus of concern. Examples of this theoretical or conceptual pluralism will be seen in Chapter 4.

Appendix G and later chapters present a general set of functional health patterns. These represent basic areas of nursing concern, irrespective of the nurse's theoretical persuasion.

To choose one theory (self-care, adaptation, unitary person, becoming) as the focus of nursing diagnosis or as a social policy statement would be unwise. Thus a focus that would appeal to all nurses remains elusive; perhaps the answer is to live with feelings of ambiguity—at least for the time being. Other ways of clarifying the domain of nursing diagnosis can be helpful, as is the NANDA definition given below.

Soares[4] has suggested that the phrase "can be alleviated by nursing actions" differentiates nursing diagnoses from other clinical terms, and Feild and Winslow[5] have suggested that "accountable for outcomes" achieves the same goal. General terms (human responses, health patterns, problems, and life processes) may be the level at which consensus can be reached. Individual nurses can think about nursing diagnoses more specifically from the perspective of ineffective adaptations, self-care agency deficits, functional and dysfunctional patterns, or any other conceptual focus they use in practice.

The following definition will be familiar from the previous chapter as the accepted working definition of NANDA; let us consider it in some detail:

Nursing diagnosis is a clinical judgment about individual, family, or community responses to actual or potential health problems/life processes. Nursing diagnoses provide the basis for selection of nursing interventions to achieve outcomes for which the nurse is accountable.[6]

Consider some of the terms in this definition. A nursing diagnosis is a *clinical judgment.* This means that nursing diagnosis is not just one observation but rather an interpretation, analysis, and judgment of the meaning of a set of observations. Individual, family, or community *responses* to problems or life situations are described as the focus of judgment. *Responses* are observable behaviors or verbal reports. They include the way a person, family, or community reacts to a situation or the personal meaning they place on events. The responses may be physiological, psychological, social, or spiritual but most commonly are a biopsychosocial-spiritual combination. For example, crying is a response. The term *actual or potential health problems* refers to conditions that are the basis for the human responses that are observed; they are labeled with diagnoses (diagnostic concepts) that give meaning to the observed responses.[7] The definition suggests two kinds of health problems that are of concern to nurses. An *actual problem* is an existing deviation from health. Dysfunctional Grieving and Pressure Ulcer are examples. Nurses do more than treat conditions that have already occurred. Traditionally, a high value has been placed on preventing problems and on risk-factor identification. When a set of risk factors is present, the condition is referred to as a *potential problem* or *high-risk state.* High Risk for Injury and High Risk for Skin Breakdown are examples. Any listing or definition of nursing diagnoses has to include both actual and high-risk health problems.

It will be useful to highlight some of the implications of the definition given above; each idea will be discussed in detail in later sections of the book.

1. Client responses to actual or potential health problems/life processes suggest that responses are synonymous with observable signs and symptoms (verbal reports). They are indicators of an underlying problem or process (which is identified through clinical judgment).
2. Making a judgment about responses suggests that diagnoses describe not just one but a cluster of signs and symptoms.
3. Diagnoses are actual or potential health problems of individuals, families, or communities.
4. Life processes suggest patterns of knowing, relating, exchanging, and so forth viewed from a health perspective. See "Response Patterns," Appendix F.
5. Nurses use nursing diagnoses as a basis for selecting nursing interventions.
6. Nurses assume accountability for treatment and outcomes of *nursing* diagnoses, in contrast to the collaborative treatment associated with medical diagnoses. Nurses evaluate their *capability* to diagnose and treat a particular condition, whether it represents a nursing diagnosis or not.

It can be noted that the NANDA definition uses the terms *life processes* and *health problems.* Some believe that limiting the scope of nursing diagnosis to actual or potential health problems (prevention and treatment) is too restrictive.[8] Nurses also deal with clients seeking enriched personal growth in areas such as parenting, health management, and self-development. As categories were identified in the "wellness" area, the definition of nursing diagnoses was expanded beyond problem or potential problem conditions to include *responses to life processes.* It has been argued that a wellness diagnosis, such as Effective Breast-Feeding, is an *outcome,* or *goal, of nursing care* rather than a diagnosis.[9] (pp. 354-355)

Questions remain. The following are some that nurses raise when developing diagnostic categories: Assuming that a nursing diagnosis is made to guide intervention, should nursing diagnoses encompass health states and healthy processes, such as *effective breast-feeding, health-seeking behaviors,* or *effective nutritional patterns?* Or do these represent the conclusions of a health status assessment rather than a focus for intervention? Are these examples of desired outcomes or goals? If these are nursing diagnoses, should nurses charge for interventions on effective breast-feeding or health-seeking behaviors? Is the intervention periodic reassessment, and if so, is the reason a risk factor indicating a potential problem? Should all areas of wellness be documented on the client's record as diagnoses? Are these wellness diagnoses really another name for strengths? Can these be documented at the end of an assessment without resorting to a nursing diagnosis? Beyond "effectiveness" is the idea of high-level wellness. Should diagnoses be developed to encompass this area; should there be diagnoses such as Family Coping: Potential for Growth or Potential for Enhanced Family Coping to describe the potential for high-level wellness? Or is it too difficult to distinguish among clients who have the potential for growth and enhancement and those who do not? Would we want to make this judgment, considering the possibility we may reach a conclusion of "no potential"? Would judgments be reliable in this area? Would Family Coping: Desire for Growth indicate that the diagnosis was the client's choice rather than the nurse's judgment? These questions provide food for thought.

There seem to be two different types of wellness diagnoses. One is the normative description of health; for example, Effective Breast-Feeding. No need for intervention is apparent from the term. The second is the specification of a potential for growth or desire for growth, which suggests a request or need for help. Usually this occurs when there is no problem from a normative (norms) perspective, but growth toward high-level wellness is a possibility. Family Coping: Potential for Growth and Parenting: Desire for Growth are examples of suggested diagnoses. Much more thought must go into the issue of health states and wellness "diagnoses." It has been suggested that an axis of the NANDA taxonomy (Appendix C) be developed for the concept of wellness, an idea similar to that of Popkess-Vater, who sees wellness conditions "as mirror images of the problem diagnoses."[9 (pp. 367-368)] Such an axis might also be used as a classification of outcomes for high-risk and actual problems.

Aside from these debates over semantics, what to classify, and territorial issues,[10] the best way to lay claim to an area of practice expertise is to demonstrate an understanding of the health problems described by nursing diagnoses and their treatment by conducting or participating in clinical research. Another way is to use practice settings to show that nurses assume accountability for assessment, diagnosis, and treatment of these problems. A review of the literature indicates that the field of nursing is beginning to direct their clinical research toward problems nurses diagnose and treat. This approach should go far toward establishing nursing's unique domain of concern as well as benefiting clients.

Comparison with other clinical terms

A number of clinical terms used in nursing, both current and historical, are sometimes confused with nursing diagnoses.[11] There is also some question about whether several categories in Appendix A meet the NANDA definition of nursing diagnosis. Consideration of these terms should help avoid conceptual errors. In addition, *positive and negative examples are useful in clarifying a concept and drawing boundaries.* Appendix A contains positive examples. To say these categories are approved means that they are sufficiently developed for clinical testing.

The diagram in Fig. 2-1 depicts entities that are not nursing diagnoses and are thus outside the boundary of the concept. Many are mentioned by Little and Carnevali.[12] The terms in Fig. 2-1 deserve some comment. All are used in nursing practice, and it is not uncommon to confuse them with nursing diagnoses. Remember that a nursing diagnosis describes a client's health problem. It does not describe, for example, the *staff's problems* in coping with clients.[12] That nurses and physicians react to stressful or frustrating situations must be recognized, but staff problems should not be labeled as diagnostic judgments about the client.

Therapeutic needs are not nursing diagnoses; they do not describe health problems or health states. For example, "needs emotional support" or "needs suctioning" is a common way of describ-

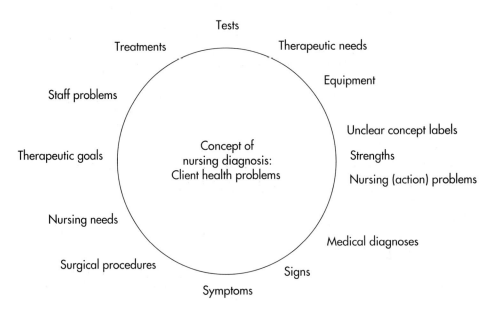

Fig. 2-1   Concept of nursing diagnosis and terms excluded from the concept.

ing needs for nursing care. These are therapeutic needs; the question arises as to why the client has these needs. In other words what is the underlying health problem, the nursing diagnosis? Once a diagnosis is established, therapeutic goals and interventions can be determined, but not before. As an example of the contrast between "needs" and diagnoses imagine that a nurse says a client "needs emotional support." The client was observed (1) pacing the room during the day before surgery, (2) commenting about being unable to sit still, and (3) stating the wish that surgery was over. A nurse might rush to provide emotional support, a diffuse nursing response. Yet in actuality the client may be having difficulty coping with the thought of disability from surgery. Perhaps a neighbor had had the same surgery and suffered paralysis two days later. The client might be identifying with this situation, although the risk of paralysis might actually be extremely low. Diffuse emotional support would probably not assist this person in handling these concerns; a problem-focused intervention is needed, as well as an empathetic manner. Using therapeutic needs as diagnoses bypasses the problem-formulation step in care planning.

The term *needs* is commonly used in another context in nursing. In Maslow's "needs hierarchy,"[13] a nonnursing theory, physiological, safety, belonging, and other needs are part of the framework. They are said to be the needs of every human being. If they are not met or conflict, these needs are the basis for the development of health problems.[4] Writing "safety needs" on a chart communicates very little; everyone needs safety. So little information is contained in this statement that one is unable to infer what the problem may be.

Just as a therapeutic need is not a nursing diagnosis, neither is a *therapeutic nursing goal,* such as "to maintain nutrition." Like "safety needs," this phrase transmits no information about the client's health problem. Everyone needs adequate nutrition; this is the question that should be asked: Is there a potential or actual nutritional deficit? The advantage of basing nursing intervention on a nursing diagnosis is the clear focus for care planning that the diagnosis provides. When a plan is based only on therapeutic goals, there is no way of knowing the client's health problem. In contrast, stating a nursing diagnosis clarifies the logical relationship that should exist between the client's problem and the proposed plan of care.

One *sign or symptom* is not a nursing diagnosis. For example, "restlessness" is sometimes given as the nursing diagnosis. Restlessness might be a sign of *pain, anxiety,* or numerous other conditions. This sign is a totally inadequate base for planning treatment and may or may not be related to a problem nurses can treat. Similarly, a symptom, such as "fatigue," is not a nursing diagnosis.[14] Its presence may signal a *chronic fatigue* syndrome and predict a client's potential self-care deficit, impaired home-maintenance management, or other problems related to decreased energy. Isolated signs and symptoms do not identify the client's health problem. A nursing diagnosis describes a cluster of signs and symptoms.

Is a nursing diagnosis the same as a *nursing problem?* The answer depends on how the latter term is being used. If it refers to a client's health problem that is amenable to nursing treatment, then "nursing problem" is synonymous with "nursing diagnosis." *Nursing problem* and *medical problem* are terms care providers use to specify who is treating a problem or to refer a client to the appropriate care provider. "Nursing problem" is not synonymous with "nursing diagnosis" when it refers to a therapeutic problem. How to promote healing may be a nursing care problem, but the health problem is pressure ulcer. A nursing diagnosis describes the client's problem, not the nurse's problem in designing and implementing care.

Little and Carnevali[12 (pp. 48-49)] take issue with the use of *concept labels* as nursing diagnoses. A conceptual term, such as *stress* or *maternal attachment,* does not indicate whether a problem exists. Yet not all signs and symptoms can be specified in the diagnostic label. If they were, the diagnosis would be too lengthy, defeating its purpose as a shorthand expression. The point Little and Carnevali make is that a diagnosis should adequately identify the problem for purposes of communication.

As seen in Fig. 2-1 and as Little and Carnevali[12 (pp. 48-49)] so clearly point out, nursing diagnoses do not describe *treatments, tests, or equipment.* For example, "catheter," "adrenalectomy," or "on heparin" clearly do not fall within the concept of nursing diagnosis. Treatments and tests do not represent health problems, nor do they represent a cluster of signs and symptoms. Possibly, further data collection would reveal a health problem and a need for nursing intervention.

The diagnosis of disease, or *medical diagnosis,* is also not part of the concept of nursing diagnosis. If a nurse makes a tentative judgment about a disease or a disease complication, that judgment is for purposes of referral; it is an important part of nursing practice but is not a nursing diagnosis.

As previously noted, *pathophysiological manifestations* of a diseased organ or system, such as *impaired gas exchange,* are not nursing diagnoses. In the collaborative or interdependent area of practice, nurses help clients monitor these conditions and carry out medical treatment until the clients can do it by themselves. Traditionally, nurses have not assumed responsibility for treatment of and research on pathophysiological manifestations of disease. The responsibility of the nurse to the client is to identify and refer problems to a physician and to prevent complications if possible. Some nurses argue that they are capable of making medical diagnoses, and indeed they may be. It is not illegal to exercise one's intellectual capabilities. Yet if the nurse's diagnosis is communicated to the patient *and* if treatment, or a lack of it, produces harm, the nurse responsible will probably find it extremely difficult to present a substantive defense against a malpractice claim in court.

There are nursing roles in which additional educational preparation legally permits diagnosis and treatment of diseases under physician supervision or protocols.[2] Nurses with these qualifications commonly practice in ambulatory care and other community-based settings and in hospitals in recent years. The portion of the nurse's role that relates to medical diagnosis is similar to the performance of medical acts by a physician's assistant. Although not to the same extent as those in ambulatory care, critical-care nurses are also responsible for making disease-related judgments and providing treatment under protocols. Judgments related to observations of disease manifestations or to treatments need not be labeled nursing diagnoses. Disease terminology is perfectly adequate. It would be ridiculous to relabel a disease with a nursing diagnosis when in fact it cannot be treated except under medical protocols. *Clearly, not everything a nurse does has to be labeled with a nursing diagnosis.* Although medical diagnoses are not referred to as nursing diagnoses, there is a connection: some nursing diagnoses can co-occur with a disease. This important point will be considered in later sections dealing with medical and nursing diagnoses in practice.

The *strengths* of a client are areas of healthy or optimal functioning. Some authors refer to strengths as nursing diagnoses.[15] However, since they are not a focus of treatment, this appears to be a misclassification. Client strengths are nursing judgments that arise out of health assessment; their importance lies in the intervention phase of care. Strengths can be mobilized to deal with problems or to move toward higher levels of human functioning.

States of health, well-being, or optimal functioning are not nursing diagnoses per se. They are goals of nursing. If a client is "healthy" and has no dysfunctional or potentially dysfunctional health patterns, it is unethical to diagnose a problem and charge for treatment. (Charges are appropriate for functional health assessment, health status evaluation, and periodic monitoring of health status.) Some clients desire help with further growth to realize their human potential and can pay for this consultation. As mentioned earlier in this chapter some nurses are interested in developing terms for wellness diagnoses. Currently clients cannot receive reimbursement for interventions directed toward "desires" or "potential for growth" from government or private insurers in the United States. Health promotion through risk-factor reduction is receiving great attention, especially in occupational and primary care. A potential problem is defined by risk factors, such as stress, sedentary life style, or nutritional excesses.

Appendix A and the previous discussion provide examples of what are and what are not nursing diagnoses. Try to apply the information in the following exercise, which contains correctly and incorrectly formulated diagnoses obtained from hospital records. Without reading further in the text, decide which are examples of correctly formulated diagnostic categories.

1. Needs suctioning
2. Inadequate insight
3. Self-bathing deficit (level II)
4. Nausea
5. Altered parenting

6. Chronic lung disease
7. Difficulty taking medicine
8. Altered neurological status

It might be inferred that Ineffective Airway Clearance is the problem in item 1, but we shall never know. The nurse has stated a need rather than a problem. Thus, "needs suctioning" is not a clinically useful diagnostic category. In item 2, the client's insight may be inadequate in some situations, but which ones, and why? The modifier "inadequate" is too judgmental; what amount of insight is adequate? There may be a health problem here, but it is not well expressed. In contrast, item 3, self-bathing deficit, is a functional problem. It directs thinking toward nursing care designed to help the client compensate for the deficit.

Nausea (item 4) is a symptom, not a diagnosis; it should lead the nurse to collect further information. Altered parenting (item 5) is an accepted diagnosis but is a broad category that requires further breakdown and definition. Entering this item on a chart would be the equivalent of a physician writing a diagnosis such as "cardiovascular disease." The question would be: Which one? Although Altered Parenting describes an area of concern to nurses, the diagnosis encompasses a number of distinct problems, and the type of Altered Parenting must be specified.[16]

Chronic lung disease (item 6) is obviously a medical diagnosis. No doubt a client with this diagnosis has problems amenable to nursing therapy. Perhaps the nurse lacked the appropriate language to express nursing diagnoses, or perhaps chronic lung disease was the diagnosis used to organize the care ordered by the physician and was erroneously labeled as a nursing diagnosis. Item 7, difficulty taking medicine, is an observation, not a nursing diagnosis. It discloses nothing about the nature and cause of the difficulty. The problem might be caused by the nurse's method of administration, the nature of the medication (pills versus liquid), development of impaired swallowing (a nursing diagnosis), and so on. Item 8, altered neurological status, is not a nursing diagnosis. Even considered as a collaborative problem, there is no hope of using this as a basis of nursing intervention. Yet frequently this type of diagnosis appears on patient records as "alterations in . . . ." Why do many nurses use such inclusive diagnoses?

Why is the medical diagnosis not used as a collaborative problem, for example, multiple sclerosis, making it a more specific focus for assessment and for reporting changes?

A useful summary of this discussion on differentiating between nursing diagnosis and other clinical terms, is the list of four important characteristics shown in the box below. Now let us define nursing diagnosis from a structural perspective. What does a nursing diagnosis look like?

STRUCTURAL DEFINITION OF NURSING DIAGNOSIS

One of the simplest ways to grasp the concept of nursing diagnosis is to ask, How would I know if I saw one? To build on the ideas already discussed, consider how a nursing diagnosis may appear on various record forms. There are three essential components of a nursing diagnosis; they have been referred to as the PES format.[1] The three components are:

1. The health problem (P)
2. The etiological, or related, factors (E)
3. The defining characteristics or cluster of signs and symptoms (S)

This does not mean that every time a diagnosis is written it must have a trailer of all the signs and symptoms. These are documented only the first time the condition is diagnosed. After they have been so documented observations are recorded in progress notes.

CHARACTERISTICS OF CONDITIONS LABELED NURSING DIAGNOSES

1. Nurses can obtain the critical assessment data necessary for making the diagnosis independently.
2. The condition can be resolved primarily by nursing interventions.
3. Nurses assume responsibility for patient/client outcomes related to the condition.
4. Nurses assume responsibility for research on the condition—its prevention, diagnosis, and treatment.

The problem

The first component of a diagnosis is the problem, a health-related state or process, manifested by the individual, family, or community. The problem is expressed in clear, concise terms, preferably in two or three words. Diagnostic categories such as those in Appendix B and others that may need to be created because of the incomplete system are used to label the nurse's judgment about the health problem. For example, *ineffective family coping* and *activity intolerance (specify level)* are concise terms that represent a cluster of signs and symptoms. The term *specify level* refers to the degree of intolerance that is observed; some diagnoses have the word "specify," which directs the user of the category to state the area in which the problem occurs. For example, the term *noncompliance* may be applied to medication regimen, dietary prescription, or any other health management practices that the client has previously agreed to carry out. Each diagnostic category describing a problem has a definition similar to a dictionary definition. It concisely summarizes the theoretical base of knowledge underlying the category and serves to discriminate it from other categories. The observable characteristics, called *defining characteristics,* serve to operationalize the definition; they will be discussed below.

Accuracy in identifying the problem is important because outcome projection and evaluation of care are based on indicators of problem resolution. In later chapters, accuracy will be related to uncertainty-geared decision making.

Syndromes

In 1982 NANDA approved Rape Trauma Syndrome as a diagnosis. Potential Disuse Syndrome and Relocation Stress Syndrome were approved in 1988 and 1992, respectively. These conditions describe a cluster of co-occuring *problems* with at least one common etiological factor, usually specified in the title. Syndromes nearly always occur as a cluster of related problems, in contrast to all other diagnoses, which represent a cluster of signs and symptoms. McCourt's[17] extensive review of the literature across many disciplines reveals two interesting definitions. A dictionary definition of a syndrome is a group of related or coincident things, events, or actions; or a predictable pattern of behavior. This definition is similar to that implicitly underlying NANDA diagnoses: co-occurring problems related by a primary causative factor and viewed as a predictable pattern. Medically a syndrome is described as as a cluster of signs and symptoms that almost always occur together and represent a distinct clinical picture. (Here the word *picture* is close in meaning to the word *pattern* used in the NANDA definition.) It would be very interesting to determine whether the terms *signs* and *symptoms* are similar in level of abstraction to what nurses call *problems.* Results might reveal a consistency between the medical and nursing definitions. A summary of syndrome characteristics drawn from McCourt's review[17] are shown in the box below.

Syndromes, because of their explicit biopsychosocial (and perhaps spiritual) dimensions, appeal to many who suggest nursing diagnoses should describe holistic, rather than reductionistic (parts), states or processes. As McCourt[17] suggests, use of the concept of syndromes can reduce the number of documented problems that share a common causative factor and repetitive interventions. Nurses should be sensitive to all problems within the cluster when planning interventions. Other conditions that meet the criteria of a syndrome will probably be tested clinically and submitted. Long-term chronic pain may be a central causative factor defined by a cluster of biopsychosocial-spiritual problems. Chronic or long-term activity intolerance is another possible causative factor.

COMMON CHARACTERISTICS OF SYNDROMES

1. Syndromes represent a cluster of nursing diagnoses.
2. Their labels give a clue to their causes.
3. Syndromes have initial and long-term phases.
4. Syndromes have emotional, social, and physical components.
5. Syndromes represent complex clinical conditions requiring expert nursing assessment and expert nursing intervention.

Specification of phases or stages may also be important in constructing syndrome concepts.

Syndromes do not have separately listed causative or related factors. This is because the primary causative factor is part of the concept. Rape, relocation, and disuse are examples of causative factors. In a typology such as that in Appendix B, syndromes are classified by their primary etiology. Potential problems (high-risk states) do not logically have a cause; rather, they have risk factors that define the high-risk state. All actual problems have causative factors listed.[18] In the next section these factors will be discussed.

Etiological or related factors

The second component of a nursing diagnosis comprises the probable factors causing or maintaining the client's health problem. These factors may be behaviors of the client, elements of the environment, or an interaction of both. As an example, impaired reality testing may be a factor that contributes to nutritional deficit in a client with psychosis who thinks all food is poisoned. Another example is decreased activity tolerance as a causative factor in impaired home-maintenance management.

Probable causes of a problem should be stated clearly and concisely, using a concise category name, when possible, to summarize the signs and symptoms observed. *Appendix A or B can be used as a dictionary of terms to describe probable causes, as well as problems.* The etiological or related factors in this component of a diagnostic statement are the basis for interventions to resolve the problem. For example, Self-Care Deficit (Level IV) Related to Activity Intolerance is treated very differently from the same deficit related to Severe Situational Depression. Clients may share the same problem but exhibit signs and symptoms indicating different etiological factors. It is important to realize that a different diagnosis exists and different treatment is required when the causative factors are different. Consider Fig. 2-2, which contains two diagnoses and some common etiological factors, each of which requires a different nursing intervention. For example, in the first diagnosis, an etiological factor is combined with the common signs and symptoms of Self-Care Deficit (Level IV) (where the person is totally dependent and does not par-

ticipate in bathing, feeding, dressing, grooming, and toileting). There is an additional set of signs and symptoms peculiar to the specified etiological factor. When a Self-Care Deficit (Level IV) is judged to be present, a differentiation among the possible reasons for the problem is required. This is an example of *differential diagnosis.* Differentiating among various contributing factors is critically important, because interventions can differ radically, as is indicated by the examples of etiological factors shown in Fig. 2-2. A different mode of treatment obviously would be required for each. A person's ability to feed, bathe, dress, groom, and toilet is not going to improve with assistive devices if the cause is *impaired reality testing.* In fact, the problem may worsen if incorrect treatments are used.

The term *related factors* has been recommended by NANDA to describe the conditions or situations that are the focus for intervention. Listed among the related factors are conditions or situations that cannot be influenced by nursing intervention and thus are not clinically useful factors, for example, groups at high risk for developing the problem. This information is useful for diagnosis, but is not the focus for intervention. For example, age is a related factor in some diagnoses; history of early abuse and pregnancy are related factors in others. These factors do not respond to nursing intervention and thus are not clinically useful in planning care.

There has been much debate over the concept of etiology and its connotation of a single cause or its traditional association with medical causes. Usually multiple factors cause a health problem. These factors should be identified and evaluated. Which changes will give the greatest "payoff" in resolving the client's problem? Which will have the highest cost (psychological or monetary)? In Chapter 10, factors influencing a problem will be analyzed as a basis for therapeutic decision making. In Chapter 8 the topic of how to state etiological factor(s) in a useful way for guiding intervention will be discussed.

Defining characteristics

A diagnosis listed in a textbook or manual has a set of defining characteristics (signs and symptoms) that are indicators of the condition. Some are

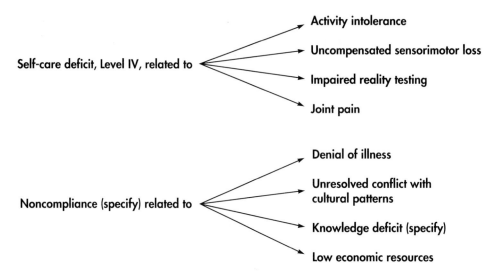

Fig. 2-2 Examples of two health problems and their possible etiological factors.

present in nearly all clients with the problem; these are called critical, or major, characteristics. Critical characteristics *must be present* to make the diagnosis. The remaining characteristics listed in a diagnostic category support or confirm the diagnosis and increase confidence in a particular judgment; these are called supporting, or minor, characteristics.

Now let us reverse the coin and consider the use of textbook information—a manual of nursing diagnosis—in a clinical setting. A nurse observes a postoperative patient crying. One of the possibilities is that the patient is in *pain.* Knowing that one critical characteristic of pain in the textbook is "verbal report of pain," the nurse should check if the patient indeed will speak of pain. If there is a verbal report of pain, the critical characteristic is present. The nurse may want to observe additional supporting characteristics (restlessness, postoperative phase, five-hour time lapse since last pain medication, and crying) to increase confidence in the judgment. This example illustrates how the textbook information on a diagnostic category is used to identify a problem and to increase the diagnostician's confidence in his or her diagnostic judgment. It also emphasizes the need to know the critical characteristics of diagnoses. The characteristics critical for diagnostic judgment must be

learned so that they will be recognized if present or can be elicited when the diagnosis is a possibility.

Critical defining characteristics (diagnostic criteria)

Critical defining characteristics are the criteria for making a diagnosis. They are fewer in number than the supporting characteristics, as was demonstrated in the pain example. They are almost always observed when the diagnosis is present and are usually absent when the diagnosis is absent. Thus the critical characteristics of each category permit diagnosticians to discriminate among diagnoses.

When a client manifests signs and symptoms that correspond to the critical defining characteristics, it is appropriate to use the diagnostic category. For example, clients who report (1) being afraid and can identify the source of their fear and (2) have observable manifestations of discomfort while experiencing muscle tension as well are exhibiting the critical defining characteristics of *fear.* In a national study of defining characteristics, these two behaviors were rated as highly characteristic of the fearful patient by the highest percentage of 212 critical-care nurses. Feelings of dread and sleep pattern disturbances were also among those identified as characteristic of *fear* and its source.[19] The first characteristic, verbal reports of fear, must be present. To increase confidence, nurses usually make use of other relevant, observable signs. Note that for the category of *fear (specify)*, the most critical datum is the verbal report of the client. *Verbal reports are necessary when diagnosing a subjective state or process.* This is an important point to remember; doing so will decrease the rate of diagnostic errors.

Supporting characteristics

Supporting, or minor, characteristics have two uses. In many instances the problem is not overt, but some cue to the condition is present. For example, a client may be restless or having sleepless nights. When questioned about these cues, the person may verbally express being "scared" or make other revealing comments. A verbal report of fear or the perception of a threat to the self, coupled with restlessness and sleep pattern disturbances, "fit the picture" of *fear.* These cues support the diagnosis.

The second use of supporting cues is to see if the client's report can be confirmed by observations; nurses search for supporting data. The client's reports and the nurse's observations are put together to increase confidence in the diagnosis. Note the importance of knowing the defining characteristics, which led to the idea of investigating the possibility of fear. Questioning and seeking information are usually also influenced by a nurse's caring, interest, and intellectual curiosity. In the above instance, it was necessary to know what observations to make to support the diagnosis of fear. Much time can be consumed searching for information on a possible diagnosis if a knowledge of what information is needed to accept or reject a diagnostic possibility is lacking.

It was stated that patients' verbal reports are necessary to diagnose a subjective state. But to every rule there is an exception, so the saying goes. Consider a situation in which the client is unable to speak. How would you know whether a state of fear was present? Since a verbal report is impossible, observations of several signs and the context of the client's situation would have to afford cues. *One reason professional judgment is needed in nursing diagnosis is that client's conditions do not always match the "textbook picture."*

Most nurses contributing to the development of diagnostic categories believe that identification of the critical defining characteristics (signs and symptoms) of approved diagnoses needs a great deal of attention. Yet this identification cannot be completed until diagnoses are used clinically and the signs and symptoms most frequently present are described. If each person who saw the same characteristics of a particular object called it by a different name, communication about the object would be impossible. The definition of the medical diagnostic category of myocardial infarction is standardized internationally, so that in journals or other forms of communication no erroneous interpretation will occur. As in medicine, or science in general, terms used in nursing diagnosis have specific definitions. It is the responsibility of the person using diagnostic terms to use them correctly.

Risk factors

High-risk states are conditions that are predicted but have not occurred. The diagnostic indicators of these conditions are called *risk factors.* They may represent historical or current information that is contextual (situational or environmental) or state-of-the-person factors, such as age. Sometimes one risk factor is such a powerful influence on problem development that its presence places a person, family, or community at high risk for a health problem. Drunken driving an example of a risk factor in High Risk for Accidental Injury. In most instances, a cluster of risk factors determines a high-risk state. All of us are at risk many times during daily activities but do not require constant nursing intervention. It is the client whose risk is greater than "normal" who represents a concern to nurses.

Interventions in high-risk states are directed at reducing the risk factors. The desired outcome is the absence or reduction of the risk. It is important to remember in developing these categories that some of the risk factors listed must be amenable to nursing intervention. Diagnosis is merely an intellectual exercise unless it is followed by nursing care designed to reduce the risk. If nursing intervention is not the primary method of reducing the risk, the problem should be referred on; the condition is probably not a nursing diagnosis.

In the discussion of problem identification in Chapter 9, more will be said about the nature and use of diagnostic categories; their development will be considered in Chapter 12.

Theoretical basis of a diagnostic category

Having just examined the structure of a diagnostic category, it is time to raise the question: Where do these categories come from? Or, more pointedly, what is the knowledge base for problems, conceptual definitions, defining characteristics, and so forth? Actually, the diagnostic category structure just described is the *last* in a series of developmental activities.

Each of the diagnostic categories in Appendix A may be thought of as a diagnostic concept. Concepts are guides to action.[20] They are ideas created to describe or explain observations. Each has a theoretical base. Theoretical knowledge is the basis for constructing a diagnostic category. Hinshaw,[21] in her keynote address to the 1988 NANDA Conference participants, remarked:

Ultimately, it will be important to have a body of knowledge surrounding and undergirding each nursing diagnosis in order to justify the use of the information in practice. Without it, the reliability, validity, and accuracy of the information will remain questionable.[21]

When nurses began to classify the problems they diagnosed and treated, there was a large store of clinical knowledge to be formulated into concepts and categories. New ideas for new diagnoses are created by attending to clinical observations and paying attention to what cannot be explained. Through a process of concept development, analysis, study, and restructuring, a category that can be tested clinically will emerge. Then:

If the diagnostic concept is a useful approximation of reality, it will be used in clinical practice—it will "survive in the marketplace" of ideas. If nursing knowledge, purpose, or values change, the concepts will change. Webster urged classifiers to categorize their world but to maintain an "openness to new formulations, realizing that there is not just one truth or one perspective," and especially to avoid "hardening of the categories."[22]

In addition and contrary to what many textbooks claim, assessment, monitoring, referral, and calling the physician are not nursing interventions to resolve a problem, as a few authors have noted.[22,23]

They are important, but they are assessment and evaluation procedures. If the only interventions for a diagnosis are watching and notifying, it is highly likely the condition is not a nursing diagnosis and is not theoretically based in nursing.

DIAGNOSIS DEFINED AS A PROCESS

As previously stated, the word *diagnosis* has two meanings. First, it may refer to a name for a health problem found in a classification system of nursing diagnoses—the meaning that was explored in the previous section. The second meaning, a process leading to a clinical judgment, is the topic introduced in this section.

It is important to appreciate the various cognitive operations involved in acquiring and using clinical information. It is equally important to understand that clinical information is acquired through nurse-client interaction. The quality of this interaction directly affects what information is obtained and, subsequently, what diagnostic judgment is made. Let us first consider some general characteristics of the diagnostic process and its components.

The diagnostic process is, essentially, a way of determining a client's health problem and evaluating the etiological factors influencing the problem. Is it ever possible to truly know the state of another person, a family, or a community? Most philosophers who deal with such questions would say no. What the diagnostician seeks is sufficient understanding of clients and situations to evaluate health, predict future health, and provide assistance when needed. One definition of diagnosis is "an analysis of the nature of something."[24] In clinical practice that "something" is a client's health status.

To diagnose is to distinguish or discriminate. As information is collected, the first discrimination that occurs is between indicators of a problem and indicators of health and well-being. This is a two-way discrimination task. If signs point toward a judgment of health, they are described and recognition is given to the client's health-promoting practices. Identifying and acknowledging healthful practices serves to support behavior that maintains health.

On the other hand, signs may point toward an actual or potential problem. Search strategies are required to identify the problem clearly. Additionally, the cluster of signs and symptoms must be labeled with the correct diagnostic category. This process represents much more than a two-way differentiation between the presence and absence of health.

Diagnostic process components

Within the diagnostic process are actions, and within these actions are other, more specific operations involving reasoning and judgment. In its broadest sense, diagnosis involves four activities:

☐ Collecting information
☐ Interpreting the information
☐ Clustering the information
☐ Naming the cluster

From this list it appears that the four activities are a sequence of steps and that the diagnostician has only to collect all the information available, analyze and arrange it, and apply category names to the health problems identified. If diagnosis were this uncomplicated, any nurse's aide could be taught the steps. Instead, what occurs in the diagnostic process is a cycle of certain perceptual and cognitive activities. Observations lead to inferences, and inferences lead to further observation. This cycle continues until the diagnostician feels confident in naming the problem.

Information collection

The admission nursing history and examination begins the process of information collection, or assessment. (Actually, information collection never ends.) In adding a person, family, or community to his or her caseload, the nurse assumes the responsibility for collecting health-related data. Skillful collection of information, which is critically important in the diagnostic process, is influenced by clinical knowledge. One perceives what one expects to perceive (on the basis of stored knowledge). Clinical knowledge stored in memory provides the expectations that make one sensitive to cues.[25] Knowing how to frame a question or measure a pulse is a basic skill. *The independent judgment of when the question or measurement is* *appropriate is influenced by one's clinical knowledge.*

Information interpretation

Collecting information is pointless if the meaning behind it is not derived. Interpretation of cues to a client's health status allows one to predict or explain the findings. Two mental operations are involved: inferential reasoning and judgment.

Information clustering

In clinical practice, nurses collecting and interpreting information are heard to remark, "It fits the picture," "I'm getting a picture of . . . ," or "No, that doesn't fit the picture." What seems to be occurring is the clustering of information in a meaningful way based on its interpretation (a diagnostic hypothesis; a hunch). Nurses know "what goes with what." How do they know this? Probably, memory stores are searched for previously learned, meaningful ways of clustering the clinical cues within diagnostic categories. The "picture" referred to is probably the memory cluster of signs and symptoms that defines a diagnostic category.

Naming the cue cluster

Information collection, interpretation, and clustering occur over and over during the diagnostic process. When observations seem to "fit" a diagnostic category, the category name is applied to the cluster of cues. For example, the client may (1) have excessive perspiration due to a fever, (2) be too weak to turn and reach for a drink of water, (3) express concern that her children are not getting good care during her hospitalization, and (4) have dry mouth. Cues 1, 2, and 4 fit the critical defining characteristics of the diagnostic category of Potential Fluid Volume Deficit. Thus this name is given to the client's problem. The verbal report, cue 3, does not fit but is possibly a cue to another problem; it requires further investigation. Identification, or naming a health problem, is an act of judgment that says, "It is this and not that." *Diagnostic reasoning and judgment are important because they are the basis for care planning.*

The goal in health evaluation and diagnosis is to arrive at correct and reliable judgments. Attaining this goal requires refinement of the commonsense approach that serves so well in everyday living. Refinement proceeds in a particular direction, toward critical reflection and curiosity. These two abilities increase the reliability of diagnostic judgments and differentiate professional expertise from the lay person's commonsense approach. Thus far this chapter has provided information about nursing diagnosis as a category and a process. For implementing diagnosis in practice, it is important to know that:

1. Nursing diagnoses are made by professional nurses.
2. Nursing diagnoses describe actual or potential health problems that are amenable to nursing intervention. Nurses assume accountability for the outcomes of nursing diagnoses.
3. Nursing diagnoses are names that refer to a cluster of cues indicating a health problem (see Appendix A).
4. Each nursing diagnosis has a small set of critical defining characteristics that represent the major signs and symptoms of the health problem. These characteristics represent the diagnostic criteria for making the diagnosis.
5. Each problem has etiological or related factors that contribute to or maintain the problem; their resolution or modification serves as a focus for nursing intervention. In the case of potential problems, risk factors are identified. When sufficient risk factors are present, the diagnosis is stated as "high risk for . . . ."[18]
6. Within the diagnostic process there is information collection, information interpretation, information clustering, and naming the cluster.
7. Commonsense reasoning may be helpful in the diagnostic process, but a diagnostician's reliability depends on critical reasoning (reflective analysis and the curiosity to ask why).

DIAGNOSTIC RESPONSIBILITY

It will probably be clear after reading this chapter that nursing diagnosis is not just the use of labels. It requires professional knowledge and skill. National standards of practice, educational preparation, and licensing laws make it clear that the re-

sponsibility for nursing diagnosis belongs to professional nurses. Who are considered professional nurses? Currently, whoever is licensed by the state to practice as a registered nurse. Yet many would argue that the baccalaureate nursing curriculum best prepares clinicians to assume this responsibility. Other nursing personnel may contribute information or carry out specified care, but registered nurses make nursing diagnoses. *Diagnostic and therapeutic decision making is never delegated to the less prepared or given over by referral.* This principle protects both the client and the nurse.

The belief that registered nurses are responsible for making nursing diagnoses was evident at the NANDA Business Meeting, Seventh Conference on Classification of Nursing Diagnoses, St. Louis, Missouri, March 1986. The General Assembly passed a motion that NANDA support the concept that only registered, professional nurses be responsible and accountable for identifying the nursing diagnoses for their patient population.

Saying that professional nurses are responsible for treating nursing diagnoses does not mean that nonnursing consultants cannot be used. Aspects of treatment may require consultation with other specialized personnel whose professions emerged from nursing. These professions include occupational therapy, physical therapy, social work, and respiratory therapy. Each offers specialized skills related to parts of the client situation. Although the term *referral* is used, nurses are responsible for coordinating treatment of nursing diagnoses. Responsibility and accountability in nursing diagnosis are important issues and will be considered in later chapters.

SUMMARY

Diagnosis as a process and diagnosis as a category can be separated for purposes of discussion, but they are inseparable when used in practice. When the term *nursing diagnosis* is used to refer to a category or concept, it presumes a specific structure, a conceptual or theoretical base, and its use within a particular context, such as nursing process. Work on diagnostic-category development and refinement is ongoing. As new knowledge is acquired, concepts and the categories derived from the conceptual knowledge base are restructured. The diagnostic process is the segment of nursing process that deals with assessment and diagnostic judgment. It includes the collection, interpretation, and clustering of information. Then a name is given to the health problem.

Because nursing diagnoses are not made in isolation and because nurses need to increase their participation in joint planning, an appreciation of other professions is needed. When participating in a joint-care planning conference, it is important to know the perspectives of other professions (just as they need to understand the nursing perspective). Chapter 3 provides information on this subject. It also provides an opportunity to see how nursing's perspective and the focus of diagnosis evolved.

NOTES AND REFERENCES

1. Gordon M: Nursing diagnosis and the diagnostic process, *Am J Nurs* 76:1298, 1976.
2. Protocols are guides for analyzing and treating a disease process or symptom complex. A protocol may be highly organized and directive or it may be general and flexible, depending on the situation, education, and experience of the users and the availability of physician supervision and support. Hudak CM: *Clinical protocols: a guide for nurses and physicians,* Philadelphia, 1976, Lippincott.
3. Hammond KR: Clinical inference in nursing: a psychologist's viewpoint, *Nurs Res* 1 5:27, 1966.
4. Soares CA: Nursing and medical diagnoses: comparison of variant and essential features. In Chaska NL, editor: *The nursing profession: views through the mist,* New York, 1978, McGraw-Hill, p 276.
5. Feild L, Winslow EH: Moving to a nursing model, *Am J Nurs* 85:1100, 1985.
6. North American Nursing Diagnosis Association: *NANDA Taxonomy I, Revised,* 1992. Philadelphia: Author.
7. Some interpret this definition to mean that nursing diagnoses are responses to actual or potential health problems. If so, what are health problems? Medical diagnoses/diseases? The scope of nursing diagnosis is severely limited to apply only to illness if we define these responses as responses to diseases. A person who is "disease-free" may still have a nursing diagnosis. The NANDA interpretation of these words is unclear. First it states that health problems may be diabetes, trauma, or surgery and later that nursing diagnosis refers to, among other things, a health problem. Carpinito LJ: The NANDA definition of nursing diagnosis. In Carroll-Johnson R, editor: *Classification of nursing diagnoses: proceedings of the ninth conference,* Philadelphia, 1992, Lippincott, pp 67, 70.
8. There is an active interest group within NANDA comprising nurses working on "wellness diagnoses." Publications on this subject include Gleit CJ, Tatro S: Nursing diagnosis for healthy individuals, *Nurs Health Care* 2:456, 1981; Gottleib LN: Small steps toward the development of a health classification system for nursing. In Kim MJ, Moritz DA, editors: *Classification of nursing diagnoses: proceed-* ings of the third and fourth national conferences, New York, 1982, McGraw-Hill.
9. Carroll-Johnson R, editor: *Classification of nursing diagnoses: proceedings of the ninth conference,* St Louis, 1991, Mosby.
10. Territorial issues are those conflicts and controversies that arise among care providers regarding domains and scope of practice. Underlying the issues are expertise and monetary concerns.
11. Silver SM et al: Identification of clinically recorded nursing diagnoses and indicators. In Kim MJ, McFarland G, McLane A, editors: *Classification of nursing diagnoses: proceedings of the fifth national conference,* St Louis, 1984, Mosby.
12. Little D, Carnevali D: The diagnostic statement: the problem defined. In Walter B, Pardee P, Molbo DM, editors: *Dynamics of problem-oriented approaches: patient care and documentation,* New York, 1976, Lippincott.
13. Maslow A: *Motivation and personality,* New York, 1970, Harper & Row.
14. As may be seen in Appendix A, fatigue is an approved nursing diagnosis, as is activity intolerance. The diagnosis that seems to be preferred is activity intolerance, which describes the functional problem.
15. Martens K: Let's diagnose strengths, not just problems, *Am J Nurs* 86:192, 1986.
16. Clinical testing will probably reveal two or more health problems in some of the current diagnostic categories, each of which will be treated differently. Alterations in parenting is such an example.
17. McCourt A: Syndromes in nursing a continuing concern. In Carroll-Johnson R, editor: *Classification of nursing diagnoses: proceedings of the ninth conference,* Philadelphia, 1991, Lippincott, pp 79-82.
18. See Gordon M: *Manual of nursing diagnosis,* St Louis, 1993, Mosby, or North American Nursing Diagnosis Association: *Taxonomy I, Revised,* 1992, Philadelphia, 1992, Author.
19. Gordon M: Critical defining characteristics of high-frequency nursing diagnoses in critical care nursing practice. Study in progress.
20. Dickoff J, James P: Theoretical pluralism for nursing diagnosis. In Carroll-Johnson R, editor: *Classification of nursing diagnoses: proceedings of the eighth conference,* Philadelphia, 1989, Lippincott, pp 98-125.
21. Hinshaw AS: Nursing diagnosis: forging the link between theory and practice. In Carroll-Johnson R, editor: *Classification of nursing diagnoses: proceedings of the eighth conference,* Philadelphia, 1989, Lippincott, p 7.
22. Gordon M: Toward theory-based diagnostic categories, *Nurs Diag* 1:1, 1990.
23. McCluskey J, Bulechek G: *Nursing intervention classification,* St Louis, 1992, Mosby.
24. Morris W, editor: *American heritage dictionary of the English language,* Boston, 1978, Houghton Mifflin, p 363.
25. "Cue" is a word that will be used frequently in this text and is synonomous with "defining characteristic," "sign," or "symptom." It is a term borrowed from cognitive psychology and means a signal to action; initially, a cognitive action. A client behavior exists; it becomes a cue only if it is perceived and interpreted by the diagnostician.

Chapter 3

Clinical Diagnosis in the Health Professions

P lacing the adjective *nursing* before the term *diagnosis* merely identifies the area of health care problems being addressed. Just as nurses use the term *nursing diagnosis* to refer to health problems within their scope of practice, physicians use the term *medical diagnosis* and social workers, *casework diagnosis.*

The client problems addressed by the various professions differ. Yet the overall method of identifying and using diagnostic categories is the same. An appreciation of these similarities and differences should enhance interprofessional communication as well as clarify some issues in nursing diagnosis. Usually we can better understand our own domain of practice when it is viewed in the context of overall professional health care delivery. In this chapter clinical diagnosis in nursing, medicine, and social work will be examined according to five interrelated elements that are relevant to diagnosis:

1. *Professional focus:* Describes the purpose or social mandate of a profession and influences its conceptual framework for practice.
2. *Conceptual framework:* A set of general ideas, or concepts, that are logically interrelated. The one concept examined here is the profession's conceptual model of the client that guides the naming of diagnostic categories (health problems).
3. *Concept of causality:* The probable reasons for health problems. Etiological or related factors are commonly used to denote these reasons.

4. *Classification systems:* Names and classes of health problems that represent the phenomena of concern to the profession.
5. *Diagnostic process:* The method of identifying client's problems.

The significance and meaning of each of these five terms is discussed below.

NURSING

Professions arise to fulfill a particular need of society. Having been created by society, they assume responsibility and accountability for that social need. The nursing profession arose out of needs associated with human suffering. First seen as a religious calling to care for the injured, ill, or infirm, nursing was practiced within religious orders. Today religious nursing orders exist, but the majority of practitioners are secular.

Nursing has passed through historical phases parallel to those of social or religious movements. Similar to Western society in general, nursing had its "dark ages," coinciding with periods of general social neglect of human suffering. "Renaissance" periods paralleled periods of humanitarianism and social reform. In contemporary society nursing has taken an increasingly active role in health care policy formation and health care delivery.

Public attitudes and values sanctioned the nursing profession in its early days and are still favorable, even in the general atmosphere of criticism of health care that currently prevails. Sometimes, in striving for ideals, nurses are more critical of nursing than is the general public.

In public surveys of various professions, nursing is usually held in high regard. In recent years higher salaries and the greater visibility of nurses' independent judgment and responsibility make the profession more attractive to high school graduates. Society sanctions a profession through state licensing laws. In recent years these laws have expanded or clarified nurses' social responsibility in health care. In many states laws include statements about nursing diagnosis as a professional function. Delegated medical diagnosis and treatment are also permitted under some degree of supervision by the physician.

Florence Nightingale's concept of nursing was formulated when she founded the profession, and it is still current. It emphasized helping both the sick and the well perform activities that contribute to health and recovery. A definition of contemporary nursing is found in the American Nurses' Association (ANA) Model Practice Act:

The practice of nursing means the performance for compensation of professional services requiring substantial specialized knowledge of the biological, physical, behavioral, psychological, and sociological sciences and nursing theory as the basis for assessment, diagnosis, planning, intervention, and evaluation in the promotion and maintenance of health; the casefinding and management of illness, injury, or infirmity; the restoration of optimum function; or the achievement of a dignified death. Nursing practice includes but is not limited to administration, teaching, counseling, supervision, delegation, and evaluation of practice and execution of the medical regimen. . . .[1]

As generalists or specialists, nurses are involved in all levels of health care. These levels include (1) primary care, focusing on health maintenance and preventive care in clinics or community settings; (2) secondary care, which may or may not require hospitalization for common illnesses; and (3) tertiary care, requiring the sophisticated technology of specialized units. In each level the focus is on individuals and families. Primary care may also include the health of communities. Recognized areas in which nurses specialize include (1) settings, such as community health; (2) age groups, such as geriatrics and child health; and (3) health problems, or health states, such as mater-

nal, medical-surgical, and psychiatric–mental-health specialties.

Some nurses have private practices. This is most common in the psychiatric–mental-health specialty. Reimbursement to clients through insurance payments may increase private practice in this and other specialties in the future. Most nurses are employees of health care institutions. This arrangement may sometimes present a dilemma to practitioners because of conflicts between institutional and professional values. In fact this conflict is experienced to some extent by members of all the health professions.

Professional focus

All health professions are concerned with human behavior. Differences exist in the way health problems are conceptualized and labeled and in the level of understanding sought. For example, medicine's predominant focus is on human biological phenomena, conceptualized as disease states. Understanding is sought at the cellular or subcellular level.

Historically the focus of nursing has been individual, family, or community needs relevant to health and welfare. These needs have ranged broadly, from sanitation in a community to energy conservation in an individual. Generalizing across specialties and practice settings, the concern has consistently been human beings' optimal functioning in their environment.

Although expressed in various terms, the specific phenomena nursing addresses are potential or actual functional problems. Potential problems may result from health-related practices and predictably contribute to future illness in an individual, family, or community. Actual problems occur in association with illness or with social, occupational, or maturational changes.

Each of the professions seeks a certain level of understanding of the phenomena with which it deals. As new knowledge becomes available, the level may change. For example, physicists once sought to understand the nature of matter at the atomic level; as a result of advances in knowledge and theory, subatomic particles are now the level of interest. Nurses seek to understand health-related behavior at the level of human organism–environment interaction. Clinical problems are viewed as holistic, or whole-person, expressions of this interaction, and diagnosis and intervention are performed within this holistic model. As we shall see in a later chapter, nursing theorists deal in different ways with the inherent complexity of this focus.

Underlying and supporting the focus of a profession are the art and science of practice. Theories, concepts, principles, and methods of treatment compose the science of a profession. The *art* is the way knowledge is used, especially in human interactions, and reflects attitudes, beliefs, and values. Yet there can never be a clear separation of art and science. Attitudes, beliefs, and values, whether internal or external to the profession, influence its science—particularly in the selection of methods, focus, and interpretations. Some interesting historical examples of the influence of changing beliefs and values on the naming and interpretation of diagnostic entities in regard to medicine are discussed below.

As would be expected in a profession with such a diverse practice focus and broad, holistic perspective, the body of clinical knowledge in nursing is extensive. Nursing science, as Rogers[2] states, is only beginning to be identified. Currently the knowledge base for practice rests to a large extent on the application of biological, psychological, and social science theory. Extending this knowledge in a way that is relevant to nursing concerns will aid in developing the science of nursing.

The body of knowledge in a profession must be descriptive, explanatory, and predictive. The increasing emphasis on clinical research in recent years has served to increase the science base of practice. Nursing diagnoses, because they isolate phenomena of concern to the profession, provide direction and focus for research and the development of nursing science.

Conceptual frameworks for practice

Each person views the world from a particular perspective, and this viewpoint affects the way the person explains and predicts events. Similarly, in the professions, the *focus of concern* in practice is described and explained from a particular perspective or frame of reference.

A conceptual model is a simplification, a cognitive construction that ignores as irrelevant some aspects of the phenomenon being considered. It narrows attention to the area of concern and purpose. For example, some psychologists find a game theory model useful in describing interpersonal relations; the model helps explain and predict one phenomenon of concern—human interaction—although (perhaps *because*) it disregards some factors to focus on others. The conceptual models of the client discussed in Chapter 4 are merely approximations of reality. They currently provide practitioners with a useful way of thinking about clients. If knowledge, purpose, or values change in the profession, the models will be subject to change.

One component of a framework is the conceptual model of the client that guides assessment and diagnosis. A brief consideration of the historical models of the client may help to clarify the background of contemporary frameworks for nursing. Out of the belief that gods, demons, or evil spirits caused suffering arose the sanatoriums of ancient Greece. The priest-physicians and attendants of these temples of healing were the forerunners of the religious nursing orders that arose when Christianity spread through the world. From Kalisch and Kalisch's[3] review of nursing history, it appears that nursing and Christian charity were interwoven. The "client" was seen as a "child of God," whether aged, infirm, orphaned, a casualty of war, or lacking relatives and friends to provide care. Devotion to religion motivated men and women of the Middle Ages to nurse the helpless in an evidently excellent manner.[4] (p. 296)

Industrialization and urbanization in the eighteenth and nineteenth centuries were accompanied by crowded living conditions, poverty, and devastating epidemics. The capacity of the religious hospitals and asylums was strained, and secular nursing began.

In the eighteenth and nineteenth centuries, both in America and Europe, the religious, devotional model of client care was lost in the public hospitals. Nurses were hired attendants who used alcohol and snuff as means of psychological escape from the poor conditions. They were portrayed in all their depravity by Dickens's description of Sairy Gamp in mid-nineteenth-century England.[5] (pp. 312-313) The physicians of that day were not much better. In America, "a common saying was that 'a boy who's unfit for anything else must become a doctor.'"[3] (p. 25) Interestingly, war provided the impetus for change.

The internationally recognized contributions of Florence Nightingale to the improvement of British military hospitals during the Crimean War and the postwar humanitarian concern in Europe combined to change these conditions. In America the Civil War brought about great changes in nursing. The changes of the late nineteenth and early twentieth centuries occurred in the social context of reform; women's rights; and advances in health care, particularly the concept of asepsis and the beginning of control of infectious disease. It must be remembered that these were the days when "common law and biblical tradition bound women to an inferior status."[3] (p. 71)

When modern nursing began, illness was believed to be nature's *remedy* for removing the effects of conditions interfering with health. Neither nurses nor physicians "cured"; that was nature's realm. Out of Nightingale's experience with the horrendous conditions in the Crimean War hospitals came the idea that a person had to be considered in interaction with the environment.[6] (p. 26) Nature could not cure if sanitation, diet, and living conditions were not improved.

Nightingale described the nursing care of her day as little more than the administration of medicines and applying poultices. She argued that it ought to be concerned with fresh air, light, warmth, cleanliness, quiet, and the proper selection and administration of diet. All these things were to be accomplished with the least drain on the energy of the person.[6]

The emphasis in the client-environment model was clearly on the environment. The person was viewed from the perspective of a "dependency model." This perspective seemed logical when common practice dictated that the sick or injured be put to bed. The rationale was to conserve "vital power"[6] (p. 6); rest and good living conditions constituted the major therapy for *all* illnesses. Ideally, the "rest cure" was provided at home. It was the poor and uneducated of the cities, the travelers, and the casualties from the battlefields who were brought to the hospital.

Clara Weeks Shaw, a contemporary of Nightingale, stressed the dependency model of the client

and the complementary "maternity model of nursing": The "sick person is, for the time being, as a child and looks to his nurse for a mother's care."[7] (p. 19) This conception of nursing emphasized personal care, environmental comfort, and cleanliness.

More changes occurred in the first half of the present century. The dependency model was beginning to wane, influenced by society's focus on education of the masses, the mental hygiene movement, and advances in medical treatment. Nursing's participation and leadership in the public health movement of the late nineteenth century was also influential.

The nursing literature began to place stress on clients regaining independence; this emphasis was reflected in discussions about teaching hygienic practices, preventing illness, and using available community resources.[8] (p. 3) This self-responsibility theme was further extended by Harmer[9] (p. 4) and Henderson.[10] She wrote of the individual's physical strength, will, or knowledge to perform activities related to health and recovery; nursing was required when these factors were absent.

From the textbooks of the time it appears that the biomedical model of the human being, used by medicine, was adopted by nursing. There were nurses who independently determined the nursing care needed, but generally the physician was responsible for identifying medical problems. Nurses were supposed to know how to provide comfort, observe disease complications, and report observations. The frequent mention in the literature of "needs" and "needs for help" suggests that a human needs model of the client predominated about midcentury but focused on disease-related needs.

Orlando[11] published a model of practice referred to as the dynamic nurse-patient relationship. Included was a distress-coping model of the client. Her method of assisting the client and of judging the client's need for help had a great impact and is still pertinent today. Orlando's model,[11] and later Orem's self-care model,[12] (pp. 5-6) emphasized self-direction and individual responsibility. Nursing was to do only what the person and his or her resources could not do unaided.

The complexity of the nursing model for practice has increased during the twentieth century. If people were to learn responsibility for self-care and prevention of illness, nurses had to do more than carry out physicians' orders and administer routine personal care. They had to make judgments about what was needed and what was not.

Lydia Hall[13] used the term *nursing process* in the early 1950s, and through the years her approach has evolved into the accepted method of delivering nursing care. The basic tenets of the Nightingale model—client-environment interaction and religious traditions of wholeness, self-direction, and will—were retained in twentieth-century nursing.[9 (p. 4);12 (pp. 5-6)] Rogers'[2] theory of nursing placed emphasis on the client rather than on tasks; this approach began to clarify nursing's science and focus. Currently human response patterns, functional patterns, and other models are used to guide assessment and diagnosis within nursing process. The focus of nursing as a professional discipline is the subject of a paper in which the author traces the development of the profession's focus:

Historically, we seem to have moved from addressing primarily the health of the body as affected by environmental factors to interplay of body-mind-environment factors in health, and more recently, to health as an experience of the unitary human field phenomena embedded in a larger unitary field.[14 (p. 11)]

The terms *energy* and *field phenomena* were introduced by Rogers[2] to describe human beings and their environmental fields. The term *unitary field,* or *unitary person,* stresses the idea that a human being is a whole, not a set of biological or psychological parts, a concept discussed further in Chapter 4.

The idea of caring has always been associated with nursing; in recent years it has received much attention as a philosophy of practice. As nursing moves into the twenty-first century, it is likely that work on the dimensions of a nursing philosophy will continue. Will a unified perspective on nursing evolve in the twenty-first century? Northrup[15] suggests that such an outlook is needed:

A unified perspective provides the starting point from which to derive and accommodate multiple and diverse theoretical concepts and/or models. Indeed, nursing theories must be placed within a larger context that is consistent with a philosophical foundation that reflects our values and our methods of knowing. The relevant quest before nursing, then, is the development and articulation

of a coherent philosphy that reflects our values and our moral ideals within the larger context: a unified perspective.

At midcentury the term *nursing diagnosis* appeared in the literature.[16] Bonney and Rothberg[17] employed the term *nursing diagnosis* in a client evaluation instrument to predict needs for nursing service. The objective was to use clients' nursing diagnoses as predictors of nurse staffing needs in long-term care facilities. Their report defined *diagnoses* as a "listing of factors" that affected the client's condition. The list was divided into strengths and liabilities. Lists, rather than problems, were formulated, yet this change in emphasis contributed to shifting the focus of description from nursing actions to client conditions.

In 1980 the ANA published a social policy statement that identified the phenomena of concern to nurses as "human responses to actual or potential health problems."[18 (p. 9)] Human responses were viewed as:

1. reactions of individuals and groups to actual problems (health-restoring responses), such as the impact of illness-effects upon the self, family, and related self-care needs; and
2. concerns of individuals and groups about potential problems (health-supporting responses), such as monitoring and teaching in populations or communities at risk in which educative needs for information, skill development, health-oriented attitudes, and related behavioral change arise.[18 (pp. 9-10)]

These two areas of human responses are similar to the focus of nursing diagnosis identified in Chapter 1: problems in health management and problems secondary to illness, medical therapy, developmental changes, or life situations. The social policy statement reflects the current focus on clients' conditions (rather than nurses' actions) and social responsibility.

In the 1970s and 1980s many nursing theorists proposed conceptual frameworks to guide diagnosis and treatment. A few current conceptual frameworks will be reviewed in detail in Chapter 4. The basic tenets of the Nightingale model—client-environment interaction and religious traditions of wholeness, self-direction, and free will—were retained in twentieth-century nursing frameworks. As the twenty-first century approaches consumers will assume more independence in personal health management, prevention of early onset of chronic disease and disability, and environmental control. The conceptual framework for nursing practice is consistent with the health services that will be needed. The degree to which nurses assume responsibility for health services will depend on choices by individual practitioners, resolution of "territorial" issues with physicians,[19] and consumer reimbursement for nursing services.

Concept of causality

A profession's concept of causality is the way its members view the cause-and-effect relationships existing between health problems and the factors that interact to produce them. Some philosophers argue that the concept of causality should be abandoned; others say it is so implicit in human thinking that it cannot be discarded. The notion of causality in nursing practice is rarely addressed, although Field[20] has provided a review of this concept in science. This is not to suggest that the idea is not used in nursing. Clinically, one hears explanations of the causes of clients' problems that range from single to multiple factors. Simple reasons and single causes may be valued for their noncomplexity. Yet when asked to explain the cause of a patient's clinical problem, nurses tend to respond with explanations that include complex, multifactor chains of events. In Chapters 6 and 9, causality and the concept of *etiology* will be considered further.

Classification systems

Diagnosis and systems for classifying the health problems addressed by nurses did not receive widespread attention in nursing until the 1970s. Considering the way modern nursing evolved, this lack may be difficult to understand. During the Crimean War, Florence Nightingale, 24 nuns, and 14 other women diagnosed and treated health problems so effectively that the mortality rate in British military hospitals showed an overall drop from 42 percent to 2.2 percent.[3] (p. 42) Well before this, in the twelfth century, when women studied nursing and obstetrics at the University of Salerno, the famous treatise *Tortula on the Cure of Diseases of Women* was written by a midwife.[3] (p. 5)

At the end of the first century of modern nurs-

ing, concepts of practice emphasized procedures, tasks, and nursing functions. The first classification of nursing problems was for the purpose of education. A subcommittee of the National League for Nursing, while revising student record forms, perceived the need to describe generic nursing practice in terms of a client-centered, as opposed to a task-centered, focus. From a survey of more than 40 schools of nursing, the first classification—of 21 problems—was completed.[21] (pp. 83–88) As the box on p. 38 shows, these now-famous "problems" were therapeutic goals of nursing. This was consistent with the emphasis at the time on client needs (therapeutic needs) and nursing problems (therapeutic problems).

Nursing was commonly described as a set of functions. In fact the numerous studies of nurses and nurses' functions caused Abdellah to comment that "as valuable as such studies are, they portray what the nurse is doing, not why she is doing what she is, nor if she should be doing what she is."[21] (p. 74) Fifteen years would elapse before a change in the focus of nursing diagnosis would begin to provide answers to the questions she posed.

In 1966 Henderson[10] identified a list of 14 basic human needs that comprised the components, or functions, of nursing. This formulation further supported the functional needs approach. These basic needs, listed in the box on p. 39, address not health problems of the client but areas in which actual or potential problems might occur. Both Abdellah's and Henderson's lists were widely used in education and practice. Their contributions stimulated nurses to go beyond routine functions and tasks to identify therapeutic problems. This shift in focus set the stage for the next step—nursing diagnoses, or client problems, as the focus of care.

The shift from care organized around therapeutic problems, such as "to facilitate the maintenance of effective verbal communication," to care organized around client problems, such as "impaired verbal communication," began in the early 1970s. This change was facilitated by the First National Conference on Classification of Nursing Diagnoses in 1973. The conference provided a beginning language with which to express judgments and to organize nursing care.

National conferences have been held approximately every two years since 1973. Hundreds of

---

MASTER LIST OF NURSING PROBLEMS PRESENTED BY CLIENTS

To facilitate the maintenance of oxygen to all body cells

To facilitate the maintenance of nutrition of all body cells

To facilitate the maintenance of elimination

To facilitate the maintenance of fluid and electrolyte balance

To promote safety through the prevention of accident, injury, or other trauma and through the prevention of the spread of infection

To facilitate the maintenance of regulatory mechanisms or functions

To facilitate the maintenance of sensory function

To promote optimal activity: exercise, rest, and sleep

To maintain good body mechanics and prevent and correct deformities

To maintain good hygiene and physical comfort

To recognize the physiological responses of the body to disease conditions—pathological and compensatory

To identify and accept interrelatedness of emotions and organic illness

To identify and accept positive and negative expressions, feelings, and reactions

To facilitate the maintenance of effective verbal and nonverbal communication

To promote the development of productive interpersonal relationships

To facilitate progress toward achievement of personal spiritual goals

To accept the optimum possible goals in the light of limitations, physical and emotional

To use community resources as an aid in resolving problems arising from illness

To create or maintain a therapeutic environment

To understand the role of social problems as influencing factors in the cause of illness

To facilitate awareness of self as an individual with varying physical, emotional, and developmental needs

From Abdellah FG: Improving the teaching of nursing through research in patient care. In Heiderken LE, editor: *Improvement of nursing through research,* Washington, DC, 1959, Catholic University of America Press.

---

nurses have participated in the conference objective: to develop diagnostic nomenclature (a system of category names) and classify nursing diagnoses. The evolution of the current classification system may be seen in Appendix U, which shows the changes, deletions, and additions that occurred in diagnostic categories between 1973 and 1992.

What are nurses classifying? An examination of the diagnostic category names (Appendix A) suggest that alterations in functions or functional patterns predominate. Ineffective, impaired, or altered human functions occur frequently in the listing. There is nearly a balance between physiological areas and psychosocial-spiritual areas. This division, of course, is invalid, since the signs and symptoms defining each category in many cases are biopsychosocial.

The very broad focus, human responses, is the current concept used in accepting and rejecting diagnoses. Recently the NANDA board and the membership have accepted "diagnoses" that describe life processes, such as effective breast-feeding or health-seeking behaviors. These health or wellness categories have raised questions about the focus of the classification system. Some argue that health-seeking behavior is a nursing goal, not a diagnosis. In contrast, others argue that nursing diagnoses describe more than problems and potential problems. In Chapter 1 the same question was raised: Do nursing diagnoses describe everything nurses assess? Or do nursing diagnoses describe only those conditions resolved by nursing care and for which nurses assume accountability for outcomes? How inclusive the classification of nursing diagnoses should be is controversial. The subject of classification is worth pursuing because not all the issues have been resolved. They mirror the larger issues related to the profession's pluralistic, conceptual focus. Other relevant questions will be addressed in Chapter 11, such as, What is the purpose of the system and how is it to be used (e.g., practice or reimbursement)?

A developing classification system requires some conceptual focus to ensure consistency in

FOURTEEN BASIC NEEDS

Breathing normally
Eat and drink adequately
Eliminate body wastes
Move and maintain desirable postures
Sleep and rest
Suitable clothes—dress and undress
Maintain body temperature within normal
    range by adjusting clothing and modifying
    the environment
Keep body clean and well groomed and pro-
    tect the integument
Avoid dangers in the environment and avoid
    injuring others
Communicate with others in expressing emo-
    tions, needs, fears, or opinions
Worship according to one's faith
Work in such a way that there is a sense of
    accomplishment
Play or participate in various forms of recre-
    ation
Learn, discover, or satisfy the curiosity that
    leads to normal development and health
    and use the available health facilities

From Henderson V: *The nature of nursing,* New
York, 1966, Macmillan.

classifying so that, for example, apples, dogs, and chairs do not get classified together. Consistency among the diagnoses classified is provided by this focus or framework. The development of a classification system is discussed in Chapter 12.

Diagnostic process

Basic textbooks rarely mentioned nursing diagnosis or the process of diagnosing to any great extent before the 1970s. Yet assessment, with emphasis on information collection, has received widespread attention in the literature of the last 30 years.

As nursing practice became more clearly defined, assessment became important in determining clients' needs for nursing care. Today diagnostic process skills are recognized as critical if clinical practice is to be maintained at an acceptable professional level. Professional standards mandate that nursing diagnoses be derived from health sta-

tus data,[22] and the American Association of Colleges of Nursing's document *Essentials of College and University Education for Nursing* views clinical judgment as an "essential ability."[23]

Assessment and problem identification are components of the diagnostic process in nursing. Assessment for purposes of diagnosis requires history taking as well as examination of the client. Skill in observation and clinical interviewing are stressed as basic to adequate assessment. Carnavali and Thomas[24] present a good overview of problem formulation, including the need for logical reasoning. Gordon [25] and Tanner[26] stress the complexity of diagnostic judgments in nursing, error-avoidance, and the probabilistic nature of judgments. Doona[27] emphasizes the importance of the cognitive skill of judgment in nursing.

Little research has been done on the diagnostic process actually used by nurses, but it may be expected to adhere to general principles of cognition and problem identification. In the last few years a number of studies on diagnostic judgment have been done and are considered in Chapters 6, 7, and 8. Increased visibility of clinical judgment within a nursing model of professional practice will encourage studies to identify successful diagnostic and treatment strategies.

MEDICINE

Medicine's view of diagnosis is of interest because of the many myths that surround disease and because of the interrelatedness of nursing and medical care, especially in acute care settings. Background information about the profession will provide a context for viewing physicians' assumptions, concepts, and practices in regard to diagnosis.

People naturally seek explanations for experiences that have an impact on their lives. So it has been with illness and disease. When people explained illness as being caused by evil spirits, they called upon medicine men for therapy. When illness was viewed as the result of transgressions against the gods, the priest acted as physician; medicine and theology were one. When people themselves and the environment began to be implicated in disease and illness, medicine began to emerge as a science, and healing became a profession.

Medicine has been a highly influential health profession during most of this century, although it has also had its "dark ages."[28] (p. 136) Although there are fewer physicians than some other types of health professionals, society has looked to physicians for direction in health care and related policies. As a result, physicians share both society's adulation because of the advances in health care and its scorn because of the current deficiencies in health care provision. Physicians traditionally have assumed responsibility and authority in health care matters. They have been protective of their professional boundaries, seeming to assume a paternalistic role toward other health professionals.

Clinical medicine is concerned with the diagnosis and treatment of disease. Its practice is based largely on knowledge gained from the biomedical sciences. These sciences seek to describe, explain, predict, and control events associated with pathophysiology or psychopathology. Understanding of illness is sought at the molecular level. For example, medical researchers in the area of congestive heart failure are attempting to describe chemical and physical derangements in the metabolic process of failing myocardial cells, and biochemical changes in the brain are being studied as a means to understanding psychiatric disorders.

Medicine places a high value on scientific explanation. Scientific generalizations about patterns of disease and general responses to treatments are being sought. These generalizations, derived from medical research, are applied to individuals and used in clinical judgments about the care of patients; this is the task of the medical practitioner. The ideal practitioner can combine the scientific aspects of medicine with compassion and understanding of the individuality of human beings.[29] (p. 66)

Diagnosis is an accepted part of the clinical practice of medicine. Both physicians and the public wish to avoid diagnostic error. The consequences of error may be death, disability, or unwarranted expense. Society has high expectations of physicians, as the frequency of malpractice claims and the size of compensations awarded indicate. When "injury" in the legal sense results from poor judgment, carelessness, or ignorance, society awards compensation through the judicial system.[30] Thus the physician, in making a diagnosis and determining treatment, is faced with a moral and humanitarian concern for the individual patient as well as a concern about personal legal liability.

The value placed on diagnostic expertise in the medical profession is reflected in the clinical training of medical students. They are repeatedly involved in diagnosis and treatment planning, review of decisions, and case conferences. Practicing physicians are expected to keep on expanding their diagnostic skills continually. Hospital rounds and conferences provide opportunities for colleague review.

In medicine it is assumed that physicians never cease being students. This attitude is reflected in this passage from a medical textbook[31] (p. 1051):

A fine method of continuing education is to place one's self in a situation where he will be continuously checked on, where his diagnoses are questioned daily and his treatments frequently modified. This is done best in a teaching hospital where young physicians and old mutually teach and learn. It takes courage and it takes humility for the established practitioner to do this, but it pays tremendous rewards. The physician who is afraid to have his opinions scrutinized is already out of date.

Professional focus

The professional focus of medicine is the diagnosis and treatment of disease. Since late in the eighteenth century physicians have studied and labeled pathophysiological and psychopathological phenomena. Disease has been conceptualized as a lesion. The predisposing factors, historical course, morbidity, and mortality of disease have been studied extensively.

The concept of all disease as a lesion has often been challenged. Obesity is an example; it is a deviation from a statistical norm, not a disease per se. In fact, in many instances it is considered a behavioral problem similar to drug addiction or alcoholism. Considering medicine's professional focus on disease and its conception of disease as a lesion, how are these challenges faced?

Blaxter[32] observes a contemporary trend toward expanding the boundaries of medicine to include the social, psychological, and behavioral fields; she sees this trend as a return to the Hippocratic idea of "the whole person in his environment." Card and Good,[33](p. 60) medical educators, have broadened the definition of disease to include the "displacement from the normal state of [a] dynamic, self-regulating system."

The observations of these British authors possibly reflect the large and well-established family practice component of British medical care. Many of the health problems encountered by physicians in family practice are psychosocial. On the other hand, even American medical literature is beginning to reflect the need for a broader professional focus.[34] It will be interesting to see whether this broader focus becomes a reality in practice. If medicine expands its current professional and diagnostic focus, will it be expanding into other professions such as nursing or social work? With the predicted future oversupply of physicians, practice boundaries will continue to be an issue.

Conceptual frameworks for practice

As stated earlier, a conceptual model, or framework, for practice is a mental construction. It is used to derive meaning and understanding; that is, to make sense of phenomena that are puzzling or disturbing. In addition, conceptual models of practice in the professions reflect the culture and milieu of the times. Early medicine, in particular, had strong ties to philosophy and theology.

Throughout history people have observed, in themselves and others, deviations that produce discomfort or disability. These deviations have been explained and treated in various ways. In primitive times few differences existed between medicine, magic, and religion.[35,36] Illness was thought to be produced by sorcery or a higher power such as a deity. Something was in the body that did not belong there, or something had been removed! This simple dichotomous model was associated with a logical approach: The diagnostic problem was to find the seat of disease. The model guided the search for the demon possessing the person, the sin committed, or the witch involved.

Rational elements existed side by side with magical thinking in primitive times. The idea that symptoms occurred in discrete combinations (anticipating the present-day notion of symptom clusters, or syndromes) was deduced from observations of people experiencing illness. However, it was

thought that the symptoms, for example, fever, *were* the disease.

Scientific medicine began in ancient Greece. Hippocrates, who is considered the father of modern medicine, and his students and followers at Cos believed illness was due to a state of disequilibrium. Health was a condition of perfect equilibrium. The Hippocratic model for practice emphasized the wholeness of the person as opposed to the mind-body dualism (separation) that arose later. Habits, life-style, pursuits, thoughts, sleep, and dreams were all proper areas of concern.[32] This model was consistent with the philosophy of the times; the Greeks believed equilibrium and harmony with nature were fundamental to life.

The medical scholars of ancient Greece developed the *humoral model* to guide medical practice. Instead of being a consequence of sin or demonic possession, illness was seen as a disequilibrium in the humors: blood, black bile, yellow bile, and phlegm. For example, in discussing convulsions (which were referred to as the "sacred disease" and associated with divine visitation), Hippocrates described the symptom cluster of the inability of speak, choking, foaming at the mouth, clenching the teeth, and convulsive movements. These symptoms, he thought, came about because the normal flow of phlegm from the brain to the mouth was blocked and the phlegm consequently entered the blood vessels.[37] Although this explanation of grand mal epilepsy sounds primitive today, it represented a dramatic departure from the previous explanatory model that combined theological and medical thought. One of the Hippocratic school's major influences on models for the practice of medicine was the idea that *disease could be explained by natural causes* such as the "humors," rather than by supernatural or magical forces.

Building on the work of the Hippocratic school and influenced by Aristotelian philosophy, Galen, in the second century A.D., introduced the idea that nature was a dynamic, active process directed toward the restoration of health. Interestingly, this is the root of the commonsense notion of the "healing power of nature." The Galenic concept of vitalism was based on a model of purposeful, goal-directed activity inherent in humans and attributed to a psyche, soul, or life force.[37,38] The search for the cause and cure of disease was beginning to focus on outside influences rather than on factors within the person and the environment.

In the fifth and sixth centuries there were few challenges to the accepted explanations of events or to models of disease and medical practice. Most medical care continued to be based largely on models of mysticism, magic, and a few scientific elements. Like other disciplines, the fledgling science of medicine almost disappeared during the Dark Ages.

In contrast to the marked influence of theology and philosophy in earlier times, after the Renaissance biological and physical science influenced medical thought and models of practice. Scientific investigation of disease processes predominated. Use of the scientific method led to rational rather than magical thinking about illness. The alliance between medicine and the biological sciences became firmly established and formed the basis for the biomedical model used in medical practice today. In part, this alliance was the result of theological influences.

The influential Christian church of the fifteenth century supported a mind-body dualism in regard to the study of humans. This position, a response to physicians' and scientists' anatomical dissections, mandated that the investigation of physical and mental processes be undertaken by two different groups. The body was viewed as "a weak and imperfect vessel for the transfer of the soul from this world to the next"[39]; therefore, in Christian thought, it could be studied objectively as a machine and subjected to scientific and medical investigation. The mind and soul were left to the philosophers or theologians, who used noninvasive study techniques. The assumption was that the whole human could be understood as a sum of the parts.[39] (p. 131) An implicit agreement existed between the church and those wishing to perform dissection to increase medical and biological knowledge: The mind and the soul would be ignored. According to Engel's analysis,[39] this agreement was largely responsible for the anatomical and structural model from which Western scientific medicine was to evolve.

Stimulated by knowledge gained from autopsies, a scientific revolution in medicine occurred in the early nineteenth century. Diseases were described after meticulous studies, and the biological concept of disease gained acceptance. During this century French pathologists developed an ana-

tomical theory of disease and identified diagnostic categories, such as gastric ulcer. Other advances led to a physiological theory of disease and to categories such as hyperthyroid or arterial hypertension. The new field of microbiology had a distinct influence on the description of diseases between 1850 and 1900; *Mycobacterium* tuberculosis is an example of a diagnostic category generated under this model. In the 1900s immunological diseases were added to the anatomical, physiological, and microbiological entities in the 200-year-old classification system.

Medicine is committed to advancing knowledge of disease and treatment. It employs the scientific method, which has procedural rules for concept formation, the conduct of experiments, and validation of hypotheses by observations and experimentation. The less manageable behavioral or psychosocial dimensions of disease are generally ignored (psychiatry is an exception) so that observations can meet the standards of objectivity required by the scientific method.

The current biomedical model combines this dualistic separation of mind and body with a mechanistic model. Clients' diseases are viewed from the perspective of biophysical or biochemical processes. Thus, in the biomedical model the body is conceptualized as a machine; disease represents the breakdown of the machine, and treatment consists of repair of the machine.[39]

The reader may wonder whether a purely scientific approach to clinical care is possible, since physicians deal with people rather than with inanimate objects or machines. The disease is an entity in itself; in a sense, it is abstracted from the person with the disease. Other implicit models of psychosocial behavior are probably used to interpret the *behavior* of the person and to plan therapy. Subjective comments of patients are not ignored in the biological model but are regarded as secondary phenomena. With access to laboratory reports and other tests, patients' reports are not always necessary elements for the diagnosis of disease. The biological model is indispensable to medical practice but does not offer a complete picture of illness and disease.[40] (pp. 55-59)

The components, or subsystems, of the biomedical systems model are listed in the box on p. 43. Except in psychiatry, the personal and social system is generally limited to structural factors such as the patient's place in the family network and the number of siblings. This segregation and limitation is typical of the dualistic framework employed during diagnosis, which separates the biological from the psychosocial.

Engel[39] (pp. 129–136) describes the shortcomings of this conceptual focus on biological (physiological) systems and argues that full understanding of the patient requires additional concepts and models. McWhinney[41] recommends a general systems theory approach that would deal with different levels of organization, such as molecular, organ, system, person, and family levels. This approach, he argues, would provide a more holistic way of viewing the phenomena of concern in medical practice.

The current biomedical model of the client reduces the body of knowledge with which the physician has to deal. This narrowing permits the clinician to focus on the already vast body of knowledge in biomedical diagnosis and therapy and to use a commonsense approach to the psychosocial aspects of disease.

The secondary position given to human psychosocial behavior in medical diagnosis has produced controversy, particularly in medical specialties such as psychiatry and family practice. According to Lazare,[42] psychiatry in fact frequently uses a combination of conceptual models; although the combination remains implicit, biomedical, psychological, behavioral, and social models are included. Thus the search continues for a conceptual framework that combines objective scientific knowledge with wisdom and understanding. Bursztajn and colleagues[43] suggest that the scientific, biological focus must be combined with empathetic understanding and moral responsibility.

Concept of causality

Various explanations of disease have dominated medical thinking through the centuries. Ruesch[38] (pp. 506-507) comments that notions about the causes of illness have remained relatively simple. Only five origins of illness are mentioned in the medical literature:

1. Coercive intrusion into the organism of evil spirits, foreign objects, bacteria, or viruses.
2. Deficient, excessive, or faulty intake of food, fluid, gases, poisons, or information.
3. Deficient, excessive, or faulty output as it occurs in disordered elimination, excessive work and strain, inability to express feelings and thoughts, atrophy or hypertrophy of certain physical structures, or one-sided development of social and psychological functions.
4. Loss of, or deficiency in, essential parts; for example, mental deficiency, castration, abortion, sensory defects, mutilation, loss of love objects, or loss of hope.
5. Disintegration of orderly structures as in cancer, toxic states, senile psychoses, or breakdown of social relations and patterns of communication.

The search for the causes of disease has always been based on the need to understand, prevent, and treat them. Indeed, there have been historical relationships between the prevailing notion of cause and the methods of treatment. A good example is the "removal" of disease by bleeding and purging the patient, which later was supplanted by "building up" the patient with iron and diet supplements.[43]

In general the etiology of disease (the theory of causation) and its effect (disease state) have been viewed as having a linear, or direct, relationship—that one basic main cause, known or unknown, exists for each disease. This single-causation hypothesis has dominated scientific medicine since the demonstration that a particular microorganism caused a particular infection. The goal was and is to find a single cause for each disease entity: When the cause is known, control can be instituted.

Science in general has moved to multicausation (many interacting causal factors) hypotheses. Multicausation is currently under discussion by physicians but not fully accepted in medical practice. Walter[45] (p. 3) states that "the doctrine of one cause for one disease has certainly failed to be a profitable concept in the search for the etiology of many common diseases, such as cancer, arteriosclerosis, emphysema, and chronic bronchitis." According to Thomas,[46] (p. 462) the multifactorial approach to the cause of human illness is now "in fashion"; infectious diseases are the exception. He groups current notions of causality into two classes, environment and life-style. Facetiously he describes the ultimate unified theory of causality that would appeal to the entire "political" spectrum:

At the further right, it is attractive to hear that the individual, the good old freestanding, free-enterprising American citizen, is responsible for his own health and when things go wrong it is his own damn fault for smoking and drinking and living wrong (and he can jolly well pay for it). On the other hand, at the left, it is nice to be told that all our health problems, including dying, are caused by failure of the community to bring up its members to live properly, and if you really want to improve the health of the people, research is not the answer; you should upheave the present society and invent a better one. At either end you can't lose.[46] (p. 463)

In everyday clinical practice, the possibility of multifactorial causes is probably ignored. The simplified view prevails—that there is one cause of a disease, whether that cause is known or unknown. Contributing or predisposing factors such as lifestyle may be considered but tend not to receive as much attention as metabolic derangements. Vaisrub[47] describes the current divergent viewpoints this way:

Suspended between the polarities of the known and completely unknown, multifactorial etiology can be interpreted in two ways. It can be regarded as a combination of factors, each contributing its share to the causation of a disease. Although one or more of these factors predominate in an individual case, none can be regarded as a single, specific cause. In fact, it can be assumed tacitly or explicitly that no single specific cause exists, and the pursuit of such cause would be futile.

On the other hand, multifactorial etiology can be viewed as a temporary ad hoc concept, which will do

until a specific cause, *the* cause, will be discovered. Presenting this view, Thomas[46] cites tuberculosis as an example of a disease that might have been easily consigned to a multifactorial etiology before the tubercle bacillus was identified as its cause. Like cancer, tuberculosis involves many organs and is influenced by environmental factors. Fortunately, the causative organism was discovered, and the disease escaped the multifactorial label before it was invented.[47] (p. 830)

Classification systems

Discrimination among types of illnesses existed in primitive spiritual medicine; names were assigned to such conditions as loss of consciousness and convulsions. Many of the present labels for diseases are inherited from the Greeks and Romans.[48] (pp. 52-53)

The beliefs and values of a society influence societal concepts of what is classified as health and illness. Leavitt and Numbers[49] (p. 3) comment, "Ideas, like individuals and institutions, have their own histories, and concepts of sickness and health are no exception. What one generation of Americans may have considered an illness, another regarded as perfectly normal." Normality, they point out, is socially defined and in part rests upon familiarity. The more familiar a condition is, the less likely it is to be labeled abnormal. For example, childbirth and malaria, once considered normal, now are generally thought to require medical attention. On the basis of social beliefs and values, some conditions have shifted from sin to sickness and from sickness to normality.

Masturbation has had quite a history; once it was classified as a sin, then it was considered a sickness, and now it is thought of as normal.[50] Alcoholism, drug addiction, and obesity, at one time crimes and vices, are now considered illnesses.[49] (p. 13) "Nervousness," hysteria, and other so-called self-indulgent female maladies were legitimized as illnesses when they were labeled *neurasthenia*. Neurasthenia also provided a reasonably respectable label for these symptoms when they were experienced by men. The relabeling of neurasthenia served to establish a clientele for the new specialty of neurology in the early twentieth century.[51]

Nosography, the systematic description and classification of diseases, began in the eighteenth century. Nosography arose because of a need to analyze the causes of death in the population. A model for classification existed; 100 years earlier botany had established its taxonomy (classification). By the year 1893, an international classification system for mortality statistics was developed. It had 161 diagnostic titles and was referred to as the *International Classification of Diseases* (ICD).

Today the ICD contains 1040 categories and is the official international code for reporting morbidity and mortality statistics. Its periodic review is sponsored by the World Health Organization (WHO).[52] The *American Hospital Adaptation of International Classification of Diseases—Adapted* is the official code in the United States. It is used for discharge analysis of hospital records by the Committee for Professional and Hospital Activities of the Joint Committee on Accreditation of Hospitals.

In the specialty of psychiatry, mental disorders are classified in the *Diagnostic and Statistical Manual of Mental Disorders (DSM III-R),* developed by the American Psychiatric Association.[53] This manual "contains a multiaxial system emphasizing psychosocial factors."[54] (p. 25) The manual presents the first classification system that codes five client dimensions:

Axis I: Clinical syndromes and V codes (conditions not attributable to a mental disorder)
Axis II: Developmental and personality disorders
Axis III: Physical disorders and conditions
Axis IV: Severity of psychosocial stressors
Axis V: Highest level of adaptive functioning[53]

A complete psychiatric evaluation includes the five axes and provides a broad perspective. It is suggested that some axes will also be relevant to evaluations done by activity therapists, social workers, nurses, and psychologists.

A number of psychiatric diagnoses are based on the intensive study of single-client cases in a prescientific era. This historical fact led to criticism of the American Psychiatric Association's *DSM II,* particularly because of the overlap in various diagnostic classifications. There is generally thought to be little support for specific clinical diagnoses, such as paranoid schizophrenia or anxiety reaction, and only general support for broad categories, such as functional psychosis, psychoneurosis, or organic psychosis. The re-

cently published *DSM III-R* addresses some of these earlier concerns.

Many other classification systems are in use in medicine and medical specialties. They vary depending on their purpose. As Engle and Davis[55] (p. 517) have observed, problems exist because there is no unified concept of disease that can be used as an organizing principle. Disease and diagnosis may be based on "gross anatomical defects, microscopic changes, so-called specific etiological agents, specific deficiencies, genetic aberrations, physiologic or biochemical abnormalities, constellations of clinical symptoms and signs, organ and system involvement, and even just description of abnormalities."[55] (p. 517) Another problem is that diagnoses are not always well defined, often lacking specific etiologies.

Vague definitions of diagnostic categories decrease accuracy and reliability. As the understanding of diseases improves, the uncertainty in diagnosis decreases. The levels of uncertainty associated with the use of diagnostic categories in medicine identified by Engle and Davis[54] are still quoted. The uncertainty is associated with a lack of knowledge and is reflected in (1) the ambiguity of a category's definition, (2) unclear etiology, and (3) variations in the clinical picture from person to person and from environment to environment. Sickle cell anemia (abnormal hemoglobin) is at the first and highest level of certainty in diagnosis. The collagen diseases and some immunological disorders are at the fifth, or lowest and most uncertain, level. The ability to make judgments under conditions of uncertainty is a skill diagnosticians develop. We will return to this topic in later chapters.

Diagnostic process

In medicine, diagnostic skills are highly valued. Accordingly, much attention has been directed toward understanding and teaching the diagnostic process. Here it suffices to consider briefly the elements of the process as it is used in clinical medicine.

The physician's purpose during diagnosis is to observe any manifestations of disease and summarize the manifestations in terms of diagnostic categories. The information physicians collect during the medical history and physical examination is standardized. Each physician uses essentially the same format, which leads to consistency in the clinical data base and among physicians.

Interpretation, analysis, and utilization of the information is facilitated because classifications of diseases correspond to the history and examination categories. For instance, one category of the history format relates to the gastrointestinal system. A physical examination of organs within this system is also done. Correspondingly, a set of gastrointestinal disease categories exists. From a cognitive perspective, clustering information according to an area of concern aids in diagnosing disease in that area if one is present.

Additionally, the basic information collected in each category is delineated in the standard data base. For instance, as part of taking the history, a client is asked about the following gastrointestinal functions: appetite, digestion, nausea, vomiting, hematemesis, abdominal pain, food idiosyncrasies, jaundice, bowel habits, constipation, diarrhea, stools, hemorrhoids, hernia, and use of cathartics. These inquiries screen for the major diseases of the system. If the client's complaint suggests a pathologic condition, a further review of symptoms is done. Laboratory tests supplement the clinical data.

This detailed description serves two purposes. First, it provides an overview of the process of collecting information in medicine. Second, it provides an example of a system that conserves cognitive capacity and facilitates information processing. We will return to these points in a later chapter.

Physicians use a hypothetic-deductive method in diagnosis.[56] This method is effective, according to research on how human beings identify things. Hypothetic-deductive thinking involves careful observation and the generation of diagnostic hypotheses about what early clinical data indicate. It is reasoned that if a hypothesis is true, certain cues should be present. Information is collected to test the hypothesis. On the basis of this information, diagnostic hypotheses are retained, discarded, or altered.

The emphasis on clinical reasoning and diagnosis in medicine has provided a fertile field for research by psychologists. Traditionally "bedside diagnosis" was considered an art involving a large component of clinical intuition. In recent years there has been greater acceptance of the fact that

this "intuition" is not a mysterious skill; it is learned through experience.

SOCIAL WORK

Social work, in contrast to medicine and nursing, has had a relatively short history. It arose out of nineteenth-century charitable societies, which were designed to relieve poverty and suffering, reform the maladjusted, and especially, relieve the community of the burden and unpleasantness of poverty.[57] (p. 36)

The profession's traditions lie in social causes and a concern for the helpless members of society. Its practitioners have been influential in the formulation of social policy at governmental levels by focusing attention on social conditions that influence the quality of life.[58] Social work has been referred to as the conscience of society, prodding it to recognize and deal with social problems.[59] Through the social services it delivers, it is also the profession that reflects and implements contemporary social attitudes and values.[60]

This twofold purpose can present a dilemma to the social work practitioner, especially one who is employed by a public social welfare agency. In one sense the social worker is an agent of society, obliged to carry out its public programs and enforce conformity to the existing social environment, attitudes, and values. On the other hand, the profession is committed to improving social services, the social environment, and the quality of life; these objectives may not always be consistent with current values or financial commitments.

As might be expected from the diversity of social problems among different age groups, social work deals with a variety of problems in a variety of settings. The unifying factor in the profession is its primary commitment to people, to society, and to the interrelationships between people and society. Differing views of professional purposes either emphasize the individual in interaction with society or focus on the society and its impact on people.[61]

These viewpoints are reflected in the diverse areas of practice in which social workers engage. A large number are involved in social planning activities, but the majority are social workers who deliver direct care to individuals and families.[62] (p. 392) One example of practitioners who focus on the individual are clinical caseworkers who provide psychotherapy through private practice or as part of mental health teams. Others who develop, modify, or administer social service programs focus on the larger society and its impact on people. Carroll[63] has developed a three-dimensional model to encompass all the diverse areas of social work practice. As seen in Fig. 3-1, the model incorporates the phenomena that are of concern, that is, social problems; the units that are of concern, from individuals to societies; and the technologies characteristic of social work practice, such as family therapy, social planning, or case work.[63] (p. 431)

Currently, social workers are seeking licensure by the states in which they practice; a few states have licensure for clinical activities (nonmedical psychotherapy). A clear definition of social work practice is specified in the National Association of Social Workers Model Licensing Act, defines social work practice as[61] (p. 390):

Service and action to effect changes in human behavior, a person's or persons' emotional responses, and the social conditions of individuals, families, groups, orga-

nizations, and communities, which are influenced by the interaction of social, cultural, political, and economic systems.

It is within these areas of practice that the social caseworker, who treats individuals and families, interacts most frequently with physicians and nurses. Thus we will examine this area of practice most closely.

The typical pattern of casework practice in health care institutions (hospitals, clinics, and community health care agencies) is to assist clients and families with social problems referred by nurses or physicians. For example, a client with a medical illness may have a problem, such as unsatisfactory living conditions, which contributes to the illness. Referral to the medical social worker in the social service department of the institution can provide the client with assistance and specialized knowledge of community resources. If a team concept is employed in a health care setting (e.g., long-term or rehabilitative care), social workers participate with nurses and physicians in planning a client's care.

In another situation, a multiproblem family may require the coordination of social services in the

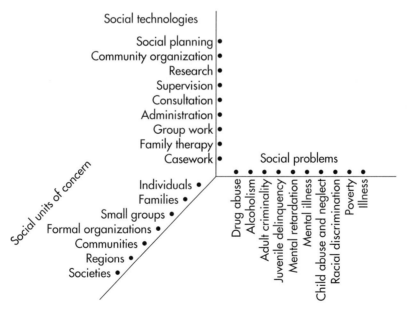

Fig. 3-1 A three-dimensional model of social work practice. (From Carroll NK: Three-dimensional model of social work practice, *Social Work* 22:428, 1977.

community, such as child care, vocational counseling, and welfare. The social worker can coordinate these services on a long-term basis and help the family learn how to deal with their problems. Through client contacts, the need for programs may also become evident to a worker in the community, and efforts may be made to engage the community in developing services, such as social programs for the elderly.

Professional focus

In contrast to medicine, which seeks to understand the clinical problems of clients at the molecular or physiochemical level, social casework emphasizes the intrapsychic, interpersonal, and social level of understanding. It draws heavily on psychological, psychiatric, and sociological theory in its practice.

According to Reid,[64] the problems addressed by the profession are "social" in two senses:

1. The problem behavior has social consequences for the individual or family.
2. The problem is troubling society.

Reid identifies broad problem areas, such as mental illness and emotional distress, difficulties in interpersonal relationships, dysfunctional and deviant behavior, and inadequate resources (unsuitable living arrangements, insufficient income, lack of health care, and the like).

Diagnosis was introduced into the practice of social work in its early years and influenced the development of casework. Also influential was an alliance with psychiatry and psychoanalytic thought.[65] (p. 13) Today, consistent with the profession's modern focus, diagnoses describe problems, or social dilemmas, in the context of the client's interaction with the world.

Some schools of thought within the profession do not rely heavily on diagnostic categorization of clients' problems but do use a narrative type of problem identification as part of practice. Each of the four major approaches to casework (psychosocial, functional, problem solving, and behavioral) defines the concept of the social problem differently.[65] (pp. 33–218) Some suggest that the diversity in practice negates a unified approach. Others argue that a uniform conceptualization of the problems addressed by social work is needed to clarify professional objectives.[64] (p. 374)

Conceptual frameworks for practice

It seems that as long as human beings form relationships in groups or societies, problems will arise. In noncomplex societies these problems are usually handled within families, tribal communities, or religious groups. When societies undergo rapid social and technological changes, as did Western society with the advent of the Industrial Age, social problems arise that overtax the known ways of handling them. This was the situation in the nineteenth century, when changes caused by industrialization produced stresses in the social order.

Charitable associations began to supplement the efforts of families and religious groups; "friendly visitors," the volunteers from these organizations, were dispatched to the homes of the poor. As an example, in Boston in 1884 there were 600 volunteer workers who visited "drunkards and their families and the poor widows with dependent children."[57] (p. 36) To relieve the conditions of poverty, they used advice, persuasion, and exhortation, as dictated by the 1883 *Handbook for Friendly Visitors Among the Poor.*

The model for practice at that time, if it can be called such, rested firmly on society's belief that hard work, thrift, and a belief in the Almighty would lead to individual success, thereby eliminating poverty and degradation.[57] (p. 36) In the early twentieth century voluntary charity workers, as well as the associations for which they worked, became organized, and the newly paid workers began to seek professional status. That was the beginning of the social work profession and of the development of conceptual models for practice. For these new workers to differentiate themselves from nurses in institutions and to implement the scientific commitment inherited from the philanthropy movement, caseworkers adopted the medical process: study, diagnose, treat.[65] (pp. 16–24)

Richmond[67] greatly influenced this new profession with a book on social diagnosis. It emphasized the "scientific" collection of information about the client as a basis for diagnosis. The approach to practice that used Richmond's ideas was referred to as the diagnostic school of thought.

Conceptual models were borrowed from medicine, particularly psychiatry, and from psychoanalytic theory, probably because of the events of that era. Caseworkers were needed to handle not only the demands of the poor in society but also the large numbers of emotional problems of veterans and their families after World War I. The birth of the mental health movement in the second decade of the twentieth century also influenced the practice models that developed in social casework.[64] (p. 16)

The model for practice during the 1930s and after was derived from personality theory, particularly Freudian. Patients' conscious, preconscious, and unconscious thoughts were examined in order to understand problem behavior.[64] (p. 18) The use of the medical process model and psychoanalytic theory brought with it an emphasis on problems of the individual. This focus on individuals represented a change from the earlier emphasis on social problems and social causes. It produced controversy in the profession for many years, and the issue is still debated.

Currently some conceptual models of social work practice emphasize the service aspect and focus on the therapeutic method of practice, that is, what social workers do in handling clients' problems. In contrast, the diagnostic model (now referred to as the psychosocial model of practice) still strongly advocates the need for diagnostic classification, particularly clinical diagnosis.[68]

The growth of sociological knowledge, particularly of role theory, broadened the concept proposed by Richmond[67] in 1917. Theoretical constructs are derived from the behavioral sciences and include anthropological and cultural theories. Theories of these behavioral sciences in addition to theories developed in the profession are used to identify the problems of clients, such as character disorders, alcoholism, and drug addiction. Traditionally, medical and psychiatric caseworkers have used the psychosocial model.

Within this model of practice the client is viewed from a systems perspective and diagnosis is directed toward the "person-situation gestalt."[68] (pp. 33–76) This client model includes the individual and the social environment as the entity of concern. Included in the concept of the social environment are social roles (family, work, social groups) and the educational milieu.

Consistent with a systems theory approach, it is assumed that changes in one part of the mutual interaction between person and social environment, such as a role change, changes the equilibrium of the entire system. In the use of this model, the phenomena of concern to the social caseworker are *interadaptational problems* such as those that arise in the subsystems of the client-situation complex; that is, the individual, the situation, or the interaction between the individual and the social environment. These problems of equilibrium or adaptation of the person-situation complex are the focus of social intervention in the psychosocial approach to casework.[68] (pp. 50–51)

Other conceptual models of social casework either bypass the diagnostic step in the clinical process or use a different concept and utilization of diagnosis. In some approaches diagnosis is seen as part of treatment, with treatment conceived as the client-therapist relationship process. This viewpoint results in an emphasis on diagnosis as a process for specifying the problem, rather than a basis for categorization prior to treatment. For example, the functional approach to casework described by Smalley[69] uses the term *diagnosis* but views it as an insight the client arrives at in relation to his or her problem. The "diagnosis" constantly changes with the client's progress during the relationship.

The problem-solving model of casework uses the term *diagnosis* to refer to the specification of the problem to be worked on at a particular time; diagnosis is an ongoing process as the client and caseworker together define the client's perception of the objective problem and subjective involvement in the problem. In this model the caseworker identifies the client's motivation and ability to solve the problem and the social means or resources available to the client.[70] As the name of the model implies, the focus is on guiding the client in problem solving. The social problem is not the major concern, rather it is the person's problem-solving motivation and ability.

All models for practice include a diagnostic statement, although some do not label it as such. Because there is no concensus on nomenclature for summarizing the clinical assessment, or because of the low value placed on specific problem identification and diagnostic classification, the caseworker usually writes a paragraph or more describing the problem(s). There is no generally accepted structure or format for the diagnostic statement.

Concept of causality

At the turn of the century, still under the influence of the seventeenth-century mechanistic physics of Newton, cause and effect were viewed as directly related: each effect has one cause. It was believed that if the cause of a social problem could be found, the cure would be obvious.[6] (pp. 10-11)

Today the high degree of complexity of social problems is recognized in the profession. Within the model of person-situation complex, the cause of a problem may reside in either the person or the situation. Actually, it is more likely to be found in the relationship pattern or transaction between the two.[6] (p. 29) Thus these three main elements have to be considered in determining causality; usually multicausation is found.

In addition, all three aspects of the person-situation complex demonstrate growth, change, and potentiality. *Potentiality* refers to emergent capabilities such as new behaviors. Germaine[65] (p. 29) suggests that to be "in accord with the modern scientific viewpoint, this requires that casework view and handle phenomena in terms of directions, flow, action and transaction, rather than in terms of cause."

Classification systems

In social work, then, there is no generally accepted typology, or classification, of social problems. An attempt was made early in the history of the profession to specify the domain of problems addressed. With Richmond's concept of social diagnosis[67] as a stimulus, in 1929 an alphabetical listing of casework problems was developed. The problems ranged from alcoholism to vagrancy.[71]

Recent authors addressing the subject of a diagnostic classification system appear to agree with Reid's argument[64] (p. 376):

The compelling advantage of formulating social work's objectives in terms of the problems it seeks to solve is that this formulation provides a clear basis for organizing and interpreting professional efforts, a basis that can be precisely explained and generally understood.

Classifications cited in the literature[72,73] are specific for certain problem areas; for example, family therapy. Reid.[64] (p. 374) proposes four areas of social work practice that may guide the conceptualization of specific problems: intrapersonal, interpersonal, personal-environmental, and environmental. Lowenberg[74] (pp. 53–54) specifies a set of three: interpersonal relationships, formal relationships, and role transaction. The examples given these typologies range from symptoms to broad problem areas.

It is obvious from the literature in this field that a number of issues must be resolved before a diagnostic classification system can be developed. The need for decisions about the domain of practice, a theoretical system to organize diagnostic categories, and the determination of the unit of classification (individual, family, or community) is stressed by authors who advocate a classification system.[75,76]

Irrespective of whether the social work profession will undertake development of a classification system, the value of doing so has been recognized. Finestone[76] (p. 139) views this task as providing rich rewards for building systematic theory for organizing knowledge for teaching, and for making practice more effective.

Diagnostic process

As may be recalled from the discussion of the diagnostic processes of other professions, information collection, analysis, and synthesis are broad common steps necessary to arrive at a concept of the state of the client and to label that state for purposes of treatment. In all the conceptual models of practice in social work, collection of information is stressed as an important clinical activity. It is viewed as a means of understanding the client's problem and is an ongoing process. The information-collection process is referred to as casework assessment and incorporates history taking.

All the models of practice emphasize the dual purpose served by information collection—the simultaneous establishment of a relationship with the client and acquisition of useful clinical information. Both these purposes are probably of crucial importance in this profession, considering the focus of concern—social problems—and the psychosocial nature of the clinical data required. It is logical to expect that only after the caseworker has established trust and communicated empathic concern will the client share this type of personal information.

Some practice models stress that treatment begins immediately. No doubt this is true. Psychosocial information collection requires careful listening. Therapeutic outcomes may result as clients verbalize the feelings and perceptions that comprise the clinical data. In addition, clients may gain insights by relating a problem to another person. For all these reasons, social casework emphasizes the importance of the initial phase of interaction with the client, during which assessment and problem identification occur.

Hollis,[68] who advocates the psychosocial approach to casework, states that the purpose of assessment is to deduce, from the information available and background knowledge of human behavior or social situations, the client's problem and what contributes to it. This deduction can then be used to determine the need and focus for change as well as the casework methods to be applied.

The data-collection method that is advocated is consistent with the psychosocial model. Hollis[68] (p. 51) states that assessment focuses on the client-situation complex, which "must be viewed repeatedly against a series of approximate norms of average expectancies (A) concerning behavior of the client and others, (B) concerning pertinent aspects of his social situation, and (C) concerning concrete realities."

The client-situation complex is viewed from sociological and psychological perspectives to collect information in problem areas and to identify the scope of etiological factors involved.[68] (p. 52) No one generally agreed-upon systematic format (history form) for collecting a clinical data base is used in casework.

In social work, as in other professions, analysis of clinical data is emphasized. To make a decision about treatment, the caseworker must have an accurate and precise understanding of the problem(s). Hollis[68] (p. 52) recommends that alternative conceptions of the client and his or her situation be considered by examining the clinical data within various frames of reference. Middleman and Goldberg[77] (pp. 88–89) suggest social workers have three areas for analysis: (1) patterns of interaction in the client's various social roles, (2) content themes that point to areas of concern, and (3)

metamessages (usually nonverbal) underlying overt expression.

Caution is suggested in case analyses to avoid (1) stereotyping, which results from faulty deductive thinking; (2) overgeneralization from experiences that may not be representative; and (3) oversimplification of cause, such as single-focused explanations. The last two items represent faulty inductive thinking.[74] (p. 261) Any of these three practices may lead to diagnostic errors.

Concise diagnostic classification is not generally found in social work except when terms borrowed from psychiatry can be used. This situation exists even among caseworkers using the psychosocial (diagnostic) approach. Hollis[68] (pp. 51-52) in her review of this model of practice, states that three types of diagnostic inferences are employed:

These inferences will be mainly of three types: dynamic, etiological and classificatory. (A) In the *dynamic* diagnosis we examine, among other things, how different aspects of the client's personality interact to produce his total functioning. We look at the interplay between the client and other people and at other systems and the interactions within them to understand how change in one part of a system may affect another. The dynamics of family interaction are particularly important here and form a large part of what is often referred to as a family diagnosis. (B) *Etiological* factors are looked for, whether these lie in the current interactions or in preceding events which still actively affect the present and are among the causes of the client's dilemma. Usually, causation is seen as the convergence of a multiplicity of factors in the person-situation configuration. The dynamic and etiological aspects of the diagnosis together provide both a "linear" and an interactional, or "transactional," view of causation. Where antecedents exist they are noted; they are usually seen as multiple. At the same time the continuous action between and among the various causative components in the transactional sense is an integral part of understanding the nature of the client-situation gestalt. (C) Effort is made to *classify* various aspects of the client's functioning, including, where pertinent and possible, a clinical diagnosis.

SUMMARY

Neither nursing diagnosis nor client care is done in isolation. Nurses, physicians, social workers, and others have to collaborate if clients are to receive coordinated care. Understanding one's own and others' viewpoints is the first step toward collaborative practice. To take this first step was one of the purposes of this chapter.

The second purpose was to help the reader further define nursing diagnosis. Various concepts of diagnosis were compared and contrasted to promote understanding. The discussion stressed that nursing traditionally has been concerned with individuals, families, and communities. Social work and medicine also have this broad area of concern. Actually, the three professions evolved because individuals, families, and society could not meet particular needs by themselves. Needs are expressed as societal mandates to the professions.

Although each profession follows essentially the same process in determining clients' needs, the information processed differs. Nurses, physicians, and social workers determine the need for professional services by collecting information and defining problems. Good judgment is valued in each profession and each sees itself as a helping profession. The three groups' distinctiveness lies in their social mandates and the models of practice developed from those mandates.

Nursing, in contrast to the other two professions, has traditionally taken a holistic view of clients and their situations. Nurses are concerned with the broad range of human functional responses to life situations. Both physicians and social workers specialize in discrete areas of the client's situation—disease and social problems, respectively.

Each profession uses conceptual frameworks for practice that are consistent with its mandate and concerns. If psychosocial problems are the focus of concern, logically the model of the client should promote the collection of psychosocial information; if disease is the phenomenon of interest, attention is directed toward pathophysiological or psychopathological manifestations. Focusing attention leads to the naming and classification of conditions the profession can address. Thus there is consistency between a profession's focus and its classification systems.

Essentially the same cognitive processes are applied by each profession, but the focus of their application differs. The information collected, the concepts used to interpret information, and the problems addressed vary. Generally, these differences are reflected in care activities.

The reader may not be sure of having gotten a clear understanding of nursing's focus. General aspects of a belief system have been emphasized, but the topic of specific conceptual frameworks for diagnosis has been skirted. Chapter 4 will be devoted to this topic; as previously stated, a specific conceptual focus for diagnosis is crucial for its definition.

REFERENCES

1. *The nursing practice act,* Kansas City, Mo, 1980, American Nurses' Association.
2. Rogers, M: *Introduction to the theoretical basis of nursing,* New York, 1970, Davis.
3. Kalisch PA, Kalisch BJ: *The advance of American nursing,* Boston, 1978, Little, Brown.
4. Tappert TG, Lehman P, editors: *Luther's works,* Philadelphia, 1967, Fortress Press.
5. Dickens C: *Martin Chuzzlewit,* New York, 1910, Macmillan.
6. Nightingale F: Sick nursing and health nursing (1893). In Hampton I, editor: *Nursing of the sick,* New York, 1949, McGraw-Hill.
7. Shaw, CSW: *A textbook of nursing,* New York, 1855, Appleton-Century-Crofts.
8. Frederick HK, Northam E: *A textbook of nursing practice,* ed 2, New York, 1938, Macmillan.
9. Harmer B: *Textbook of the principles and practice of nursing,* ed 5, revised by Henderson V, New York, 1955, Macmillan.
10. Henderson V: *The nature of nursing,* New York, 1966, Macmillan.
11. Orlando IJ: *The dynamic nurse-patient relationship,* New York, 1961, Putnam.
12. Orem DE: *Nursing: concepts of practice,* St Louis, 1985, Mosby.
13. Hall LE: Quality of nursing care, *Public Health News* (New Jersey State Department of Health) 36:212, 1955.
14. Newman M: Prevailing paradigms in nursing, *Nurs Outlook* 40:10, 1992.
15. Northrup DT: Disciplinary perspective: unified or diverse? *Nurs Sci Q* 5:154, 1992.
16. McManus L: Assumptions of functions of nursing. In Teachers College Division of Nursing Education: *Regional planning for nursing and nursing education,* New York, 1950, Teachers College Press.
17. Bonney B, Rothberg J: *Nursing diagnosis and therapy,* New York, 1963, National League for Nursing.
18. *A social policy statement,* Kansas City, Mo, 1980, American Nurses' Association.
19. Andrews L: Health care providers, *J Prof Nurs* 2:60, 1986.
20. Field M: Causal inferences in behavioral research, *Adv Nurs Sci* 2:81, 1979.
21. Abdellah FG: Improving the teaching of nursing through research in patient care. In Heidgerken LE, editor: *Improvement of nursing through research,* Washington DC, 1959, Catholic University of America Press.

22. *Standards for clinical nursing practice,* Kansas City, Mo, 1991, American Nurses' Association.
23. *Essentials of college and university education for nursing,* Washington DC, 1986, American Association of Colleges of Nursing.
24. Carnavali DL, Thomas MD: *Diagnostic reasoning and treatment decision making in nursing,* Philadelphia, 1993, Lippincott.
25. Gordon M: Nursing diagnosis and the diagnostic process, *Am J Nurs* 76:1300, 1976.
26. Tanner CA: Teaching clinical judgment. In Fitzpatrick JJ, Taunton RL, editors: *Annual review of nursing research, 5,* 153, 1987.
27. Doona ME: The judgment process in nursing, *Image* 8:27, 1976.
28. Duffy U: The changing image of the American physician, *AMA* 200:136, 1967.
29. Tumulty PA: What is a clinician and what does he do? In Bulger RT, editor: *Hippocrates revisited: a search for meaning,* New York, 1973, Medcom.
30. Cassell EJ: Error in medicine. In Englehardt HT, Callahan D, editors: *Knowledge, value, and belief,* New York, 1977, The Hastings Center.
31. Keefer CS, Wilkins RW: *Medicine: essentials of clinical practice,* Boston, 1970, Little, Brown.
32. Blaxter M: Diagnosis as category and process: the case of alcoholism, *Soc Sci Med* 12:10, 1978.
33. Card WI, Good IJ: A logical analysis of medicine. In Passamore R, editor: *A companion to medical studies,* vol 3, sec 60, London, 1974, Blackwell.
34. Baron RJ: An introduction to medical phenomenology: I can't hear you when I'm listening, *Ann Intern Med* 103:606, 1985.
35. Rivers WHR: *Medicine, magic, and religion,* New York, 1927, Harcourt, Brace and World.
36. Engle RL Jr: Medical diagnosis: present, past, and future: II. Philosophical foundations and historical development of our concepts of health, disease and diagnosis, *Arch Intern Med* 112:521, 1963.
37. King LS, editor: *A history of medicine: selected readings,* Baltimore, 1971, Penguin, p 13.
38. Ruesch J: The helping traditions: some assumptions made by physicians. In Galdston I, editor: *Man's image in medicine and anthropology,* New York, 1963, International Universities Press.
39. Engel GL: The need for a new medical model: a challenge for biomedicine, *Science* 196:129, 1977.
40. Wulff H: *Rational diagnosis and treatment,* ed 2, Boston, 1981, Blackwell.
41. McWhinney IR: Beyond diagnosis: an approach to the integration of behavioral science and clinical medicine, *N Engl J Med* 287:384, 1972.
42. Lazare A: Hidden conceptual models in clinical psychiatry, *N Engl J Med* 288:346, 1973.
43. Bursztajn H et al: *Medical choices, medical chances,* New York, 1990, Routledge.
44. Berman A: The heroic approach in 19th century therapeutics, *Bull Am Soc Hosp Pharm* 11:320, 1954.
45. Walter JB: *An introduction to the principles of disease,* Philadelphia, 1977, Saunders.
46. Thomas L: Notes of a biology watcher: on magic in medicine, *N Engl J Med* 299:462, 1978.
47. Vaisrub S: Groping for causation, *AMA* 241:830, 1979.
48. Fejos P: Magic, witchcraft, and medical theory in primitive cultures. In Galdston I, editor: *Man's image in medicine and anthropology,* New York, 1963, International Universities Press.
49. Leavitt JW, Numbers RL, editors: *Sickness and health in America: readings in the history of medicine and public health,* Madison, 1978, University of Wisconsin Press.
50. Englehardt T Jr: The disease of masturbation: values and the concept of disease. In Leavitt JW, Numbers RL, editors: *Sickness and health in America,* Madison, 1978, University of Wisconsin Press.
51. Sickerman B: The uses of diagnosis: doctors, patients and neurasthenia. In Leavitt JW, Numbers RL, editors: *Sickness and health in America,* Madison, 1978, University of Wisconsin Press.
52. *International classification of diseases,* Geneva, 1977, World Health Organization.
53. *Diagnostic and statistical manual of mental disorders, DSM-IIIR,* Washington, DC, American Psychiatric Association.
54. Talbott J: An in-depth look at *DSM-III:* an interview with Robert Spitzer, *Hosp Comm Psychiatry* 31:25, 1980.
55. Engle RL Jr, Davis BJ: Medical diagnosis: present, past and future: I. Present concepts of the meaning and limitations of medical diagnosis, *Arch Intern Med* 112:512, 1963.
56. Elstein AS, Schulman LS, Sprafka SA: *Medical problem solving: an analysis of clinical reasoning,* Cambridge, Mass, 1978, Harvard University Press.
57. Robinson VP: Changing psychology in social casework. In Robinson VP editor: Development of a professional self. In *Teaching and learning in professional helping processes: selected writings,* 1930–1968, New York, 1978, AMS Press.
58. Morris R: Caring for vs caring about people, *Soc Work* 22:353, 1977.
59. Cooper S: Social work: a dissenting profession, *Soc Work* 22:361, 1977.
60. Dean WR: Back to activism, *Soc Work* 22:369, 1977.
61. Simm BK: Diversity and unity in the social work profession, *Soc Work* 22:394, 1977.
62. Morales A: Beyond traditional conceptual frameworks, *Soc Work* 22:390, 1977.
63. Carroll NK: Three-dimensional model of social work practice, *Soc Work* 22:428, 1977.
64. Reid WJ: Social work for social problems, *Soc Work* 22:374, 1977.
65. Germaine C: Casework and science: a historical encounter. In Roberts RW, Nee RE, editors: *Theories of social casework,* Chicago, 1970, University of Chicago Press.
66. Roberts RW, Nee RH: *Theories of social casework,* Chicago, 1970, University of Chicago Press.
67. Richmond M: *Social diagnosis,* New York, 1917, Russell Sage.
68. Hollis F: The psychosocial approach to casework. In Roberts RW, Nee RH, editors: *Theories of social casework,* Chicago, 1970, University of Chicago Press.
69. Smalley RE: The functional approach to casework practice.

In Roberts RW, Nee RH, editors: *Theories of social casework,* Chicago, 1970, University of Chicago Press, pp. 77-128.

71. Perlman HH: The problem-solving model in casework practice. In Roberts RW, Nee RH, editors: *Theories of social casework,* Chicago, 1970, University of Chicago Press, pp 129-180.
72. *The Milford conference report,* New York, 1929, American Association of Social Workers.
72. Ackerman NW: *Psychodynamics of family life,* New York, 1958, Basic Books, p 329.
73. Ripple L, Alexander E: Motivation, capacity and opportunity as related to the use of casework service: nature of the client's problem, *Soc Rev* 30:38, 1956.

74. Lowenburg FM: *Fundamentals of social intervention,* New York, 1977, Columbia University Press.
75. Selby LG: Typologies for caseworkers: some considerations and problems, *Soc Serv Rev* 32:341, 1958.
76. Finestone S: Issues involved in developing diagnostic classifications for casework. In *Casework papers, 1960: papers presented at the 87th Annual Forum, National Conference on Social Welfare, Atlantic City, June 5-10, 1960,* New York, 1960, Family Service Association of America, pp 139-154.
77. Middleman RR, Goldberg G: *Social service delivery: a structural approach to social work practice,* New York, 1974, Columbia University Press.

CHAPTER 4

FRAMEWORKS FOR THE DIAGNOSTIC PROCESS

T he diagnostic process begins with the collection of information and ends with an evaluative judgment about a client's health status. To carry out this process in nursing, one must make decisions about what information is important and what areas are of nursing concern. A conceptual framework for nursing process supports these decisions. As the term implies, a *conceptual* or *theoretical framework* is a set of interrelated concepts. The concepts are abstract ways of looking at:

Client-environment
Nursing goal
Nursing intervention

These three areas are taken-for-granted essentials in practice. When nurses think about practice, they are dealing with these three areas of knowledge.[1] For conceptual frameworks to be applicable in diverse nursing situations, these three interrelated concepts must be abstract and must provide a useful way of thinking for practice. It is the conceptual framework that helps answer questions regarding what to assess, what problems are of concern, what the nursing goals are, and what should be the general focus of intervention. A framework provides a focus for nursing process (diagnostic and therapeutic judgment). There has been some discussion suggesting that nursing diagnoses be used as a framework for practice and curricula instead of as a conceptual framework. These entities are not interchangeable. A framework is a broad perspective of nursing. Nursing diagnoses are concepts used to explain a cluster of cues (observations). Both are necessary. In fact, without a nursing perspective, it would be difficult to use nursing diagnoses.

In this chapter four conceptual frameworks are reviewed: the *life process, adaptation, self-care agency,* and *behavioral systems models.* Discussion within each framework will be limited to client-environment concepts, view of diagnosis, and nursing's goals.

One purpose of reviewing selected conceptual frameworks is to discover *what* to assess and *why.* The conceptual perspective of clients and of nursing's goals that are chosen strongly influences what kinds of things are assessed. Everyone has a perspective, whether or not one is aware of it. Problems may arise if the perspective "in the head" is inconsistent with the actions taken during assessment. Information collection must be logically related to one's view of nursing. A second purpose of reviewing selected frameworks is to further define nursing diagnosis within a theoretical perspective.

Conceptual frameworks specify the focus of nursing and thus of nursing diagnosis. For example, one framework specifies that nursing diagnoses are actual or potential *self-care agency deficits*[2]; another specifies *ineffective adaptations* as problems of concern to nurses. The two concepts in a framework that are relevant to the diagnostic phase of nursing process are the concepts of the client and of nursing goal. The concept of the client provides guidelines for the logical deduction of what is to be assessed; the concept of the nursing goal describes a general idea of the health outcome that assessment, diagnosis, and care planning are to achieve. While studying conceptual frameworks, it is important to appreciate that the frameworks cause one to see different things. When observing a client, one nurse may pay attention to self-care agency. To this nurse a nutritional deficit would be viewed as a self-care agency deficit. Another nurse, using an adaptation framework, would view this problem as an ineffective adaptation during a weight reduction program. All nursing frameworks specify optimal health as the goal of nursing, but ways of looking at health differ. Concepts of the client also differ, but they all focus on health-related behavior. The conceptual view of the client and of the goal of nursing are logically related[3]; a review of several frameworks will demonstrate this logical relationship.[4]

CONCEPTUAL FRAMEWORKS

A conceptual framework provides a model or perspective; in turn, a model provides an abstract guide to judging what is to be assessed. For example, rarely do nurses assess the stock market investments of a client; they just are not within the model nurses use. In contrast, a broker places high priority on this information. There are a number of ways to arrive at guidelines for information collection (assessment) and for diagnostic judgments. One approach is to start with the abstract question: What is nursing? Then the nurse tries to reason "down" to the clinical level. A number of frameworks that have been proposed by nursing theorists can be used to do this. A deductive process of reasoning is involved, beginning with assumptions and beliefs and ending with applications to specific situations.

A second way of deciding what is to be assessed is to examine the assessment formats in current use. In nursing there is no lack of proposed assessment tools; they are numerous in the literature, especially of the 1970s and early 1980s. A review would show how items could be grouped into broad categories for guiding information collection. This would be an inductive process of reasoning, from particular to general areas.[5] The assumptions of persons constructing each tool influ-

ence the end product—the assessment data—that result from use of the tools.

There is still another approach to determining what information to collect: Why not look at the clients themselves? What health problems amenable to nursing intervention do they have? A list of these problems would yield broad assessment categories. A related method would be to ask clients a simple question: Which health problems can nurses assist you with? Asking this of many clients would provide items to categorize. Now the assumptions have been shifted to the client—assumptions about nursing and what nurses do.

All the above methods are encompassed to some extent in the conceptual frameworks of nursing that have appeared in the literature. The theorists who developed these frameworks are nurses, and their beliefs and experiences in nursing are incorporated. During the discussion of selected frameworks (the life process model, the adaptation model, the behavioral systems model, and the self-care agency model), the reader may wonder why there is more than one way of viewing the client. (Actually, theories have proliferated and authors rarely address the similarities or differences between the theories they propose and those in any previously published works.) There are more than a dozen nursing frameworks. Philosophical differences exist, there are strong vested interests, nurses are creative, and the profession should not close off development of ideas at too early a point. This is not unlike other disciplines where the all-encompassing unified theory remains elusive; for example, the "theory of everything" in physics:

> In the 1980s many leading physicists thought they had a glimpse of their finish line—they believed they were closing in fast on a final, all-encompassing theory that would serve as a fundamental framework for physics. They even went so far as to talk of a "theory of everything." But now, like all marathoners who have "hit the wall" they are . . . wondering whether the finish line is in fact an illusion. As physicists envisioned eight years ago, this finish line was made of superstrings—a single fundamental entity said to make up all of the diverse particles and forces recognized by traditional physics.[6]

Life process model

A framework of the life process that encompassed a philosophy of wholeness and presented a world view of human beings evolving was proposed by Martha Rogers in 1970.[7] In Rogers' framework, life is viewed as a creative, formative process. It is characterized by the human species' evolution toward greater diversity and innovation. The life process is an interaction between the human energy field and the environmental field. Both fields are characterized by wholeness of life pattern, and both are continuously and simultaneously repatterned as person and environment interact. This means that nursing focuses on the whole person-environment complex, not the sum of the psychological, biological, or social parts. Further, it means that the client and environment are continuously affecting each other. Individuals, families, and communities are viewed as energy fields that have pattern, organization, and openness to constant interaction with the environment.

With simultaneous and continuous client-environment interaction, new life patterns emerge. Nursing seeks to help the client maintain a pattern of living that coordinates, rather than conflicts, with the emerging pattern. Although assessment and diagnosis focus on the life process at a particular point in time, the probability that new behaviors will emerge must be considered. Nursing promotes the attainment of emerging potentialities by its focus on the means—maximum health potential—to the end—continuing development and becoming.

The ideas in this model need to be carefully considered from a broad, world view perspective. For example, do you think new human and world patterns are developing? Is this happening sequentially, such that the human race is never what it was, only what it is becoming? Is emergence goal-directed? Is life pattern and organization getting more complex? Are the changes innovative and spiral (something like the Slinky toy with its cyclic spirals)? Is there order to evolutionary development? If your answer is yes to these questions, you share the same assumptions about human beings as Rogers[7] (pp. 43-77):

1. Man is a unified whole possessing his own integrity and manifesting characteristics that are more than and different from the sum of parts.
2. Man and environment are continuously exchanging matter and energy with one another.
3. The life process evolves irreversibly and unidirectionally along the space-time continuum.

4. Pattern and organization identify man and reflect his innovative wholeness.
5. Man is characterized by the capacity for abstraction, imagery, language, thought, sensation, and emotion.

Nursing goal

Nursing can promote a client's progress toward his or her maximum health potential by (1) strengthening the mutual interaction of the human and environmental patterns, (2) recognizing the potentialities of the client and the environment, and (3) helping the client to use conscious personal choice in goal seeking. Is change orderly? Yes. Is it predictable—that is, can we ever predict client health outcomes? Yes, but only in terms of probabilities and only by looking at the holistic, rhythmical pattern of the person and the environment.[7] (pp. 89-102) Needless to say, highly probable predictions are few and far between unless the most influencing factors are identified. This, Rogers would say, requires research in nursing science.

Client focus

Rogers' conceptual model of the client focuses on unitary human beings and particularly on the life process of human beings. The individual is thought of as an energy field that extends into space. Part of the field, the body, is visible. Pattern and organization of life (1) provide personal integrity, individuality, and wholeness and (2) reflect the life process, which is creative, formative, and evolving. The person and the environment affect each other's pattern, organization, and creative-formative evolution. The life process model therefore represents a holistic concept of the unity of person-environment. Neither the client nor the environment can be understood separately, a factor that influences practice within this world view.

To understand the holistic life pattern, one must consider a configuration of events both within and external to the person's awareness. Examples are client-other interactions (some of which are perceptible) or radiation levels in the environment (imperceptible). In assessing the client's life pattern, the holistic concept must be at the forefront. At a point in time the nurse describes the extent to which the client is emerging toward maximum health potential. This emergence is assessed by (1) observing the pattern and organization of the creative, formative process (life process) and (2) determining the degree to which the environment permits the achievement of maximum health potential. More specifically, the nurse assesses two aspects: (1) the client and environment pattern and (2) organization and preceding patterns (configuration of events) that led up to the present.

Patterns that do not permit movement toward maximum health potential require nursing attention. Behavioral manifestations of unified human functioning are the assessment data.[7 (pp. 124-127)] It is to this extent that Rogers' publications specify what to assess. Data are synthesized to reveal a view of the client's life process (creative, formative). The life process model does not include a set of categories for guiding assessment; only principles are delineated. Nurses using the life process model face the challenge of developing holistic assessment parameters.

Theorist's view of diagnosis

Rogers[7 (p. 125)] states, "The total pattern of events at any given point in space-time provides the data for nursing diagnosis." She refers to the "diagnostic pattern" and adds that nursing diagnosis encompasses "man-environment relationship" and seeks to identify "sequential cross-sectional patterning in the life process." Health problems have multiple causes, and relationships between cause and effect are always probabilistic rather than absolute.

In summary:

1. The concept of the client in Rogers' life process model is unitary human being.
2. Diagnosis focuses on the pattern of client-environment interaction.
3. The goal of nursing is to help clients repattern toward healthful behaviors (maximum health potential) in order to realize their creative-formative potentials.

Adaptation model

Roy[8] and her colleagues[9] have proposed that an adaptation model provides a useful way of thinking about nursing. Adaptation is seen as a process necessary to (1) maintain human integrity and (2) free energy for healing and for attaining higher levels of wellness. This conceptual framework includes the view of adaptation as a state of dynamic equilibrium.

Nursing goal

Within this framework the goal of nursing is to promote responses that lead to adaptation. In turn, adaptation is a "response to the environment which promotes the person's general goals including survival, growth, reproduction, self-mastery, and self-actualization."[9 (p. 53)] *Adaptation* is a term that refers to both a process and a state: the client may be either in the process of effectively coping with stressors or in the adapted state that results from effective coping.

Client focus

Consistent with the goal of nursing, the client is viewed as an open, adaptive system. The adaptation level reflects the system's ability to cope with environmental interaction. Coping may be adaptive or ineffective in maintaining human integrity. Ineffective coping behaviors require nursing attention. Two coping mechanisms are identified: the *cognator* and the *regulator*. The cognator mechanism consists of (1) perceptual information processing, (2) learning, (3) judgment, and (4) emotion. Coping with stressors also occurs through the regulator mechanism, which has "(1) neural, (2) endocrine and (3) perception-psychomotor" processes.[9 (p. 60)] The processes of the cognator and regulator are manifested in four modes of adaptive behavior: the physiological, self-concept, role function, and interdependence modes. These are defined in the box on p. 59.

The four adaptive modes provide a format for nursing assessment. In each mode behaviors are assessed and any stressors in the client-environment interaction are identified. Behaviors may be judged "adaptive" or "ineffective" relative to (1) the client's goals and (2) the maintenance of human integrity.[9 (p. 57)]

Theorist's view of diagnosis

In the adaptation framework, a nursing diagnosis is defined as a "judgment about ineffective or potentially ineffective behavior within a mode and identification of the most relevant influencing factors" causing the behavior.[9 (p. 286)] It is suggested that influencing, or etiological, factors can be focal stimuli (stressors) or ineffective cognator and

---

FOUR ADAPTATION MODES IDENTIFIED BY ROY

Physiological mode

Exercise/rest
Nutrition
Elimination
Fluids and electrolytes
Oxygen and circulation
Regulation of temperature
Regulation of senses
Regulation of endocrine system

Self-concept mode

Physical self
Personal self

Role function mode

Expressive, instrumental
Role identity
Role expectations
Role interactions

Interdependence mode

Cognitive/affective
    parameters in relation to independency-
    dependency needs
Affection achievement (love/support)

Adapted from Roy C, Roberts SL: *Theory construction in nursing: an adaptaton model,* Englewood Cliffs, NJ, 1981, Prentice-Hall.

---

regulator processes. The latter are discussed in relation to cross-modal diagnoses.[9] (pp. 286-287) This notion of etiology raises the question of whether intervention is facilitated by (1) specifying the stressor that produces ineffective adaptation or by (2) describing the client's ineffective, or maladaptive, response to the stressor. If the nursing goal is to promote adaptation, the identification of ineffective adaptive responses appears more useful for directing intervention. It is important in diagnosis that it be clear whether (1) the coping response to the stimulus or (2) the stimulus itself is specified as the cause(s) of the problem. The former dictates a typology of maladaptive coping responses (cognator and regulator processes) and the latter, a typology of stressors and the needs or deficits they produce. This issue may be resolved as the adaptation model is developed further and tested in practice.

In summary, in the adaptation model:
1. Four categories (see the box above) and two coping mechanisms (cognator and regulator) are provided as a framework for assessment.
2. Diagnoses are viewed as problems in adaptation.
3. The probable cause, or etiology, of problems is stressors or responses to stressors occurring during client-environment interaction.
4. The goal of nursing is to promote adaptive

responses so that higher levels of wellness can be attained.

Behavioral systems model

The behavioral systems model was initially proposed by Johnson.[10] In recent years it has been extended by Grubbs.[11] Although the framework contains the term *systems,* the focus is different from the focus of the biomedical systems framework used in medicine.

Nursing goal

Health, the goal of nursing, in the behavioral systems framework is viewed as a behavioral balance or stability. This stability is seen as the moving state of equilibrium with the ability to adjust and change but still maintain purposeful, orderly, predictable behavior.[11] (pp. 222-223)

Client focus

Using the behavioral systems model, the nurse views the client as an organized, interrelated complex of interacting subsystems. Each subsystem, for example, affiliation, has a pattern. The patterns the client develops determine and limit interaction with the environment.[11] (pp. 223-224)

Development of efficient and effective behavioral patterns requires the "sustenal imperatives" of protection, nurturance, and stimulation. Drives explain goal-directed behavior, choice, predispositions to act, and the repertoire of actions developed to sustain each subsystem. Interrelationships among the subsystems are monitored and controlled by biophysiological, psychological, and sociocultural mechanisms.[11] (p. 235)

Stress can disturb the client's patterns and lead to disequilibrium. Factors that cause disturbances in the regularity and orderliness of behavior patterns threaten the integrity and function of the entire behavioral system. Disturbances may be due to:

1. inadequate drive satisfaction,
2. inadequate fulfillment of the functional requirements of the subsystems, and
3. fluctuations in environmental conditions which exceed the system's capacity to adjust.[11] (p. 224)

Stress may also result from changes in sustenal imperatives (protection, nurturance, stimulation). As may be obvious from deductive reasoning, if the client is viewed as a system with behavioral subsystems, the latter are assessed in order to determine health status.

Assessment focuses on (1) behavioral patterns, (2) interrelations, and (3) sustenal imperatives. The assessment of subsystems may be directed by questions such as: Is there an actual or perceived threat to loss of pattern stability? Are there changes in behavioral patterns? Are there sufficient "sustenal imperatives"? What abilities does the client possess to adapt? Problems in subsystem behavior, if identified, are further assessed in order to plan intervention; nine areas of problem analysis have been identified and include client actions, predispositions, and choice.[11] (pp. 239–240)

The behavioral subsystems that lend structure to assessment when this model is used are listed in the box at right. The goal is behavioral stability; therefore, present behavior is compared with past behavior to judge whether change has occurred and to evaluate the contribution of the change toward stability.

Theorist's view of diagnosis

Within this model, the meaning of *diagnosis* is to determine "underlying dynamics of the patient's problematic behaviors in a situation."[11] (p. 240) (A recent interpretation of the model ignores the concept of diagnosis.[12] A problem is defined as an ac-

---

EIGHT BEHAVIORAL SUBSYSTEMS OF JOHNSON'S FRAMEWORK

Achievement subsystem: To master or control oneself or one's environment; to achieve mastery and control

Affiliative subsystem: To relate or belong to something or someone other than oneself; to achieve intimacy and inclusion

Aggressive protective subsystem: To protect oneself or others from real or imagined threatening objects, persons, or ideas; to achieve self-protection and self-assertion

Dependency subsystem: To maintain environmental resources needed for obtaining help, assistance, attention, permission, reassurance, and security; to gain trust and reliance

Eliminative subsystem: To expel biological wastes; to externalize the internal biological environment

Ingestive subsystem: To take in needed resources from the environment to maintain the integrity of the organism or to achieve a state of pleasure; to internalize the external environment

Restorative subsystem: To relieve fatigue and/or achieve a state of equilibrium by reestablishing or replenishing the energy distribution among the other subsystems; to redistribute energy

Sexual subsystem: To procreate, to gratify or attract, to fulfill expectations associated with one's sex; to care for others and be cared about by them

From Grubbs J: The Johnson behavioral system model. In Riehl JP, Roy C, editors: *Conceptual models for nursing practice,* ed 2, New York, 1980, Appleton-Century-Crofts.

---

tual or potential instability in the system. As discussed below, the problem may be either functional or structural. Problem, etiology, and problem source are all included in the statement of the diagnosis. The problem source is stated as an adjective that classifies the problem.

Diagnostically, a health problem originating in one subsystem is classified as an insufficiency or a discrepancy relative to the subsystem goal. Incompatibility and dominance are the two classifi-

Table 4-1 Diagnostic Classifications of Disorders in the Behavioral Systems Model

Single-subsystem disorders	*Insufficiency:* Exists when a particular subsystem is not functioning or developed to its fullest capacity because of an inadequacy of functional requirements
	Discrepancy: Exists when a behavior does not meet the intended goal
Multisubsystem disorder	*Incompatibility:* The goals or behaviors of two subsystems in the same situation conflict with each other to the detriment of the individual
	Dominance: The behavior in one subsystem is used more than any other subsystem regardless of the situation or to the detriment of the other subsystem(s)

From Grubbs J: The Johnson behavioral system model. In Riehl JP, Roy C, editors: *Conceptual models for nursing practice*, ed 2, New York, 1980, Appleton-Century-Crofts (pp. 240–241).

Table 4-2 Etiological Classification in the Behavioral Systems Model

Etiology of health problem	Definition of etiological type
Structural stress	That which occurs within the subsystems; involves internal control mechanisms and reflects inconsistencies among goals, sets, choices, or actions
Functional stress	An overload or insufficiency of any of the sustenal imperatives, results in functional disorders; usually arises externally from the environment

From Grubbs J: The Johnson behavioral system model. In Riehl JP, Roy C, editors: *Conceptual models for nursing practice*, ed 2, New York, 1980, Appleton-Century-Crofts (p. 241).

cations for multisubsystem problems. These classes are defined in Table 4-1 and help identify intervention, according to Grubbs.[11] Grief is an example of a problem or behavioral pattern instability. The problem source is classified as insufficiency in the affiliative subsystem. The cause, or etiology, of the instability in the subsystem pattern may be either internal or external stress. In addition, the client may be an active or passive participant. The instability is classified etiologically on the basis of two possible causes: structural stress and functional stress. These stresses are defined in Table 4-2. Grubbs'[11] classification places the source of structural stress within the subsystems (client). Functional stress is most often caused by factors in the external environment. The active or passive participation of the client as the cause of stress rests on the assumption in the model that the client has a choice of alternative behaviors. An example of an etiology of structural stress is the "de-

liberate avoidance of achievement situations" (p. 241)[11]; the cause lies within the person and, more specifically, within the achievement subsystem. The goal of the subsystem is to master and control, but the chosen behavior is not meeting this goal. Thus the reason lies in the client's behavior: choosing not to achieve.

Grubbs compares this example to functional stress. The etiology might be a "lack of achievement opportunities." In this case "the patient is essentially a passive victim of his environmental situation."[11](p. 241) Note the dichotomous judgment the diagnostician must make regarding internal or external stressors when using this classification. The dichotomy will not appeal to those who support the concept of multicausality or who believe that problems result from the interaction between person and environment.

According to Grubbs,[11] (p. 241) identifying whether the stress is structural or functional is helpful for diagnostic purposes. Even if this dichotomy of the probable sources of stress is accepted, value-laden statements (with or without sufficient clinical data) should be avoided. In Grubbs' example, the term *deliberate avoidance* has a negative connotation. Also, it does not seem that with this level of formulation "the intervention course becomes clear."[11] (p. 241) A nurse who thinks "avoidance" is "deliberate" needs to go further to understand why this is so.

The specification of etiology requires an in-depth assessment. It also requires an analysis of the clinical data to gain an understanding of the probable factor(s) that precipitate or maintain less-than-optimal states. Explanatory concepts (etiology) are helpful in care planning if they are formulated at a level that suggests nursing interventions. For diagnostic purposes, Table 4-2 is useful as a structure to organize thinking. It ensures that neither the client's behavior nor external circumstances and events are ignored in the attempt to understand the probable contributing, predisposing, or precipitating factors.

In summary, in the behavioral systems model:
1. The client is viewed as having a set of interrelated behavioral systems that form the framework for assessment.
2. Diagnoses are problems of instability that occur because of structural or functional stress.
3. The goal of nursing is behavioral balance and consequently optimal function, as evidenced by the ability to adjust to change.

A number of guidelines are offered for identifying problems and etiologies.[11]

Self-care agency model

Orem's[13] new formulations of her self-care agency framework contain three interrelated concepts: self-care agency (operations and abilities), self-care, and nursing. The capacity of clients to manage their own health and that of their dependents, such as children, is emphasized. Nurses help them achieve this goal.

Nursing goal

In discussing the goal of health care, Orem[14] (p. 173) defines health as a "state of wholeness or integrity of the individual human being, his parts and his modes of functioning." This framework has always stressed the importance of helping the client move toward independent self-care. This goal is achieved when the client's actions (in regard to self and dependents) regulate "internal and external conditions necessary to maintain life processes and environmental conditions supportive of life processes, integrity of human structure and function-

ing, and human developmental processes."[14] (p. 24)

Orem's underlying view of clients is that they are responsible and engage in deliberate choice and action. In accordance with this view, clients are expected to be socially responsible agents of their own self-care and the care of their dependents. Deficits or limitations in self-care actions, relative to requisites, require nursing attention.

Client focus

People are viewed as having universal, developmental, and health deviation self-care requisites, which are described below:

1. *Universal* self-care requisites are common to all human beings during all stages of life. They are associated with life processes and with the maintenance of the integrity of human structure and functioning. Universal self-care requisites include sufficient intake of air, water, and food; elimination; a balance between activity and rest and between solitude and social interaction; prevention of hazards; and the promotion of human functioning and development relative to potentialities.

2. *Developmental* self-care requisites vary with age and condition, such as pregnancy. There are two categories of developmental requisites:

   The bringing about and maintenance of living conditions that support life processes and promote the processes of development, that is, human progress toward higher levels of the organization of human structures and functions and toward maturation . . . [and] provision of care either to prevent the occurrence of deleterious effects of conditions that can affect human development . . . or to mitigate or overcome these effects.[13]

   Like universal self-care requisites, these developmental needs are met either through one's own abilities (if one is an able adult) or by another (as in the case of dependent children).

3. *Health deviation self-care requisites:* Orem[14] (p. 37) identifies and summarizes six categories:

   Health deviation self-care requisites are associated with genetic constitutional defects, human structural and functional deviations and their effects, and medical diagnosis and treatment.

Using these areas, the total "therapeutic self-care demand" of any individual can be determined. Also, self-care actions can be examined for their "therapeutic value."[14 (pp. 39-40)] If therapeutic, the person's actions contribute to "(1) support of life processes and promotion of normal functioning; (2) maintenance of normal growth, development, and maturation; (3) prevention, control, or cure of disease processes and injuries; and (4) prevention of, or compensation for, disability."[14 (pp. 42-44)]

When self-care is lacking or is carried out in a nontherapeutic manner, deficits exist. Self-care deficits are determined by examining:

1. An individual's therapeutic demands (required actions) in the areas of universal, developmental, and health deviation.
2. The self-care actions currently being carried out.
3. The therapeutic value of current actions. In addition, potential decreases in self-care abilities or increases in demands may be predicted.

Theorist's view of diagnosis

It clearly follows from this model of the client that the focus of nursing diagnosis is deficits in self-care agency (abilities); that is, when clients cannot manage their health, developmental, and therapeutic self-care needs. This inability may be the result of the client's lack of knowledge or skill, limitations in capacity (transitory or permanent), or lack of resources.[14 (p. 141)] The diagnostic judgment of deficits or limitations is related to (1) universal self-care requisites and the quality and type of present self-care activities and (2) actual or predicted abilities or actions. Essentially, *diagnosis involves a comparison of current actions and potential for action with actual or potential demands. If deficiencies are found, a problem in self-care agency is diagnosed.*

Orem[14] does not explicitly discuss a concept of etiology. She makes comments on the underlying cause of the inability to perform self-care actions, such as the client who can not use a fractured leg. Limitations in self-care "may be caused by the effects of the disease process, the therapy used, the lack of necessary knowledge and skills, or a lack of resources."[14 (p. 141)] In addition, the lack of motivation to alter self-care actions may also cause limitations in therapeutic self-care or care of dependents.[14 (p. 62)]

In summary, Orem's framework views the client as a self-care agent. The goal of nursing is the client's independence in self-care actions. As a framework for the diagnostic process, this model directs assessment toward data related to self-care demands and self-care capabilities. *Self-care agency* deficits, actual or potential, are the focus of diagnosis.

The models reviewed above provide a sampling of various conceptualizations of the client from a nursing perspective. Recall that the purpose of reviewing these models was to demonstrate answers to the questions of what information to collect and in what areas responsibility exists for diagnostic judgments. In this discussion of frameworks for the diagnostic phase of nursing process, the emphasis was on concepts of the client, diagnostic focus, and causality. These conceptual frameworks are summarized in Table 4-3. Although some overlapping can be seen, these ideas are essentially different views based on different assumptions about clients.

To implement any framework for nursing process, the nurse must understand the entire model and its philosophical assumptions. The reader is encouraged to review a number of models and their interrelated concepts of client, intervention (nurse-client interaction), and nursing goal. Several of the references listed at the end of this chapter pertain to the conceptual frameworks just discussed. Other nursing conceptual frameworks focus on human needs,[16] needs-conservation-adaptation,[17 (pp. 1-33)] needs-distress,[18] needs-social systems,[19] existential becoming,[20] stress,[21] Parse's man-living-health model[22] (an extension of Rogers' unitary human beings model), and Watson[23] (a model of caring).

ACQUIRING AND USING A CONCEPTUAL MODEL

Now the question arises as to how to choose a model that can give purpose and direction to nursing process and, particularly, to diagnosis. For students, the conceptual framework of the curriculum should provide guidance. The framework includes the faculty's concept of the client, nursing goal, and nursing intervention. For example, Orem's self-care agency framework[13,14] can guide a student to assess self-care agency and self-care deficits. If they are sufficiently developed, use of the

Table 4-3 Four Frameworks for the Diagnostic Process

Framework	Assessment focus	Diagnostic focus	Causality
Rogers' life process model[7]	Behavioral manifestations of events in the human and environmental field Holistic patterns of functioning (total pattern of events at a given point in space-time)	Pattern and organization of the life process which does not support maximum health potential and the creative-formative process (No diagnostic classification)	Multicausality found in human and environmental field interaction

Roy's adaptation model[8,9]	Adaptive responses to need deficits or excesses:
	Physiological mode
	  Rest/exercise
	  Nutrition
	  Elimination
	  Fluids and electrolytes
	  Oxygen and circulation
	  Regulation of temperature
	  Regulation of senses
	  Regulation of endocrine system
	Self-concept mode
	  Physical self
	  Personal self
	    Moral-ethical
	    Self-consistency
	    Self-ideal
	    Self-esteem
	Role function mode
	  Primary/secondary/tertiary roles
	  Expressive/instrumental:
	    Role identity
	    Role expectations
	    Role interactions
	Interdependence mode
	  Cognitive/affective, parameters in relation to independency-dependency needs:
	    Affection achievement (love, support)
	Influencing factors: focal, contextual, and residual stimuli
		Potential problems in adaptation; actual maladaptation problems
		(Diagnostic classification according to four adaptation modes: physiological, self-concept, role function, and interdependence modes)
			Causality lies in need deficits or excesses produced by stressors (focal stimulus) or in coping mechanisms (cognator and regulator)
			Multicausality concept, but intervention focus is on primary cause

Johnson's (Grubbs') behavioral system model[10,11]	Structural and functional level of behavioral system and the behavioral subsystem:
	  Achievement
	  Affiliative
	  Aggressive/protective
	  Dependency
	  Eliminative
	  Ingestive
	  Restorative
		Instability in the system; behavior at variance with the desired state; behavior that does not maintain equilibrium:
		Intrasubsystem insufficiency
		Intrasubsystem discrepancy
		Intersubsystem incompatibility
		Intersubsystem dominance
		Inadequate coping/adaptation
		(Diagnostic classification ac-
			Etiological classification according to source of stress/instability
			Etiology used in singular sense

Table 4-3 Four Frameworks for the Diagnostic Process—cont'd

Framework	Assessment focus	Diagnostic focus	Causality
	Sexual Coping effectiveness	cording to eight subsytems, intrasub system or intersub system problem)	
Orem's self-care agency model[13,14]	Eight universal self-care requisites, two developmental self-care requisites, and six health deviation self-care requisites (as well as interrelationships among these) Current repertoire of self-care practices (self and dependent): Degree of development Degree of operability Adequacy relative to demand	Presence of a deficit between existing powers of self-care agency and the demands on it Actual or potential deficits in type and quality (therapeutic value) of self-care actions Diagnostic classification according to self-care needs in relation to (1) development, (2) health deviation, and (3) universal	Cause may be disease process; therapy used; or lack of knowledge, skills, resources, interest, or motivation

concepts that structure the curriculum as a framework for nursing process provides consistency between classroom theory and clinical practice and makes learning easier.

The learner who is currently practicing nursing is already assessing, diagnosing, intervening, and evaluating on the basis of some framework, possibly without full awareness of what that framework is. It may be a rewarding experience to discover one's own professional point of view by reflecting on one's own practice. Examining personal assumptions about clients and about nursing leads to consciousness raising.

Sometimes nurses find they are using a medical or social work model to guide *nursing* practice. Although it seems illogical, it may occur. The reviews in this chapter and further reading about conceptual frameworks may assist in formulating a model for nursing practice.

Some nurses claim, "I don't need all that theoretical stuff to give nursing care," or, "I don't need that, I just look at what the patients need or tell me they need." These nurses are deluding themselves. *All* nurses act on some of their observations and make referrals on the basis of others. Beneath these actions and referrals is a personal concept of nursing and some idea of what "should" receive attention.

Even implicit, unrecognized models influence

perception and judgment. In the second statement quoted above, the nurse has a model but doesn't know it. A human needs model is obviously being used and probably only requires some conscious organization.

Testing a model in practice

Conceptual models or frameworks of nursing can be elegant designs with logical relationships between the concepts that are spelled out and diagrammed. The crucial test, however, is whether a framework works in clinical practice. Does it provide a useful way of viewing clients? Does it capture the essence of the special contribution nursing makes to health care delivery? Does the concept of what nurses should do with and for clients (intervention concepts) seem realistic?

The only way to answer these questions about a model is to try it in practice. The concept of the client should be used in assessment and diagnosis. The nurse should try to state and then evaluate client outcomes that are developed from the framework's concept of the nursing goal. The concept of intervention in the model should be used as a guide for planning and implementing nursing care. After a number of months of this kind of testing, the strengths, weaknesses, and areas needing further development become apparent. Undoubtedly the nursing theorist who developed the model would welcome a thoughtful critique and ideas for further development. These critiques and comments may be published in the nursing literature or relayed through personal communication. That is how conceptual models become refined. Clinicians have to test them in practice and identify their clinical usefulness.

Why the emphasis on models of the client? To reiterate, because *nursing* diagnosis cannot be done without a *nursing* focus that provides clear guidelines for the collection of clinical information: It is as simple as that.

THE SEARCH FOR A UNIFIED MODEL

At this point, if not earlier, the reader may be asking why nurses do not agree on just one model of the client. Riehl and Roy[24 (p. 392)] state that having a single model would facilitate communication, help develop a body of knowledge, and form one common nursing approach to practice. This model would still allow diversity in concepts of, and approaches to, nursing intervention. On the other hand, Riehl and Roy cite disadvantages and barriers: basic philosophical differences exist, frameworks have not been sufficiently tested, and there are strong vested interests. These authors note that with unification, the question of which model to select would arise. They point out that such a selection might inhibit creativity and close off new and more productive conceptualizations.

There are areas of agreement among the theorists, although, as Zderad[25] has suggested, these areas of agreement would be more explicit if, when a new model was proposed, similarities and differences were addressed. When new conceptual models are published, theorists rarely compare their respective perspectives with previously published models.

The idea of a unified model is not foreign to other disciplines. In the general scientific community, theories have been proposed to unify the sciences. In many sciences, there is a great deal of knowledge gained from research that can be integrated into a unified model. Nursing science is just beginning, and perhaps efforts should go into forming middle-range theories. For all the reasons

discussed, it is unlikely that a unified model (client, goal, intervention) will be accepted in the near future. It might be well to examine the problems this situation presents for nursing diagnosis and look for potential solutions.

For nurses who each day confront clients, students, or research data, the issue of a unified model of the client to guide assessment and diagnosis is not just an "ivory tower" idea. It has implications for nursing care delivery, nursing education, research, and our ability to market our services outside the institutional setting. The implications are critical for developing commonly agreed-upon diagnostic nomenclature. For example, diversity now exists among nursing care delivery settings: clients may have different aspects of their health status assessed, depending on the hospital they go to, the level of care they receive (primary, secondary, or tertiary), and the particular nurse they happen to encounter. From the nurse's own perspective, every time there is a change in employment settings, the nurse usually faces a different format for assessment. Similarly, it is not unusual for a student to be introduced to a different assessment tool by each different clinical instructor or in each area of practice. This variation certainly does not facilitate learning or the development of nursing practice expertise, nor does it facilitate clinical nursing research. How can continuity of nursing care in various settings and with various nurses be provided if there is no basic clinical assessment data base? How can there be studies of common health problems nurses treat? There is no assurance that assessment and diagnosis are done comprehensively. Nor can a consumer of nursing care be reasonably assured that all his or her actual or potential health problems will be detected.

Components of nursing practice have been agreed on and standardized nationally. From the consumer's perspective, nurses are expected to do assessment, diagnosis, intervention, and evaluation. Pressuring for unification at the abstract level of the models, which may remain diverse, may not be the solution. Maybe what is needed for practice, education, and research is a unification at the concrete level of assessment (information collection) and, as the American Nurses Association (ANA)[26] has suggested, a uniform language. Then more abstract concepts of the models could be applied to the basic data and to intervention.

Unification of assessment structure

Is agreement possible, at a concrete level, about the information needed for nursing assessment? Are there common areas of information about clients that are needed to implement *any* of the models of nursing? For example, regardless of the model used in clinical practice, is every nursing clinician interested in information about dietary patterns? Remember that the focus of this discussion is on structural aspects of assessment: that is, what information to gather (what to pay attention to). Differences are expected in the way the information is interpreted and used.

Let us consider some of the models. Take, for example, the clinician who believes with Orem that the goal of nursing is to facilitate self-care agency. The nutritional pattern is decidedly an aspect of self-care, so nutritional patterns are assessed. The approach includes a nutritional pattern description, but self-care actions underlying the pattern are emphasized. The nurse clinician who has adopted Roy's adaptation framework also wants to know the basic nutritional pattern. This nurse will approach the analysis of clinical data by determining the client's or family's adaptation of nutritional patterns under certain situations. The clinician concerned with patterns of living coordinated with environmental changes (Rogers' life process model) is interested in nutritional patterns as they relate to other rhythm changes; for example, during hospitalization. Information about diet would be considered specific data to be included in synthesizing a holistic view of the life process. The dietary pattern would be evaluated in terms of the goal of maximizing health for the creative-formative process of evolution (becoming).

Diversity in nursing models does not prevent standardization of assessment structure. Standardization does not imply a standardized interpersonal *approach* to assessment or to analysis and synthesis of clinical data. Neither does it suggest that the profession should have a standardized concept of the goal of nursing and of nurse-client interaction.

Although diversity is the watchword, at a concrete level there must be some uniformity in practice. In organizations theory-based practice is important, but whose theory should be used? Every client deserves to know that, minimally, certain health-related patterns will be assessed for potential or actual problems. This idea is certainly not new. Dorothy Smith[27] started prodding the profession at least 25 years ago and recently the ANA has suggested the same.

Standardization of assessment areas requires thoughtful consideration of related issues and consequences. In addition, proposed formats for standardized assessment must be evaluated, both initially and periodically, in all settings and specialties of nursing practice. The profession must take action to delineate the basic areas of assessment applicable to all clients. Then (1) the domain of responsibility and accountability would be clear; (2) the focus for clinical studies would be identified; and (3) the foci for development of expertise in assessment and diagnosis would be clearly delineated for teachers, students, and practitioners. The typology of assessment categories proposed in Chapter 5 is a step in the direction of unification of assessment areas. As stated previously, each nurse's approach to these areas is dictated by the conceptual framework used.

SUMMARY

This chapter contains important ideas for using nursing diagnosis and the diagnostic process. There is an ethical responsibility in diagnosis. One aspect of that responsibility is to have a consciously defined purpose and a systematic approach. Clients should not be subjected to an unorganized set of questions, and the reasons for collecting information should be clear. Hence a nursing focus is necessary when using the diagnostic process.

Several current conceptual frameworks were described to demonstrate a nursing focus for diagnosis. Particular attention was given to concepts of the client and of nursing's goal. These concepts are particularly relevant to the focus of information collection for diagnosis. No unified framework for nursing—one that is accepted by all—exists or can be predicted to exist in the near future. It was suggested that at a basic level, all frameworks require similar assessment data.

NOTES AND REFERENCES

1. These areas of knowledge are sometimes named *person, environment, health,* and *nursing* (used as a verb) and are the taken-for-granted perspective. These latter concepts make up a *metaparadigm,* which is the generally accepted structure or perspective of the profession. A conceptual framework, in contrast, is more specific and states what is of concern about the client-environment from a nursing viewpoint; for example, an adaptation model. This is similar to other sciences where there are multiple philosophical perspectives of important dimensions of a phenomenon.
2. Self-care agency deficit should not be confused with self-care deficit, the diagnostic category in Appendix A. The former is an abstract way of thinking about all diagnoses, whereas the latter is one particular diagnosis.
3. The logical relationship between the goal and client focus (also intervention focus) is referred to as the *internal consistency* of a conceptual framework.
4. Frameworks will not be discussed comprehensively here; certain concepts have been selected because of their pertinence to diagnosis. The reader is encouraged to read the original sources and the reviews listed in this bibliography.
5. In the early 1970s the author used an inductive process as one of the methods for identifying common areas of assessment in nursing as a basis for the functional health patterns of Chapters 5 and 6.
6. Flam F: The quest for a theory of everything hits some snags, *Science* 256:1518, 1992.
7. Rogers M: *An introduction to the theoretical basis of nursing,* Philadelphia, 1970, Davis.
8. Roy C, Roberts SL: *Theory construction in nursing: an adaptation model,* Englewood Cliffs, NJ, 1981, Prentice-Hall.
9. Andrews HA, Roy C: *Essentials of the Roy Adaptation Model,* Norwalk, Conn, 1986, Appleton-Century-Crofts.
10. Johnson D: *One conceptual model of nursing.* Paper presented at Vanderbilt University, Nashville, Tenn, April 25, 1968.
11. Grubbs J: The Johnson behavioral system model. In Riehl

JP, Roy C, editors: *Conceptual models for nursing practice,* ed 2, New York, 1980, Appleton-Century-Crofts.
12. Loveland-Cherry A, Wilkerson SA: Dorothy Johnson's behavioral system model. In Fitzpatrick J, Whall AL, editors: *Conceptual models of nursing,* ed 2, Norwalk, Conn, 1991, Appelton & Lange, pp 147–163.
13. Orem DE: *Nursing: concepts of practice,* ed 3, St Louis, 1985, Mosby.
14. Orem DE: *Nursing: concepts of practice,* ed 2, St Louis, 1980, Mosby.
15. Yura H, Walsh M: *Human needs and the nursing process,* Norwalk, Conn, 1978, Appleton-Century-Crofts.
16. Putt AM: *General systems theory applied to nursing,* Boston, 1978, Little, Brown.
17. Levine ME: *Introduction to clinical nursing,* ed 2, Philadelphia, 1973, Davis.
18. Orlando J: *The dynamic nurse-patient relationship: function, process and principles,* New York, 1961, Putnam.
19. King IM: *Towards a theory for nursing: general concepts of human behavior,* New York, 1971, Wiley.
20. Patterson JG, Zderad L: *Humanistic nursing,* New York, 1976, Wiley.
21. Neuman B: The Betty Neuman health care systems model: a total person approach to patient problems. In Riehl JD, Roy C, editors: *Conceptual models for nursing practice,* ed 2, New York, 1980, Appleton-Century-Crofts.
22. Parse RR: Parse's man-living-health: a theory of nursing. In Parse RR, editor: *Nursing science: major paradigms, theories, and critiques,* Philadelphia, 1981, Saunders.
23. Watson J: *Nursing: human science and human care,* Norwalk, Conn, 1985, Appleton-Century-Crofts.
24. Riehl JP, Roy C: Discussion of a unified nursing model. In Riehl JP, Roy C, editors: *Conceptual models for nursing practice,* New York, 1974, Appleton-Century-Crofts.
25. Zderad L: *Future directions in nursing theory.* Paper presented at Nurse Educator Conference, New York, Dec 4–7, 1978. (Cassette available from Nursing Resources Inc, Wakefield, Mass.)
26. Saba VK: ICN to review nursing diagnosis, *American Nurse* 24:24, 1992.
27. Smith DM: A clinical nursing tool, *Am J Nurs* 68:2384, 1968.

CHAPTER 5

FUNCTIONAL HEALTH PATTERNS: A STRUCTURE FOR ASSESSMENT

C hapter 4 included various ways of thinking about nursing from various conceptual viewpoints. It was stated that frameworks that guide practice must be abstract. Otherwise they would not be useful in a variety of nursing care settings or in dealing with diverse client populations. Yet specific guidelines for assessment are also necessary. This chapter presents a set of health patterns that specify areas of basic information to be collected no matter what framework is used. The objectives of the chapter are to (1) discuss the concept of functional health patterns, (2) define the 11 patterns proposed, and (3) help the reader understand how these patterns provide a structure for assessment and a basic data base for nursing diagnosis.

The term *assessment* means evaluation. In nursing the term is used to describe initial and continued health evaluation of a person, family, or community. *Deliberative and systematic assessment* is an intentional process based on a plan for collecting and organizing information. The typology of functional health patterns proposed in the next section provides this plan. Information collection is organized in a way that facilitates health evaluation and nursing diagnosis. Health pattern areas provide a standard assessment format for a basic data base, regardless of a client's age, level of care,

or medical disease. The pattern areas have additional advantages:

1. They need not be continually relearned. Their application is expanded as clinical knowledge accumulates within the nursing setting or specialty or, in the case of students, across nursing specialties.
2. They lead directly to nursing diagnoses (Appendix B).
3. They encompass a holistic approach to human functional assessment in any setting and for any age group at any point in the health-illness continuum. They incorporate the concepts of client-environment interaction, age-developmental level, health-illness, and culture in the holistic idea of dynamic life patterns.
4. They guide the collection of information on the client's, family's, or community's life world and their experience of events and problems related to health and health management.

All human beings have in common certain functional patterns that contribute to their health, quality of life, and achievement of human potential. These common patterns are the focus of nursing assessment. Description and evaluation of health patterns permit the nurse to identify functional patterns (client strengths) and dysfunctional patterns (nursing diagnoses). Both traditional and contemporary ideas of nursing practice are represented in a concise, easily learned set of categories. Before further discussion of functional health patterns, consider the abbreviated definitions contained in the box on the right. The 11 patterns are fully defined in Appendix G. Functional health patterns can be used in a number of ways:

1. As a format for organizing assessment data (Appendix H) and as a corresponding structure for grouping nursing diagnoses (Appendix B).
2. As a system for organizing clinical knowledge. Courses or curricula using these patterns have been organized in a number of educational programs.
3. As a system for organizing clinical literature. Reports on the classification of conference papers and literature reviews.
4. As topics for clinical research on health patterns.[1]

At this point let us concentrate on grasping the idea of functional health patterns and then decide if this framework constitutes a basic data base for arriving at a holistic understanding of a client's life pattern.

FUNCTIONAL HEALTH PATTERNS: A FRAMEWORK FOR ASSESSMENT

The list of assessment areas above uses the term *pattern,* which is defined as a configuration of behaviors that occur sequentially across time. Sequences of behavior, rather than isolated events, are the data used for clinical inference and judgment. For example, a nurse observes a hospitalized client having an argument with her husband. What does the nurse conclude? Nothing, one hopes! Is the quarrel a sign of the client's general pattern of relationships, including marital? Maybe or maybe not. Obviously, information about interactions with her husband across time is needed to determine whether relationships are a problem for the client. Suppose additional information about this couple reveals the marital relationship has problems. The nurse is still at an elementary level of understanding. Other relationships must be assessed to see

---

TYPOLOGY OF 11 FUNCTIONAL HEALTH PATTERNS*

Health perception–health management pattern: Describes the client's perceived pattern of health and well-being and how health is managed

Nutritional-metabolic pattern: Describes the client's pattern of food and fluid consumption relative to metabolic need and pattern indicators of local nutrient supply

Elimination pattern: Describes patterns of excretory function (bowel, bladder, and skin)

Activity-exercise pattern: Describes patterns of exercise, activity, leisure, and recreation

Sleep-rest pattern: Describes patterns of sleep, rest, and relaxation

Cognitive-perceptual pattern: Describes sensory-perceptual and cognitive patterns

Self-perception–self-concept pattern: Describes the client's self-concept pattern and perceptions of self (e.g., self-conception/worth, body image, feeling state)

Role-relationship pattern: Describes the client's pattern of role engagements and relationships

Sexuality-reproductive pattern: Describes the client's patterns of satisfaction and dissatisfaction with sexuality pattern; describes reproductive pattern

Coping–stress-tolerance pattern: Describes the client's general coping pattern and the effectiveness of the pattern in terms of stress tolerance

Value-belief pattern: Describes patterns of values, beliefs (including spiritual), and goals that guide the client's choices or decisions

*The pattern areas were identified by the author in the mid-1970s to teach assessment and diagnosis at Boston College School of Nursing. Colleagues have suggested some minor changes in labels and content. Faye E. McCain's and Dorothy Smith's assessment concepts were particularly influential, as were the comments of clinical specialists and students who reviewed and tried out the categories in practice.

whether this relationship problem can be generalized to other areas of life and times or is specific to this relationship at this point in time. These components of the total relationship pattern may include parent-child, work, and social interactions. When these data have been collected, the diagnostician can move toward understanding the overall role-relationship pattern and the client's perception of the pattern. Further discussions may reveal why the marital stress exists and what remedies the couple has tried.

As information is collected, the nurse begins to understand the functional area being assessed. Gradually, a pattern emerges. It is important to recognize that what occurs during information collection is the *construction of a pattern* from a client's descriptions and the nurse's observations. An observer does not *see* a pattern; the observer's mind constructs the pattern by "putting things together." How is this done? Let us begin with a concrete example and then consider more complex behavioral patterns. A client has a normal temperature every 4 hours except for the 4 PM measurement, which is 101° F. This occurs 3 days in a row and suggests a pattern of afternoon elevation. Recognizing a pattern involves (1) attention to observations or verbal reports of behavior, and (2) noticing repeated instances of a particular behavior across time or repeated instances of a type of event or behavior. For example, a client who is receiving counseling from a nurse about relationships with a boyfriend may describe difficulties in relationships at work and within her family. Connecting these data, the nurse thinks: Is it possible a general pattern of relating exists that is not productive for this person? In some cases during assessment the client may connect events or behaviors and put them together as a pattern; the client may say, for example, "I'm not coping well in any part of my life." This is called insight and is probably the same phenomenon a nurse experiences when connecting behaviors. Note that connections are constructed. Recognizing that patterns are constructed:

1. Avoids the collection of superficial data that can lead to errors in diagnosis.
2. Reminds the nurse that patterns are not observable. They are *constructed* by cognitive

operations on the assessment data and are always open to challenge by new information. When they are no longer supportable, they are discarded.
3. Emphasizes a point that will be repeated frequently: Patterns must be validated.

Consider some examples of assessments from which a pattern emerges (is constructed). In the first example a 50-year-old construction worker reports the following sleep pattern.

Sleep-Rest Pattern. He feels rested after his usual 6 to 7 hours of sleep and ready for day's work. There is no delay in sleep onset, interrupted sleep, early awakening, or use of sleep medications. He dreams occasionally; reports no nightmares.

This information indicates an optimal adult sleep pattern. You can "see" the client's pattern from the data: restful, undisturbed sleep without the use of medications. In contrast, what pattern is evident in this report for another client 1 day prior to heart surgery?

Sleep-Rest Pattern. States he always was a "good sleeper": 6 to 7 hours regularly, would be well rested on awakening. Reports "insomnia" and delayed sleep onset 2 to 3 hours during last 3 weeks. Lies awake "worrying" about the success of the heart surgery. Is "scared" at night when there is "no one to talk to."

The reported change in sleep pattern is very apparent. Historically this client had a normal sleep pattern, but a change has occurred. The abrupt change, combined with the scheduled heart surgery, suggests the change may be due to fear or anxiety. If the underlying problem is not diagnosed and treated, his sleep pattern may not improve. In the next example try to identify the client's pattern.

Sleep-Rest Pattern. Says he has not slept well for the last few months. Did not sleep first night in the hospital. Sleeping pill ineffective. Uses three pillows.

This assessment is superficial. Although there is information to support a dysfunctional sleep pattern, the information is incomplete. For example, "three pillows" suggests a breathing problem. Is that why the client has not slept well? What does the vague statement, "not slept well," mean? We are left with these questions because the pattern was not evident in the minimal data recorded on the chart. This lack of an identifiable pattern may have led to a delay in diagnosis and, most important, to a delay in treatment.

Even with adequate information to describe a pattern, understanding it may be elusive until all functional patterns are assessed, because the 11 functional patterns are an artificial division of integrated human functioning. (Our limited cognitive capacity cannot easily grasp the complexity of the whole in one glance.) *Patterns are interrelated, interactive, and interdependent.* Reasons for a dysfunctional pattern (etiological factors) may be found within this composite, as well as the strengths needed to solve problems. This is true for each of us: no single pattern can be understood in isolation.

An example may clarify the idea of the interrelatedness of patterns. During a home visit a community health nurse collected the following information as part of a data base:

> Sixty-five-year-old man, recently retired after selling the grocery store that previously occupied his time from 8 AM until 6 PM. States he has little to do now and gets into arguments with his wife: "She doesn't like me around the house; it interferes with what she wants to do. I just want to spend more time talking to her and doing things together." Wife states she has the house to keep up, meals to cook, and her volunteer activities at a day care center every afternoon. Complains she can't get things done because "he's in the way" and "he mopes around the house."

The nurse collected two types of data: previous patterns and current patterns that show a change has taken place. Even with this minimal information it can be seen that the problem may be in the area of roles and relationships; family conflict is a tenable diagnostic hypothesis at this point.

Look again at the list of functional health patterns in the box on p. 70. In which categories might the reasons (etiological factors) for this problem be found? Is it not probable that data about the coping pattern, activity pattern, and value-belief pattern would help the nurse identify the etiological factors and perhaps also refine the problem in this situation? For example, is the husband's activity tolerance low, and if so, what meaning does it have for him? Is that why he does not engage in activities in or outside the home? Are the wife's and

husband's values, relative to their relationship, divergent? Is there a lack of resources for retired persons in their community, or has a choice been made not to use them? Certainly questions can be raised regarding the contribution of all other pattern areas to this problem.

This example makes two points. First, the functional patterns provide a structure for analyzing a problem *within* a category, as in this husband-wife conflict about family roles and relationships. Second, a structure is provided to focus the search for causal explanations that usually lie outside the problem category; in the example of the grocer, activities, values, and coping patterns would be explored. To make information processing even easier, the current list of approved diagnoses is classified into functional health pattern areas (see Appendix B). As discussed in another chapter, a nurse can move horizontally from data in a pattern area to problem identification and then vertically through the patterns to identify etiological factors. Diagnosis is facilitated if information is gathered and organized in a way relevant to problem identification.

Does the process just described sound foreign? Consider that it is usually not possible to make a judgment about data, such as heart rate or blood pressure, unless baseline data are available. Even one baseline measure and one current measure describe an elementary pattern across time, *if the nurse puts the data together.* In another example, think of a friend's behavior that has come to your attention recently. Did you expect the particular behavior, or was it unexpected? Why did you have any expectation at all?

Knowledge of your friend's previous behavioral patterns caused you to notice, or not to notice, a difference. Further, to understand the meaning of different behavior, you compared the friend's historical pattern (baseline) and current behavior. Many pieces of information were brought together to gain understanding. The process is not unusual; human beings process information this way every day. When it is important for the life or comfort of another person that the correct synthesis and judgment are made, the process is conscious and systematic.

This discussion of pattern leads to a second question: What is a health pattern? This question should be answered in terms of a definition of health. *Health,* defined within the context of functional health patterns, is the optimal level of functioning that allows individuals, families, or communities to develop their potential to the fullest. Health is measured by parameters and norms (statistical, cultural, etc.) combined with a subjective client description. Ideal health is consistent with individual potential and allows intervention to be individualized.

Functional focus

There may be a question about the use of the term *functional patterns.* Since *functional* is a term used in other professions as well, it is helpful to consider the differences and similarities of its use in various fields. Traditionally "ways of living," or functional patterns, have been an important focus of nursing's health promotion, assistance, and rehabilitation activities. In medicine the word *function* is used to describe a physiological process, such as respiratory, cardiac, or brain function. The diagnostic focus is on the functions of cells, organs, and systems, not on the integrative function of the whole individual. *Functional performance* and *functional disability* are commonly used terms but usually refer only to mobility and other physical parameters.

Biological systems (neurological, cardiac, and so forth) support health patterns and provide one type of assessment information. In caring for a person who is unable to monitor his or her own heart rate or pupil dilation, nurses collect information for two purposes: to understand or predict changes in functional health patterns and to report complications and disease progression to a physician when the client lacks the expertise or ability to do so. In fact, a dysfunctional pattern (nursing diagnosis) may be a cue to an underlying disease and the reason a nurse guides the patient to see a physician.

Organs and systems are at a lower level of complexity than the functional health patterns, which represent integrative, human functioning. For example, cardiac, respiratory, and neuromuscular systems are important factors in any activity-exercise pattern. Yet the pattern is more than the supporting parts; the health pattern is a manifestation of the whole. It is incorrect to call certain functional health patterns "physiological" and others

"psychosocial." Each pattern is a biopsychosocial-spiritual expression.

Functional patterns, health, and disease

Pathological conditions and their treatment can alter patterns. In Fig. 5-1 arrows depict the secondary functional effects of disease or treatment on patterns. Examples are the changes disease causes in customary coping patterns and stress tolerance, changes in elimination patterns and metabolism that occur with bed rest, and the not uncommon readjustment of value-belief patterns after a life-threatening illness. Consider a common case: A person is hospitalized for weight loss, frequent urination, thirst, and an elevated blood glucose level. Medical tests support a diagnosis of diabetes mellitus. Nurses familiar with the typical client with newly diagnosed diabetes can attest to the fact that the secondary effects of the disease are widespread. The pathological condition, its treatment, the personal response of the client and family, and the long-term management of the condition influence all functional patterns, as illustrated in Fig. 5-1 by the arrows leading from medical diagnosis outward to pattern areas. Certainly there will be effects on client-environment interaction, particularly in the role-relationship pattern.

In addition to disturbances in functional patterns secondary to disease, dysfunctional patterns may occur when no clinical evidence of disease is present. A client may be found to be medically healthy but still require nursing care. This phenomenon is also illustrated in Fig. 5-1. The arrows proceeding from functional patterns to medical diagnosis represent the idea that unresolved dysfunctional patterns may increase susceptibility to various diseases, stressors, and microorganisms. Almost everyone is exposed to the media messages that life patterns can predispose an individual to illness. People are told to walk or jog (exercise-activity pattern), cut down on saturated fats (nutritional-metabolic pattern), stop smoking, lose weight, get regular physical checkups (health management pattern), learn to handle stress (role-relationship pattern), set priorities and ignore inconsequential annoyances (value-belief pattern), and remember "number one" (self-perception–self-concept pattern). This list of mes-

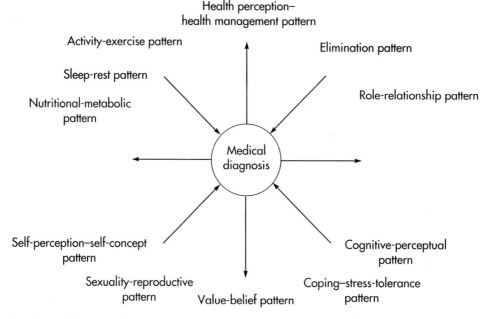

Fig. 5-1 Effect of disease on functional patterns and of functional patterns on the development of a disease.

sages is meant only to prevent cardiovascular disease.

Many people need help to work out productive health patterns. Nurses have always assumed responsibility for health promotion and health maintenance. Systematic, early identification and treatment of actual and potential problems (dysfunctional patterns) would probably have demonstrable positive effects on the health of the population. Consider, for example, coronary heart disease. List the patterns in Fig. 5-1 that increase a person's risk of a heart attack.

If nurses helped clients change dysfunctional patterns, the positive impact on illness and death statistics for many disease conditions would be great. This premise is supported by the U.S. Department of Health and Human Services' report on a health strategy for the nation, *Healthy People 2000*.[4] The report outlines the areas that must be addressed to impact the rates of coronary heart disease, cancer, obesity, spinal cord and head injury, suicide, and teenage pregnancy. Risk evaluation and risk reduction objectives center around functional patterns. The areas in which health recommendations are made are:

  Physical activity and fitness (activity-exercise pattern)
  Nutrition (nutritional-metabolic pattern)
  Cigarette smoking and alcohol consumption (health perception–health management pattern)
  Teenage pregnancy (sexuality-reproductive pattern)
  Suicide and depression (self-perception–self-concept pattern)
  Violent and abusive behavior (role-relationship pattern)

Who are the high-risk populations? In one area nearly all of us, according to the following quote:

Few Americans engage in regular physical activity despite the potential benefits. Currently, only 22 percent of adults engage in at least 30 minutes of light to moderate physical activity 5 or more times per week and only 12 percent report that they are this active 7 or more times a week. Less than 10 percent of the population exercises 3 or more times a week at the more vigorous level necessary to improve cardio-respiratory fitness. Nearly 25 percent of adults report no leisure-time physical activity, and the prevalence of sedentary behavior increases with advancing age.[4] (p. 55)

As Fig. 5-1 suggests, dysfunctional patterns can cause disease and the reverse is also true.

Client-environment focus

Interaction between the client and the environment is an essential, common thread running through all functional patterns. From this interaction patterns develop. For example, patterns of role-relationships and self-concept are influenced by the environment, particularly by people and culture. This influence begins at birth and is more pronounced as language and nonverbal expression are learned. Taking and giving emotional support is another example of client-environment interaction; in this instance the interaction influences coping patterns.

Crop production, food additives, and environmental temperature all influence a nutritional-metabolic pattern. As another example much has been said in news reports about human activities that degrade the natural environment, such as a pattern of industrial waste elimination. This example illustrates a change in the natural environment produced by human beings that then in turn influences human patterns. Client-environment interaction is an integral part of information collection in each pattern area.

Consider the example of environmental influences on the role-relationship pattern of an institutionalized elderly client confined to a wheelchair:

> **Role-Relationship Pattern.** States she is the "last" of nine brothers and sisters; husband dead: no children; elderly friends are unable to visit. Doctor (family friend) suggested she enter a nursing home 1 month ago after her stroke. Reports, "What else could I do?" Prior to stroke was active socially. Currently is apathetic and withdrawn. States, "Everything is on schedule here; you're supposed to talk to people on schedule, go to this, go to that. Never before have I been told who I have to talk to. There is no way out; I can't do anything about it." States she asked to visit on another floor "where the clear-headed ones are" but "they're too busy or they come to take me when I'm tired." States, "They told me I had to live on this floor

because I'm in a wheelchair." Appearance sad and withdrawn. Roommate and majority of other patients are confused.

The client's pattern of socialization and choices regarding socialization are dramatically influenced by her environment. Her social isolation is evident, and when it was combined with data from other pattern areas, an underlying problem of powerlessness was diagnosed. The basic problem illustrated by this example is the influence of the environment on functional patterns. Previously the patient had been considered "depressed" and given drugs—a superficial evaluation.

Age-developmental focus

Nurses are concerned with the human development of children, adults, families, and communities. Consequently any structure for nursing assessment must take development into account. What is human development? Can it be conceived as the development of the functional patterns? Human growth and development are reflected in each pattern area. Elimination patterns change, particularly in the area of control. Maturation toward adult norms occurs in role-relationship, cognitive-perceptual, and other patterns as the years go by. Patterns are a product of developmental factors; thus a developmental focus is built into the functional typology and into assessment guidelines (see Appendix H). *The 11 functional patterns are always judged against age or developmental norms, if useful norms are available.*

Cultural focus

Culture is an important personal and social-environmental influence on the development of health patterns. Similar to the age-developmental focus, health patterns are a product of environment and culture. More specifically, culturally based age, developmental, and gender norms may be important in understanding health patterns.

Increasing attention is being given to cultural diversity. One definition of cross-cultural nursing care, that of the American Academy of Nursing Expert Panel, is "care delivered to individuals, families, or groups that are considered (by self or others) a minority because of race, culture, heritage, or sexual orientation."[5] (p. 278) Competent care is sensitive to cultural issues. The panel suggested that cultural norms, values, and communication/time patterns must be identified and used as the knowledge base for a clinical model of competent care. This sensitivity is particularly relevant in the collection and interpretation of assessment information.

Studies of the cultural adequacy of some current diagnostic categories have been attempted.[6] It is important not to label cultural factors as problems or as reasons for problems (intervention focus) in a society that encourages diversity. For example, labeling behavior as social dissonance indicates a social disparity, discord, or variance (versus consonance, which is defined as agreement, harmony, and accord). This "social dissonance" may be a contextual factor that should be recognized (and sometimes applauded) as a characteristic of a person outside the dominant culture but is not a "problem" situation, per se, to be changed unless the client requests help in doing so. An individual client may wish to tolerate a social and language dissonance and its consequences because a higher value is placed on heritage and cultural practices. Some people born into a culture are also at variance with some of the prevailing mores and values.

Studies that focus on care, rather than on diagnoses, have been advocated.[7] Knowledge gained from "care" studies applied outside the context of diagnostic judgments about a situation will not lead to culturally competent care. Clinical judgments are interpretations. The cultural or meaningful character of signs and symptoms and the clinical task of interpreting those cues within a person's reality is a central task. What is needed first and foremost are studies (in various cultural contexts) of behaviors that define a particular diagnosis and its cultural meaning. If this information were available for diagnoses, it would encourage cultural sensitivity. Yet this information still does not substitute for a philosophy of practice that is sensitive to the underlying personal and cultural reality of a client's problems. The personal and cultural meaning of situations add much to the understanding of a client's experience. For example, the diagnosis of obesity is frequently made. MacKenzie[8] comments that in American culture a

diagnosis of obesity means (1) social condemnation for loss of self-control and lack of competence, (2) the shame of being the fat (slow, ugly) kid in the gym class, (3) embarrassment in dating situations or when buying clothes, (4) low status or social class, and (5) Weight Watchers. The current definition of obesity (the intake of nutrients that exceeds body needs) and its current diagnostic label, Altered Nutrition: More Than Body Requirements, give no clue to the meaningful context in which obesity may be culturally embedded. Diagnoses should not be expected to serve this role. Not all persons the nurse encounters or all cultures place such meanings on being fat. *The key is to appreciate that a personal meaning is attached to conditions and to elicit this personal meaning when appropriate.* The information may influence interpretations, interactions, and interventions.

Use in practice

What makes an assessment format usable and useful in practice? *Usability* means that the format matches the competencies and time constraints of the users. *Usefulness* refers to the consistency between the format and the user's role-responsibilities.

Professional nurses are competent to assess the 11 functional health patterns. These areas are stressed in nursing textbooks and nursing education. In fact, the functional areas do not represent any totally new ideas; they are only a format for directing and organizing assessment in a systematic way. Higher levels of expertise develop with continued use. The interest of clinicians in this format is accompanied by some questions regarding its use in practice:

1. Doesn't a functional pattern assessment take too much time?

The answer might be formulated in relation to the moral issue of the *allocation of resources.* What are the high priorities for the use of nurses' time? The question relates to usability relative to the time available in a clinical setting. The time issue is important to nurses; it is often said that nurses never have enough time! And it cannot be automatically assumed that nurses do not organize their time efficiently; sometimes clients' care needs exceed the staff time available. The length of time required to complete an admission assessment varies greatly. The amount of time required depends partly on the ability of the nurse to zero in on the pertinent data and partly on the client. The more health problems a client has, the more time is needed to identify the underlying dysfunctional patterns. From a moral perspective, the nurse assumes the responsibility of protecting the client from harm ("moral duty") when an assignment is accepted. From the consumer's perspective and because of the high costs they are paying for health care, there must be enough time. If lack of time is a constant theme, staffing patterns and other factors should be changed. Hints on how to increase nurses' efficiency will be offered in other chapters.

2. Should all patterns be assessed or just those that are relevant?

An interesting question. How does one know which patterns are relevant until the assessment is done? It might be said that if you know the medical diagnosis, you know the nursing diagnoses. Many diagnostic manuals list nursing diagnoses that occur with each medical diagnosis. Using these standard listings without careful assessment is risky. Some nursing diagnoses can be predicted, but generally medical diagnoses are not reliable predictors of nursing diagnoses; the person with the disease, not the disease, is the focus of *nursing* assessment.

It is hard to say which functional health patterns are not important to assess when a nurse is "too busy." Value-belief patterns? That sounds abstract, so can it be sacrificed? To do so is risky; it may later be found that all nursing care efforts have been in vain because the client's values or beliefs were ignored. Sexuality-reproductive pattern? In the author's experience, if nurses exclude any of the 11 patterns from an assessment, it is these two. Possible explanations for this behavior are: screening questions are inadequate and nurses are uncomfortable using them, and treatment priority in these areas is low priority, or the interventions are highly specialized and not generally known. Yet none of these reasons is sufficient to justify eliminating screening of these two health patterns.

Is some information needed in all categories? Every client entering the health care system should have a basic functional health assessment; otherwise an administrative problem exists. If assessment is important, then it must be done; if valued, it will be done. Nurses find it difficult to deprive clients of something they (the nurses) feel is needed. When assessments are not done, usually it is because of the value-belief system of the nurse. Yet when other valued activities cannot be carried out, the problem is referred to administration.

The practical response to the time dilemma can be problem screening in each pattern area. For example, a new client might be asked, "Most mornings when you wake up, do you feel rested and ready for the day's activities?" This screening question for the sleep-rest pattern may provide sufficient information to make a judgment about whether or not a problem exists. Six additional questions on sleep patterns are probably not of high priority. Other client health problems, age, or the nurse's observations may provide cues to help the nurse decide when the risk of screening, rather than full health assessment, can be taken. The full assessment can be done later, perhaps along with daily care delivery.

3. When is the full functional assessment appropriate?

Logically a full assessment is appropriate before deliberative nursing care begins, usually at admission to the unit or to a nurse's caseload. No other professionals begin interventions without assessment. Again there are exceptions to the "rule." In emergency situations only certain patterns may be screened for problems; Corrigan[9] (p. 167) describes different levels of assessment in an emergency room setting and presents ideas that may be useful for other short-term contact situations. She also suggests that while nurses are interacting with patients, they begin to "think in pattern areas" and do the documentation at a later time. "Pattern area labels help to recall and then to cluster important information."

A full functional assessment is nationally mandated by law in long-term care (e.g., nursing homes) on admission and periodically thereafter. The rationale for this ruling is that "the provision of high-quality care requires careful assessment,"[10] (p. 294) a rationale applicable to assessment in other nursing settings as well. The National Resident Assessment Instrument[10] is discussed later in the chapter because it is very similar to the data required in a functional health pattern assessment in that it includes all functional health patterns except sexuality.

4. In what settings is a functional assessment useful?

A brief answer is: Wherever nursing care is delivered. In the preceding sections the usefulness of the functional assessment was discussed in regard to developmental and client-environment assessment. The usefulness for individual, family, and community assessment will become clearer later in this chapter. If the central focus of nursing is human functioning, the format is useful in all specialties and settings, such as psychiatric, gerontological, cardiac, and neurological nursing, and with all age groups and all levels of acuity. The patterns are useful when the focus is on health and progress toward higher levels of wellness. In ambulatory-care settings, medical history and examination may be integrated into a functional pattern assessment. In general a functional assessment is useful when care is person-, family-, or community-focused rather than just disease-focused.

5. Do the functional health patterns "take into account" the disease?

Yes. The patterns are a product of person-environment interaction. Listed below are the important factors that are "taken into account" in every assessment:

Age
Developmental level
Gender
Culture

If health patterns are always an expression of the influence of these factors, the factors must always be taken into account.[11] In contrast, a disease or mental disorder is not always present and thus is a different type of influencing factor. When either is present and if a holistic philosophy of care is used, the disease should be taken into account and added to the list above. The next question may be: What is meant by "taking into account?" Briefly, because this will be a subject of considerable discussion later, "taking into account" refers to two activities: collection of information and its interpretation. One component of assessment is examination, during which many physical characteristics are as-

sessed. It is up to the nurse to decide which characteristics need screening and which should be assessed in depth because of the disease or mental disorder.

6. Do functional health patterns facilitate nurses' ethical judgments?

Functional health assessment may provide data useful in making ethical judgments about issues that arise. For example, data from the cognitive-perceptual pattern are useful in determining the need for a substitute decision maker. Clinical data from the health perception–health management pattern may reveal a lack of understanding in decision making, and information from the value-belief pattern may be used in determining, at a later date, the client's wishes about life-sustaining and other treatments. Weiler[12] describes the functional approach that is useful in determining a person's decision-making capacity:

The functional approach centers on a more complex analysis of the patient's ability to interact with the environment and participate in the decision-making process. Four tests have been proposed to determine the patient's functional ability:

1. Evidence of a choice
2. Understanding the relevant issues
3. Manipulating information
4. Appreciating the situation[12 (p. 329)]

Functional health pattern assessment provides clinical data on each of these tests.

Whether the nurse's framework is adaptation, self-care agency, life process, or another model, functional patterns provide the basic data base. Perhaps the greatest argument for their value is that the format is being used in diverse settings and with diverse client populations and age groups in the United States and other countries. This argument also supports the validity of the functional health patterns; they seem to represent realities of assessment in clinical practice.

Specific items that are assessed within each pattern are discussed in the next section. It will become clear that the functional pattern assessment format contains items required by most assessment tools. The format also screens for all current nursing diagnoses. Functional health pattern assessment makes it easy to move from data to diagnosis.

In summary, functional health patterns describe

a set of 11 areas related to health. They have a functional, developmental, and cultural focus that allows their application to all settings, specialties, and age groups. Patterns are configurations of behaviors constructed from client descriptions and nurse observations that have some stability over time. Even with adequate information to describe a pattern, understanding may be elusive until all functional patterns are assessed, because of the interdependent nature of the patterns.

ASSESSMENT OF FUNCTIONAL HEALTH PATTERNS

An initial assessment of a client's functional health patterns is obtained through a nursing history and examination. Let us briefly consider the history and examination so that the question "What to assess?" will be more meaningful. Whenever a client is added to a nurse's caseload, an initial assessment is made of the 11 functional health patterns. This assessment establishes the nursing data base. Initial assessments are referred to as a data base because (1) basic historical and current information about all health patterns is collected, and (2) the information is used as baseline criteria against which any future changes are evaluated.

An admission assessment consists of a nursing history and an examination. The former is done by interviewing the client or others; the latter, by observation and other examination techniques. Generally a comprehensive assessment is necessary. If a client's condition is critical (i.e., if physiological or psychological instability exists), only a very brief assessment of patterns may be warranted. Information collection in the admission nursing history permits a systematic description of the 11 functional health patterns and the client's perception and explanation of any problems. The explanations that clients provide for particular behaviors or situations are important. They can be diagnostic of knowledge deficits and health management deficits, among other things.

In primary care (ambulatory care) settings a functional health pattern assessment and a biomedical systems assessment can be integrated. In these settings the history and examination are designed to (1) detect dysfunctional health patterns *and* diseases (tentative diagnoses of disease are referred to a physician or treated under protocols) and (2)

identify life-style and health promotion be-haviors.

In home care a complete assessment is done when a family is initially visited. Similarly, community nurses responsible for program planning do a community assessment to reveal environmental and other problems influencing the health patterns of groups. For example, in community assessment the history may include the general dietary patterns of an elderly population; hazardous-waste elimination patterns within a geographic area; the community's self-image pattern; and its level of activity as indicated by patterns of participation in work and political or recreational activities. Examination of the community may include observations of people on busy streets or on buses and observations of resources and facilities. (The local barber or bartender is the source of a wealth of community information.) The examination follows the nursing history. Physical characteristics such as gait and mobility, skin integrity, heart rate, and range of joint movement are observed. Cues obtained during history taking provide impressions of the client's speech (its tone, rate, and quality) and, possibly, interactions if another person is present (parent-child or client-other relationship). Assessment in the home provides opportunities to observe living conditions, safety hazards, and the client's neighborhood. At this point, it is useful to review the nursing history and examination that appears in Appendix I. The appendix provides an overview of the "end product." While reading the assessment in each of the 11 pattern areas, notice the type of information collected in each area and the method of recording the admission interview. Underlying the history and examination is a structure for interviewing and observation. Screening questions and observations, planned in advance by the nurse, help the client describe functional patterns and help the nurse do a systematic assessment.

Let us now consider an assessment format for each functional health pattern.[11] Depending on the practice setting, health screening may be limited to only one type of client: individuals, families, or communities. Yet the identification and solution of a specific problem may require further information about a family or community to determine the factors contributing to an individual's problems. Many times in family assessment, dysfunctional patterns of a particular member are detected, which may then require the use of the individual format.

In community assessment it may be necessary to interview a set of selected families if a high-risk group is detected. For these reasons it is important to be familiar with formats for assessing various types of clients.

While reviewing the following assessment formats,[13] note the following:

1. Each pattern is defined. The history (questions) and examination (observations) are derived from the definition.
2. Questions and observations are used for screening. If the information obtained suggests that problems are present (dysfunctional or potentially dysfunctional patterns), further questions and observations will be necessary. The critical defining characteristics of the diagnoses under consideration direct further assessment (see Chapters 7 to 9).
3. Questions in the history format are stated concisely. Individualize the interview by framing the question in your own way and in a way suitable to the particular client and situation.
4. Combine information from the history and examination for all patterns to identify diagnoses and etiological or contributing factors.

1. Health perception–health management pattern

Definition

Describes the client's perceived pattern of health and well-being and how his or her health is managed. Includes the client's perception of his or her health status and its relevance to current activities and future planning. Also included is the general level of health care behavior such as health promotion activities, adherence to mental and physical preventive health practices, medical or nursing prescriptions, and follow-up care.

Discussion

The goal of nursing is to promote health. Yet it is clients who actually perceive and manage their health. Clients' perceptions of their health status and the practices they use to maintain health can be assessed. This information may indicate a dysfunctional pattern or influence decisions about interventions for other problems. Clients may be-

come despondent about changes in their health and believe they have no control over events. They may view "fate" rather than their behavior as the main determinant of health. Teaching health practices in these situations will be to no avail. Perceptions and beliefs must be dealt with first.

The objective in assessing the health perception–health management pattern is to obtain data about clients' general perceptions, general health management, and preventive practices. Specific details are explored in other relevant pattern areas. For example, if a client takes laxatives for constipation, this information is noted. The question that follows may be, "Do you find you can solve most of your health problems yourself?"

In this pattern area, cues to potential health hazards in client practices, clients' potential or actual noncompliance, and their unrealistic perceptions of health or illness should not be overlooked.

Individual assessment

I. History
   A. How has *general* health been?
   B. Any colds in past year? If appropriate: any absences from work?
   C. Most important things you do to keep healthy? Think these things make a difference to health? (Include family folk remedies, if appropriate.) Use of cigarettes, alcohol, drugs? Breast self-examination?
   D. Accidents (home, work, driving)?
   E. In the past, has it been easy to find ways to carry out doctors' or nurses' suggestions?
   F. If appropriate: What do you think caused this illness? What actions did you take when you perceived symptoms? Results of action(s)?
   G. If appropriate: What things are important to you while you're here? How can we be most helpful?

II. Examination
   A. General health appearance.

When asked, each of us can offer a generalization about our health pattern. Sometimes we refer to recent years; for example, "I've really felt good these last few years." Other statements may refer to childhood, such as, "I was a sickly child and ever since. . . ." or, "I never paid much attention to what I did; this illness has really taught me a lesson." The client's health perceptions can be used as a basis for understanding his or her past practices, including preventive measures, and for predicting the client's future motivation in promoting health.

Questions about health perceptions and health management may also elicit descriptions of illness. As the client talks about illness, listen for health perceptions and health management practices. For example, an adult client says, "After about a month of . . . (symptoms), I tried to find a doctor who would see me." Listening would cause the nurse to think, "Delay in seeking help? No established resource for health care? Knowledge of community resources? Routine checkups?" Perceptions, meanings, responses, and practices comprise the nursing data.

Although the client is generally examined after a history, his or her general appearance can be observed during the interview. Observation of an individual's actual health practices is difficult. Usually a nurse must rely on clients' reports unless information is available from home visits or unless a client in a hospital can be given responsibility for certain treatments.

Family assessment

I. History
A. How has the family's general health been (in last few years)?
B. Colds in the past year? Absence from work/school?
C. Most important things you do to keep healthy? Think these make a difference to health? (Include family folk remedies, if appropriate.)
D. Family members' use of cigarettes, alcohol, drugs?
E. Immunizations? Health care provider? Frequency of checkups? Accidents (home, work, school, driving)? If appropriate: storage of drugs and cleaning products, scatter rugs, etc.
F. In the past, has it been easy to find ways to carry out doctors', nurses', social workers' (if appropriate) suggestions?
G. Anything important in family's health that I might help with?
II. Examination
A. General appearance of family members and home.

B. If appropriate: medicine storage, cribs, playpens, stove, scatter rugs, other hazards.

The family's perception of their health as a group is usually expressed in "we" statements such as, "We've always been a healthy family because I see to it that. . . ." Usually one question phrased to obtain the group perception elicits both a perceived health pattern and explanations for the pattern. When individual members' health and health management (as perceived by the family representative speaking) are described, the nurse should cluster data. A generalization about the family must be made if each member's pattern and practices are described specifically. Listen to learn who seems to be the influential member in health-related decisions. This information may be useful if health practices need improving. Problems in the areas of general health management, risk-factor control, use of a health care system, and safety should not be overlooked.

Community assessment

I. History (community representatives)
A. In general, what is the health/wellness level of the population on a scale of 1 to 5, with 5 being the highest level of health/wellness? Any major health problems?
B. Any strong cultural patterns influencing health practices?
C. People feel they have access to health services?
D. Demand for any particular health services or prevention programs?
E. People feel fire, police, safety programs sufficient?
II. Examination: (community records)
A. Morbidity, mortality, disability rates (by age group, if appropriate).
B. Accident rates (by district, if appropriate).
C. Currently operating health facilities (types).
D. Ongoing health promotion-prevention programs (utilization rates).
E. Ratio of health professionals to population.
F. Laws regarding drinking age.
G. Arrest statistics for drugs, drunk driving, by age groups.

Listening to residents of a community, a nurse may hear, "The drug problem here is terrible; this used to be a good community to raise children in"; "We need a stop sign here for the children's crossing"; "They closed the clinic and now we have to go to the city"; or "Everybody's got the flu and it spreads through the schools; I can't remember a worse winter for sickness." Some of these statements provide cues to how people perceive the community's health pattern. Others provide cues about health management in the community. Sampling key groups can usually elicit historical patterns of "then and now" or "we've always been. . . ." The perceived reasons for patterns and practices usually are given without prodding. If a problem is identified by a community group, the first step in health promotion is already accomplished. Other groups may have to be helped to gain insight into problems that exist.

Objective data on the health pattern of a community may be obtained from mortality and morbidity statistics, accident rates, and other data of public record. Assessing the use of health facilities and examining health legislation may also provide cues to a community's management pattern. Even more basic, do such services as home care, school health, and care of the aged exist?

2. Nutritional-metabolic pattern

Definition

Describes patterns of food and fluid consumption relative to metabolic needs and pattern indicators of local nutrient supply. Includes the individual's patterns of food and fluid consumption, daily eating times, types and quantity of food and fluids consumed, particular food preferences, and use of nutrient or vitamin supplements. Reports of any skin lesions and general ability to heal are included. The condition of skin, hair, nails, mucous membranes, and teeth and measurements of body temperature, height, and weight are included.

Discussion

Clients' nutritional patterns and underlying dietary habits have always been of concern to nurses because of nurses' recognition that all life functions and well-being depend on adequate intake and the supply of nutrients to tissues. The focus of assessment in the nutritional-metabolic pattern area is food and fluid consumption relative to metabolic need.

The assessment objective is to collect data about the typical pattern of food and fluid consumption.

Additionally, gross indicators of metabolic need are assessed, such as growth states (child growth, pregnancy, and tissue healing). Subjective reports are obtained regarding food and fluid consumption, problems perceived by the client or others, the client's explanations of problems, actions taken to solve problems, and the perceived effect of those actions. Examination provides data on the observable effects of nutrient intake and supply relative to metabolic need.

Individual assessment

I. History
   A. Typical daily food intake? (Describe.) Supplements (vitamins, type of snacks)?
   B. Typical daily fluid intake? (Describe.)
   C. Weight loss/gain? (Amount.) Height loss/gain? (Amount.)
   D. Appetite? Breastfeeding? Infant feeding?
   E. Food or eating: Discomfort? Swallowing? Diet restrictions? Able to follow?
   F. Heal well or poorly?
   G. Skin problems: lesions, dryness?
   H. Dental problems?

II. Examination
   A. Skin: bony prominences? Lesions? Color changes? Moistness?
   B. Oral mucous membranes: color, moistness, lesions.
   C. Teeth: general appearance and alignment. Dentures? Cavities? Missing teeth?
   D. Actual weight, height?
   E. Temperature.
   F. Intravenous/parenteral feeding (specify).

The assessment of individual clients includes an account of a typical daily intake of food, fluids, and nutrient supplements such as vitamins. Change(s) in nutritional-metabolic patterns may be discovered through interview or observed during examination. Physical examination focuses on the skin, bony prominences, hair, oral mucous membranes, teeth, height and weight relative to age norms, and temperature. Physical indicators may provide validation of client reports regarding nutrient intake, nutrient supply to tissues, or metabolic need.

The assessment of the skin provides important data about the quality of nutrient intake and the supply of nutrients to this tissue. Indicators of nutritional pattern include tissue healing after injuries; skin integrity; and integrity of mucous membranes, hair, and nails. Skin and mucous membranes in particular are highly metabolic organs. Cell duplication is rapid and, accordingly, so is utilization of nutrients. Because of the significant requirements of these tissues, changes can be observed when problems exist in food or fluid consumption. Also, growth and physical development depend on nutrition and metabolism. As a minimum approach, the nurse should screen for patterns indicating nutritional and fluid deficits, excess intake, and skin alterations or breakdown.

Family assessment

I. History
  A. Typical family meal pattern/food intake? (Describe.) Supplements (vitamins, types of snacks, etc.)?
  B. Typical family fluid intake? (Describe.) Supplements: type available: fruit juices, soft drinks, coffee, etc.?
  C. Appetites?
  D. Dental problems? Dental care (frequency)?
  E. Anyone have skin problems? Healing problems?
II. Examination
  A. If opportunity available: check refrigerator contents, meal preparation, contents of meal, etc.

Family or household patterns of food, fluid, and supplement consumption are especially important. Many of our habits, as well as likes and dislikes, are learned in the family setting. The family member who does the shopping and cooking is most important to the assessment (as well as to subsequent intervention); this may be the family member who makes the nutrition-related decisions. Again the aim is to obtain general patterns; if the need arises, a nurse may shift to individual assessment of one or more members.

Community assessment

I. History (community representatives)
  A. In general, do most people seem well nourished? Children? Elderly?
  B. Food supplement programs? Food stamps: rate of use?
  C. Foods reasonably priced in this area relative to income?
  D. Stores accessible to most? "Meals on Wheels" available?
  E. Water supply and quality? Testing services (if most have own wells)? If appropriate: water usage cost? Any drought restrictions?
  F. Any concern that community growth will exceed good water supply?
  G. Heating/cooling costs manageable for most? Programs?
II. Examination
  A. General appearance (nutritional appearance; teeth; clothing appropriate to climate)? Children? Adults? Elderly?
  B. Food purchases (observations of food store check-out counters).
  C. "Junk" food (machines in schools, etc.).

Groups of people living in the same geographic area share common nutritional-metabolic patterns. You have heard comments to substantiate this: "All these people are on food stamps, and you should see what they buy." "Look at the elderly in this place; they're all thin; never enough money for food." "Just sitting in the park you see all the pink-cheeked, healthy babies and kids; you know, our schools have thrown out all those junk food machines." Through interviews, observation of people, and checking community resources, a nurse can obtain an overview of the qualitative and quantitative aspects of a community's pattern of food and fluid consumption.

3. Elimination pattern

Definition

Describes patterns of excretory function (bowel, bladder, and skin) of individuals. Includes the individual's perceived regularity of excretory function, use of routines or laxatives for bowel elimination, and any changes or disturbances in time pattern, mode of excretion, quality, or quantity. Also included are any devices employed to control excretion. Includes family or community waste disposal pattern when appropriate.

Discussion

Regularity and control of elimination patterns are important in most people's lives. Perhaps culturally based toilet training and media commercials about body odor and waste disposal emphasize this functional health pattern. It is an important area about which to assess clients' concerns.

The assessment objective is to collect data about regularity and control of excretory patterns (bowel, bladder, skin, and wastes). Subjective descriptions, problems perceived by the client or others, the client's explanations of problems, remedial actions taken, and the perceived effects of those actions are the data of concern. Examination includes gross screening of specimens, inspection of prostheses (devices such as ostomy bags), noting any odors, and observing family or community patterns of waste disposal.

Individual assessment

I. History
   A. Bowel elimination pattern. (Describe.) Frequency? Character? Discomfort? Problem in control? Laxatives, etc.?
   B. Urinary elimination pattern. (Describe.) Frequency? Problem in control?
   C. Excess perspiration? Odor problems?
   D. Body cavity drainage, suction, etc. (Specify.)
II. Examination
   A. If indicated: Examine excreta or drainage color and consistency.

The individual client's descriptions of regularity, control, quantity, and other characteristics of bowel, bladder, and skin excretory patterns are assessed. If problems are perceived by the client or others, the nurse obtains explanations, learns what remedial actions have been taken, and asks about the perceived effect of the actions.

The excretory pattern indicators (quantity, regularity, etc.) are applicable even if a client cannot use the normal route of excretion; there is still a bowel or urinary elimination pattern.

Laypeople have many misconceptions about regularity and control. Dependency on laxatives or enemas may mean that the client does not understand bowel regulation. The diagnosis Knowledge Deficit should not be overlooked. Waste disposal, as discussed below, is also a component of excretory pattern that may be relevant to individual assessment during a home visit. Minimally, the nurse screens for patterns of incontinence and irregularity. Habits in regard to elimination and data from other pattern areas (nutritional, for example) may explain a dysfunctional pattern.

Family assessment

I. History
   A. Family use of laxatives, other aids?
   B. Problems in waste/garbage disposal?
   C. Pet animals' waste disposal (indoor/outdoor)?
   D. If indicated: Problems with flies, roaches, rodents?
II. Examination
   A. If opportunity available: Examine toilet facilities, garbage disposal, pet waste disposal; indicators of risk for flies, roaches, rodents.

When asking about family excretory patterns, the nurse focuses on waste disposal and related hygienic practices. Thus in a home visit, the nurse may inquire whether garbage disposal is a problem. Observation should include sanitary practices related to waste disposal. These components of the excretory pattern are also pertinent to an individual living alone.

Community assessment

I. History (community representatives)
   A. Major kinds of wastes (industrial, sewage, etc.)? Disposal systems? Recycling programs? Any problems perceived by community?
   B. Pest control? Food-service inspection (restaurants, street vendors, etc.)?
II. Examination
   A. Communicable disease statistics.
   B. Air pollution statistics.

Communities are aggregates of individuals, households, and industries. Each of these social units has an excretory pattern of waste disposal that can influence the community. In recent years much attention has been given to hazardous waste disposal and air pollution. These topics, as well as common sanitation or disposal practices, are included in community assessment. Usually data can be collected from community leaders and from statistics on specific infections, diseases, and radiation or pollution levels.

4. Activity-exercise pattern
Definition

Describes pattern of exercise, activity, leisure, and recreation. Includes activities of daily living requiring energy expenditure, such as hygiene, cooking, shopping, eating, working, and home maintenance. Also included are the type, quantity, and quality of exercise, including sports, which describe the typical pattern. (Factors that interfere with the desired or expected pattern for the individual, such as neuromuscular deficits and compensations, dyspnea, angina, or muscle cramping on exertion, and, if appropriate, cardiac/pulmonary classification, are included.) Leisure patterns are included and describe the recreational activities undertaken with others or alone. The emphasis is on activities of major importance to the client.

Discussion

Movement is one of the most important functional patterns. It permits people to control their immediate physical environment. Assessment of activity patterns can lead to the detection of poor health practices, prevention of major functional losses and may help compensate for such loss. The object of assessment is to determine the client's pattern of activities that require energy expenditure. The components are daily activities, exercise, and leisure activities. Subjective descriptions of these pattern components, problems perceived by the client or others, the client's perceived reasons for any existing problems, actions taken to solve the problems, and perceived effects of those actions are elicited. Observation is an important aspect of assessment in this pattern area.

Individual assessment

I. History
  A. Sufficient energy for desired/required activities?
  B. Exercise pattern? Type? Regularity?
  C. Spare time (leisure) activities? Child: play activities.
  D. Perceived ability (code for level) for:

Feeding ___ Grooming ___
Bathing ___ General mobility ___
Toileting ___ Cooking ___
Bed mobility ___ Home maintenance ___
Dressing ___ Shopping ___

Functional level codes:
Level 0:   Full self-care
Level I: Requires use of equipment or
Level II: Requires assistance or supervision from another person

Level III: Requires assistance from another person (and equipment or device)
Level IV: Is dependent and does not participate

II. Examination
  A. Demonstrated ability (from code listed above) for:
Feeding ___ Dressing ___
Cooking ___ Bathing ___
Grooming ___ Shopping ___
Toileting ___ Bed mobility ___
General mobility ___
Home maintenance ___
  B. Gait ___ Posture ___
     Absent body part? (Specify) ___
  C. Range of motion (joints) ___
     Muscle firmness ___
  D. Hand grip ___ Can pick up a pencil?
  E. Pulse (rate) ___ (rhythm) ___
     (strength) ___
  F. Respirations (rate) ___
     (rhythm) ___ Breath sounds ___
  G. Blood pressure ___
  H. General appearance (grooming, hygiene, energy level)

The nurse must assess the client's routine daily activities. These include the client's perceived capabilities for movement, self-care (feeding, bathing, dressing, grooming, and toileting) and, if relevant, home management. Each can be classified using the functional levels 0 to IV. Classifications also exist for assessing the activity tolerance of clients with cardiac or pulmonary problems.

Irrespective of the client's mobility level, some degree of either active or passive exercise is needed. During assessment the type, amount, and frequency of exercise should be determined. People also need leisure activities. Assessment of the activity-exercise pattern includes the type of recreational activities and the amount of time spent pursuing them.

The screening examination of the client may be limited to gait, posture, muscle tone, absence of a body part, and prostheses or assistive devices employed. If indicated, assessment of the client's range of motion in joints, hand grip, and ability to pick up a pencil provides additional data. Pulse rate and rhythm and respiratory rate and depth may explain the client's subjective reports about activity tolerance.

Minimally, screening assessment should reveal

any actual or potential dysfunctional activity patterns. In particular, deficits in mobility, self-care, home management, and diversional activity should not be overlooked. The client's potential for joint contractures and ineffective airway clearance are also problems within nurses' scope of diagnostic judgment. These two conditions may predispose clients to activity pattern dysfunctions. In general, if a client has a cardiac, neurological, or respiratory disease, in-depth assessment is warranted. Also, developmental problems in children may be revealed by assessment of their specific motor skills.

Family assessment

I. History
   A. In general, does the family get a lot/little exercise? Type? Regularity?
   B. Family leisure activities? Active/passive?
   C. Problems in shopping (transportation), cooking, keeping up the house, budgeting for food, clothes, housekeeping, house costs?
II. Examination
   A. Pattern of general home maintenance and personal maintenance.

Families may exhibit activity patterns. Some households operate at a hectic level; others seem almost lethargic. The pace of activities is a characteristic of family activity; it may or may not be related to the number of family members.

Other than clichés, such as "The family that plays [leisure pattern] together, stays together," little information exists in nursing about family activity patterns. Doing things together and sharing recreational interests appears to increase family solidarity. No diagnoses have been identified in the area of family activity patterns. Problems in home maintenance, general self-care, and exercise or leisure patterns should not be overlooked.

Community assessment

I. History (community representatives)
   A. Do people in the community find transportation convenient? To work? To recreational areas? For health care centers?
   B. People have/use community centers (seniors, others)? Recreation facilities for children? Adults? Seniors?
   C. Is housing adequate (availability, cost)? Public housing?

II. Examination
   A. Recreation/cultural programs.
   B. Aids for the disabled.
   C. Residential centers, nursing homes, and rehabilitation facilities relative to population needs.
   D. External maintenance of homes, yards, apartment houses.
   E. General activity level (e.g., bustling, quiet).

Communities have rhythmic activity patterns. Some "roll up the sidewalks" at 9 PM and other are bustling night and day. In communities, activity may be associated with noise and crowding and may elicit complaints from residents who wish for more peace and quiet. Community activity patterns are also often beneficial, such as scheduled recreation. These resources permit individuals and families to socialize and enjoy leisure. Any community may be described in terms of its diversional activities, both recreational and cultural.

Evidence of generalizations at the community activity level include statements such as "There is nothing to do in this town," or "I'm so busy since I retired, with all the senior citizen activities going on." Because political, recreational, and cultural activities fulfill the lives of people, community assessment should include this pattern area.

Communities also have mobility patterns—public transportation systems. Information about this area is important for understanding the accessibility of facilities for health care, recreation, or socialization.

5. Sleep-rest pattern
Definition

Describes patterns of sleep, rest, and relaxation. Includes patterns of sleep and rest-relaxation periods during the 24-hour day. Includes the perception of the quality and quantity of sleep and rest and the perception of energy level. Also included are aids to sleep such as medications or nighttime routines.

Discussion

Preoccupation with sleep arises only when it eludes us; otherwise it is something taken for granted. In today's busy world, rest and relaxation may also elude a lot of people.

The objective in assessing a sleep-rest pattern is to describe the effectiveness of the pattern from the client's perspective. Some are well rested after

4 hours of sleep; others need much more. Rest and relaxation are also assessed in regard to client perceptions. What may be relaxing to some is considered work by others. If problems are perceived by the client or others, explanations, previous actions taken, and perception of the effect of actions should be assessed.

Individual assessment

I. History
  A. Generally rested and ready for daily activities after sleep?
  B. Sleep onset problems? Aids? Dreams (nightmares)? Early awakening?
  C. Rest-relaxation periods?
II. Examination
  A. If appropriate: Observe sleep pattern.

The nurse screens the client's sleep-rest pattern by finding out about the person's general feeling of readiness for daily activities after sleep. If problems are perceived, the dysfunctional pattern is described. Rest and relaxation comprise a second component to be assessed in this pattern.

If problems are present, assessment should include sleep onset, sleep interruption (including dreams), or early awakening patterns. Sleep pattern reversal (day-night reversal) is another problem that should not be overlooked. Use of sleeping aids, both prescription and nonprescription, should be elicited during pattern assessment. As previously stated, the client's perception of a dysfunctional pattern provides valuable cues. Clients who appear to sleep normally but report sleep deprivation may not be getting sufficient deep sleep.

Family assessment

I. History
  A. Generally, family members seem to be well rested and ready for school/work?
  B. Sufficient sleeping space and quiet?
  C. Family finds time to relax?
II. Examination
  A. If opportunity available: Observe sleeping space and arrangements.

There may be a general pattern of sleep within a family. Some adhere to "early to bed, early to rise." Rest and relaxation patterns also are frequently built into family patterns, which can be assessed. Sometimes the family pattern is disturbed because of one member's sleep problem. This situation may require a shift to individual assessment.

Community assessment

I. History (community representatives)
  A. Generally quiet at night in most neighborhoods?
  B. Usual business hours? "Round-the-clock" industries?
II. Examination
  A. Activity-noise levels in business district; in residential district.

Communities usually have patterns of sleeping, resting, and relaxation. Some towns are described as "never shut down." Disturbances in the community sleep-rest pattern may be inferred from residents' comments about continuous highway noise or airplanes going over all night. Such disturbances produce health concerns and may increase levels of stress.

6. Cognitive-perceptual pattern

Definition

Describes sensory-perceptual and cognitive pattern. Includes the adequacy of sensory modes, such as vision, hearing, taste, touch, or smell, and the compensation or protheses used to deal with disturbances. Reports of pain perception and how pain is managed are also included when appropriate. Cognitive functional abilities, such as language, memory, judgment, and decision making are described.

Discussion

Thinking, hearing, seeing, smelling, tasting, and touching are human functions taken for granted until deficits arise. Preventing deficits and helping clients to compensate for losses are important nursing activities.

The objective of assessing the client's cognitive-perceptual pattern is to describe the adequacy of his or her language, cognitive skills, and perception relative to desired or required activities. Subjective descriptions, problems perceived by the client or others, compensations for deficits, and the effectiveness of efforts to compensate for them are elicited during the history.

During the examination, cognitive and sensory capabilities are observed. Data in this pattern area are critical for future nursing intervention. For example, if a client's judgment capabilities are inadequate, that client may need supervision. If the person is blind, safety may be a problem.

Individual assessment

I. History
  A. Hearing difficulty? Hearing aid?
  B. Vision? Wears glasses? Last checked? When last changed?
  C. Any change in memory concentration?
  D. Important decisions easy/difficult to make?
  E. Easiest way for you to learn things? Any difficulty?
  F. Any discomfort? Pain? If appropriate: How do you manage it?
II. Examination
  A. Orientation
  B. Hears whisper?
  C. Reads newsprint?
  D. Grasps ideas and questions (abstract, concrete)?
  E. Language spoken.
  F. Vocabulary level. Attention span.

Cognitive and perceptual pattern components are assessed. Cognitive functions include language capability, memory, problem solving, and decision making. These are basic functions but should be evaluated relative to the complexity of the environment chosen by the client. A mentally retarded person may function quite independently in a sheltered environment. An active business executive in the same type of environment may exhibit symptoms of sensory or cognitive deprivation.

Cognitive patterns are examined during the history. The nurse observes the client's language skills, grasp of ideas and abstractions, attention span, level of consciousness, reality testing, and any aids required for communication. Some problem the client describes during assessment may be selected to measure problem solving and decision making. In fact, in each pattern area the client's perception of problems, reasons for problems, actions taken, and perceived effectiveness of actions provide a wealth of information about cognitive functions.

The subjective report of the client regarding patterns of vision, hearing, touch, taste, and smell may be supplemented by actual testing. For example, keep some newsprint in your pocket and use it to screen the client for visual difficulties. Don't forget to assess prostheses such as glasses or hearing aids.

The ability to feel pain or discomfort is another sensory capability of human beings. If pain is present, especially chronic pain, ask the client how he or she manages it. The answer may reveal deficits in pain management that require intervention. Nurses have many ways of helping people deal with pain.

In assessing cognitive functions and sensory modes, be alert to compensating actions or behaviors clients may use that mask basic dysfunctions. The safety of the client may be jeopardized if such problems are not detected. Remember that at times we all have memory lapses, make illogical statements, and fail to recognize a familiar object or person. It may be necessary to elicit impressions from family members to differentiate between common, temporary lapses and progressive deficits.

Cues to sensory deficits, sensory deprivation or overload, and pain management problems must not be overlooked. Impaired reasoning, knowledge deficits related to health practices, and memory deficits are additional problems that may exist and may even be the basis for other dysfunctional patterns. If problems are perceived by the client or others, explanations of previous actions taken to relieve the problem and perceptions of the effect of these actions should be elicited.

Family assessment

I. History
  A. Visual or hearing problems? How managed?
  B. Any important decisions family has had to make? How made?
II. Examination
  A. If indicated: Language spoken at home.
  B. Grasp of ideas and questions (abstract/concrete).
  C. Vocabulary level.

The cognitive-perceptual pattern of a family becomes evident by seeing how family decisions are made, by the concreteness or abstractness of thinking, and by whether decisions are oriented to the future or present. Data in these areas may be the basis for understanding other problems, such as family disorganization and stress. Nurses have a number of ways of helping families in the cognitive-perceptual area of health functioning.

Community assessment

I. History (community representatives)
   A. Most groups speak English? Bilingual?
   B. Educational level of population?
   C. Schools seen as good/need improving? Adult education desired/available?
   D. Types of problems that require community decisions? Decision-making process? What is the best way to get things done/changed in the community?
II. Examination
   A. School facilities. Drop-out rate.
   B. Community government structure; decision-making lines.

A nurse can obtain data on decision making while assessing a community, especially regarding health-related matters. Are the school board and parent-teacher association effective? How are community decisions made? Sitting in on meetings of committees dealing with health issues usually provides a wealth of information. Do all groups participate, and are their voices heard regarding health matters? Is future planning done, or are crisis reactions the pattern? These questions can elicit data about the cognitive processes operating in a community.

7. Self-perception–self-concept pattern

Definition

Describes self-concept pattern and perceptions of self. Includes attitudes about self, perception of abilities (cognitive, affective, or physical), image, identity, general sense of worth, and general emotional pattern. Pattern of body posture and movement, eye contact, and voice and speech patterns are included.

Discussion

Many psychologists have tried to describe the consciousness of being, or awareness of existence, that all humans have. This sense of being is commonly referred to as the self. Clients have perceptions and concepts of themselves, such as body image, social self, self-competency, and subjective mood states. Negative evaluations of the self can produce personal discomfort and also can influence other functional patterns. Change, loss, and threat are common factors that may impinge on self-concept.

The objective of assessment in this pattern area is to describe the client's pattern of beliefs and evaluations regarding general self-worth and feeling states. Problems the clients or others identify, explanations or reasons they give for the problem, actions taken to try to solve the problems, and effects of those actions are also described.

Assessment of self-concept and self-perception usually is not effective (accurate and thorough) unless the client has a sense of trust in the nurse. People tend not to share personal feelings unless the nurse has already established an empathic and nonjudgmental atmosphere. As Powell reminds us, "But, if I tell you who I am, you may not like who I am, and it is all that I have."[14] (p. 12)

Individual assessment

I. History
   A. How do you describe yourself? Most of the time, feel good (not so good) about self?
   B. Changes in body or things you can do? Problem for you?
   C. Changes in way you feel about self or body (since illness started).
   D. Things frequently make you angry? Annoyed? Fearful? Anxious? Depressed? Not being able to control things? What helps?
   E. Ever feel you lose hope?
II. Examination
   A. Eye contact. Attention span (distraction).
   B. Voice and speech patterns. Body posture.
   C. Client nervous (5) or relaxed (1); rate from 1 to 5.
   D. Client assertive (5) or passive (1); rate from 1 to 5.

A person's self-perception–self-concept pattern may be screened by obtaining data about (1) general feelings of self-worth and personal identity and (2) general emotional pattern. If cues or situations warrant it, more in-depth assessment can be done.

Observation during an admission interview can reveal nonverbal cues about self-concept and self-perception. It is important to observe body posture and movement, eye contact, and voice and speech patterns. Cues to identity confusion, altered body image, lowered self-esteem, perceptions of powerlessness, situational depression, and fear should not be overlooked.

Family assessment

I. History
  A. Most of the time the family feels good (not so good) about themselves as a family?
  B. General mood of family? Happy? Anxious? Depressed? What helps family mood?
II. Examination
  A. General mood state: nervous (5) or relaxed (1); rate from 1 to 5.
  B. Members generally assertive (5) or passive (1); rate from 1 to 5.

Families have perceptions and concepts about their image, their status in the community, and their competency as a unit to deal with life. Emotional patterns tend to be shared because of the close relationships in a family or household. Situations that affect one member usually produce an effect on the entire family group. To help a family realize its potential, the nurse needs to assess how family members perceive their family.

Community assessment

I. History (community representatives)
  A. Good community to live in? Going up in status, down, about the same?
  B. Old community? Fairly new?
  C. Any age group predominant?
  D. People's moods in general: Enjoying life? Stressed? Feeling "down"?
  E. People generally have the kind of abilities needed in this community?
  F. Community/neighborhood functions? Parades?
II. Examination
  A. Racial, ethnic mix (if appropriate).
  B. Socioeconomic level.
  C. General observations of mood.

Just as families and individuals have patterns of self-worth and personal identity, so do communities. Image, status, and perceived competency to deal with problems are characteristics that can be assessed.

The image of a community may be reflected in its housing conditions, buildings, and cleanliness. Community perception of self-worth may relate to school systems, crime rates, accidents, and whether residents and outsiders consider it "a good place to live." Competency in dealing with social and political issues and community spirit cause self-evaluation to be positive. Knowing the level of community "pride" may assist a nurse in innovative health programs. The emotional tone (fear, depression, or a generally positive outlook) can usually be related to findings in other pattern areas. For example, tensions in the community relationship pattern may explain a general feeling of fear in the residents.

8. Role-relationship pattern

Definition

Describes pattern of role engagements and relationships. Includes perception of the major roles and responsibilities in client's current life situation. Satisfaction or disturbances in family, work, or social relationships and responsibilities related to these roles are included.

Discussion

Much has been written about relationships, including the human need for others and the influence of relationships on personal and group development. People engage in many levels of relationships. Some are very close, such as family relationships. Others are superficial and without any true sharing, as described in the lyrics of "The Sounds of Silence" by Paul Simon:

> And in the naked night I saw
> Ten thousand people, maybe more,
> People talking without speaking,
> People hearing without listening,
> People writing songs that voices never shared.
> No one dared
> Disturb the sounds of silence.*

The objective of role-relationship pattern assessment is to describe a client's pattern of family and social roles. The client's perception about his or her relationship patterns (satisfactions and dissatisfactions) is also a component of this pattern area. If problems are perceived by the client, the perceived cause, actions taken, and effects of these actions are elicited.

---

*© 1964, 1965 by Paul Simon. Used by permission.

Individual assessment

I. History
   A. Live alone? Family? Family structure (diagram)?
   B. Any family problems you have difficulty handling (nuclear/extended)?
   C. Family or others depend on you for things? How well are you managing?
   D. If appropriate: How family/others feel about your illness/hospitalization?
   E. If appropriate: Problems with children? Difficulty in handling them?
   F. Belong to social groups? Close friends? Feel lonely (frequency)?
   G. Things generally go well at work? School?
   H. If appropriate: Income sufficient for needs?
   I. Feel part of (or isolated in) neighborhood where you are living?

II. Examination
   A. Interaction with family member(s) or others (if present).

The major role-taking and relationship patterns in a person's life situation are the components of the role-relationship pattern. Family roles, work or student roles, and social roles are some of the major aspects assessed. Clients' satisfactions and dissatisfactions with role responsibilities and relationships are elicited. If the client perceives problems in this pattern area, assess the perceived reasons for the problems, actions that have been taken to remedy the problems, and effects of those actions.

Family roles are usually particularly important in the individual's life. Discussion with a client in this area discloses how many are in the family group or household, including both children and adults, and whether there is a nuclear or extended family. Roles and relationships are usually reviewed before the sexuality-reproductive pattern. This sequence permits a natural transition in the discussion.

Loss, change, and threat produce the major problems in the role-relationship pattern. The cues that should not be missed are related to problems such as grieving, conflict, social isolation, impaired verbal communication, and potential for violence.

Working roles and relationships are an important area to assess. Statistics indicate that many people (nurses included) suffer occupational role stress.[15] Assessment should include whether the client perceives the work environment to be safe and healthy. Does the work role leave time for rest and leisure? Because work has the potential to contribute to self-fulfillment, the client's satisfaction with work roles and the organization of work activities is assessed. Financial concerns, unemployment, and other issues related to work are identified. Assessment of the school-aged client or college student should elicit any problems related to the roles and relationships in these settings.

Family assessment

I. History
   A. Family (or household) members? Ages of members and family structure (diagram).
   B. Any family problems that are difficult to handle (nuclear/extended)? Child rearing?
   C. Relationships good (not so good) among family members? Siblings? Support each other?
   D. If appropriate: Income sufficient for needs?
   E. Feel part (or isolated) from community? Neighbors?

II. Examination
   A. Interaction among family members (if present).
   B. Observed family leadership roles.

Roles and relationships of a particularly close kind are a fundamental aspect of family life. Relationships can be supportive and growth-producing. At the opposite extreme, violence and abuse can permeate relationships of families under stress.

As with individual assessment, structural aspects of the family are assessed. These include living space, number of members, their ages, and their various roles.

There are a number of ways the dynamics of family relationships can be assessed. One is in terms of interdependence, dependence, and independence. Another approach is based on the ways relationships influence the family's developmental tasks. Family developmental tasks, according to Duvall,[16] include (1) physical maintenance; (2) resource allocation; (3) division of labor; (4) socialization of members; (5) reproduction, recruitment, and release of members; (6) maintenance of order; and (7) maintenance of motivation and morale.

Community assessment

I. History (community representatives)
   A. People seem to get along well together here? Places where people tend to go to socialize?
   B. Do people feel they are heard by government? High/low participation at meetings?
   C. Enough work/jobs for everybody? Wages good/fair? Do people seem to like the kind of work available (happy in their jobs/job stress)?
   D. Any problems with riots, violence in the neighborhoods? Family violence? Problems with child/spouse/elder abuse?
   E. Get along with adjacent communities? Collaborate on any community projects?
   F. Do neighbors seem to support each other?
   G. Community get-togethers?
II. Examination
   A. Observation of interactions (generally or at specific meetings).
   B. Statistics on interpersonal violence.
   C. Statistics on employment, income/poverty.
   D. Divorce rate.

The basic function of a community lies in its collaborative relationships and allocation of role responsibilities. Nursing assessment is particularly concerned with whether a community structure of roles and relationships permits residents to realize their health-related potentialities. Patterns of crime, racial incidents, and social networks are indexes of human relationships in a community.

9. Sexuality-reproductive pattern

Definition

Describes patterns of satisfaction or dissatisfaction with sexuality; describes reproductive pattern. Includes the perceived satisfaction or disturbances in sexuality or sexual relationships. Included also is the female's reproductive state, premenopause or postmenopause, and any perceived problems.

Discussion

Sexuality is the behavioral expression of sexual identity. It may involve, but is not limited to, sexual relationships with a partner. Just as in other functional patterns, cultural norms regulate its expression.

Currently in Western society the norms for sexuality are in a state of flux. The distinction between what is masculine and what is feminine is sometimes blurred, and the scope of acceptable sexual expression is widening within some groups. Yet society still imposes limits. Sexual abuse of children and incest are not tolerated. When clients choose modes of expression that are marginally acceptable, problems may arise. Individual problems may also arise when discrepancies exist between the expression of sexuality the person has attained and the expression he or she desires.

Reproductive patterns involve reproductive capacity and reproduction itself. The cultural norms that affect reproduction are also undergoing change. The number of children in families is smaller than in past generations, and in many cases pregnancies and births are planned.

The objective of assessment in the sexuality-reproductive pattern is to describe perceived problems or potential problems. If problems exist the client is asked about contributing factors, actions taken, and the perceived effect of these actions.

Individual assessment

I. History
   A. If appropriate to age and situation: Sexual relationships satisfying? Changes? Problems?
   B. If appropriate: Use of contraceptives? Problems?
   C. Female: When did menstruation start? Last menstrual period? Menstrual problems? Para? Gravida?
II. Examination
   A. None unless a problem is identified or a pelvic examination is part of full physical assessment.

Screening assessment of a client's expression of sexuality is focused on developmental patterns and perceived satisfactions or dissatisfactions. If problems are perceived, the nurse obtains the client's explanation of the problem, a history of any remedial action taken, and the client's opinion about the effectiveness of those actions. It is important not to miss problems related to the expression of sexuality in clients of any age.

Assessment of reproductive patterns involves collecting information about the client's stage of reproductive development in relationship to developmental milestones such as menarche or climacteric. The number of pregnancies and live births provides information about a female client's reproductive pattern. The development of reproductive capacities (secondary sex characteristics and genital development) should be assessed in young clients. It is important not to miss problems associated with contraceptives, reproduction, menstruation, or climacteric.

Family assessment

I. History
  A. If appropriate (sexual partner is in household or part of the situation): Sexual relations satisfying? Changes? Problems?
  B. Use of family planning? Contraceptives? Problems?
  C. If appropriate (to the age of the children): Feel comfortable in explaining/discussing sexual subjects?
II. Examination: None

The information collected in the assessment of a family's sexuality pattern includes a couple's level of satisfaction with their sexual relationship, any problems they perceive, how the problems are managed, and the results of actions taken to resolve the problems. When there are children in the household, the nurse should be interested in what information about sexual subjects is taught to the children as well as when and how this information is communicated. If the adults feel uninformed or uncomfortable in discussing sexual subjects with children, the nurse who is aware of the problem can provide important assistance. Although previously considered a very personal matter, sexual relationships and feelings related to sexual identity are now more openly discussed. This trend toward freer discussion may not affect all clients; thus the nurse should obtain information in a sensitive manner.

The reproductive pattern assessment includes any problems the couple perceives, the explanations they offer for the problems, the actions they have taken to deal with the problems, and the result of the actions. The number and ages of children, number and outcomes of pregnancies, and birth control methods being used are included in the family data base.

Community assessment

I. History (community representatives)
  A. Average family size?
  B. Do people feel there are any problems with pornography or prostitution? Other?
  C. Do people want/support sex education in schools/community?
II. Examination
  A. Family size and types of households.
  B. Male/female ratio.
  C. Average maternal age. Maternal mortality rate. Infant mortality rate.
  D. Teen pregnancy rate.
  E. Abortion rate.
  F. Sexual violence statistics.
  G. Laws/regulations regarding information on birth control.

Community attitudes toward sexuality are assessed. Do educational programs exist in schools or churches? Does the community desire such programs? If the residents view sex education as a function of the family, are there programs for parents?

Crime in general was assessed in the area of relationships. In the sexuality-reproductive pattern it is useful to note the incidence of sex-related crime or sexual abuse of children in the community. A high incidence of either or both may indicate the need for increased community awareness and action.

The reproductive pattern of a community is reflected in birth, miscarriage, and abortion rates. Maternal and fetal mortality rates are also very important indicators. The accessibility of health services as well as the availability of childbirth education programs should be assessed. Access to family planning and abortion services is assessed in terms of the community's desire for such services. In areas with high rates of adolescent pregnancies, the availability of programs for continued schooling is assessed.

Compiling such information enables the nurse to evaluate community needs and available services. Problems are identified when needs and health services do not match. The sexuality-reproductive pattern of individuals, families, and communities may be viewed as a component of the role-relationship pattern. It is listed separately so that sexual and reproductive assessment are not neglected. An additional reason for separating the two is that sexuality and reproduction involve a different level of relationships than those established in social or work groups. The assessment interview should flow smoothly from self-concept pattern to relationships with others and then on to sexual relationships.

10. Coping–stress-tolerance pattern

Definition

Describes general coping pattern and effectiveness of the pattern in terms of stress tolerance. Includes the reserve or capacity to resist challenges to self-integrity, modes of handling stress, family or other support systems, and perceived ability to control and manage situations.

Discussion

Stress is a part of living for any person at any age. In fact, many say that without stress there would be no growth. For example, learning to walk places stress on bones, a necessary factor for their integrity and development. Separating from the security of home also produces stress but leads to social development.

Stressor, coping, and *stress tolerance* are three terms whose definitions are intertwined. A stressor is an event that threatens or challenges the integrity of the human being. It produces a psychophysiological response that can lead to growth and further development or to disorganization manifested as anxiety, fear, depression, and other negative changes in self-perception or roles and relationships.

People respond to events differently. To know if a particular event is stressful for a person, family, or community, the nurse should ascertain the client's perception or definition of the situation. Community disasters, loss of a family member, illness, and hospitalization are usually perceived as threats to the integrity or the usual pattern of life activities; thus these are stressors. The meaning of potentially stressful events to the client and the perceived degree of control over the events influence the amount of stress induced.

The way in which people generally respond to events perceived as a threat is their coping pattern. Clients' general patterns of coping may or may not be effective in handling stressful situations. Some clients employ problem-solving techniques; others respond with denial or other mental mechanisms.

All these are learned behaviors for dealing with stress. The more effective the coping pattern, the greater the sense of control the client can exert over the threat to integrity.

The stress-tolerance pattern describes the level of stress the client has handled effectively. This, of course, is related to the amount of stress previously experienced and the effectiveness of the client's coping patterns. A client's stress-tolerance pattern predicts, to some extent, the potential for effective coping; however, people can mobilize resources and withstand levels of stress that exceed their previous experience.

The objective of assessment in this pattern area is to describe the stress-tolerance and coping pattern of a client. Not to be overlooked are changes in the effectiveness of a coping pattern, which can occur if a threat to integrity is perceived as beyond personal control (personal coping capacity). This type of situation should lead the nurse to make a more in-depth assessment of the support systems available to the client.

Individual assessment

I. History
- A. Any big changes in your life in the last year or two? Crisis?
- B. Who is most helpful in talking things over? Available to you now?
- C. Tense or relaxed most of the time? When tense, what helps?
- D. Use any medicines, drugs, alcohol to relax?
- E. When (if) there are big problems (any problems) in your life, how do you handle them?
- F. Most of the time, is this (are these) way(s) successful?

II. Examination: None

The nurse asks the client to recall stressful life events, briefly tell how they were managed, and evaluate the effectiveness with which he or she coped with those situations. This history provides information about the stress-tolerance and coping pattern.

Data from other pattern areas may indicate that the client perceives a current or anticipated threat to his or her integrity. If such a threat is perceived, assessment proceeds to an examination of perceived control; that is, the nurse inquires how the client plans to deal with the situation and has the client evaluate the likelihood that the proposed coping pattern will be effective.

Why the emphasis on the individual's perception of events? As Selye[17] says, "It is not what happens to you, but the way you take it [that matters]." The surgical mortality rate may be less than 1 percent, a low probability of death, yet if the client perceives that the threat of death is high, surgery will be a stressor. Clients' personal concepts, constructed from the knowledge they have, determine their reactions. In a sense it is irrelevant what the reality is; reality "is" whatever the client perceives. This explains why subjective data are so important. Intervention begins with the way the client views the situation.

Family assessment

I. History
  A. Any big changes within family in last few years?
  B. Family tense or relaxed most of time? When tense what helps? Anyone use medicines, drugs, alcohol to decrease tension?
  C. When (if) family problems, how handled?
  D. Most of the time is this way(s) successful?
II. Examination: None

The dimensions of family assessment in this pattern area are similar to those in individual assessment. It is well to remember that family life revolves around a set of interrelationships. These relationships can be the supportive structure of a coping pattern but can also be a source of stress.

Community assessment

I. History (community representatives)
  A. Any groups that seem to be under stress?
  B. Need/availability of phone help-lines? Support groups (health related, other)?
II. Examination
  A. Delinquency, drug abuse, alcoholism, suicide, psychiatric illness, statistics.
  B. Unemployment rate by race/ethnicity/sex.

Stressors are sometimes experienced by a whole community. These are usually revealed in the data of previous pattern areas and may include such problems as unemployment, racial or ethnic tensions, drug problems, and accident rates. Natural disasters may threaten community integrity and require outside support for coping patterns.

A pattern of coping with community-wide stressors is usually revealed by interviews with community members. Leaders are quick to evaluate the effectiveness of community coping and "what works in our town." A community's stress tolerance depends on supportive relationships between community groups.

11. Value-belief pattern
Definition

Describes patterns of values, goals, or beliefs (including spiritual) that guide choices or decisions. Includes what is perceived as important in life and any perceived conflicts in values, beliefs, or expectations that are health related.

Discussion

A pattern of valuing and believing is found in people of all ages. As people develop, the emerging pattern of values and beliefs becomes more complex and, generally, more conscious. Beliefs and values include opinions about what is correct, proper, meaningful, and good, in a personal sense. Collective value and belief patterns also exist within a society or culture. These group norms may or may not be consistent with the personal pattern of a particular client or health care provider. Conflicts may arise. When important alternatives present themselves, values help determine choices. Choices deal with what is right or wrong for the person. *Right* and *wrong* relate to action; *good* and *bad* refer to outcomes or goals.[18]

Belief patterns describe what people hold to be true on the basis of faith or conviction. They are arrived at by inference and form the basis for attitudes or predispositions. Beliefs are the philosophical and theological dimensions of personal knowing. They include explanations at a very abstract level, including explanations of life, existence, and why certain things are valued. Common day-to-day actions may not require this level of thought and explanation. Illness and other significant events provide the time and motivation to review life, goals, and what is important.

Patterns of valuing describe the importance or worth accorded to goals, actions, people, objects, and other phenomena. The client's value pattern can influence his or her health-related decisions about personal practices, treatments, health priorities, and even life or death.

The objective in assessing clients' value-belief patterns is to understand the basis for health-related decisions and actions. This understanding increases sensitivity to value-belief conflicts that may arise if preventive action is not taken.

Individual assessment

I. History
   A. Generally get things you want from life? Important plans for the future?
   B. Religion important in life? If appropriate: Does this help when difficulties arise?
   C. If appropriate: Will being here interfere with any religious practices?
II. Examination: None

Life requires making decisions. Thus, as human beings develop they construct a system of beliefs and values—in fact, a philosophical system. This system provides guidelines for making important decisions and for ways of behaving. It may or may not be tied to theological and religious beliefs and values.

The assessment of value-belief patterns focuses on what is important to clients in their lives. Beliefs and values may be regarded as spiritual in the broadest sense of "human spirit." Nurses usually assess more specific areas, such as religious preference or religious practices. This broader view of "what is important" includes, but is not limited to, religious practices.

Understanding a client's personal value-belief pattern can increase the nurse's sensitivity to potential conflicts and help clients examine how their belief system can assist them in decision making. Clients' use of philosophical or theological values and beliefs as a predominant coping strategy has not been systematically studied in nursing. The nurse who understands the client's spiritual beliefs (including, but not limited to, religious beliefs) may be able to support coping strategies of this type.

Family assessment

I. History
   A. Generally, family members get things they want out of life?
   B. Important plans/goals/hopes for the future?
   C. Any "rules" in the family that all members believe are important?
   D. Religion important in the family? Does this help when difficulties arise?

II. Examination: None

Families have value-belief patterns. Some say sharing values and beliefs is one of the important characteristics of a successful marriage. Dissimilar value-belief patterns within a marital or family relationship usually produce conflicts in other pattern areas, such as role-relationships. Conflicts also arise when family members, such as teenagers, are in the process of developing a conscious awareness of values and beliefs. Because of the potential for family disorganization, value-belief pattern conflicts should not be overlooked during assessment.

Community assessment

I. History (community representatives)
   A. Community values: What seem to be the four most important things to people living here (note health-related values, priorities)?
   B. Do people tend to get involved in causes/local fund-raising campaigns (note if any are health related)?
   C. Religious groups in community? Churches available?
   D. Do people tend to tolerate/not tolerate differences/socially deviant behavior?
II. Examination
   A. Zoning conservation laws.
   B. Scan community government health committee reports (goals, priorities).
   C. Health budget relative to total budget.

Communities have values and beliefs, including health-related values; understanding these values and beliefs is critical in diagnosing conflicts when working with community groups. Value patterns underlie decisions about where tax money should be spent and whether or not the community should have an abortion clinic, sex education in the schools, senior citizen centers, and special education for the handicapped. These and many other community issues that affect health ultimately rest on the predominant value-belief pattern of a community.

Other concerns (individual, family, community)

In individual, family, or community assessment it is important that the nurse ask the client about other concerns when concluding the admission interview. There may be areas not previously discussed that the client wishes to mention or has questions about specific things. Further information may be elicited by asking the client the following:

1. Any things we haven't talked about that you'd like to mention?
2. Any questions?

The functional health pattern format guides the collection of a basic data base. If verbal responses to questions (history) or the nurse's observations (examination) signify a dysfunctional or potentially dysfunctional pattern, *it is necessary to collect further information to identify the problem:* The nurse should assess behaviors that are characteristic of the diagnoses being considered. As the client's problem becomes clear, assessment is guided by the *conceptual framework* of the nurse. Having considered each pattern, the reader may wish to refer to the composite of assessment items in Appendix H before considering special cases of functional assessment.

ADAPTING THE ASSESSMENT FORMAT
Infant and child assessment

The functional health pattern format for assessment requires adaptation of questions to and observations of infants, children, and early adolescents. Also, their patterns must be judged according to developmental norms. For example, nocturnal bed-wetting is expected in an infant but not in older children. Items assessed during a nursing history and examination reflect developmental considerations. Examples of questions and observations for infancy and early childhood are found in Appendix H. A nursing history is obtained from (1) a parent (or guardian) or (2) the child *and* a parent or guardian. As their communication skills develop, it is important to include children's viewpoints. Adolescents usually can provide information for individual assessment (see format in previous section).

A further consideration in infant, child, and early adolescent assessment is the influence of the environment on development. In particular, parents and the family's functional patterns greatly influence child development. These patterns should be briefly assessed using previously discussed formats for adult assessment. If problems are present, a further assessment of environmental factors is necessary (home, school, etc.).

Assessment of the critically ill

Clients who are critically ill, such as those with severe respiratory, cardiac, neurological, or psychological instability, are unable to respond to a full functional health pattern assessment. It is also not appropriate to obtain a full history in a recovery room, operating room, or emergency room. (Some clients come to an emergency room with a nonemergency problem; nursing judgment dictates the extent of assessment that is needed prior to clinic referral or discharge to home.)[9]

During the critical phase of an illness, the major objectives of nursing and medical care are to stabilize physiological or psychological processes and to prevent further complications, injury, and emotional distress. *Examination and observation are the major data collection methods used during the critical phase of an illness when the client does not have the energy, capacity, or attention span to provide a health history.* Family or close friends, if present, can supply historical information that may be appropriate to critical care. (When the client is transferred from intensive care nursing, a full assessment should be completed.)

Upon the client's admission to an intensive care unit, assessment should include screening for high-incidence nursing diagnoses and pathophysiological or psychiatric (in psychiatric intensive care) cues related to the disease and its complications. Anticipation of family responses to the crisis and attention to cues are also necessary. Any of the following conditions, which are listed under the appropriate functional health patterns, may be present during the critical phase of care; thus it is important that the nurse be sensitive to cues to these conditions. A full listing is in Appendix H.

Health perception–health management pattern

1. High Risk for Infection: Risk factors should be assessed frequently, especially in clients with depressed immunological systems, trauma, general debilitation, or surgical incisions.
2. High Risk for Physical Injury or Suffocation: Risk factors for this condition should be assessed if the client is confused or disoriented. Any client who demonstrates the capacity and intention to get out of bed or remove

tubes and equipment should also be evaluated for these diagnoses. It is especially important to evaluate the risk of suffocation in an infant or child.

Nutritional-metabolic pattern

1. High Risk for Altered Nutrition: Less than Body Requirements; Fluid Volume Deficit: This condition may occur in psychiatric intensive care. Even in medical-surgical intensive care, prevention of these problems may not be integrated into the treatment of the medical problem.
2. High Risk for Pressure Ulcer: This risk factor should be of prime concern in clients immobilized by equipment (including casts or traction) or restraint and in those who are on bed rest. Attention to this risk factor will prevent decubitus or other pressure ulcers.

Elimination pattern

1. High Risk for Constipation (leading to impaction): Daily observations are required to prevent this condition, especially when clients spend a number of days in intensive care. Certain drugs used in psychiatric intensive care may predispose clients to this problem.

Activity-exercise pattern

1. High Risk for Activity Intolerance: Most clients receiving intensive care manifest activity intolerance; assessment is directed toward those who have risk factors for low tolerance but are beginning to assume some independent self-care.
2. Total Self-Care Deficit (Levels III to IV): While a client is experiencing severe physiological or psychological instability and immobility, assessment is directed toward the client's capacity to participate in some aspects of self-care (except, of course, in the case of children who have not attained these skills). Depending on staffing and reimbursement procedures, this diagnosis may be recorded for every client in intensive care or, because all have this problem, it may be *understood* that nursing time is spent in compensating for Self-Care Deficits and recording the diagnosis is not required.
3. High Risk for Joint Contractures: These risk factors are usually present in clients who are immobilized for more than two days.
4. Ineffective Airway Clearance: This is a common condition that should be assessed especially in clients with illnesses affecting the respiratory system or who are comatose or semicomatose.

Sleep-rest pattern

1. Sleep-Pattern Disturbance: Sleep-wake cycles should be assessed in all clients in critical care units. Sleep-onset disturbances and sleep-pattern interruption are two conditions that occur frequently.

Cognitive-perceptual pattern

1. Pain: This is a diagnosis nearly always present in critical care.
2. Uncompensated Sensory Deficit (Specify): Assessment of vision and hearing disturbances is essential. These conditions can precipitate anxiety or cognitive disturbances in clients in critical care units.
3. Sensory Deprivation or Overload; High Risk for Cognitive Impairment: Verbal reports of or cues to hallucinatory experiences or nightmares should be assessed.
4. Decisional Conflict: Assessment for cues to this condition is important when clients or families are faced with certain treatment decisions.

Self-perception–self-concept pattern

1. Fear (Specify); Anxiety: Cues to these conditions should not be overlooked in clients or families. Fear (death) is common during the crisis phase of an illness.
2. Powerlessness: Clients who are conscious but have minimal control of their body and treatment decisions often feel powerless.
3. Self-Esteem Disturbance: If a client is conscious, disturbances in self-esteem or body image may be noted, especially following extensive, disfiguring surgery, trauma, burns, or debilitating medical illnesses.

Role-relationship pattern

1. Anticipatory Grieving: Perception of the future consequences of an illness may cause clients to grieve as soon as they begin to regain consciousness after an injury, surgery, or a disease.

2. Unresolved Independence-Dependence Conflict: As the crisis of an illness begins to resolve, clients may manifest cues to conflict over dependency either verbally or by independent activities that are contrary to the treatment regimen.
3. Altered Family Processes: Guilt, anxiety, or role disturbances that are associated with a client's illness may be manifested in family conflict or disorganization.
4. Weak Parent-Infant Attachment: Cues to this condition should not be overlooked in neonatal intensive care units, where parents and infants are separated for long periods of time.
5. Impaired Communication: This condition should not be overlooked, since it may be the etiology of anxiety, fear, or powerlessness.

Coping–stress-tolerance pattern

1. Avoidance Coping: Psychological abandonment of a dying client may be a cue to ineffective family coping strategies. However, Avoidance Coping can be beneficial during a crisis and should not be diagnosed as a condition requiring treatment; denial in the early stages of a crisis may be used by either clients or families to provide the time necessary to integrate the event.

Value-belief pattern

1. Spiritual Distress: Distress over the ideas of suffering or death may be manifested by some clients during the crisis period of an illness.

The conditions above are a sample of the health problems amenable to nursing intervention during the intensive care phase of a life-threatening illness. Altered Cardiac Output, Impaired Gas Exchange, Altered Tissue Perfusion, Excess Fluid Volume, and many other disease-related conditions may also be present. These conditions are treated collaboratively by physicians and nurses. During a physiological crisis, the physician has primary responsibility for their treatment plans. Implementation of the medical plan, 24-hour observation, and reporting are collaborative areas of nursing practice that require a high level of clinical judgment. These collaborative activities are combined with nursing diagnosis–based care during the crisis phase of an illness.

SUMMARY

The purpose of this chapter has been to present a structural format for assessment of clients who are considered healthy or have various diseases or types of mental illness. The usefulness of this assessment format extends through all phases of the health-illness continuum and all settings where nursing is practiced. Its usefulness in practice supports its broad applicability to human beings of any age.

The assessment categories are not new to nurses; however, the format's major contribution is the organization of assessment data for purposes of identifying nursing diagnoses. The categories also provide a useful format for nurses wishing to switch from a purely medical model to a nursing model for practice. Diseases influence functional patterns; therefore, it is logical that the assessment of pathophysiological processes should be incorporated into the examination phase of assessment. What physiological processes should be assessed? That depends on the disturbances anticipated from knowledge of the disease. What developmental processes should be assessed? That depends on the client's developmental phase. What cultural patterns should be assessed? Clearly, culture influences all functional patterns; assessment data should be evaluated in the cultural, developmental, and illness context of the client situation, and further data should be collected when needed.

This chapter focused on the description and use of functional health pattern assessment in clinical situations. Assessment items, or parameters, were presented that can be used to assess individuals, families, or communities. How extensive should the assessment be when a new client is added to a nurse's caseload? The answer has two parts:

1. The nurse must decide the extent of personal resources (time) that can be allocated to the client. This decision must be balanced against the amount of risk that can be tolerated. The risk involves missing diagnoses or a misdiagnosis because of insufficient information and the possibility that the client may suffer discomfort, distress, or harm. In many instances, when the professional staffing of units is low, the decision becomes a moral dilemma and even a legal (malpractice) concern for nurses.
2. Consideration of the client situation helps

determine the extent of the assessment on admission. Clients having surgery or delivering a baby in the next several hours or the next day may not be able to focus their attention on topics they perceive to be unrelated to the impending experience. Critically ill clients may have neither the energy nor the level of consciousness to provide a history. Obviously, "rules" regarding the extent of an admission assessment cannot be set; nurses must use their professional judgment for each particular situation.

Having considered what information is useful to collect when screening for nursing diagnoses, we next move to an overview of current diagnoses, or dysfunctional patterns. The functional health pattern assessment format is designed to screen for these diagnoses. The information from Chapters 4 and 5 will then be used in examining the process of diagnosis: information collection, interpretation, and clustering and giving a name to the client's health problem or potential problem.

NOTES AND REFERENCES

1. The various uses of functional health patterns are reflected in the "Annotated Bibliography" at the end of the book. Comments on organizing literature or conference papers can be found in Rossi L: Organizing data for nursing diagnoses using functional health patterns. In McLane A, editor: *Classification of nursing diagnoses: proceedings of the seventh conference,* St Louis, 1987, Mosby.
2. McCain F: Nursing by assessment—not intuition, *Am J Nurs* 65:82, 1965.
3. Smith D: A clinical nursing tool, *Am J Nurs* 68:2384, 1968.
4. U.S. Department of Health and Human Services: *Healthy people 2000: national health promotion and disease prevention objectives*, Washington, DC, 1992, U.S. Government Printing Office.
5. American Academy of Nursing Expert Panel: Culturally competent health care, *Nurs Outlook* 40:277, 1992.
6. Geissler E: Nursing diagnoses: a study of cultural relevance, *J Prof Nurs* 8:301, 1992. Further work on the three diagnoses studied is necessary, since the cultural additions are limited by the lack of a definition of the culturally based related factors, nonmeasurable defining characteristics, and terms, such as *unacceptable behavior,* used to describe a reason for a problem.
7. Leininger M: Leininger's brief rejoinder to Feild's response, *J Transcult Nurs* 3:29, 1991.
8. Eisenberg L, Kleinman A, editors: *The relevance of the social sciences for medicine*, New York, 1980, Reidel.
9. Corrigan J: Functional health pattern assessment in the emergency department, *J Emerg Nurs* 12:163, 1986.
10. Morris J et al: Designing the National Resident Assessment Instrument for nursing homes, *Gerontologist* 30:293, 1990.
11. Examination of hundreds of functional health pattern assessments suggests that health patterns are *always* an expression of the influence of age/development, gender, and culture. Logical analysis supports this conclusion if it is assumed that patterns are a product of person-environment interaction. This assumption has not been systematically studied.
12. Weiler K: Functional assessment in the determination of the need for a substitute decision maker, *J Prof Nurs* 7:328, 1991.
13. Community assessment items are adapted from Gikow F, Kacharski P: *Functional health pattern assessment of a community*. Paper presented at the 112th annual meeting of the American Public Health Association, Anaheim, Calif, November 13, 1984. The association used the assessment to evaluate the health-related needs of a community served by its agencies.
14. Powell J: *Why am I afraid to tell you who I am?* Chicago, 1969, Argus Communication, p 12.
15. McLean A, editor: *Reducing occupational stress: proceedings of a conference*, Westchester Division, New York Hospital–Cornell Medical Center, White Plains, NY, May 10-12, 1977.
16. Duvall E: *Family development*, Philadelphia, 1967, Lippincott.
17. Selye H: Stress without distress. In Garfield CA, editor: *Stress and survival*, St Louis, 1979, Mosby.
18. Steele S, Harmon V: *Values clarification in nursing*, New York, 1979, Appleton-Century-Crofts, pp 1-4.

CHAPTER 6

DYSFUNCTIONAL HEALTH PATTERNS

H ealth patterns can be functional, dysfunctional, or potentially dysfunctional. As discussed in Chapter 4, when health patterns are functional, they signify health and wellness, provide a basis for continued development of human potentialities, and are strengths to be recognized and mobilized in dealing with health problems. In contrast, dysfunctional or potentially dysfunctional health patterns do not meet expected norms and are defined as *health problems.*

A dysfunctional pattern generates therapeutic concern on the part of the nurse, client, family, friends, or community. In other words, the situation is viewed as a problem requiring therapeutic measures. Diagnostic categories are currently being developed to describe these health problems (Appendix B). To be clear about the terms in current use, it should be kept in mind that two types of health problems are described by diagnostic categories:

1. Actual health problems, which describe dysfunctional health patterns
2. High-risk health problems, which describe the high risk for a dysfunctional health pattern

Therapeutic concern is a term used by Taylor[1] to refer to a client's desire to receive treatment or a professional's desire to provide it.

RECOGNIZING HEALTH PATTERNS

The distinction among the types of health patterns seen in nursing practice is important, because each type of health problem requires a different kind of nursing intervention. Interventions for functional patterns that describe health, wellness, or optimal level of functioning are intended to encourage clients in their healthy life-style and their growth to higher levels of wellness. Treatment for dysfunctional patterns (actual problems) is directed toward factors that contribute to or maintain the problem, whereas for potentially dysfunctional patterns (high risk), the objective is to prevent the problem by reducing the risk factors.

Functional patterns

A functional pattern is different from an expected norm. Norms are developmental, social-cultural, and personal baseline values. The first two norms are learned in the study of the sciences, arts, and humanities; the last is learned by nursing assessment. A biological range of values specifies the "normal" heart rate response to activity; the person's age group norm is taken into account.[2] In every culture, parenting processes that are deemed by that culture to provide a safe, nurturing environment and enhance growth *and* the parents' values constitute a "standard" for recognizing a healthy parenting pattern. In the United States, people were shocked by a news report of a couple who left their two children (both under 12 years old) at home unsupervised while they went off on vacation for a week. This behavior was viewed as "culturally unacceptable" by the public; it had violated norms.

Functional patterns imply health; thus it is important to consider a definition of health. The definition should be consistent with the conceptual framework being used. Kim[3] captures the functional view in summarizing Naegel's[4] comments:

Health as a state allows one to do what one wants to do and to be what one wants to be. . . . A moral good that is desired by all. . . . [A] person is able to participate in the affairs of the world and the affairs of self with the freedom of the individual. . . . Autonomy is the basic functional requirement for an individual's freedom of pursuit. . . .[3 (p. 60)]

In contrast to functional patterns, dysfunctional patterns and illness limit the autonomy of the individual, family, and community. Individual freedom is valued in American culture, but it may not be a dominant value in other cultures that emphasize the individual's responsibility to the group. Personal baseline values need to be applied in conjunction with culture or population norms in judging patterns. Indeed only a tentative judgment about a pattern is made until it is viewed in the context of the full pattern assessment. For example, food and fluid intake may meet the female adult norms but may not be normal for a particular woman. Why? The woman is pregnant (sexuality-reproductive pattern)!

Dysfunctional patterns

A *dysfunctional pattern,* or actual problem, describes a set of behaviors that do not meet norms or the client's healthy, personal baseline and that negatively influence overall functioning. Patterns may change or development may be delayed; either may lead to the following three types of dysfunctional patterns observed in clinical practice:

Change from a functional to a dysfunctional pattern

Is the change unhealthy for the whole client situation? Is it an acute or recent change?

Stabilized dysfunctional pattern

Is there a long-term history of a dysfunctional pattern? A chronic change over time?

Stabilized dysfunctional developmental pattern

Is the development (of child, adult, elder) delayed or interrupted?

The first pattern may come to the nurse's attention when a change from the client's functional baseline occurs. An example of a recent change in a client's activity pattern might be:

Reports he has had to "slow down in the last month." Cleaning his apartment used to be easy but now causes shortness of breath and greater fatigue. "Cleaning is too much for me since my heart can't be improved."

The judgment that change has occurred is based on historical data, "used to be easy," and current data, "now causes shortness of breath and fatigue." Compare the historical and current data of the client's state to determine change. Consider norms and the client situation as a whole to judge whether the change is functional or dysfunctional.

In the second type of health problem, the stabilized dysfunctional pattern, no recent change has occurred, but the pattern is unhealthy for the client's developmental level. Historical and current data may provide support for this diagnostic judgment, as the following example shows:

A geriatric clinical specialist found that her clients, elderly residents of an inner city housing complex, were restricting their outdoor activities. Many confined themselves to the buildings they lived in, except for arranged bus trips, because of a high incidence of violent crime in their neighborhood.

Although the activity-exercise pattern of these elderly clients was adaptive in the particular environment, it was judged dysfunctional. The judgment of a chronic dysfunctional pattern is made by comparing historical and current data with developmental norms.

When assessing patterns of functional development, the third type of dysfunctional pattern, the stabilized, dysfunctional development pattern, or chronic developmental lag, should also be considered. A number of theories and milestones (norms) of development may be used in evaluation. Underdeveloped potential may exist in individuals, families, and even in communities or regions of the world. Nurses are concerned when underdevelopment results from or leads to health problems:

A child already in school had not yet developed self-care abilities consistent with his age, such as tying his shoe laces or dressing independently. His parents did not want him to "strain" himself because they feared his asthma might get worse. Some of the other children referred to him as a "baby"; gradually and silently he became sullen and withdrew from play activities in the neighborhood and in school.

The diagnosis of a dysfunctional developmental pattern is based on a comparison of developmental norms with current developmental achievements, capabilities, and potentials. In the situation described above, the child's developmental lag might be caused by his parents' fear and misunderstanding of activity tolerance; the social isolation is secondary. The problem is described as a developmental delay to distinguish it from the loss of an ability, which may occur in an adult. A useful and concise way of stating this idea in the problem/etiology format would be: Developmental Delay: Self-Care Skills Related to Parental Misunderstanding (Activity Tolerance). This diagnosis would be a subcategory of Altered Growth and Development.

The purpose of discussing the various types of dysfunctional patterns is not to make diagnosis more complex; rather it is to provide some concrete guidelines. When clients describe their patterns (what is eaten, how they cope with stress, perceptions of their health state, and so forth), data should be obtained to evaluate whether change has occurred in a pattern area, when it occurred, and if the change has led to higher levels of functioning or overall dysfunctioning.

Relationships among dysfunctional patterns

There are usually relationships among the health problems identified by the nurse and patient during assessment. Of particular interest for nursing intervention are causal relationships, which provide answers for the following questions:

Why does the problem exist?

What factors have contributed to the development of the problem?

What factors are maintaining the problem?

The answers to these questions are critical. They will direct nursing care designed to help the person reduce or remove the probable cause. Background nursing knowledge and experience can suggest theoretical links among problems. For example, if Self-Care Deficit and Activity Intolerance have been identified in the assessment, they can be linked theoretically and the linkage supported: activity intolerance is an inability to tolerate large-muscle, energy-consuming tasks. Self-care includes bathing and dressing, which are energy-consuming tasks. It is logical and demonstrable that activity intolerance may be a reason for self-care deficit; thus it is a probable cause.

Factors that are probable causes of a health problem and that contribute to or maintain the problem are called *etiological* or *related factors*. When they can be identified, they are the focus of nursing intervention. In practice settings, the reasons for a problem may be referred to as "the etiology." This expression should not necessarily convey that only one factor is involved; many factors influence the client situation. However, nurses may select, from among multiple contributing factors the most probable etiological or related factor that can be influenced by nursing intervention at a particular time. Explanations of why a problem exists are based on assessment data and theory stored in memory. Let us now consider how the functional health patterns format can be used to identify these factors.

Functional health patterns are interdependent and interactive. Human beings function as a whole within their environment, and behavior is a product of the person-situation complex. Thus explanations, reasons, or probable causes of a health problem usually lie in one or more functional health patterns. For example, a dysfunctional sleep-rest pattern, such as delayed sleep onset, may be primarily caused by a dysfunctional self-perception–self-concept pattern, that is, fear of surgical anesthesia. In addition, assessment of one client may reveal that his or her anxiety is related to sleep deprivation, whereas another client's assessment may reveal that sleep deprivation is related to anxiety. In the problem/etiology format the etiology represents the focus for nursing care activities. The formulation of problems from assessment data is discussed in Chapter 9. To summarize:

1. Look for probable causes of a health problem (etiological or related factors) within the 11 pattern areas. Appendix B may be helpful in regard to terms.

2. Assessment data and clinical reasoning determine the problem/etiological or related factors in particular situations. There need not be "prepackaged," or "fixed," problem/etiology sets, although sufficient research may suggest the probability of relationships.
3. Clinical reasoning is based on theoretical knowledge and experience that suggests probable linkages between problems.
4. Use diagnostic category labels (Appendix B) to describe either a problem or etiological factors.
5. Etiological or related factors focus nursing interventions.

Potentially dysfunctional patterns

Since modern nursing began, health promotion and preventive intervention have been an integral part of clinical practice. Thus the identification of potentially dysfunctional patterns (potential problems) is as important as diagnosing patterns of dysfunction. As with actual problems, potential problems may arise in the absence of a medical disease or appear in conjunction with disease, surgery, or treatment. A potential problem or high-risk nursing diagnosis describes a set of risk factors for a dysfunctional pattern. The focus of nursing intervention for potential problems is risk-factor reduction. During assessment, be aware of two types of potential problems:

High risk for change from a functional to a dysfunctional pattern

Diagnoses in this area describe a high risk for change toward a less functional pattern, indicating that risk factors are present in the client's behavior, the situation, or both. Risk factors predispose to an actual problem; for example: High Risk for Fluid Volume Deficit or High Risk for Health Management Deficit (Medication Regimen).

High risk for a dysfunctional pattern of growth and development

Diagnoses in this area describe a high risk for problems related to the biopsychosocial growth of an individual or family. When entering a new phase of human development, a child, adult, or family may not have the developmental background or situational resources for continued personal growth and development; for example: High Risk for Developmental Delay (Social Skills) or High Risk for Family Conflict (Child-Rearing Practices).

For a client to be susceptible to (or at risk for) a health problem, risk factors must be present. Usually the historical or current data include a combination of signs in one or more patterns. For example, if an elderly woman at home (1) has a fever, (2) has no energy to reach to her bedside table for a pitcher of water between meals, and (3) it is summertime with the temperature hovering around 90° for several days, she will be at high risk for fluid volume deficit if no intervention is undertaken to change any of the three risk factors.

High Risk for Injury is another example of a risk state. Of hospital admissions for burns 40% are due to scalding from excessively hot water in showers or bathtubs; 56% of fatal residential fires are cigarette-related, many due to smoking in bed, according to the U.S. Surgeon General's report. Having this information, the nurse doing an assessment should evaluate risk factors in highly susceptible people.

An example of a potential problem secondary to disease and its treatment is High Risk for Noncompliance. Multiple prescriptions and other factors increase the risk that a client may not follow the treatment regimen even when the desire and intention to do so were initially present.

The diagnosis of potential problems is limited to those individuals who have a greater number of risk factors than the population as a whole. For example, everyone is at risk for injury while crossing a city street, slicing vegetables in the kitchen, or shaving. Most clients are not at any greater risk than the rest of the so-called normal population carrying on everyday activities. But persons in particular subpopulations who have sensory-perceptual problems, a mobility deficit, or a tendency to bleed may be at substantial risk while performing these everyday activities.

A comparison of two groups in a population of clients on a surgical service will clarify this idea. For example, a person who is of normal body weight, does not smoke, has no chronic lung disease, and has been reasonably active physically is going to have surgery to remove his gallbladder. Compare this person to another scheduled for the same operation who smokes heavily, has chronic bronchitis, is 60 pounds overweight, and has relatively poor muscle tone because of a sedentary activity pattern. Which client is at risk for postoperative atelectasis? Stated differently, which client should have intensive nursing treatment to prevent this pulmonary complication after surgery? Clearly the second client is at high risk for atelectasis. (The risk increases if, postoperatively, because of incisional pain, neither of these clients carries out deep breathing and coughing exercises.)

This comparison illustrates the idea of a population at risk. The first person is representative of the normal population who undergo a cholecystectomy (gallbladder removal). The second client facing this surgery represents a different population whose characteristics of heavy smoking, chronic bronchitis, and weak muscle tone greatly predispose them to atelectasis after upper abdominal surgery.

As discussed in the preceding section, when a problem is present, the question of the probable cause of the problem is addressed. However, such a question does not apply here. High-risk states do not have "probable causes" in the same sense. The reason for the risk state is determined when risk factors are identified. All that is needed to formulate a potential problem is a cluster of risk factors and the diagnostic label to describe them. Specifying causal factors would require restating the risk factors that are already specified as signs of the high-risk state. Also, how can there be a probable cause for something that is potential but does not yet exist? In diagnosing a high-risk state, the historical and current data in one or more functional patterns must be considered.

In conclusion, it may be said that from a nursing perspective a problem is a dysfunctional health pattern. A problem represents a dysfunctional change in a pattern or an unhealthful pattern that has stabilized. Developmental problems exist when development is stabilized at a dysfunctional level relative to the client's potential. A risk state indicates the presence of factors that predispose a client to a dysfunctional health pattern. High Risk for Impaired Skin Integrity, High Risk for Altered Parenting, and High Risk for Noncompliance are diagnoses that describe dysfunctional nutritional-metabolic, role-relationship, and health perception–health management patterns, respectively. A potential state is a predicted state, not an actual state with an actual cause; thus the etiology

is not specified and intervention is directed toward reducing risk factors.

DIAGNOSTIC CATEGORIES

In the previous section dysfunctional and potentially dysfunctional health patterns were defined and some examples of diagnostic category labels were given. Now let us briefly review some diagnostic concepts and their category labels as developed by nurses in the United States and Canada. Initially, diagnostic categories are learned in the same manner as the concepts and category labels that describe the signs and symptoms of medical conditions, such as hemorrhagic shock, congestive heart failure, or tetralogy of Fallot. This review provides an introduction only; the in-depth study of these diagnoses continues throughout a nurse's professional career.

Most concepts and their category labels currently identified by the North American Nursing Diagnosis Association (NANDA) are in an early stage of development (see Chapter 11). Their evolution into scientific concepts within nursing science rests with the practitioners, theorists, and researchers who are working toward validating the phenomena and improving the precision of diagnostic categories. Continued development is a characteristic of any classification system. Not too long ago "dropsy" was an accepted medical diagnosis, diabetes was a single entity, and acquired immune deficiency syndrome (AIDS) was not labeled.

Further research is needed to determine if the defining characteristics of the currently identified categories are valid descriptions of the realities encountered in practice. In addition, studies of the incidence of nursing diagnoses in particular age, sex, cultural, or medical disease populations are needed.

We will now consider the current categories listed in Appendix B.

Health perception–health management pattern

Twelve conditions have been grouped under this pattern, which in a sense is an "umbrella pattern." It describes general health management and usually elicits a perception of health or illness during assessment as well as major concerns. The other

10 functional patterns may be viewed as specific areas of health management.

Health perception–health management patterns are influential in moving individuals, families, and communities toward their optimal level of human functioning. Two dimensions of this pattern interact to produce health management practices: the way clients perceive their general health and their health goals. Person-environment factors that place a client at risk for infection, injury, and other conditions are grouped in this pattern area. One category describes health-seeking behaviors. Six actual problems and five high-risk conditions have been identified in this pattern area:

Health-Seeking Behaviors (Specify)
*Health Management Deficit (Total)
*Health Management Deficit (Specify)
Ineffective Management of Therapeutic Regimen
Altered Health Maintenance
Altered Protection
Noncompliance (Specify)
*High Risk for Noncompliance (Specify)
High Risk for Infection
High Risk for Injury (Trauma)
High Risk for Poisoning
High Risk for Suffocation

The diagnoses in this pattern area may be used as a basis for designing nursing interventions to improve clients' health promotion and health management practices. Health-Seeking Behaviors is a term used to describe the behavior of clients in stable health who actively seek out ways to move toward a higher level of health.

There is little difference between the definitions of Health Management Deficit and Altered Health Maintenance. Generally it is assumed that an altered health maintenance results from poor health management; thus management practices should be of primary concern in diagnosis. The characteristics of Altered Health Maintenance overlap with those of Knowledge Deficit, Impaired Adjustment, and Health-Seeking Behaviors. The diagnosis of Altered Health Maintenance should not be used indiscriminately to label all patients with a disease, a practice sometimes reflected in charts.

---

*Not currently on NANDA-approved list.

Diagnoses with the word *altered* in the title are usually not clinically useful for planning intervention. They are too abstract and include many conditions that may require different interventions. It would be the equivalent of entering *neurological disease* on the record as the patient's diagnosis; both terms are too general to direct treatment. Broad categories (such as Altered Parenting, Impaired Skin Integrity, Sleep Pattern Disturbance) are useful in a classification system but not helpful in practice.[5] The "alterations" and "disturbances" that remain unspecified are probably the clinically useful diagnoses.

The term *Specify* in Health Management Deficit and Noncompliance indicates that the diagnostician should cite particular management areas, such as medication or exercise regimen, dietary prescription, follow-up care, or health-promoting practices. If a client is unable to assume responsibility for any health management practices, Total Health Management Deficit would be used. The term *health* in this category label may include the inability to manage a disease regimen that may be observed; for example: High Risk for Health Management Deficit (Diabetes) or Health Management Deficit (Diabetes) in a community setting. Generally the actual problem is not observed in a hospital or nursing home, where there is higher control over regimens.

The term Ineffective Management of Therapeutic Regimen refers to the management of illness and its sequelae to meet health goals. This diagnosis and the diagnosis of Noncompliance have been criticized. Noncompliance particularly is a diagnosis that has received a lot of attention in the literature. Some view this category label as value-laden and believe it does not address the real problem or reflect mutual decision making between the client and nurse.[6] Definitions of this term vary. If an author views Noncompliance as the failure to carry out doctors' or nurses' orders, it is judged to be a negative label.[7] Those who define Noncompliance as nonadherence after informed decision and expressed intention[8] or as nonadherence associated with adverse effects[9] see the term as a point of departure for determining why the client is noncompliant. Regardless of how Noncompliance and Ineffective Management are defined, there is a culturally embedded definition: does not follow the care provider's orders. The use of the term Health

Management Deficit (Specify) may be a clearer way of expressing the problem. The reasons the client is unable to handle health or disease management are stated as factors contributing to the problem. The term High Risk for Health Management Deficit (or for Noncompliance) is used when data indicate risk factors are present but the client has had no opportunity to implement the recommendations (e.g., a hospitalized person).

High Risk for Infection, Injury, Poisoning, and Suffocation are categories that describe risk factors for specific areas of health management. Only clients who are at high risk should be diagnosed, since all human beings have some risk for these problems. It should also be noted that clients may be at risk for infection in a general sense or for infection in a particular body part or system. It is more precise and gives a clearer base for preventive treatment if this distinction is specified. A study and analysis of critical care nurses' ratings of defining characteristics of High Risk for Infection[10] revealed four diagnoses embedded in this category:

High Risk for Urinary Tract Infection
High Risk for Respiratory Infection
High Risk for Skin Infection
High Risk for Postpartum Infection

All shared the general risk factors for infection but each had particular defining characteristics. Clinical testing would determine if this level of specificity is important for directing intervention.

The same type of specification might add precision to High Risk for Injury. For example, High Risk for Slips and Falls appears to be an important diagnosis in some settings. Caution should be exercised to ensure that sufficient data are present to support a judgment of high risk, and other professionals should be informed of the high-risk state so that their treatment plans take it into consideration.

Developmental Health Management Deficit (Specify) may be useful in describing a condition in which a child does not have the ability to assume the responsibility for health promotion, disease prevention, or disease management that he or she is expected to have at a particular developmental level. This delay may be related to a lack of opportunities for learning. High Risk for Infection, Injury, and Suffocation are useful diagnoses for describing conditions encountered in pediatric as well as adult health care.

Altered Protection refers to the decreased ability to guard against internal or external threats such as illness or injury. The condition is inferred from defining characteristics, such as altered clotting, impaired healing, or neurosensory alterations. As are other "altered" states, it is a very general category.

Nutritional-metabolic pattern

Twenty-one diagnostic categories have been identified in the nutritional-metabolic pattern area. Diagnoses describing dysfunctional nutritional patterns are biopsychosocial conditions related to nutrient intake and supply. Nutrients are necessary for cellular metabolic processes, such as energy production and the synthesis of substances used in cellular function, growth, and repair. Four diagnoses describe conditions related to breastfeeding and infant feeding. Seven diagnoses describe dysfunctional food and fluid patterns, three describe possible reasons for the patterns, four describe local metabolic problems in nutrient supply to the skin, and four describe metabolic problems in body temperature regulation.

Nutritional patterns are influenced by (1) maturation; (2) family, social, and cultural patterns; (3) learned psychological associations between food and basic needs; and (4) environmental availability of foods. For example, as growth and maturation proceed, the type of foods ingested, the method of ingestion, and the social-psychological milieu of eating change. Bottles and high chairs are replaced by family silverware and social dining. Biopsychosocial factors (including cultural and spiritual factors) may lead to dysfunctional patterns, such as exogenous obesity and nutritional deficits.

Consider first the set of categories describing food and fluid patterns. (The terms in brackets in the lists in Appendix B are more concise labels, in the opinion of this author, than these NANDA-approved diagnostic labels.)

Altered Nutrition: More Than
  Body Requirements
Altered Nutrition: Less Than
  Body Requirements
Altered Nutrition:
  High Risk for More Than
  Body Requirements

Fluid Volume Deficit

Fluid Volume Excess

High Risk for Fluid Volume Deficit

Nutritional Deficit and Obesity are more concise names for the nutritional diagnoses specifying more, less, and the potential for more than body requirements. Unless a total nutritional deficiency is present, the nutrients that are deficient should be specified so that intervention and teaching can be focused. For example, less than the daily requirement for protein intake would be labeled Nutritional Deficit (Protein Intake). High Risk for Fluid Volume Deficit usually responds to nursing treatment at early levels. Significant Fluid Volume Deficit or Excess Fluid Volume usually requires medical treatment.

Effective Breastfeeding, Ineffective Breastfeeding, and Interrupted Breastfeeding are three types of breastfeeding concerns within the nutritional-metabolic pattern. Ineffective Infant Feeding Pattern is grouped as a category in this pattern rather than with Self-Feeding Deficit.

Effective Breastfeeding

Ineffective Breastfeeding

Interrupted Breastfeeding

Ineffective Infant Feeding Pattern

This grouping of diagnoses includes one "health" diagnosis (Effective Breastfeeding); that is, the condition is not a problem. Some maintain this is an outcome or goal. Others suggest that effective breastfeeding requires periodic observation and support to maintain the behavior. Three additional diagnoses in this pattern area are listed below:

Impaired Swallowing

High Risk for Aspiration

Altered Oral Mucous Membrane

The latter two categories are useful in describing possible reasons (etiologies) for nutritional deficits, such as Nutritional Deficit Related to Uncompensated Swallowing Impairment. Inserting the word *uncompensated* makes the intervention focus clear; the client is taught how to compensate. These two diagnoses are also risk factors for a nutritional or fluid intake deficit. Avoid using a medical diagnosis, such as cerebrovascular accident (stroke), as an etiological factor contributing to a swallowing impairment. Also avoid, for example, using Altered Oral Mucous Membrane (problem) Related to Stomatitis (etiology), because stomati-

tis is a type of alteration, not a reason for the alteration. It would be clearer to name the specific oral membrane condition that is amenable to nursing intervention and delete the word *altered,* in the broad classification category. The conditions listed below pertain to the highly metabolic organ, the skin, or to metabolism:

High Risk for Impaired Skin Integrity	Hyperthermia
Impaired Skin Integrity	Hypothermia
Impaired Tissue Integrity	Ineffective Thermoregulation
*Pressure Ulcer (Specify Stage)	High Risk for Altered Body Temperature

The accepted diagnoses Impaired Skin Integrity, Impaired Tissue Integrity, and High Risk for Impaired Skin Integrity are very general; they include too many conditions to be useful as a focus for definitive nursing intervention. Impairments may range from a surgical incision to blisters. The treatment plan is unclear when a surgical incision is labeled "Impaired Skin Integrity"; if the concern is to prevent infection and if the client is at high risk, use High Risk for Wound Infection. High Risk for Skin Breakdown and Pressure Ulcer (Specify Stage) describe specific skin impairments and are added to increase clarity and precision. When using Pressure Ulcer to describe observations, consult a manual[8] or articles on the stages of ulceration to make the diagnosis precise. Also note that certain stages of ulceration require surgical treatment, so that the problem is temporarily referred to a physician. The diagnosis Impaired Tissue Integrity is extremely broad; it is defined as damaged or destroyed tissue such as cornea, mucous membrane, integumentary (skin), or subcutaneous. Thus the diagnoses discussed above, as well as Altered Oral Mucous Membrane, are included. In treatment planning it is more useful to specify the area of damage for conditions that can be resolved by nursing actions.

High Risk for Altered Body Temperature describes risk factors for hypothermia, hyperthermia, or ineffective thermoregulation. When this diagnostic category is used, the type of alteration

---

*Not currently on NANDA-approved list.

should be specified before interventions can be determined. High Risk for Hyperthermia, High Risk for Hypothermia, or High Risk for Ineffective Thermoregulation are more useful categories. The actual conditions of hyperthermia, hypothermia, and ineffective thermoregulation may or may not respond to nursing treatment. If nursing can provide only palliative care, or if there is any question about the reason for these conditions, they should be referred for medical diagnosis and treatment.

Altered Growth and Development is a NANDA nursing diagnosis that may be used to classify specific dysfunctional developmental patterns, such as developmental delays. Development is an inherent characteristic of functional patterns; thus developmental delays may occur in any pattern area. As will be seen in other pattern areas, three common types of delay have been added. In this pattern, growth delays may result from inadequate nutrition. Diagnoses might be developed to describe the conditions that can be resolved through nursing action. Metabolic (endocrine) problems manifested in delayed growth are referred to a physician.

Elimination pattern

The 12 diagnostic categories within this pattern area describe bowel and urinary elimination patterns. No high-risk conditions have been identified. We will consider bowel elimination first:

    Intermittent Constipation Pattern
    Colonic Constipation
    Perceived Constipation
    Diarrhea
    Bowel Incontinence

Each of the conditions listed in the bowel elimination pattern is within the scope of nursing practice, but the diagnostician should be cautious: constipation, diarrhea, or incontinence may be a symptom of a disease that requires medical treatment. For example, an intermittent constipation pattern usually is due to inadequate roughage and fluids in the diet and poor bowel routines but may also be a symptom of cancer of the bowel.

The set related to urinary elimination contains the broad category Altered Urinary Elimination Pattern and six specific types of alterations: Retention and five types of incontinence, each of

which has a specific definition. Precise assessment is necessary to differentiate among the types of incontinence, and specific interventions are required to assist the client in managing each problem.

    Altered Urinary Elimination Patterns
    Urinary Retention
    Functional Incontinence
    Reflex Incontinence
    Stress Incontinence
    Urge Incontinence
    Total Incontinence

Developmental delay may occur in any functional pattern area. In this pattern the NANDA-approved nursing diagnosis Altered Growth and Development may provide a focus for clinical identification of specific diagnostic categories to describe, for example, delays in the development of bowel and bladder control. Etiological or related factors that can be resolved by nursing should also be identified. In addition, pediatric nurses are concerned with providing anticipatory guidance to prevent dysfunctional patterns; they need to describe and classify the high-risk states encountered in their clinical practice.

Activity-exercise pattern

The 24 diagnoses in this area describe dysfunctional patterns of activity, exercise, and leisure and dysfunctional supporting processes. The diagnoses in this area differ. Dysfunctional patterns are concerned with activity and exercise abilities and describe the client's ability to engage in energy-consuming activities such as play (child), work, exercise, self-care, and leisure. The loss of the ability to engage in the activities of daily living is associated with feelings of dependency and lack of control over the immediate environment. Diagnoses related to daily activities include:

    High Risk for Activity Intolerance
    Activity Intolerance (Specify Level)
    Fatigue
    Impaired Physical Mobility (Specify Level)
    High Risk for Disuse Syndrome
    Impaired Home Maintenance Management (Mild, Moderate, Severe, Chronic)
    Diversional Activity Deficit
    Total Self-Care Deficit (Specify Level)
    Self-Bathing/Hygiene Deficit

Self-Dressing/Grooming Deficit
Self-Feeding Deficit
Self-Toileting Deficit
*Altered Growth and Development: Self-Care Skills (Specify)

High Risk for Activity Intolerance is a useful category to describe the presence of risk factors for an abnormal response to energy-consuming activities. Clients who have been inactive or on prolonged bed rest are frequently at high risk for this problem. In cardiac rehabilitation this category may be used to describe the risk factors associated with increasing activity after an acute myocardial infarct; it alerts nurses to observe the client's activity response carefully. Activity Intolerance (Specify Level) is useful in describing a common etiology for problems such as self-care deficit, perceived sexual dysfunction, impaired home maintenance management, or social isolation; for example: Self-Care Deficit (Level III) Related to Activity Intolerance, or Sexual Dysfunction Related to Activity Intolerance. It would be incorrect to use Activity Intolerance (Level II) Related to Cancer or Activity Intolerance (Level II) Related to Peripheral Arterial Disease. As with other diagnoses, avoid stating the medical disease as the etiology for activity intolerance. Etiology or related factors are the focus for nursing intervention; physicians design the interventions for medical conditions.

It is important not to miss signs and symptoms of Activity Intolerance in hospital care and home care of the frail elderly; to do so might produce a number of problems. It may be noted that a number of diagnoses in this pattern area require specification of a functional level. Activity Intolerance can be specified by levels of endurance such as:

Level I: Walks at a regular pace on level ground but becomes more short of breath than normal when climbing one or more flights of stairs.
Level II: Walks one city block (500 feet) on level ground or climbs one flight of stairs slowly without stopping.
Level III: Walks no more than 50 feet on level ground without stopping and is unable to climb one flight of stairs without stopping.

---

*Not currently on NANDA-approved list.

Level IV: Dyspnea and fatigue at rest.
Using these levels, the degree of activity tolerance might be specified as Social Isolation/Activity Intolerance (Level III) using the problem/etiology format.

Fatigue and Activity Intolerance appear to be similar; indeed, fatigue is a sign of activity intolerance. Close examination of the definitions[11] and the defining characteristics of these two categories suggests that fatigue is an all-encompassing, sustained feeling of exhaustion not necessarily related to activity. People with cancer sometimes experience this type of fatigue. Whereas activity intolerance is fatigue that is experienced with activity. Persons with cardiac and respiratory conditions experience fatigue with activity.

Impaired Mobility (Specify Level) is a frequently identified diagnosis. It can severely restrict a client's control over his or her environment and is frequently due to pain self-management deficit (as commonly occurs in chronic arthritis) or an uncompensated sensory-motor deficit (as occurs with hemiplegia). Used as an etiology the term describes a reason for problems such as self-toileting deficit or social isolation. Different levels of impairment require different nursing interventions; thus the level should be included in the diagnostic statement. The client's mobility may be described using levels of dependency. Level 0 is included below to show the range used in a health status evaluation but would not be used in stating a diagnosis because it indicates that no problem is present:

Level 0: Is independent in movement
Level I: Requires use of equipment or device
Level II: Requires help from another person(s) in the form of assistance, supervision, or teaching
Level III: Requires help from another person and equipment or device
Level IV: Is dependent and does not participate in movement

Mobility includes more specific diagnoses related to transfer, locomotion, ambulation, and bed mobility used in specialized care settings. The second set of diagnoses in this area describes dysfunctional activity patterns:

Impaired Home Maintenance Management describes the inability to carry on energy-consuming activities related to shopping, cooking, cleaning, laundering, and general home maintenance. This dysfunctional pattern is often caused by Activity Intolerance or Impaired Mobility. Other etiological factors that may contribute to Impaired Home Maintenance Management are Uncompensated Short-Term Memory Deficit or General Cognitive Impairment, Knowledge Deficit, Reactive Situational Depression, or Family Stress. It is important in hospital discharge planning to anticipate this problem, as it may delay discharge if the person has no support services. In many cases inability to manage household activities is diagnosed in a home visit.

Diversional Activity Deficit may be found in high-risk populations such as hospitalized clients (adults and children) with "nothing to do," newly retired persons without preretirement plans, or frail elderly confined to their homes. The overstressed "workaholic" may have a deficit because of lack of planning for recreation and leisure time.

For precision in the diagnosis of Self-Care Deficits[11] use the previously listed levels of dependency to classify the client's ability. If assessment data suggest that the client performs all but one self-care activity, a subcategory is used. In hospital and community nursing, Self-Care Deficit is a common problem that is usually produced by Activity Intolerance, Impaired Mobility, Uncompensated Short-Term Memory Deficit (as in Alzheimer's disease), and Uncompensated Cognitive or Sensorimotor Deficits. Hyperactive or withdrawn psychiatric clients or children who have mastered self-care skills may also exhibit this problem.

The client's response to self-care deficits may be fear of continued dependency, which is described by the following diagnostic statement: Fear (Dependency) Related to Self-Care Deficit (Level IV). Increasing the self-care ability of the client by teaching compensatory methods should begin to resolve his or her fear. This is a more clinically useful way of stating the diagnosis than Fear (Dependency) Related to Stroke and provides a basis for a nursing treatment plan to increase self-care ability.

Altered Growth and Development: Self-Care Skills (Specify) describes delays in bathing/hygiene, dressing/grooming, feeding, or independent toileting. The term *specify* requires that the diagnostician identify the specific skill that deviates from norms for the age group. Developmental de-

lays in crawling, walking, and other activities should also be described and labeled as the development of the diagnosis Altered Growth and Development proceeds. Careful consideration needs to be given to the description and labeling of various types of altered growth and development so that a consistent nomenclature results. Perhaps the term Developmental Delay: Self-Care Skills is more precise.

Supporting processes describe conditions that impact on the activity and exercise patterns just discussed. Ability is influenced by the development of coordination, strength, skill, endurance, and nutrient supply to tissues (cardiovascular and respiratory reserves). The following list describes broad dysfunctional patterns that influence all energy-consuming activities:

*High Risk for Joint Contractures
Dysfunctional Ventilatory Weaning Response (DVWR)
Ineffective Airway Clearance
Ineffective Breathing Pattern
Dysreflexia
High Risk for Peripheral Neurovascular Dysfunction
Decreased Cardiac Output
Altered Tissue Perfusion (Specify Renal, Cerebral, Cardiopulmonary, Gastrointestinal, Peripheral)
Impaired Gas Exchange
Inability to Sustain Spontaneous Ventilation

These diagnostic categories describe conditions that influence energy-consuming activities, such as mobility, self-care, activity intolerance, and other problems previously discussed. Most of the diagnoses listed above respond to nursing intervention. High Risk for Joint Contractures occurs when movable joints are kept immobile. Tendons at the joints shorten and the joints move into a flexed position. Independence in walking, feeding, and other body motions require movable joints; thus it is important to recognize the risk factors for contractures, make the diagnosis, and institute preventive nursing interventions. High Risk for Peripheral Neurovascular Dysfunction is a broad category dealing with disruption in circulation (tissue perfusion), sensation (sensory-perceptual alteration), and motion of an extremity (impaired mobility)

---

*Not currently on NANDA-approved list.

and overlaps with other diagnoses. Considering the risk factors,[11] the condition describes compression of the vessels in an extremity. An example would be the risk factor of pressure from a cast. Further development may allow the concept to be expressed more concisely and descriptively.

Ineffective Airway Clearance is a condition in which the client is unable to clear secretions or an obstruction from the respiratory tract, which may produce a state of fear or panic about not being able to breathe. The condition occurs in clients who have reduced awareness of secretions, impaired cough reflex, and debilitation. Ineffective Breathing Patterns require education about compensatory behaviors; it occurs with other conditions, such as chronic obstructive pulmonary disease (COPD). Without such education, the client's compensatory behaviors may be inadequate to maintain a sufficient oxygen supply for cell requirements. This diagnostic category would be more useful for nursing if it were defined by characteristics describing ineffective patterns of breathing under the voluntary control of the client (rather than the hypoxic results). The client with a chronic respiratory condition whose ineffective breathing pattern contributes to a self-care deficit or to other problems (e.g., Self-Care Deficit/Ineffective Breathing Pattern) should be helped to learn ways to increase vital capacity and air exchange. In contrast, after upper abdominal surgery, pain may cause a breathing problem and the diagnostic statement is formulated as: Ineffective Breathing Pattern/Incisional Pain.

Based on the definitions[11] of the diagnostic categories Decreased Cardiac Output and Impaired Gas Exchange, these two conditions do not respond to nursing intervention and do not meet the criteria listed on page 23. If these conditions are judged to be present, a physician should be informed and care under protocols or palliative care instituted, with nursing assessment for co-occurring nursing diagnoses.[13] The conditions are within the collaborative or interdependent domain of nursing practice. Frequent observation is a major nursing role in the treatment of these conditions. It is also important to recognize that clients with these conditions usually also have conditions described by nursing diagnoses. If these conditions are documented by the physician using medical diagnoses, nurses can use the medical diagnoses as a focus for the disease-related care they (the nurses) design and for documentation.

Sleep-rest pattern

The only approved diagnostic category in this pattern area is Sleep Pattern Disturbance, a common condition diagnosed by nurses. All sleep disturbances are not treated the same way; therefore, it is more useful to identify the various types of sleep-pattern disturbances such as Delayed Sleep Onset, Interrupted Sleep Pattern, or Sleep Pattern Reversal. Delayed Sleep Onset is a dysfunctional pattern that may occur with fear, anxiety, conflict, or presleep activities that are not conducive to relaxation. Sleep Pattern Reversal describes the condition wherein a client remains awake at night and sleeps or naps in the daytime. This condition is sometimes seen in elderly clients and produces difficulties for both clients and their families. A hospitalized client may experience an Interrupted Sleep Pattern when he or she is awakened for medications or treatments. It is also common in the postpartum period when the mother of the newborn is awakened frequently. Another sleep disturbance, early awakening pattern, may be a symptom of depression and should be investigated further. No diagnostic categories have been identified for dysfunctional rest/relaxation patterns.

Cognitive-perceptual pattern

Of the 12 diagnostic categories in this pattern area 8 have been approved by NANDA. All describe dysfunctional sensory-perceptual and cognitive patterns. Information from the internal and external environment is channeled through sensory receptors and relayed to centers in the brain concerned with perception and cognition. Deprivation or an excess of sensory information may affect both perception and cognition. Dysfunction or retarded development of cognitive processes, such as attention, orientation, memory, problem solving, and decision making, may produce dependency on others. Consider this set of diagnostic categories:
  *Uncompensated Sensory Deficit (Specify)
   Unilateral Neglect

*Not currently on NANDA-approved list.

Sensory-Perceptual Alterations: Input Deficit
[or Sensory Deprivation]

Sensory-Perceptual Alterations: Input Excess
[or Sensory Overload]

Pain

Chronic Pain

*Pain Self-Management Deficit (Acute, Chronic)

The diagnostic category Uncompensated Sensory Deficit requires that the deficit be specified. Some examples of diagnostic statements are: Impaired Mobility Related to Uncompensated Visual Deficit and Impaired Socialization Related to Uncompensated Hearing Deficit. The modifier *uncompensated* directs the nurse to help the client compensate for the loss. Care may range from full assistance to helping the client obtain simple or complex assistive devices. Unilateral Neglect describes a condition in which a client gives no attention to the side of the body that has a sensorimotor loss and to objects on the affected side; this condition may occur with a stroke. This perceptual deficit may be an etiological factor in self-care deficit and a high-risk factor for injury. Sensory Deprivation describes signs and symptoms resulting from a low level of sensory input. This condition may occur in homebound or hospitalized elderly who already have sensory deficits, in intensive care settings, in newborns in incubators, and in other situations in which the level of sensory input is reduced. The possibility that this problem will occur should also be recognized. In contrast to deprivation, Sensory Overload describes a condition in which the level of sensory input is greater than the person can handle. Clients with cognitive impairments may experience overload in an environment that has high, sustained sensory stimulation.

Three diagnostic categories describe pain conditions. Pain is a highly utilized diagnosis. In clinical situations, an added modifier such as *chest, joint,* or *incisional pain* is useful. Such modifiers provide a base for more definitive interventions. Usually, acute pain is treated collaboratively and resolved quickly; when the pain experience becomes chronic, clients must have support in their management of this condition. More important to the focus of nursing treatment is the category Acute or Chronic Pain Self-Management Deficit. Nursing intervention is directed toward helping a client manage and control

his or her pain by encouraging such actions as notifying the nurses when he or she experiences pain, needs help in positioning, or needs some distraction for relaxation. Clients with Chronic Pain Self-Management Deficit must learn to choose the medication that matches the severity of their pain. *Discomfort* is a frequent hospital nursing judgment. Clearly, clinical studies are needed to see if discomfort is separate and distinct from the category of Pain.

Dysfunctional cognitive patterns currently described by diagnostic categories are:

High Risk for Cognitive Impairment

Altered Thought Processes

*Uncompensated Memory Deficit

Knowledge Deficit (Specify)

Decisional Conflict

The first three diagnostic categories provide labels for dysfunctional or potentially dysfunctional cognitive patterns. High Risk for Cognitive Impairment describes the risk factors for impairment in memory, reasoning ability, judgment, and decision making. These risk factors include low sensory input, hearing and visual deficits, and tranquilizers or sedatives. A combination of these factors, such as is sometimes found in the elderly, places the client at high risk for cognitive impairment.

The diagnostic categories of Impaired Thought Processes and Uncompensated Memory Deficit are useful in describing etiological factors causing problems in self-care, home maintenance, and activities of daily living. It is sometimes possible to improve a client's nonreality-based thinking, help the client compensate for memory deficits, and increase his or her attention span by focusing nursing intervention on these etiological factors.

Health education and counseling are professional activities valued highly by nurses and have repeatedly been documented as nursing responsibilities. The category Knowledge Deficit (Specify) describes the inability to state or explain information or the inability to demonstrate a skill that is necessary for health (or disease) management. The term *Specify* requires that the particular area of knowledge deficit be included when this category is used. Such specification might apply to medica-

---

*Not currently on NANDA-approved list.

tion, diet, activity, or health practices such as exercise or relaxation.

Decisional Conflict (Specify) describes a state of uncertainty about a course of action when the choice involves risk, loss, or challenge to personal life values. Clients may experience this condition when faced with surgery, certain therapies, divorce, or other life events. The treatment of this condition involves helping clients resolve the conflict while respecting their autonomy in making the decision.

Developmental delays may occur in the cognitive-perceptual pattern. These may be described and classified in the current taxonomic category Altered Growth and Development. Nurses in pediatric settings frequently encounter conditions in which an infant's or child's development of cognitive abilities is not consistent with the norms for his or her age group. A child's cognitive development may be delayed in a low-stimulus environment or because of parental overprotection. Potential developmental problems and the risk factors they describe also need to be described and classified.

Self-perception–self-concept pattern

This pattern includes 12 diagnoses related to mood and perception and to ideas or attitudes about the self and self-competency (cognitive, affective, or physical). All the categories describe clients' subjective feelings and thus require verbal reports for diagnosis. The currently identified dysfunctional patterns of self-perception–self-concept are:

Fear (Specify Focus)
Anxiety (Mild, Moderate, Severe)
Anticipatory Anxiety (Mild, Moderate, Severe)
*Reactive Situational Depression
Hopelessness
Powerlessness (Severe, Moderate, Low)
Self-Esteem Disturbance
Chronic Low Self-Esteem
Situational Low Self-Esteem
High Risk for Self-Mutilation
Body Image Disturbance
Personal Identity Disturbance

---

*Not currently on NANDA-approved list.

Fear and anxiety are two conditions encountered in all nursing settings. A distinction must be made between these two conditions, which share many of the same defining characteristics. (This type of discrimination is referred to as *differential diagnosis*.) Fear is a focused feeling of dread, threat, or danger to the self; the focus of the fear must be specified. Intervention is directed toward helping the client deal with the specific fear. In contrast, Anxiety is nonspecific in focus. The client may express feelings of dread, threat, or danger but cannot identify a specific reason for these feelings. One of the first steps in treatment is to help the client identify the focus. Anticipatory Anxiety describes an increased level of arousal associated with the perception of a future threat (unfocused) to the self or to significant relationships. Both fear and anxiety may be seen at various levels of severity. Designating the level of severity is helpful in making treatment decisions. If a client is in a panic state, it may be necessary to obtain a medication order before nursing treatment of the condition can begin.

Reactive Situational Depression describes feelings of sadness, despair, or dejection regarding a particular situation. Usually the condition is transitory and responds to nursing intervention. A distinction must be made between this condition and hopelessness; in the latter the problem is an all-pervading sense of no hope, choices, or alternatives. Powerlessness describes a subjective feeling of lack of control over a situation and that one's actions will not significantly affect the outcome. This condition is frequently seen as a factor contributing to the client's reactive situational depression. Hopelessness describes a subjective state in which an individual sees either very limited or no alternatives or personal choices. When in a state of hopelessness, clients are passive and cannot mobilize resources in their own behalf. Discrimination is required between this condition and reactive situational depression, since hopelessness may also be symptomatic of depression.

Self-Esteem Disturbance is a category used to describe negative feelings or conceptions of the self. Defensive self-esteem may mask a Self-Esteem Disturbance. A self-report of high self-esteem may be a defensive reaction to negative feelings about the self. This category is useful in describing adolescents and adults with such a problem; in pediatric settings Developmental Self-Esteem Disturbance may be a more useful diagnosis. Body Image Disturbance is closely related to disturbances in self-esteem. This category describes negative feelings or perceptions about characteristics, functions, or limits of a client's body or body parts. It may arise with the loss of a body part or function, with underdevelopment, or after a large weight loss. Some clients who are dependent on machines for long periods of time will suffer body image distortions. Personal Identity Disturbance describes the inability to distinguish between the self and others and feelings of "not knowing who I am." This condition is also seen in adolescents in psychiatric settings.[14]

Delays may occur in the development of a functional pattern of self-perception–self-concept. Diagnostic categories are needed to describe these delays and dysfunctional developmental patterns of self-concept, personal identity and competency, body image, and the perception and control of mood states. Delays should be suspected when behavior does not meet the norms for the age group.

Role-relationship pattern

Twenty categories for naming dysfunctional role-relationship patterns have been classified; 14 are NANDA-approved. People establish relationships to meet the human need for contact and interaction with others. Roles and relationships serve as a structure for family units, friendships, work and play, community groups, and the larger society. Dysfunctional patterns of role performance, interactions, and relationships may be the source of developmental problems or role stress in persons, families, or communities. Consider first the diagnostic categories that describe the dysfunctional patterns that influence any type of interaction:

Impaired Verbal Communication
*Altered Growth and Development: Communication Skills (Specify)
Altered Role Performance
*Unresolved Independence-Dependence Conflict
High Risk for Violence
Relocation Stress Syndrome
Language permits the communication of ideas,

---

*Not currently on NANDA-approved list.

needs, purposes, feelings, and intentions. Impaired Verbal Communication describes the reduced or absent ability to use language in these human interactions. The category is broad; currently it is used to describe clients who are unable to speak, have speech impairments, or do not speak the dominant language. It seems that when communication is impaired because a person does not speak the predominant language of the health care agency, it is usually the care provider's responsibility to obtain an interpreter. Altered Growth and Development: Communication Skills (Specify) manifested as a developmental delay is sometimes a problem in the care of young children.

Unresolved Independence-Dependence Conflict describes the need or desire to be independent (in activities of daily living or in decision making) in a situation that requires some dependence. This conflict may be present in therapeutic, maturational, or social situations. For example, the need for complete rest may be required but produces conflict because the client's desire for self-care and ambulation is equally strong. The client may have the inability to move, but this inability conflicts with the desire for mobility. Thus an adolescent may be in conflict over the wish to be independent but may also realize (or be reminded) that full maturational competency has not yet been attained. Accepting help from others when needed may generate conflict for a person who has a history of independence and a strong desire to be independent. Unresolved Dependence-Independence Conflict is also a useful category. It describes the situation in which a person or family experiences conflict between the insecurity that more independence brings and the present security in being dependent. The term *unresolved* directs nursing intervention to help the client resolve the conflict. Altered Role Performance is a broad category that includes many types of role disturbances.

High Risk for Violence describes a set of risk factors for trauma to the self or to others during periods of anger, rage, agitation, or depression. This condition is usually treated in psychiatric settings, where the aim of treatment is to reduce person-environmental risk factors. Yet in some areas, because of the high incidence of family or street violence, this category is equally useful when delivering care to communities, families, or individuals. Further specificity may be inserted to increase the category's applicability: High Risk for Family Violence or High Risk for Community Violence.

Now we will consider a set of diagnostic categories that describe patterns that involve loss of relationships or reduced human interaction relative to the client's need. Relocation Stress Syndrome describes a set of biopsychosocial problems that occur particularly in circumstances of dependency and environmental change. Common examples of environmental change are transfer from a critical care unit to a convalescent unit, transfer from home to a nursing home, and change of room and location within a long-term care facility. For a person who is dependent or whose adaptive capacity is limited, the change from familiar surroundings, routines, people, and relationships may produce dysfunction in a number of patterns. This diagnosis is grouped under the role-relationship pattern instead of the coping-stress tolerance pattern because the central factor is that relocation disrupts roles and relationships with people, things, and the environment. (Syndromes represent a cluster of diagnoses occurring in conjunction with a central etiological factor. In this case the central factor is the stress of relocation.)

    Anticipatory Grieving
    Dysfunctional Grieving
  *Social Isolation
    Social Isolation (or Social Rejection)
    Impaired Social Interaction
  *Altered Growth and Development: Social Skills
    (Specify)

Grieving is a subjective state that follows a loss or a change in a pattern of relationships. The loss may involve a person, possessions, job, status, home, ideals, or parts or processes of the body. Anticipatory Grieving describes the expectation of a disruption in a familiar pattern or in a significant relationship; sadness and sorrow are expressed in anticipation of the loss. The normal grieving process should not be confused with Dysfunctional Grieving, which describes extended length or severity of grief and mourning. When there are risk factors for delayed grieving or for severe reactions to loss, the need for preventive intervention may be based on the diagnosis of High Risk for Dys-

functional Grieving. When using any of these diagnostic categories, it is important to keep in mind that grief and mourning are culturally influenced and that observations of the person, family, or community should be evaluated in the context of their culture. Some have also suggested that the term *specify* would make the category more useful, as, for example, Dysfunctional Grieving (Loss of Spouse). It may also be noted that loss of a spouse is the focus of grieving and not an etiological factor. As discussed previously, etiological factors are the focus for intervention. Thus to be useful the primary factor should be something that responds to nursing intervention. An example would be Dysfunctional Grieving (Loss of Spouse)/Unavailable Support Systems. This etiological factor suggests interventions, such as helping the person to talk about feelings, reactions, hopes, and plans and to make contact with bereavement groups in the community. Some suggest that Grieving should be a diagnosis, but this is a human process; perhaps a nurse who intervenes is showing his or her appreciation for the client's need for support. Extended intervention may be directed by the diagnosis High Risk for Dysfunctional Grieving; the treatment objective is to prevent dysfunctional grieving.

There is an affective component to human communication that includes nonverbal sensitivity to others' facial expression, body posture, and tone and inflection of speech, as well as culturally appropriate behavior in social interactions (the so-called social graces). These components of social interaction may be influenced by a lack of knowledge and skill as well as by neurological conditions, such as cerebrovascular accident (stroke) or mental illness. Impaired Social Interaction is a diagnostic category that may be used to describe (1) an ineffective quality of social exchange that leads to discomfort in social situations and (2) an insufficient or excessive quantity of exchange. The problem that most commonly occurs because of impaired social interaction is Social Isolation or Social Rejection; thus the diagnosis may be expressed in the problem/etiology format as Social Isolation/Impaired Social Interaction. Altered Growth and Development: Social Skills (Specify) describes developmental delays in role-relationship patterns. If social skills such as those discussed above in regard to impaired social interaction do not develop according to developmental norms for the age group, the condition is described by the diagnostic category Altered Growth and Development: Social Skills (Specify). As with previous diagnoses, the taxonomic category may be dropped from clinical recordings when specific developmental delays are clearly and more succinctly described in diagnostic terms.

Social Isolation describes interpersonal interactions below the level desired or required for personal integrity. The category is useful in describing the condition that results from voluntary or therapeutic isolation from others. It may occur because of therapeutic isolation in hospitals, impaired mobility, fear, or body image disturbances. In contrast, the NANDA-accepted diagnosis Social Isolation has a different orientation; this author has relabeled it Social Rejection, based on the definition and defining characteristics.[11] This category describes a condition of aloneness perceived as imposed by others and as a negative or threatening state. Other diagnoses should be developed in this pattern area. One example might be Support System Deficit. This would describe a condition in which the client has insufficient access to or utilization of help from others during a crisis period. The help needed by a client may be instrumental, such as assistance with child care, obtaining a job, or locating a community service. In other instances the need for support may be expressive, such as caring, trust, intimacy, and empathy during a crisis period. Interventions differ for the two types of support system deficit (instrumental and expressive); thus it is more clinically useful to specify the type of support systems the client needs when developing this category.

A third set of diagnostic categories within the role-relationship pattern describes dysfunctional primary relationships:

    Altered Family Processes
    High Risk for Altered Parenting
    Altered Parenting
  *Weak Mother-Infant (Parent-Infant) Attachment
    Parental Role Conflict
  *Parent-Infant Separation
    Altered Family Processes is currently defined as

*Not currently on NANDA-approved list.

the inability of the family (or household members) to (1) meet the needs of members, (2) carry out family functions, or (3) maintain communications for mutual growth and maturation. This category is very broad and inclusive; the specific alterations need to be identified because in many instances the three components do not occur together and require different interventions. The previously given caution against using a classification category as the problem ("Altered" or "Alterations in . . .") and the specific diagnosis as the etiological or contributing factor pertains here also. Using "altered family process related to dysfunctional family communication patterns" would be similar to expressing a medical condition as "respiratory disease related to viral pneumonia."

Altered Parenting and High Risk for Altered Parenting are also broad and inclusive categories that do not focus thinking on a particular alteration and a particular treatment plan. Specific diagnostic categories need to be identified to increase clinical usefulness. One type of altered parenting is in a stage of development, Weak Mother-Infant Attachment or Weak Parent-Infant Attachment. This describes a *nonreciprocal* bonding relationship between the parent or primary caretaker and the infant. The term *nonreciprocal* refers to behaviors on the part of the parent(s) *and* the infant. Thus assessment should be concerned with (1) the parent(s), (2) the infant, (3) the interaction that exists between them, and (4) the environment, which can facilitate or inhibit attachment. If risk factors for weak attachment are observed during the prenatal period, High Risk for Weak Mother-Infant Attachment would be an appropriate focus for preventive intervention. As in some of the previously considered diagnostic categories, conditions involving family or parent-child relationships should be evaluated in the cultural context of the client. Otherwise diagnostic errors may result. Another category being developed[15] is Parent-Infant Separation. This category might be a reason for weak attachment as well as other conditions.

Early discharge after surgery, long-term care of a spouse with an uncompensated memory loss, and a disabled child can tax the resources of family caregivers and produce stress. These situations may be described by the following diagnoses:

    High Risk for Caregiver Role Strain
    Caregiver Role Strain

The role of caregiver can be demanding; role strain may result in the condition Caregiver Role Strain. Early diagnosis and treatment (risk-factor reduction) of High Risk for Caregiver Role Strain may prevent this from occurring. Caregivers may need instrumental, social, and emotional support to continue the caregiving role. This condition may also adversely affect the relationship between the caregiver and the person being cared for; in extreme circumstances role strain may lead to abuse.

Sexuality-reproductive pattern

The five diagnostic categories in this pattern area describe the clients' perceived disturbances in sexuality or reproduction. Although closely tied to the role-relationship pattern, the sexuality-reproductive pattern is considered a distinct functional health pattern for assessment. Five diagnostic categories have been identified:

Sexual Dysfunction
Altered Sexuality Patterns
Rape Trauma Syndrome
Rape Trauma Syndrome: Compound Reaction
Rape Trauma Syndrome: Silent Reaction

Sexual Dysfunction describes perceived problems in achieving desired sexual satisfaction. The term *perceived problems* is used to indicate that it is the client's perception of problems, not the care provider's personal values regarding what constitutes sexual dysfunction, that is the focus of diagnosis. The category is very broad and inclusive; thus specific dysfunctions amenable to nursing intervention need to be identified. Clients with limitations in sexual expression imposed by disease or therapy may come to the nurse's attention. In other instances sexual dysfunction may be a symptom of a relationship problem. The diagnosis Altered Sexuality Patterns, accepted in 1986, is similar to Sexual Dysfunction. The criteria for the diagnosis are less well defined. There is one defining characteristic: reported difficulties, limitations, or changes in sexual behaviors or activities. This suggests it is a higher-level taxonomic category.[11]

Developmental patterns that do not meet expected cultural or social norms for an age group should be developed. When developed, diagnostic categories may be classified under the NANDA-approved category Altered Growth and Development in the Diagnostic Taxonomy.

Rape Trauma Syndrome and the two types of reactions are diagnostic categories describing the biopsychosocial problems following rape. A compound reaction includes the reactivation of physical or psychiatric illness or of reliance on alcohol, drugs, or both. Rape Trauma Syndrome: Silent Reaction is associated with a lack of verbalization about the rape along with abrupt changes in relationships and sexual behavior, sudden onset of phobic reactions, and increased anxiety.[11]

Coping–stress-tolerance pattern

Nine diagnoses have been identified in the coping–stress-tolerance pattern. *Coping* is defined as the cognitive and emotional processes used by a person, family, or community group to manage stress. When a client perceives that an event or relationship taxes or exceeds personal resources and presents a threat to well-being, stress exists.[16] Stress-tolerance is essentially a measure of vulnerability; persons with low stress tolerance will show signs of ineffective coping. Currently these diagnostic categories describe dysfunctional patterns of coping–stress-tolerance:

Ineffective Coping (Individual)
*Avoidance Coping
Ineffective Coping
Defensive Coping
Ineffective Family Coping: Compromised
Ineffective Family Coping: Disabling
Family Coping: Potential for Growth
Post-Trauma Response
Impaired Adjustment

As currently defined by NANDA, Ineffective Coping describes the impairment of adaptive behaviors and problem-solving abilities used to meet life's demands and roles. Essentially it refers to the management of stress or anxiety. Avoid using this diagnosis to describe excess food or alcohol intake, noncompliance, or uncooperative behavior unless anxiety, perception of life stress, and inability to solve problems are also present.[16]

Avoidance Coping is a type of ineffective coping. The category is used to describe minimization or denial of information (facts, meanings, consequences) when a situation requires active coping.

---

*Not currently on NANDA-approved list.

Avoidance can be a problem if the reality of chest-pain is distorted or if denial of diabetes results in health management deficits. *In using this category it is important that avoidance coping is not confused with hope or adaptive denial.* For example, avoiding the facts or implications of a situation may be adaptive in the early stages of a severe crisis; no diagnosis should be made because a diagnosis implies treatment directed toward resolution of the denial. The NANDA-approved category Ineffective Denial is really denial. It is defined as an attempt to disavow (deny) the knowledge or meaning of an event to reduce anxiety or fear. This is a situation in which denial is detrimental.[11] Given the nature of this definition, it might be more clinically useful to drop the word *ineffective* and to call the condition Denial or Avoidance Coping.

Defensive Coping is defined as a falsely positive self-evaluation based on self-protection. This method of coping defends the client against the perception of threats to his or her positive self-regard. Two of the diagnostic categories listed above describe Ineffective Family Coping. The term *compromised* refers to the situation in which ineffective family coping results in insufficient or ineffective family support of members. The diagnosis is more concisely stated as Compromised Family Coping.

Ineffective Coping: Disabling describes neglect, rejection, abandonment, and other coping behaviors that are detrimental to family members. This term should also be more concise. The diagnostic category Family Coping: Potential for Growth describes a situation in which coping is effective and family members have the potential to grow through the experience of coping with stress. Nursing is directed toward helping the client use the experience of coping with stress to attain higher levels of personal or family development. Several diagnoses in other patterns are similar in focus. They deal with situations in which there is a possibility of moving beyond the norm to a higher level of wellness. These category names may be expressed as Potential for Growth, Desire for Growth, or Desire for Enhanced Growth.[17] The addition of the word "desire" suggests that the assessment data include the client's expressed wish or desire, a factor that is most important.

Post-Trauma Response describes a sustained crisis reaction to an overwhelming traumatic event. Such a reaction can interfere with cognitive, affective, and sensorimotor activities and is characterized by repetitive dreams or nightmares, guilt, and flashbacks. This condition may follow war experiences, disasters, epidemics, rape, assault, torture, or other events that are viewed as crises by the person. Impaired Adjustment describes the situation in which there is a change in health status but the client is unable to modify his or her life-style and behavior. As currently defined,[11] this diagnostic category is used to describe behaviors consistent with impaired adjustment to illness.

No diagnostic categories have been identified to describe the dysfunctional development of coping strategies and the ability to tolerate stress. In addition, these current diagnostic categories may describe conditions encountered in the care of children, but the defining characteristics (behaviors) sometimes pertain only to adults.

Value-belief pattern

Only one diagnosis has been identified in this pattern area. Values, beliefs, goals, and life commitments guide the choices made by a person, family, or community; they can influence the evaluation of situations in terms of personal meaning. Thus values, beliefs, goals, and commitments may explain why a situation may be stressful for one client and not another and why one person is highly motivated in a situation and another is not. Currently the one diagnostic category that has been identified by NANDA in this pattern area is Spiritual Distress (Distress of the Human Spirit). As currently defined, Spiritual Distress describes "disruption in the life principle which pervades a person's entire being and which integrates and transcends one's biological and psychosocial nature"[11] (p. 46); it is used when clients express concern about the meaning of life, death, suffering, or their personal belief system. No diagnostic categories have been developed to describe dysfunctional development in this pattern area. A number of theories exist to describe and explain children's spiritual and moral development and the evolution of ethics and values in adulthood. These theories plus clinical observation of conditions encountered in caring for children may help to identify diagnostic categories in this area.

SUMMARY

Early in this chapter a distinction was made between functional, dysfunctional, and potentially dysfunctional patterns. Data that indicate a pattern is functional in the context of the whole person's (family's, community's) functioning reveal a strength that may be mobilized to deal with health problems. Dysfunctional patterns (actual problems) and potentially dysfunctional patterns (high-risk problems) were described by diagnostic categories. Various types of patterns were discussed, including unhealthful changes from baseline and developmental delay or dysfunctional development.

When an actual problem is diagnosed, the search begins for etiological or related factors that are the focus for intervention. In contrast, when diagnosing high-risk processes or states, the nurse must delineate the contributing risk factors; intervention focuses on risk-factor reduction.

Currently identified categories that provide labels for nursing diagnoses were discussed. These are terms used to describe actual or potential problems. It was noted that while the categories are in an early stage of development, most have been shown to be useful in describing problems encountered in clinical practice and as a focus for treatment planning. The overview of current diagnostic language in this chapter should be followed by intensive study of the conceptual basis, definition, and critical defining characteristics for each diagnostic category. This brief introduction to diagnostic categories should prepare the reader to consider the diagnostic process, which employs information collection, interpretation, clustering, and naming of the condition judged to be present.

NOTES AND REFERENCES

1. Taylor FK: A logical analysis of the medico-psychologic concept of disease. I, *Psychol Med* 1:356, 1971.
2. Nurses may cite norms in judging patterns, but in actuality they combine these standards with personal baseline information. This is beginning to be demonstrated in research. Jenny J: Knowing the patient: one aspect of clinical knowledge, *Image* 24:254, 1992.
3. Kim HS: *The nature of theoretical thinking in nursing,* Norwalk, CT, 1983, Appleton-Century-Crofts.
4. Naegel KD: A model of health. In Cummings E, editor: *Health and healing,* San Francisco, 1970, Jossey-Bass.
5. In some instances a diagnostic category area is introduced in general terms in order to suggest a diagnostic area for study. Altered Parenting and Sleep Pattern Disturbance are examples; yet no diagnoses have been submitted describing alterations in parenting or the disturbances in sleep patterns that nurses diagnose and treat.
6. Bruenig K et al: Noncompliance as a nursing diagnosis: current use in clinical practice. In Hurley M, editor: *Classification of nursing diagnoses: proceedings of the sixth conference,* St Louis, 1986, Mosby.
7. Stanitis MA, Ryan J: Noncompliance: an unacceptable diagnosis, *Am J Nurs* 82:941, 1982.
8. Gordon M: *Manual of nursing diagnosis,* St Louis, 1993, Mosby.
9. Vincent K: Letters to the editor, *Am J Nurs* 33:266, 1985.
10. Gordon M: High risk nursing diagnoses in critical care nursing practice. In Carroll-Johnson R, editor: *Classification of nursing diagnoses: proceedings of the tenth conference,* Philadelphia, 1993, Lippincott.
11. North American Nursing Diagnosis Association: *NANDA nursing diagnoses: definitions and classifications, 1992,* Philadelphia, 1993, the Association; Gordon M: *Manual of nursing diagnosis,* St Louis, 1993, Mosby.
12. It is important to remember that self-care deficit and self-care agency deficit are two very different concepts. Self-care deficit refers to the inability to do the daily activities specified. Self-care agency deficit is an abstract concept within a conceptual model (see Chapter 4) and is defined as a discrepancy between self-care agency and self-care demand.
13. The reason the author recommends referring NANDA-approved nursing diagnoses to a physician will be discussed in the section on collaborative problems in Chapter 9. Briefly, when assessment reveals collaborative problems, they are referred to a physician; their treatment is outside the legal domain of nursing.
14. Oldaker S: Identity confusion: nursing diagnoses for adolescents, *Nurs Clin North Am,* 20:763, 1985.
15. This diagnosis was studied in a research project by T. Heather Herdman, Doctoral Student at Boston College School of Nursing, Chestnut Hill, MA 1991.
16. Lazarus R, Folkman S: *Stress, appraisal, and coping,* New York, 1984, Springer.
17. This was suggested to the author in a conversation with Dorothea Jacob, Toronto, Canada, a number of years ago when we were trying to find a way to label "wellness" diagnoses.

CHAPTER 7

CLINICAL INFORMATION COLLECTION

s previously described, the diagnostic process includes four activities:

Information collection
Information interpretation
Information clustering
Naming the cluster

In Chapters 4 and 5 we began the discussion of information collection. The focus was on *what* information is to be collected. This chapter continues the discussion, but the focus is on *how* information is collected during assessment.

A term used frequently in nursing, *assessment,*[1] is a health status evaluation that requires the collection and interpretation of clinical data. It continues during all professional, nurse-client interactions. Assessment never stops, but at times a diagnosis may be made, revised, or discarded as a basis for directing nursing treatment. Can assessment occur without diagnosis? Yes. When the information reveals no health problems, the clinical data are summarized and recorded as the health status evaluation. In some instances data are collected, problems are identified, and treatment is instituted under medical-nursing protocols or the problem is referred to a physician.

Professional responsibility to the client requires that diagnoses be based on assessments that are deliberate and systematic. These characteristics of data collection increase the likelihood of obtaining accurate information and thus making accurate diagnoses. *Deliberate assessment* has purpose and

direction. It is based on many of the ideas already discussed, such as:

1. Awareness of the professional domain and scope of practice responsibilities (Chapters 3, 4, and 5)
2. A clear concept of the information needed to fulfill the nurse's duty to a client (Chapter 5)
3. Use of focal questions and observations that conserve clients' and nurses' time and energy (Chapter 5)

A *systematic approach* implies organized information collection and logical sequencing of questions and observations. Three main factors may influence organization during assessment; they structure the content in this chapter:

1. *Situational context:* Includes the physical and interpersonal characteristics of the situation and how the assessment is structured
2. *Nature of the information:* Influences both how information is collected and how it is used
3. *Diagnostician's cognitive-perceptual capabilities:* Are important tools for collecting health-related information

All three factors operate simultaneously in every clinical situation in which information is being collected. For example, in a hospital room (situational context), a nurse (diagnostician) anticipating that a client may be having pain looks closely for facial grimacing related to pain (nonverbal nature of information). Information for health assessment and diagnostic judgment is collected by knowing the nature of the desired information, setting up the ideal situation for its collection, and fine-tuning the senses required for perceptual recognition.

Situational context for assessment

The context of assessment situations refers to the circumstances in which information is collected. Although information collection is the goal in all assessment situations, contexts differ in terms of the immediate purpose and scope of data to be gathered, the probability of health problems, clients' response level, and the structure of the physical and interpersonal environment. These contextual factors are examined in relation to the types of assessment that are common in clinical practice: initial assessment that a nurse conducts when a client is added to his or her caseload; problem-focused assessment that is done daily (or more frequently if needed); time-lapse reassessment in clinics and health maintenance organizations or in occupational, school, and residential settings; and emergency assessment, which is required when initial impressions indicate a life-threatening situation.

Take particular note of differences in the probability of a health problem. These differences directly influence the diagnostician's approach to information collection and the inherent difficulty of the task. Clearly if one knows what one is looking for (problem-focused assessment), the search is easier than if one does not (universe of possibilities). As described in a later chapter, nurses have strategies for quickly narrowing the universe of possibilities during initial assessments.

INITIAL ASSESSMENT

Whenever a client is added to a nurse's caseload, an admission assessment of the 11 previously described functional health patterns is done. This establishes the *nursing data base*. Initial assessments are referred to as a data base because (1) basic historical and current information (data) about all the client's health patterns is collected and (2) the information is used as baseline criteria against which any further changes are evaluated.

Purpose and scope

The purpose of the initial assessment is to evaluate a client's health status, identify any functional patterns that may present a problem, and establish a therapeutic, helping relationship. The components of the admission assessment are a nursing history of functional patterns and an examination of pattern indicators. The former is done by interviewing the client, significant others, or both. The latter requires observation and other examination techniques. Generally a comprehensive assessment is necessary. If a client's condition is critical (physiological or psychological instability exists), only a screening assessment of patterns may be warranted (see Chapter 5 for format).

The collection of data may be influenced by the psychological set of the clinician and by the client's view of a nursing history and examination. How each of these influence the purpose and scope of data collection is described below.

Psychological set: the nurse

A psychological set, or disposition, is an inclination to take certain actions or hold certain attitudes. A set influences what areas will receive attention as well as the overall motivation. Thus the nurse's psychological set directly influences the purpose and scope of the data collection as well as the nurse's expectations of the probability of health problems. The goal of any professional health care provider doing a health assessment is to understand and explain the data that are gathered. Psychologists[2] suggest that there are a number of psychological sets that influence the focus of attention during information gathering. Which of the following sets do you think is most productive in establishing a therapeutic, helping relationship?

1. *The Descriptive-Explanatory Set* is related to the questions, Why is this behavior manifested? What does it mean?
2. *The Personal Self-Maintenance Set* is related to the questions, What is the client in relation to me? Can the client help me meet my needs?
3. *The Personal Role Set* focuses on the questions, Who is the client in relation to me? What role shall I play?
4. *The Expectations of the Client-Role Set* focuses on the acceptable and unacceptable be-

havior of the client and on the question, How well does the client meet my expectations of a client?[2]

During history and examination the most productive set, or motivation, is item 1, the Descriptive-Explanatory Set. This set encourages the clinician to describe, explain, and evaluate the client's functional health patterns and subsequently to offer the client help or guidance as necessary and if it is desired. This fact should be kept in mind because it is not the common, everyday social set. Most interpersonal interactions are not descriptive-evaluative or purposefully diagnostic. Neither are they necessarily or deliberately therapeutic.

The nurse's motivation in the interaction complements the client's role set. Although sometimes disguised, the client's objective generally is to obtain help in health evaluation, problem solving, or physical activities. The nurse's first step in providing help is to describe and explain the client's current health patterns. Then professional decisions can be made regarding the mode of helping and its goals.

A psychological set to perceive and interpret greatly influences the way client behaviors are categorized. Imagine what might ensue if one's primary set in a psychiatric setting with patients who have mental disorders was self-maintenance. Clients' behavior might instantly be interpreted as potential violence. Or a nurse with a set that evaluates how a client "stays in line" with the patient role might be quick to see too much independence and "taking over" during assessment. Far too often care providers slip into nonproductive sets during interactions with clients. It is not unusual, when first doing assessments, for a learner to slip into the personal role and self-maintenance set, both of which focus on the nurse rather than on the client.

Part of socialization into professional nursing is to learn role behavior; for example, the predominant motivation in assessment is the descriptive-explanatory, or *why,* set. This is not to say that the other sets are never used. An experienced nurse may reflect on how sensitive the client is to another's (the nurse's) needs. Are social cues to roles (the nurse's role) received? How well does the client meet various role expectations? The nurse-client interaction and client-client interactions on a unit are used as the object of observation. Nurses pay attention to the affective reactions and the impressions that are generated in them by the client's behavior. These personal reactions are used as examples of how others may react to the client. This insight may provide data about role-relationships. These techniques are particularly useful in specialty areas such as psychiatric nursing assessment.

Psychological set: the client

Assessment is more successful when the assessor is aware of his or her own perspective and takes into account the motivation and perspective of the client. According to one school of social psychology behavior is greatly influenced by the way a person "defines the situation."[3] Extending this idea to assessment suggests a number of ideas. Initially both client and nurse bring past experience, expectations, and values to the situation. Each synthesizes these "predefinitions" of the situation with current perceptions. Unspoken questions may arise: What is happening? What role shall I play? How shall I behave? The nurse's personal definition of the assessment situation is one factor that influences behavior in interpersonal interaction. This idea provides food for thought. How does the nurse help the client define and understand the "situation" of assessment and health care? Before discussing possible approaches, let us extend this idea further.

Diagnosis is also a "definition of situation"; it is a way of defining the situation that prompted contact with the health care provider. The client usually has some idea of what the health problem might be when the assessment begins. This idea includes notions, expectations, and feelings that may be realistic or unrealistic. By relating his or her health history a client may even be disposed to define the situation in a new way. Simultaneously the nurse gains information that will aid in defining the situation diagnostically.

Prior to assessment the individual, family, friends, or society must define the situation as one requiring health consultation or care. Otherwise no action is taken. The client's preencounter definition of the problem, the data collection process, and the health care system need to be taken into account. Herzlich and Graham[4] identified the meanings people attribute to the terms *health* and *illness.* Of interest to our discussion are their findings concerning when and why people consult health care providers.

In these researchers' middle-class urban sample and in other studies[5-7] it was found that the clients' perception of symptoms was not sufficient to initiate health consultation. Passage from a perceived state of health to one of perceived sickness occurred when symptoms interfered with work or social activity. People then defined themselves as needing to know "what is the matter." A person viewed his or her symptoms as ambiguous; they could either mean nothing or be important. This ambiguity produced uncertainty. Most important, symptoms interfered with activity. These are the main reasons people sought help. They expected that the health care provider would define the situation and give it meaning. Routine health examinations were sought even in the absence of symptoms but for the same reasons; the care provider would reassure the client that the absence of symptoms meant health.[4 (pp. 78-87)]

In these studies interference with functional activities involved in daily living was the main concern that initiated health consultation. This aspect must be addressed in health care delivery; merely diagnosing a disease is an insufficient response. Diagnosis should also focus on how the person or family is managing their functional activities as described by the health patterns and the capabilities required; this is the province of nursing diagnosis. However, at present it is not a diagnostic area that is offered to the consumer in a systematic, organized way by nurses, especially those in joint practices with physicians.

Most clients, on their entry into the health care delivery system, expect providers to focus on medical diagnosis, medical treatment, and the prognosis for physical or mental disease. This is how people have been socialized. The details of their health management are usually left for them to work out as best they can. One result is a high incidence of noncompliance with therapeutic recommendations. Surprised reactions from clients are common when nurses begin to assess other things besides the physical aspects of a disease. One reaction is amazement that the nurse would be concerned "about me." Consumers have to become accustomed to defining the health care system as one that offers both nursing and medical consultation and that is oriented to both health and disease. People should be made aware of this distinction and of nursing's role in health care. This type of communication can be incorporated into the nursing assessment of the functional health patterns described in Chapter 5.

Consider some examples of how to initiate an assessment so as to help the client define the situation. The nurse, being purposefully vague, might say, "Ms. Klein, I'm your primary nurse. I wonder if we can talk about how you're managing your health at home and see if I can help—and if you have any questions. . . ." With a more direct approach the nurse might say, "Ms. Klein, I'd like to do a nursing assessment. There may be things you would like help with, so let's talk about the way you plan your diet and . . ." (mention a few relevant things). The latter approach clearly implies a strategy for educating the consumer about nursing. It familiarizes the client with nursing vocabulary ("nursing assessment"), definitions, and what benefits may be derived from the assessment. Either of the above statements may be used to orient the client to an understanding of and cooperation with a nursing history and examination. The first example may be beneficial when a client is frightened; the latter is a more direct approach.

When the situation is perceived clearly, the client is in a better position to respond to assessment questions. Time and again this concept has been demonstrated in psychological studies of cognition since it was first proposed by Bruner, Goodnow, and Austin.[8] Clients' responses are more appropriate when they know what is expected, and they become more involved when the benefits are clear. These points are sometimes neglected in clinical practice.

Probability of health problems

The initial assessment cannot be problem focused at the start; no current data are available, so that *the hypothesis of no dysfunctional pattern is as probable as the hypothesis that dysfunctional health patterns exist.*

The question directing assessment is: Does a health problem exist? The universe of possibilities is open. On the basis of initial cues (client's age, health concerns, nurse's initial observations or impressions), likely possibilities are generated.

Structure for information collection

The interpersonal situation in which initial diagnoses are established is important. Imagine a situation in which the person, family, or community group does not know the nurse. The nurse should concentrate on establishing trust and rapport with the client(s) during the assessment. These interpersonal factors are critical in obtaining valid information and for a future helping relationship. The environmental setting is also critical to the initial assessment. When people are asked to share information about personal "ways of living," their privacy must be ensured. Both clinician and client, trying to structure a therapeutic relationship characterized by confidence and rapport, need a comfortable setting free from interruption and distraction.

The structure for information collection during an initial assessment is provided by the nursing history and the examination. The history contains the client's subjective reports of functional health patterns, whereas the examination consists of nursing observations. A format for taking a history and examination was discussed in Chapter 5; how to do this type of assessment is discussed in greater detail in this chapter. The assessment is a complex and important nursing activity that initiates the professional relationship.

Nursing history and examination

The nursing history may be done by interview, by questionnaire, or by a combination of both.[9] Important differences exist. If the client fills out an assessment form, the responses must be taken at face value, since no interpersonal interaction occurs as the questions are answered. In contrast, during an interview branching questions may lead to further clarification. Some health care settings combine both approaches, most often when entering clients are not acutely ill or cognitively impaired, for example, in ambulatory or day surgery settings. If the client's admission is scheduled before the admission date, either an assessment form may be sent to the home for preentry completion or the admission office will distribute the form. Then follow-up questions are asked during an admission interview. The advantages of this procedure are that it saves a portion of the nurse's time and there is still an opportunity to follow through on actual or potential problem patterns. In addition, the client can relax and fill out the information at his or her own pace. The interpersonal contact in either situation is designed to clarify the issues, permit elaboration by both parties, and thus allow the nurse to arrive at an understanding of the client's responses. Currently history taking by interview is most common.[10]

A successful interview is guided, not dominated, by the nurse. Actually the client should be talking about 80% of the time and the nurse 20%. The nurse guides the interview by opening a topic (pattern area), assisting with the narrative, focusing, and closing a topic. The first decision is how to begin; the last involves termination.

Beginning an assessment

An initial assessment begins with the nursing history. Introductions are important because people consider names personal. Address the client by name, introduce yourself, and state your title—for example, student nurse, registered nurse, or clinical specialist. Explain your purpose. All the introductions described below have been observed in clinical settings: which one begins to establish a professional relationship?

1. Mr. Jones? I'm Ms. Arnold, a student nurse at the university. I'd like to talk to you about your health and how you're managing.
2. Hi, Mr. Jones. I'm Ms. Arnold, a student. I have to do a nursing assessment on you.
3. Mr. Jones? I'm Joan, but most of my friends call me Jo. I'd like to see if you have any problems.
4. Bill Jones? I'm Ms. Arnold; before I go off duty I have to do your nursing care plan.

The overly friendly approach of choices 2, 3, and 4 is not appropriate in initiating an admission assessment. Examples 2 and 4, with their "have to do" phrase, may communicate that the nurse would prefer to be involved in other activities. In the fourth choice especially, the client is made to feel that he or she is delaying the nurse from going off duty; this situation generates the expectation that it is going to be a "rush job." Rather than focus on a task to be done, focus on the client's needs as illustrated in the first choice, which is the preferred introduction. The idea of how to begin health pattern assessment will be expanded in later chapters on diagnostic strategies.

Helping the client describe health patterns

Both the knowledge of what to assess and the interpersonal skills that facilitate history taking are important in helping clients describe their health patterns. Much has been written about communication and interviewing techniques; below are a few major points.

Topic transitions. As each pattern is assessed, try to relate the next pattern area to a previous statement. Use an appropriate transitional comment; then follow with a question. Otherwise the nursing history appears to be an interrogation. Note the difference in the use of transitional comments in the following two assessments of the sleep-rest pattern of a hospitalized adult:

Assessment 1

Nurse: *You mentioned before that you felt tired during the day; when you get up most mornings do you feel rested and ready for work?*

Client: *No, not lately; I guess I'm not getting enough sleep.*

Nurse: *That certainly can contribute to being tired during the day. Has this been a few days, weeks, or longer?*

Client: *It's been about a month now.*

Nurse: *About how many hours do you sleep on the average?*

Client: *About 4; I try to go to sleep about 11:00 PM and I'm still awake between 3:00 and 4:00 AM; then I have to get up at 7:00.*

Nurse: *That can be irritating, lying awake in the dark. I'm sure you've thought about what might be causing it and what would help you get to sleep (questioning tone)?*

Client: *I start thinking about all my problems and I worry that my husband will have another heart attack at night. I guess I finally fall asleep around 3:00 AM from exhaustion. I don't take any pills.*

Nurse: *He'd been home 4 weeks when you had to come into the hospital, right? How has he been doing?*

Client: *Well, he seems to be doing well; his doctor is very pleased with his recovery. I guess*

I'm silly to worry but . . . (voice trails off).

Nurse: *Well, sometimes thinking can help work out things, but maybe we need to talk further about your concerns. I could come back this afternoon after you've had x-rays taken. Are you concerned right now about him being alone?*

Client: *No, my daughter is staying over; but you'll come back later.*

Nurse: *Yes, let's talk this afternoon; I notice you have glasses; are they for reading or . . . (nurse uses this to introduce the cognitive-perceptual pattern assessment).*

Assessment 2

Nurse: *I'd like to ask you about your sleep pattern now. When you get up in the morning, do you feel well rested?*

Client: *No, not lately.*

Nurse: *How many hours do you sleep at night?*

Client: *Not more than 4; I have to get up at 7:00 AM to go to work.*

Nurse: *When do you go to bed?*

Client: *Eleven.*

Nurse: *So you don't get to sleep until 3:00 AM?*

Client: *Yes . . . (Nurse asks the next question as the client hesitates.)*

Nurse: *How long have you had this problem?*

Client: *About 4 weeks; I just can't seem to get to sleep before 3:00 AM 'most every night. It's terrible lying awake.*

Nurse: *Do you take anything to sleep?*

Client: *No, but the doctor ordered some sleeping pills here.*

Nurse: *Well, that should help. Do you know why you have trouble sleeping at home?*

Client: *No . . . not really.*

Nurse: *Any nightmares or bad dreams?*

Client: *No.*

Nurse: *Well, maybe you'll sleep better after you've taken the pill, and after you've had your tests and go home things will be better. How's your vision? (Nurse introduces the cognitive-perceptual pattern.)*

In the first assessment the transition from pattern to pattern and from question to question is smoothly made. The interview is personalized, and the nurse exhibits interest and concern. In the second assessment one gets the impression that there is a set of questions to be asked and that the history taking is an interrogation. Generally both nurses asked the same questions and obtained data to support a sleep-onset disturbance. Which one was more effective in establishing a supportive relationship? Which obtained better data for diagnosing the probable cause of the sleep-onset problem?

Asking short, abrupt questions or reading questions one by one from a paper is not effective in establishing an interpersonal relationship that communicates caring. In fact, the nurse in the second assessment did not obtain any information about the probable cause of the sleep-pattern disturbance. At the point where the second nurse asked about nightmares, the client may have been ready to share her concerns about her husband, but the nurse continued the questioning (her agenda). Instead, when the client hesitantly said, "No, not really," the nurse might have responded in a supportive tone of voice: "Sometimes worries can keep us awake at night. Do you have any concerns?" Even without knowledge of the client's concern about her husband having a heart attack, the nurse should have considered that perhaps the client was experiencing fear and anxiety. These are two of the most common causes of sleep-onset disturbance.

Some further examples of smooth transitions may be helpful. A number of problems may be verbalized while the client reports data about his or her health perception–health management pattern. The transition to nutritional pattern can be made by saying, "Let's jot down those problems; we will want to talk further about them. I seem to need more specific information about some things. You mentioned that planning meals was difficult. What kinds of foods have you been eating at breakfast, lunch, dinner, and for snacks? Let's begin with breakfast." This leads into the nutritional pattern.

The nurse should attempt to construct a comfortable transition, especially in areas usually considered personal. For example, after inquiring about family structure and relationships, the nurse should move on to sexuality patterns: "You mentioned that you've been married nearly 10 years. Do you find your sexual relationship satisfactory?" Or, less directly, "Do any marital problems arise now and then?" Or, "Has this illness been associated with any problems in your sexual relationship?" Creating transitional statements takes practice. The main idea is to personalize the interview.

Pick up on something that has been said and relate it to the next topic for discussion.

Creating questions. The content of questions for individual, family, and community assessment was listed in Chapter 5. These questions need to be formulated in the context of the ongoing assessment; that is, they need to be individualized to the situation. In addition, branching questions are always needed to clarify, elaborate, or validate information.

Various types of questions and remarks facilitate history taking. One is the *open-ended question;* the topic for discussion is specified in a general question and usually elicits descriptions and current concerns. As an example: "What's it like for you when all the children are at home for the day?" This approach is in contrast to a direct question, which requires a specific yes or no answer; for example: "Do you get upset when all the children are home for the day?" After a client has responded to an open-ended question, *focused questions* may provide particular information. When a specific diagnostic possibility is being considered, the critical characteristics (diagnostic criteria) of the category guide the formulation of questions.

Probing questions are frequently needed to obtain clarification. These are questions that permit the client to elaborate. They are commonly used when a client employs abstract terms or offers judgments such as "nervous," "depressed," or "ulcer." Beware of accepting such words at face value: the client may define them totally differently than you do. Probe with a follow-up inquiry such as, "What feelings do you notice when you're nervous?" Sometimes this question leads to the discovery that cardiac rhythm irregularities are occurring. Similarly, "ulcer" may mean a skin abrasion. It is also not uncommon for clients to circumvent an area that is emotionally charged, such as death. They may not be sure the nurse will accept their beliefs or feelings. The nurse who suspects this must probe with care and at the same time be accepting and supporting.

Facilitating communication. Support, reassurance, empathy, and silence are methods of communication that assist the client in describing health patterns. *Support* demonstrates interest, concern, and understanding. It can enhance description or close it off, depending on whether the nurse communicates understanding. *Reassurance* communicates that the client has worth and self-reliance. *Empathy* indicates that the nurse accepts or can clarify the client's feelings or behavior. Supportive silence permits the client to continue a response when description is difficult or emotionally charged. Below are examples of these types of communication:

Support

Client: *I have a terrible time trying to get to sleep at night.*
Nurse: *That must be difficult. What seems to be . . . ?*

Reassurance

Client: *I have a terrible time trying to get to sleep at night.*
Nurse: *I think we can come up with some things you can do to make sleeping easier. What seems to be . . . ?*

Empathy

Client: *I have a terrible time trying to get to sleep at night.*
Nurse: *That can cause you a lot of worry and concern. What seems to be . . . ?*

A nurse's silence may communicate interest or withdrawal. For example, when the client uses the words "terrible time," the nurse might physically shift forward very slightly, holding eye contact. This movement indicates interest and concern. Shifting away from the client and from eye contact indicates withdrawal from the problem, regardless of what the nurse says or of the silence that intervenes. The client may be sensitive to this body language and may not elaborate, thinking the nurse is uncomfortable or not interested.

Questions and remarks may be *reflective* or *confronting*. A reflection echoes a portion of what the client has just said. For example, a child may say, "I get upset in school"; the nurse then says, in a gentle, supportive, questioning tone, "Upset?" Confrontation focuses attention on feelings or behavior. It is used to probe more deeply. A client may describe some change. Three or four sentences later it is evident that this change began 2 months after a divorce. The nurse, feeling attention should be focused on the time sequence, may say, "Do you think that was related to your feelings after your divorce?" Confrontations may be based on the need to validate an inference or an observation during the diagnostic process; confrontation during an intervention may have other objectives, such as insight development.

During the assessment of emotionally charged areas, a client may begin to cry. Accept this demonstration of feeling without feeling guilty. Feelings of guilt are a sign to the nurse that his or her focus has turned inward toward self rather than outward toward the client. Crying is a cue to depth of feelings, such as frustration or sadness. Empathy, reassurance, or silence combined with touch usually is helpful. After the client gains some composure, the nurse can ask whether he or she can help in any way. This is a better approach than suggesting that the interview stop; the only recourse then would be to leave, since the nurse's presence indicates she or he is waiting to continue.

Early indications of fatigue or increasing anxiety need to be observed. Try to validate these impressions with the client. Both fatigue and anxiety during the interview should be treated as data. Fatigue is a cue to activity tolerance. It should be noted and a decision made about whether to shift from a detailed assessment to a few screening questions. The nurse must use judgment regarding the signs of increasing anxiety. Either the topic or the discussion of the topic with a nurse who is not yet fully trusted may be producing a personal threat to the client. The client may be asked whether he or she wishes to talk further about the topic or to continue later. There are many good books about interviewing and assessment that deal with situations such as these and prepare the beginner for handling this type of situation if it arises.

Examination

Following the nursing history, an examination is done. Physical characteristics, such as gait and mobility, skin integrity, heart rate, and range of joint movement are observed. Cues obtained during history taking provide impressions of client's speech (tone, rate, and quality) and, possibly, interactions if another person is present (parent-child or client–other relationships). Assessments that take place in the home provide opportunities to observe client's living conditions, safety hazards, and neighborhoods.

Five sensory modalities (vision, hearing, cutaneous touch, smell, and kinesthesia) provide the means for obtaining clinical data during examination. (Taste, the other sensory modality, is rarely used.) The nurse is a sensitive measuring device for listening, interpersonal interaction, observation, inspection, and examination (auscultation, palpation, and percussion). An amazing amount of information can be collected through the use of the five sensory modalities and these four methods of data collection. If warranted, the areas listed under "Examination" in Chapter 5 may be expanded. (Many excellent books about physical assessment and methods of data collection are available; some are cited in the reference list at the end of this chapter.)

A synthesis of the history and examination data provides information about a client's functional health patterns. For example, a pattern of exercise-activity described in the history may be understood in the context of an observed gait impairment. A schoolchild's poor hygiene may be understood after an examination of his or her living facilities. A deeper understanding of functional patterns is acquired only if physical assessment findings are collected for this purpose. Does this seem obvious? Apparently it is not, because sometimes, when a biomedical systems format (gastrointestinal, cardiovascular, and similar categories) is used, physical examination data are separated from nursing history data. If functional health patterns are a reasonable focus for nursing assessment and diagnosis, clinical data should be considered as indicators of these patterns. What is observed during examination may be the outcome of existing or emerging functional patterns that the client described during the history. Or the observational data may explain why certain patterns exist, have changed, or are emerging developmentally. It is important to remember that the examination of the client and situation verifies or expands the understanding gained during history taking. Examination provides further data, not surprises.

Terminating the admission assessment

After information is collected through history taking and examination, termination of the initial assessment begins. The termination process has three objectives:

1. It offers the client the opportunity to add further information or express additional health concerns.
2. It summarizes the assessment.

3. It may be used to make plans for the treatment of problems.

As experience in diagnosis grows, the nurse, in most cases, is able to structure the possible diagnoses simultaneously with history taking and examination. After asking whether the client has further information or concerns, the nurse summarizes and makes plans in the context of ongoing events. Table 7-1 shows an example of the termination of an initial assessment of a 60-year-old female client admitted 1 day before gallbladder surgery; the diagnoses are Anxiety Related to Knowledge Deficit (Perioperative Procedures), Exogenous Obesity Related to Caloric Intake–Energy Expenditure Imbalance, High Risk for Atelectasis, and Social Isolation Related to Stress Incontinence.

Summarizing and planning with the client at the time the assessment ends may not always be possible, especially when the nurse is in the early stages of learning diagnosis. Also, even the experienced diagnostician may not be able to formulate diagnoses "on the spot" because of the complexity of the health problem or because of missing data. The nurse should not feel pressured to diagnose, summarize, and plan at the end of the assessment; it is better to discuss concerns at the symptom level than to share early judgments that may be incorrect. For example, a nurse might say, "We've talked about a number of things; while you're thinking about anything we've missed, I'll just look over what we've talked about." Or, when data are missing or time is needed to formulate a problem, an expression of interest and concern may be sufficient, such as, "You've mentioned a number of things; I think you can work out some solutions if we talk more about them later" or, "Let's both think about what might be causing your family to react this way."

The message behind these examples is that after assessment, clients should:

1. Perceive that something will be done with the information that has been shared
2. Have a feeling of future self-competency in handling any identified problems with (or without) assistance from the nurse.

Basically, what is being described is a sharing of interest, concern, and understanding—the nurse offers the caring response even before the actual care plan has been designed.

In summary, we have focused on how informa-

Table 7-1 Example of Termination of an Initial Assessment

Interaction		Purpose
Nurse:	You've mentioned a few things that we can help you with while you're in the hospital. Is there anything we haven't talked about that is of concern to you?	Give cues that summarization is forthcoming.
Client:	No, I can't think of anything; the worst thing is not being able to control my urine when I can't find a bathroom quickly.	
Nurse:	That can be troublesome; there are ways to manage that, and we'll also have to see what ideas the doctor may have. Is that something that will be troublesome now?	Summarization and plans for the concerns that have been expressed. (Notice that in summarization the actual diagnostic labels need not be used.)
Client:	Oh, no, the bathroom is right here and I have a bedpan in my table.	
Nurse:	You mentioned wanting to lose weight; that's another thing we can work on after your surgery. It seems your diet and fluid intake have been good. Also, you mentioned bowel movements have been regular in the past week. All these things are important for healing after surgery. Your concern about the surgery is something we'll want to talk about after lunch. I've got some ideas that might help you control what happens. This afternoon we'll go over how you can manage things like discomfort and how to prevent other problems with particular exercises. Read the little booklet; if your daughter comes in this afternoon, should we include her?	Summarization and plans for expressed concerns. (Notice that for some diagnoses the nursing care will not be started until after surgery.) Leave client with feeling of ability to cope with problems or concerns identified. Preoperative preparation plans and plans to discuss anxiety response further.
Client:	Oh, yes, she would like to know all about it too.	
Nurse:	Good. See you around 2:30. Enjoy your lunch.	

tion is collected in the admission assessment. Various terms are used to refer to this activity, including *assessment* and *data collection* and/or the *admission nursing history and examination.* A history is obtained by interview; an examination requires observation and other techniques. These techniques were described briefly and will be discussed in later chapters.

Both clients and nurses have expectations during the initial assessment. The nurse seeks information to describe and explain clients' functional health patterns. Clients expect to learn the meaning of their symptoms or to be reassured about their health and health practices. In addition to understanding the interpretations of their physiolog-

ical symptoms, clients wish to know the meaning of symptoms relative to the human functions they engage in day by day. These functions are the focus of nursing, and assessment begins the process of nursing. The client may need to be told why nurses wish particular information so that the purpose of the interview is clear.

We now consider other types of assessment with other objectives.

PROBLEM-FOCUSED ASSESSMENT

Problem-focused assessment involves collecting information on the critical defining characteristics of a previously diagnosed problem. It is used after diagnoses have been made and treatment has been initiated. It might be assumed that diagnoses are made, care is planned and carried out, problems are resolved, and outcomes of care are evaluated. This sequence, proceeding so neatly through time, is the "textbook picture" of clinical practice. In reality, people change, unexpected events occur, and diagnoses are added, deleted, or revised. When a treatment plan is implemented, the expectation is that the client's health problems will begin to resolve. To know whether or not the treatment is effective, the status of the problem is periodically assessed; this type of assessment is problem focused.

Purpose and scope

The purpose of a problem-focused assessment is to evaluate the *presence or absence of a particular diagnosis.* The scope of data collection is narrower than that in an initial assessment of a new client and, naturally, a problem-focused assessment requires less time. As described below, guidelines for information collection are based on the previously made diagnosis. The anticipation of new problems and alertness to discover missed problems or misdiagnoses accompanies this type of assessment.

Probability of health problems

As the name implies, in problem-focused assessment a health problem is assumed to exist when information collection begins. *The hypothesis that a dysfunctional health pattern exists is more likely than the hypothesis that no dysfunctional health pattern exists.* The question pursued is, Does the problem exist now, and, if so, what is the status of the problem?

The assessment task is more structured relative to the other types of assessment already described.

Structure for information collection

The structural context in problem-focused assessment differs from that of an initial assessment. Change has occurred in the interpersonal dimension; the nurse and client are no longer strangers to each other. Whereas in the first encounter trust, confidence, and rapport had to be built, successive encounters focus on extending and maintaining

them. In addition, in the admission assessment, the setting was structured to promote the sharing of information in a relaxed manner. In problem-focused assessment, the nurse is more likely to interweave assessment and care activities such as teaching, bathing, or treatment. It is still important to exercise judgment regarding the client's privacy and whether care activities are a source of distraction.

Information collection may be structured by using the assessment parameters of the problem. These parameters are derived from the defining characteristics described in manuals.[11] For example, consider the diagnosis Self-Bathing Hygiene Deficit Related to Activity Intolerance (Level III), which means the person's tolerance is quite low. Transforming the major characteristics of this diagnosis into assessment parameters is easy. During problem-focused assessment, information is collected on the following assessment parameters:

1. Ability to get to water source
2. Ability to regulate water source
3. Ability to wash upper and lower body
4. Verbal report of ease of breathing before and after bathing/hygiene
5. Heart rate and rhythm before and after bathing/hygiene
6. Use of energy conservation measures in bathing/hygiene

Parameters 3, 4, and 5 are assessed in every client with this diagnosis. If the client is known to walk to the bathroom without Activity Intolerance and has sufficient strength and coordination to turn on the faucets in a shower, then items 1 and 2 are deleted. If problem-focused assessment reveals no change in the bathing/hygiene deficit, assessment of item 6 is necessary.

Lack of improvement may indicate that the person is not using energy-conservation measures. Interventions are directed toward teaching the client both general energy-conservation techniques and those particularly related to bathing and hygiene. Therefore this assessment parameter provides a check on the effectiveness of the nursing intervention and a possible explanation of why there has been no change in items 3 to 5.

How often is a problem assessed after treatment has begun? This depends on the diagnosis and the time predicted for a treatment response. For example, the status of a client's Self-Esteem Disturbance may be checked daily. Yet a daily check may be too infrequent for a diagnosis of Severe Anxiety or High Risk for Violence, which perhaps should be checked every 15 minutes. Problem-focused assessment is multipurpose; it can reveal:

1. The validation or lack of validation of the original diagnosis and etiological factors (a recheck of diagnostic accuracy)
2. Changing levels of acuity, severity, or function that necessitate revision of the diagnosis
3. The progress of a problem toward resolution (outcome attainment)
4. The effectiveness of the treatment plan

EMERGENCY ASSESSMENT

When a client is admitted to a critical care unit, enters the emergency room, or has a life-threatening episode in any setting, emergency assessment is indicated. This must be done within seconds in order to institute immediate treatment.

Purpose and scope

A life-threatening emergency is always expressed, however subtly, in all functional patterns. Yet to determine that an emergency exists, only a few pattern indicators need to be assessed. The purpose of assessment is to:

1. Identify the situation as either an emergency or a nonemergency
2. Determine the nature of the emergency quickly
3. Intervene quickly

Although probably with little conscious recognition, a nurse scans for certain overt, perceptible cues every time she or he has an interaction with the client. This scan take approximately 2 to 7 seconds and is done in a particular order. For example, a primary scan of three indicators of change in metabolic and activity patterns (skin color, posture, and facial expression) provides a wealth of information on the client's heart-lung-brain complex in less than a second. Additional information, if indicated, includes the radial or apical pulse and feeling for the passage of air at the mouth. This information dictates whether further emergency assessment is needed.

The preliminary scan of skin, posture, and face is usually done while the client is being questioned. A verbal or even a nonverbal response may indicate changes in the client's cognitive-perceptual pattern. Environmental factors are often of major importance in the assessment. For example, if a person in a restaurant develops an inability to breathe, panics, and has a bluish cast to the skin, a "cafe coronary" may be suspected (acute strangulation from the aspiration of incompletely chewed food).

Certain crises in the life of a person, group, or community also require emergency assessment. For example, psychotic breakdown and a high risk for suicide or violence are crises requiring immediate assessment, diagnosis, and intervention. Indicators of critical changes in self-concept (which may lead to suicide) or relationship patterns (which may result in violence) are cues to whether or not a crisis exists. In community health practice, emergency assessment may be required on the rare occasions of impending mob violence, riot, epidemics, or natural disasters.

Probability of health problems: emergency assessment

Obviously, in an emergency admission of a client or in an emergency in the community, *the hypothesis of an acute dysfunctional change in a pattern is more likely than the hypothesis that no acute change has occurred*. The question is, What is the nature of the dysfunction?

Structure for information collection

Emergency assessment differs from other assessments.[12] Both the time between observation and action and the purpose of intervention are different. In emergency assessment the life-threatening "diagnosis" is usually identified as a cluster of signs and symptoms. Immediate action and thoughts about cause are simultaneous. The purpose is to preserve life. Consequently, emergency assessment may not impose as high a cognitive demand as other types of assessment. Yet emotional and situational demands may be high. Also the need for swift decisions and actions contributes to the overall perception of the situation. Human life is valued. This value contributes to the heightened emotional state of care providers when a life-threatening emergency occurs.

TIME-LAPSE REASSESSMENT

In this type of assessment the length of time since a previous assessment may be considerable. Three, six, twelve, or more months may have elapsed since the last clinic visit or since the last health status review in a residential center. The client's functional patterns and situation may have changed. Natural growth, health management practices, or long-term care can have demonstrable effects over time. Equally possible, nonproductive patterns may have emerged because of health practices or situational factors.

Purpose and scope

The basic purpose of a time-lapse reassessment is to evaluate changes in the client's functional patterns. It is similar to the problem-focused assessment in that the current status of previous problems is reviewed. Depending on the time lapse, new patterns may have emerged and require assessment; accordingly, a total screening of all patterns is done in somewhat less depth than the initial assessment. If problems are perceived, it may be necessary to elicit an in-depth history of events since the last evaluation.

Probability of health problems

When a client has not been seen for a few months, it is difficult to predict problems with any certainty before information has been collected.

The preencounter hypothesis, either that a dysfunctional change has occurred or that none has occurred, is influenced by previous knowledge of the client. The question is: Has change occurred over time, and, if so, what is its direction?

Structure for information collection

Time-lapse reassessment is common in the follow-up of clients in ambulatory care settings and in periodic assessment in residential facilities, long-term care facilities, long-term home care, and school and industrial nursing. Situational factors play a similar role in this type of assessment as in the other types of assessment discussed above. The information load and cognitive strain vary with the complexity of changes in the client's health status over time.

SUMMARY OF SITUATIONAL CONTEXT FOR ASSESSMENT

As this discussion has indicated, the structure of the assessment situation differs according to the possibility that problems are present and to the questions directing the assessment. The differences among the four types of assessments are shown in Table 7-2. This table suggests that it is important to know the purpose of assessment so that assessment procedures can be structured to obtain valid and reliable data. The section "Nature of Clinical Information" (below) should further expand the notion of just how valid and reliable data can be. Additionally, it will become evident that the nature of the information influences how it is collected.

Nature of clinical information

This section focuses on the specific nature of clinical information and how its characteristics can influence the accuracy of health assessments and diagnostic judgments. During an admission assessment a large number of cues to the health status of a client are collected. The word *cue* is defined as "a piece of information that influences decisions." Among the decisions made in assessment are whether to collect more information, diagnose a dysfunctional pattern, or judge if a pattern is functional. Cues are the "building blocks"[13] or "raw data" used to understand health patterns. Many difficulties may be avoided by understanding the nature of clinical cues and how to use them.

Psychologists classify judgment tasks on the basis of the number and complexity of the cues involved and whether or not the judgment task is structured or unstructured. Clinical judgment within an admission assessment ranks high in both the lack of structure, the amount of information to be processed, and the complexity of the information. For example, in clinical diagnosis cues have multiple values, only some of which are signifi-

Table 7-2 Comparison of the Four Assessment Situations and Their Structural Influences

Assessment situation	Preencounter probabilities	Questions directing the assessment	Structure of the environment
Initial (admission) assessment	The hypothesis of no dysfunctional pattern is as probable as the hypothesis that dysfunctional patterns exist	Does a problem (dysfunctional pattern) exist?	Establish a setting for obtaining accurate data (lighting, quiet, etc.) Establish an interpersonal atmosphere conducive to sharing thoughts, feelings, beliefs
Problem-focused assessment	The hypothesis of a dysfunctional pattern is more likely than the hypothesis that no dysfunctional pattern exists	Does the problem exist today? If so, what is the status of the problem?	Extend and maintain an interpersonal atmosphere conducive to sharing thoughts, feelings, beliefs
Emergency assessment (client classified by instantaneous perception of life-threatening cues)	The hypothesis of an acute, dysfunctional change in a pattern is more likely than the hypothesis that no acute change has occurred	What is the nature of the dysfunction?	Establish a setting for obtaining data quickly and for immediate life-sustaining action
Time-lapse reassessment	The hypothesis that no dysfunctional change has occurred or that dysfunctional change has occurred is influenced by previous knowledge of the client	Has change occurred over time? If so, what is its direction?	Establish a setting for obtaining accurate data (lighting, quiet, etc.) Reestablish interpersonal atmosphere conducive to sharing thoughts, feelings, beliefs

cant. The values take on different meaning when occurring alone or in combination with other cues. Consider the following situations:

Situation 1.   Increased heart rate of 20 beats/min when client transfers from bed to chair

Situation 2.   Increased heart rate of 20 beats/min 4 hours after cholecystectomy (gallbladder removal)

A person-characteristic, such as heart rate, may take on multiple values; only those within a narrow range are compatible with life. Also the values within this range take on different meanings when viewed in the context of other cues. In both examples above the heart rate has increased 20 beats, a cause for concern in any context. The meaning of the increase in Situation 1 is probably Activity Intolerance, but in Situation 2 the meaning of the increase is possibly hemorrhagic shock.

Generally, clinical cues to a nursing or medical diagnosis are *probabilistic*, which means they are not perfectly dependable indicators of a person's actual health state or process. Because of the nature of the available information, clinicians must deal with uncertainty-geared judgments. Collecting more and more information when that information is not 100% dependable does not increase the accuracy of judgment. It is the quality of the information, not the quantity, that is important in diagnosis or even in everyday uncertainty-geared judgments. Consider some of the characteristics of the information used in clinical judgment:

Valid-invalid
Reliable-unreliable
Relevant-irrelevant
Diagnostic-supporting
Subjective-objective
Historical-current
State-contextual

Each of these characteristics influences how data are used in making accurate diagnoses; they are discussed in this section.

If the list of characteristics seems overwhelming, be assured that most human beings already have an intuitive grasp of each of them. For example, early in life we learn to make the judgment of when it is safe to cross a busy street. The judgment is probabilistic, that is, uncertainty-geared. A probability exists that one or more drivers will not stop for a red light. The light itself is a cue that can take on multiple values (red, green, yellow), each of which has meaning. We learn that the speed of the car approaching a traffic light is relevant data, although it is a subjective rather than an objective cue. Sometimes information is available about how many accidents have occurred at a particular crosswalk (historical data), but the most valid diagnostic cue to safety is that at the moment of crossing the street, all cars have stopped. (Yet there is still the chance that a car will start up because of an irrational driver.) Supporting data help if this possibility occurs to us; looking at the driver's face as we cross provides some contextual data, such as a "behavior reading." No cue is perfectly dependable (reliable), but in combination they do increase the probability of making an accurate judgment about when it is safe to cross.

Good judgments are based on good data, and valid and reliable cues are valued as "good" data. Below are some important points about the information collected in a functional health pattern assessment (a more extensive discussion and more clinical examples are found in Appendix J):

1. A cue is valid if it represents the properties of the entity being judged. For example, the description of food and fluid intake represents one property of a nutritional-metabolic pattern; thus it is one piece of information that is valid for making a judgment about this pattern.

2. Information is reliable if it is (1) a dependable indicator of a functional pattern or of a diagnosis and (2) obtained through accurate measurement. Crying is not a reliable indicator of fear because it occurs for many reasons; for example, joy or sadness.

3. The terms *relevant* and *irrelevant* are used frequently to pertain to validity. The relevance of a cue depends on the purpose of the information collection, such as health status evaluation. Specific information about the essential properties of each pattern is considered relevant data. For example, what the client eats in a typical day is information relevant to the nutritional pattern.

4. Diagnostic cues, or criteria, are the critical characteristics of a diagnostic category. They must be present if the diagnostic label is used because they coincide with the formal definition of the category. For example, when a client repeatedly verbalizes negative feelings about an actual or perceived change in the structure or function of his or her body or body part, this provides a diagnostic cue to body image disturbance. Other cues may be present in the situation, such as anxiety, fear, or hiding/overexposing/ignoring a body part. These are supporting cues that increase the diagnostician's confidence and serve to validate a client's verbal expression of feelings. Supporting cues may be useful but are not highly reliable indicators of a diagnosis.

5. In common use *objective data* refers to care provider observations and laboratory and other tests, whereas *subjective data* refers to perceptions, feelings, and other reports by the client. Subjective data include subjective perceptions and feelings, such as self-concept or pain. In contrast are the so-called objective data the nurse observes, such as skin color, heart rate, or parent-child interaction.

6. To appreciate the distinction between historical and current information, keep in mind that current data come from "the here and now." Historical data may pertain to last night, 2 days ago, or 10 years ago (see the box on p. 136).

CUE CLASSIFICATION

1. *Historical state cues.* Include historical measures of client characteristics, such as previous blood pressure values, appetite, family roles, and body perception. In community assessment, traffic fatalities or cardiovascular death rates in previous years are historical cues.
2. *Current state cues.* Describe current data about attributes of the client, including current blood pressure values, comfort level, activity level, caloric intake, age, laboratory test values, and emotional state. In community assessment current state cues include the number of clinics and health programs or data on the community water system.
3. *Historical contextual cues.* Describe previous values of unchangeable characteristics of the person (birthdate, for example) or situation (tonsillectomy at age 4). In family assessment, past living environment or significant past family events are cues.
4. *Current contextual cues.* Derived from assessment of the client's current situation. For example, assessment usually includes the structure of the interpersonal environment. Is the person a hermit or part of a large, closely structured family network? What are the characteristics of the neighborhood and community, and what health services are available? What are the significant current events in a client's life, such as an episode of physical illness, divorce in progress, or a husband dying at home?

Historical state cues

Historical cues, which describe the state of the person, family, or community, provide an individualized baseline for interpreting the current state. A common example is blood pressure. What does a current value of 105/78 mean? If the value for the past 2 years has been 150/90, the interpretation is different than if the value has consistently been in the 100/70 to 105/80 range. To identify emerging patterns and detect changes, current state cues in combination with historical state baselines are used.

Current state cues

These cues should always be sought before making diagnoses. To determine whether a current change in pattern has been abrupt or gradual, current state cues combined with historical data are used.

Historical contextual cues

This information describes events that have already occurred and are part of one's life history. Not only are they history, they are also the context out of which current functional patterns have evolved. Historical contextual cues (situational context) are helpful in understanding functional patterns but also play an important role in prediction. Research indicates[14,15] that nurses use situational cues to predict the most probable health problems to be assessed. Diagnoses based on historical cues alone may result in errors of historical stereotyping.

Current contextual cues

These cues have two main uses in diagnosis. When examined in context, the meaning of a cue to the state of the person may become clear.

Why bother with a clinical cue classification? Mainly because cognitive operations need some checks and balances. Nurses may develop habits that affect their efficiency and accuracy. Feedback is not always available after a nurse's student days are over. The nurse may fall into a pattern of diagnosing only on the basis of the here and now, which is probably cognitively inefficient (see the discussion of diagnostic strategies). Another habit pattern is diagnosing only on the basis of historical information; this type of diagnosis is close to stereotyping and very risky. Nurses should examine the cues they habitually use so as to provide checks and balances on the needed mixture of historical and current information.

HANDLING UNCERTAIN CUES IN CLINICAL JUDGMENT

As previously mentioned, clinical judgments (diagnostic, therapeutic, and ethical) are uncertainty-geared; there is always a degree of probability, rather than full certainty, in the cue relationships.

The word *probability* means the same as chance. Nursing diagnoses are made at a level of probability, not absolute logical certainty. Sometimes a judgment that "feels certain" is a "psycho-logical" certainty about a level of confidence. This uncertainty stands in contrast to other types of categorizations, or identifications of things, in which information permits an inference with logical certainty. These latter situations are not common in the everyday world or in clinical practice.

From the time a person first notices the surrounding world, he or she learns about probabilities. These probabilities involve whether trains are apt to come on time, the possibility of a good grade or a pay raise, and the chance that a driver will stop at a stop sign. From childhood on, each person works on learning the likelihood of events and *what is a predictor of what.* For example, if an object looks like a book, it probably has printed pages.

The uncertainty-geared nature of nursing practice has been described by Hammond.[16] He argues that client conditions produce different cues, and the same cue may be produced by different conditions. In other words, the cues available for diagnosing a health problem are not always completely reliable. Consider an example: A smile is a cue to friendliness. Let us say that 80% of the time when people are friendly, they smile. On the other hand, smiling may be present 20% of the time when people are really hostile and angry. Smiling does not predict friendliness with 100% certainty. Smiling is a probabilistic cue. If these figures are correct, this cue has only 80% predictive validity. That is, the inference that a person is friendly when he or she smiles is accurate in only 80 out of 100 cases. Dependence on this cue alone results in error in 20 cases out of 100. In the ideal situation cues would be certain; then clinicians could be "sure" of their diagnoses. Yet human behavior is variable, and the ideal probably can never be reached. At least at this point no one can actually "stand in the shoes" of another person and know what the other knows, feels, or believes.

Anxiety is another example. Consider first two people. Inwardly they both feel anxious. Yet they manifest different signs (cues); that is, they express their anxiety differently. Now consider one person who is anxious. This person will not necessarily demonstrate the same signs of anxiety in two different social environments or at two different times. Thus a set of cues may be unreliable in terms of various individuals and also in terms of one individual in different situations and through time.

According to Hammond,[16] clinicians are hard-pressed to point to one set of cues that *always* indicates a diagnosis. Most textbooks reflect this lack of predictability in the way they describe the signs and symptoms of nursing or medical diagnoses. They use words such as "*usually* presents the symptoms of . . . ," "*nearly always* associated with these signs . . . ," or "*frequently* demonstrates an elevated . . ." (italics added). This "hedging" reminds one of the kind of language used in another probabilistic, uncertainty-geared profession—weather forecasting; it has the same built-in uncertainty.

Clinicians generally consider physical cues to be more reliable and valid indicators of a diagnosis than social cues. For example, either redness or blanching over bony prominences of the back is a highly reliable and valid sign of High Risk for Skin Breakdown in white- or yellow-skinned persons. However, signs of Body Image Disturbance are variable between one individual and another; thus they are less reliable predictors of the diagnosis. This difference in the reliability of signs results in a greater feeling of uncertainty in making a diagnosis related to Body Image Disturbance than in making a diagnosis related to the redness and blanching in the first example. To identify the subjective states (feeling states) or self-perceptions of clients, it is critical to obtain verbal reports from the person. Verbal reports increase the clinician's confidence in the diagnosis as well as the validity and reliability of the diagnosis. For example, consider the observable signs of restlessness and facial grimacing combined with a history of abdominal surgery 24 hours previously. One possibility is that the client is having incisional pain. How confident would you be about making this diagnosis from the observable data?

The more knowledge you have about postsurgical care, the *less* confident you will be! These cues are highly uncertain predictors of pain; they do not discriminate among three or four other conditions that are also manifested by restlessness and facial grimacing. Suppose the postoperative client says, "I've tried turning and taking the medicine;

nothing helps the pain." Does this cue increase confidence in the diagnosis of Pain Management Deficit? Yes, it does; now the other cues become supporting cues. When the cues are considered together, confidence is high enough to warrant the diagnostic judgment.

Can doubt always be erased by more information? No—not unless the cue is a more valid and reliable indicator than the information already secured. A verbal report of pain increases the validity of the cues in the example above because pain, by definition, is a subjective state really known only to the client. Note that a verbal report alone is not always sufficient data. Usually both a client's verbal report and observational data indicating the client is in pain are required to reach a level of confidence high enough to warrant giving the client a narcotic. Although feeling pain is a valid indicator, our methods of measuring feelings (assessing the client's subjective report) are not always reliable. Verbal reports are used to measure feelings and may be biased by the conscious or unconscious motives of the person reporting.

In contrast, High Risk for Skin Breakdown is an objective phenomenon. It is not critical that the client confirm the clinician's observation (that the skin is red or blanching). The cues gleaned from the history and examination have a wide range of predictive accuracy. Also, judgments often must be made with limited information and time.

The above considerations are important. Uncertainty-geared judgments are common in nursing and medical diagnosis. Good diagnostic judgments are made on the basis of the most valid and reliable cues that can be acquired in a particular situation. The more valid and reliable the cues, the less uncertainty and the higher confidence the nurse will have in his or her judgments. Of course, the better the diagnostic judgments are, the higher the probability that the care plan devised for the client will be effective.

Whitehorn,[17] commenting on education's role in training people to make uncertainty-geared judgments, states

perhaps the greatest benefit of a liberal education is to escape the tyranny of first impressions and of naive preconceptions—to learn to suspend judgment and action, not indefinitely and vaguely, but long enough and sturdily enough for the orderly review of evidence and the weighing of probabilities and values. . . . Indeed,

one cannot become aware of alternatives without some ability to tolerate uncertainty, and one cannot exercise good judgment and common sense in reaching well considered conclusions and wise action unless one can tolerate uncertainty with equanimity.[17]

Diagnosticians' basic tools

This section focuses on the diagnostician, who can be thought of as a creative user of information and a sensitive measuring device. Thinking of oneself in this way permits some objectivity in examining. Reasoning processes will be used to study reasoning the way cognitive and perceptual processes are used in information collection and analysis.

Cognitive and perceptual abilities are the basic "tools" used in information collection. Nurses have been developing these capabilities since birth. They include:

Perception
Intuition
Inference

In fact, a complex skill used in nursing diagnosis began to develop during infancy. Learning that a toy ball did not cease to exist after rolling behind the chair ushered in the development of inference. Diagnosis requires sharpening cognitive and perceptual abilities and one important additional ingredient, clinical knowledge. The discussion begins with this factor because, as will be clear later, perceptions are based on previously acquired knowledge.

CLINICAL KNOWLEDGE

Knowledge is a necessary but not a sufficient condition for expertise in nursing diagnosis. Expertise also involves the ability to access (memory) and use knowledge in thinking. In this section sources of knowledge are discussed; in Chapter 8, discussion is focused on using knowledge in reasoning and judgment.

What is an adequate knowledge base for nursing diagnosis? It is difficult to say. At a minimum, knowledge of the functional pattern areas described in Chapter 3 is needed for health status evaluation and diagnosis. Below are the specific, necessary areas of knowledge for nursing diagnosis and treatment:

1. The range of norms for the 11 functional health patterns (age norms), including the health patterns/life processes that clients exhibit
2. The natural development of functional patterns during the life-span
3. Variations in patterns related to culture, environment, disease, gender, and other influences
4. Common dysfunctional patterns (nursing diagnoses), including the factors associated with the patterns (etiological or related factors)
5. Indicators of dysfunctional patterns
6. Outcomes that can be achieved and nursing actions that have a high probability of achieving the outcomes.

The practical approach is to gain a working knowledge of the functional patterns and of high-incidence nursing diagnoses and their treatment. It is most important to use the patterns consistently in assessment. Knowledge develops with experience, but the clinician has a responsibility to see that experience contributes to knowledge development. Fulfilling that responsibility takes analysis and reflection; it does not happen automatically. The cognitive and perceptual abilities discussed later in this chapter are the means used to learn about clients; they are also the means used to continually increase and organize clinical knowledge.

Storage of clinical knowledge: memory

Humans retain information for long and short intervals. For example, nurses observe and retain information about a pulse rhythm for a minute (the usual observation period); they remember a telephone number until dialing is completed; and they recall the type of surgery a person had last year. The concepts of short- and long-term memory storage are used to explain remembering and forgetting. They are important ideas in assessment, because lost information can lead to error.

Images, thoughts, and information in a person's current awareness are the contents of short-term memory. Information can be held for seconds or for a minute or more before being stored in long-term memory. A number of interesting explanations have been suggested for how humans store information and what units are stored.[18 (p. 290); 19-22] Some say we recognize familiar patterns with minimal information using "fuzzy traces" that contain the gist or essence of the pattern, event, or idea stored in memory. Others suggest that information is represented in the brain as symbols called schemata, scripts, or frames. Condition-action pairs containing "chunks" of information in the form of "if-then" pairs are used to explain the phenomenon of intuition. Knowledge may be stored in a network of connections among neurons.

Chunking information

Short-term storage is "working memory" and consciousness. It is within this short-term memory that perceptual inference, conceptual thinking, problem solving, and decision making go on in a deliberative, conscious sense. Miller[23] suggests that the human mind can hold only about five to nine separate pieces of information in short-term storage. To overcome this limited memory capacity, "chunking" is used. Pieces of information are put into broader categories, or "chunks," by abstraction. For example, a nurse might use the basic food groups as categories in which to "hold" information as a client recites all the foods eaten in a typical day. Diagnostic concepts are chunks, or clusters, of signs and symptoms. Chunking may also explain how configurations or clusters of cues are stored in memory until activated during an intuitive insight.

Chunking prevents overload. Without chunking, pertinent pieces of information may be lost. In clinical situations the nurse must hold information in short-term memory storage until it can be recorded, processed in decision making, or understood by being compared with other past experiences retrieved from long-term memory.

If short-term memory images are lost within seconds, how does a nurse remember a pulse rate or rhythm? Indeed, how does anyone remember the last numbers of a 7- to 10-digit telephone number after dialing the first few digits? "Rehearsing" information, such as repeating a telephone number, decreases the rate at which memory of the digits and their sequence are lost. Yet if similar information, such as other numbers, enters the short-term store, forgetting occurs.[21] This is a common event everyone has experienced.

The transfer of information to long-term memory storage explains humans' ability to remember after lengthy time lapses. Long-term recall partially depends on the intentional rehearsal of the information to be remembered. (What is thought to occur in rehearsal is that neurons maintain reverberating circuits or that synapses undergo some type of structural or functional change.) In addition to intentional rehearsal, constant thinking or rumination about an event can firmly establish its memory. Note taking can also assist memory.

Note taking

New information may cause prior information to be lost if its rehearsal is interrupted. This process should be taken into account when a nursing history and examination data are being collected. Among the inventions that compensate for the limited human capacity to hold information in consciousness are pencil and paper!

Some nurses do not take notes during a history and examination. This may give the client the impression that the information he or she is providing is not important enough to write down. In addition, research findings suggest that retaining continuous information over a period of even 20 minutes is highly unlikely.[21] A period of 5 to 10 minutes is necessary for minimal consolidation in long-term memory and an hour or more for maximum consolidation.[24]

Organization and access

Another important point relevant to assessment is that remembering and forgetting seem to be influenced by information coding. Experiments have demonstrated that the ability to remember (to recall memories from long-term storage) depends on (1) the way in which the information was rehearsed and stored and (2) the retrieval probe used.[21]

Some nurses must retrieve nursing knowledge by using a disease category probe because their clinical knowledge was originally learned and stored that way. This cognitive organization around disease categories would facilitate practice if nursing comprised only disease-related care. Person-focused nursing requires knowledge to be organized within categories that describe any human being, with or without disease. The 11 functional pattern areas are an example of such organization. In long-term memory these areas are then "cross-referenced" with likely dysfunctional patterns and diseases. This method of categorization enables the nurse to organize nursing knowledge *and* medical knowledge and to integrate the two classes of information. A retrieval probe can retrieve all three bodies of knowledge (nursing, medical, and integrated) if the situation warrants. If the client is seen only for health promotion, a disease-oriented probe is not necessary to retrieve clinical knowledge of functional patterns.

The idea of memory probes and long-term memory retrieval may also be applied to assessment. Suppose one wished to get rid of those pages and pages of an assessment tool that defy memorization. Assessment items might be coded in memory under the 11 functional pattern areas. For example, a nurse learns (that is, places in long-term storage) the areas to be assessed in the nutritional-metabolic pattern (Appendix H). The specific data in each area could be retrieved and used to guide questions and observations during history taking and examination. The nurse might list relevant items on a small sheet of paper until the learning process was complete.

A set of categories, such as the functional health patterns, serve as advanced organizers for storing specific items of information. Advanced organizers are "ideational scaffolding" for the retention of details.[25] The payoff in this type of cognitive organization lies in the ease of retrieval; the succinct list of patterns may be used as quick probes for the data to be collected in each area. The key to any memory retrieval is an appropriate "search set." The key to learning is to organize and categorize details in ways meaningful for clinical practice.

PERCEPTUAL RECOGNITION

Attaching a name to a sensory event is an act of perceptual recognition and categorization. The process of recognition and categorization is evident in statements such as, "The new patient is a male" or, "His skin is warm." *Male* and *warm* are examples of concrete perceptual inferences and concrete identity categorizations. In a particular situation these kinds of perceptions may be cues to a diagnosis if the nurse uses them to go beyond mere recognition. Vast amounts of information impinge on the nurse's sense organs at any given moment. Recognition involves coding and making an inference about identity. Coding a sensory experience makes it possible to categorize it—to say, for example, that *this* is a textbook and *that* is a novel.

Sensitive observers recognize things and their meaning. There are three major requirements for becoming a sensitive observer:

1. Have *categories* available for coding relevant sensory data so that the identity and meaning of what is observed may be determined (clinical knowledge base).
2. *Anticipate,* or look for, cues on the basis of the knowledge that certain client behaviors are likely in particular situations.
3. Focus *attention* so that sensory data are not missed.

These three factors influence perceptual sensitivity to cues, prevent cues being missed, and subsequently influence the accuracy of diagnostic judgments.

Categories

A category may be a detailed discrimination (mottled skin) or a global representation ("poor" skin color). The choice of a category is determined by the interests and needs of each person and, basically, by past interactions with the environment. For example, English teachers pay close attention to grammar and sentence structure. They have categories for coding auditory or visual data about grammatical errors, such as dangling participles. When compared with nurses, English teachers may fare poorly in perceiving and categorizing heart rhythms or nonverbal messages. They lack discriminating categories and category systems in these areas. Many sophisticated discriminations are required in nursing. For example, nurses learn to discriminate among at least nine changes in skin color: jaundice, mottling, flushing, bronzing, sallowness, ashenness, glossiness, pallor, and cyanosis.

The mention of categories may give rise to the assumption that clients are being pigeon-holed. Some nurses may do this, but generally diagnoses are not used as negative stereotypes. Categorization is a basic aspect of human cognition. Without categories there would be no perceptual experience or higher levels of conceptual activities.[8,26] Categorization helps a person learn to respond to things judged as similar (things in the same category). When skin is categorized as mottled, nurses derive certain meanings from this perception. A different meaning is derived when sensory data are put into another category; for example, sallow skin.

Ways of representing the perceptual world of nursing practice are learned primarily from others. Descriptions, names for things, and meanings are part of nursing's "cultural heritage." During learning, images are constructed and stored in memory. Think for a minute; conjure up an image of a thermometer. Describe it. Presumably the reader does not have one handy; thus some mental image from past learning must be scanned. Images are also referred to as categories.[27] They are representations of entities that are stored in memory from past interactions with the world. In fact, categories and their interrelations are each individual's personal descriptions of their world. If, when verbalized, they are not reasonably congruent with other people's descriptions, the discrepancy is called madness or creativity!

Much of nursing education involves learning to use categories. The nurse learns to do the following:

1. Isolate important data and categorize observations
2. Work with the descriptive labels used in health care
3. Recognize relationships among categories
4. Plan treatment for the problems that are categorized

Most important, by learning to categorize the nurse is able to order and relate one thing to another, such as one cue to another, clusters of cues to a diagnosis, and then diagnosis to treatment to outcome. Categorization also permits anticipation of things not immediately observable.[28]

Anticipation

Sensitive observers see not only the very obvious and apparent things but also the not-so-apparent. They anticipate and predict. *Sensitivity* is a term used frequently in nursing. Clients use it in the context of "such a sensitive nurse." It is enhanced by empathy, clinical knowledge, and a sincere interest in people. It appears that sensitivity is highly valued in a nurse, because people rarely confront each other directly with accusations of insensitivity to others.

Perceptual sensitivity to client behavior depends in part on anticipation of behavior. If a particular behavior is anticipated, the nurse needs less information for coding sensory input, because categories and relationships are more accessible in memory.[29] A knowledge of the likelihood of events permits anticipation and perceptual readiness. Perception is accurate as long as what is expected corresponds to the frequency of events in reality.

An example may further clarify how anticipation increases perceptual sensitivity: Suppose a nurse knows that 3 days of bed rest can produce muscle weakness. When a client begins to get out of bed after confinement, a slight buckling of one knee may be enough to identify the possibility of muscle weakness due to bedrest. Lacking the background knowledge of the expected likelihood of muscle weakness, another nurse might miss the relatively subtle cue of the buckling knee, and the client might not be supervised as he or she begins ambulation. An impressive cue, such as falling, might be necessary.

Focused attention

In addition to having categories for coding sensory inputs and a knowledge of the likelihood of events, sensitive observers are able to focus their attention. People have the capacity to direct their attention selectively to particular aspects of their environment. The functional advantage of focused attention is that one is more apt to "see" what is important relative to the goal of the moment; distraction by extraneous stimuli is reduced. This selectivity may be lifesaving in crossing a busy street and advantageous in looking for a friend in a crowd.

During a health pattern assessment, focusing his or her attention increases the nurse's sensitivity to relevant information. For example, the functional health patterns previously discussed focus the nurse's attention on 11 areas of health-related behavior that are relevant to nursing. This focus enhances the nurse's readiness to perceive cues to these patterns.

In summary, unless appropriate categories and category systems are available for coding sensory events, perception may be delayed or inaccurate.

The inability to place sensory input into an appropriate category results in a "long, close look." This prolonged observation is common in the child or adult who pauses to stare at something of interest that cannot be immediately categorized. Learning, asking questions, and curiosity increase the availability of categories. In contrast, ignoring observations or events that cannot be classified or understood inhibits learning and may lead to diagnostic error.

Various causes of nurses' failure to recognize cues have been identified.[30] These causes and recommendations for preventing such failures are listed below.

1. Lack of categories in memory (for example, lack of clinical knowledge). Study and memorize the words used in textbooks to describe client behaviors and health problems.
2. Lack of training in discrimination (for example, discrimination of skin color changes or between fear and anxiety). Seek opportunities in clinical practice for discriminating among levels of a cue and differentiating one diagnosis from another.
3. Blocks to the retrieval of categories when needed because of fatigue or emotional upset. Avoid fatigue or emotional upset.
4. Expecting too exact a degree of fit between sensory data (cues) and categories in memory or accepting too gross a fit (insufficient data). Discuss observations and diagnoses with instructors or clinical specialists to get their feedback. Learn to grasp the subtle differences in cues among clients with the same diagnosis; seek repeated experiences (same diagnosis, different clients).
5. Lack of precise criteria for recognition (the category in memory has not been or cannot be precisely defined by observable data). Learn the criteria for recognizing cues to diagnoses.

Everyone has experienced the failure to recognize something because of the reasons listed above. In clinical practice steps must be taken to reduce the causes of such failure to a minimum. If the recognition of cues depends on stored representations of the world and their retrieval from memory, several questions arise: How is this information used in judgment? What are the "basic tools" used in making clinical judgments? Problem identification and problem solving employ perception and recognition. Beyond the information given by perception is inference. Human beings infer the meaning of things they perceive. Drawing meaning from cues is an important part of the diagnostic process.

GOING BEYOND THE INFORMATION GIVEN

The previous discussion emphasized perceptual recognition. In uncertainty-geared clinical judgment the data of perception may be ambiguous or incomplete, and the human tendency is to hypothesize and predict. Human beings go beyond the information given by their senses. They "complete the picture," extend the "picture," synthesize a "picture," or create a "picture." Nurses go beyond the information given to make inferences at different levels of complexity:

1. *Inferences about behavior* (sadness)
2. *Inferences about a problem/diagnosis* (powerlessness, nutritional deficit)
3. *Inferences about the dynamics* of a life situation or pattern

Inferences about the dynamics of client-environment interaction involve creating a picture, case dynamics, or map that encompasses all diagnoses, strengths, interrelationships, dimensions, and dynamics. These complex inferences are used in working with an individual, family, or community over time.

Inference is used in nursing judgments. Diagnoses are inferences; for example, on the basis of a cluster of cues a nurse may infer that a person is coping with job stress ineffectively. Nursing interventions are based on conditional inferences of the "if-then" type. For example, a nurse may infer that *if* attachment enhancement activities are used, *then* the parents of a premature baby may strengthen their attachment to their new baby.

Going beyond the information given to make inferences may be associated with errors or may be highly accurate impressions and creative solutions. Thus it is important to understand what is known, or surmised, about how human beings go beyond the information given in assessment.

Although the literature related to the study of human judgment has serious gaps, most researchers agree that human beings are capable of performing many types of cognitive tasks and using many thinking modes, some of which are probably not yet identified. Two ways of knowing that have been discussed in relation to clinical judgment and decision making in nursing are analytical inference and intuitive inference.

Analytical inference

Analytical inference is the understanding that results from a process of reasoning and analysis. It is sometimes viewed as a "clinical adaptation" of formal logic involved in induction and deduction.[31] Others have proposed higher-level dialectic operations that are characteristic of adult thought.[32] Those who subscribe to this school of thought would say that clinical reasoning is an interpretive rather than a deductive process.[33] The diagnostic process is usually defined within an analytical model, although this may be an oversimplification. Reasoning within the nursing process has been described as linear; that is, a step-by-step process. This is a questionable description given the inherent complexity of the nursing process.

Clinical inference has been described as deliberate, conscious reasoning leading from observations to a judgment. The judgment represents a grasp or understanding of the health problem. Reasoning is based on rules that specify the relationships among cues. At a simple level a student may learn that there are four indicators of High Risk for Pressure Ulcer. Before making the diagnosis the presence or absence of each critical indicator is confirmed. Otherwise the nurse may learn the propositional rule that not turning (change in position) a patient with impaired bed mobility every 1½ hours will result in compression of the capillaries over the bony prominences and deprivation of glucose and oxygen to the cells, which in turn will lead to tissue necrosis, a condition called pressure ulcer.

As the nurse builds a network of propositional rules, he or she begins to associate Pressure Ulcer with stages, complaints of pain, and images of decaying tissue, difficulty in healing, perhaps death and the associated negative feelings. Eventually these concepts form a chunk of information in memory and may be accessed in various ways. As seen in Fig. 7-1, the core of the chunk may be accessed by indirect cues, such as the client's decreased level of consciousness. The conscious analysis of data allows thinking to be made public

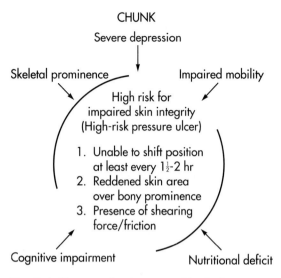

CHUNK

Severe depression

Skeletal prominence — Impaired mobility

High risk for
impaired skin integrity
(High-risk pressure ulcer)

1. Unable to shift position
   at least every 1½-2 hr
2. Reddened skin area
   over bony prominence
3. Presence of shearing
   force/friction

Cognitive impairment   Nutritional deficit

Fig. 7-1. Memory chunk accessed by indirect cues.

and affords an opportunity to learn and to correct errors. Analytical reasoning takes more time than other methods because it is careful and systematic.

It is misleading to think of analytical reasoning and intuition as a dualism; that is, two different or opposing ways of arriving at a clinical judgment. "Although intuition is the final fruit of skill acquisition, analytic thinking is necessary for beginners learning a new skill. It is also useful at the highest levels of expertise, where it can sharpen and clarify intuitive insights."[34] (p. xiv) This thinking is consistent with the views of Rew[35] and Benner[36] in nursing. The process of analytical inference or judgment within the context of diagnostic reasoning is discussed in Chapter 8. From that discussion, it will be clear that analytical reasoning must be followed by a synthesis that affords a grasp of the whole client-situation.

Intuitive inference

Intuition is also experienced as a grasp or an understanding of the whole client situation but in contrast to analytical inference it "occurs in a brief interval of time without detectable, explicit reasoning."[25] (p. 242) Intuition is going straight to the heart of a problem versus trudging toward a solution step by step. Intuition is holistic processing that results in an immediate, uncritical per-

ception of the whole rather than the parts.[37,38] This immediate apprehension results in insight that includes seeing into the inner or hidden nature of the client situation and provides a deeper understanding. It is grasping "what is crucial in any given problem and why it is crucial."[39] (p. 19) It can result in a grasp of the spirit or essence of the person.[40] According to the classical intuitionists we know the "ultimate reality" through intuition. Perhaps it is intuitive knowing that is the basis for beliefs about the dignity of human beings. In this way intuition relates to the art of nursing and the philosophy of caring that permeates many nurses' practice. Leininger[41] comments that nursing both refutes intuition and covertly uses it in practice.

Intuition is also a way of grasping the situation of particular patients, such as the client who is "going bad" or "the fighter," the baby who will survive its extremely low birth weight. When nurses know their clients well, they are able to pick up subtle changes in the client's behavior but must struggle to communicate exactly what they are detecting. This process is not to be confused with extrasensory perception; rather it reflects the nurse's familiarity with the client's life world; the nurse is able to take the client's perspective. In some clinical judgments, intuitive inference probably predominates, especially when the cues are ambiguous and uncertain.

Experienced clinicians report having more intuitive experiences than do novices. For example, in nursing homes where powerlessness is a frequent diagnosis, five indicators form the "picture." This condition is viewed as highly likely to occur in this patient population (e.g., the base rate occurrence). After making 50 to 100 diagnoses of this condition, a nurse needs only one or two cues (not five) to quickly generate the possibility of a diagnosis of powerlessness and all that it means for the client; absolutely no deliberation is needed at all. A nurse specializing in gynecology nursing would probably not think of this problem. Intuition depends on familiarity with a client population and expertise. It is important to discriminate between imagination and intuition; clinicians have to be clear on the difference. An intuitive grasp should be treated as a likely possibility to be investigated, not as truth, especially when outcomes are critical. Devine and Sherman[26] (p. 154) suggest that

Humans do engage in quick, intuitive decision making. We use simple heuristic principles, and we automatically and quickly process information in certain ways. . . . Heuristics often and typically lead to a correct (or in the ball-park) decision. More important, they save a tremendous amount of time and energy in decision making. So it is not the use of quick-and-dirty heuristic and intuitive judgments that is the problem. It is the overuse and misuse of such principles. . . . The key issue, it seems to us, is when to use heuristic and intutitive processes of judgment and when not to.

Devine and Sherman go on to say that the value of intuition lies only in its quickness and express their concern about the stereotyping that is possible with quick intuitive judgments. Stereotyping has been shown to influence the interpretation of ambiguous behavior."[26] In some cases ambiguity can be reduced by further assessment and involvement in the client situation, thus avoiding stereotypic categories.

In addition to intuitions about conditions and actions, people can make holistic inferences about another's feelings, desires, or experiences. This intuitive capability is called *empathy*. Intuitions of this type are based on a shared human understanding of common experiences. For example, nearly all human beings have lost something or someone they loved and can "appreciate" the sadness that results when this happens. Nurses use empathy to anticipate. Anticipation increases sensitivity to cues and motivates the nurse to assess further based on the possibility that the person is experiencing sadness, grief, or tension.

Empathy also influences the way an intervention is carried out. The nurse thinks: "If I had a large cut through my abdomen . . . it would be very painful for me to sit up and get out of bed." This leads to an appreciation of how the patient feels; to gentleness; and to compassionate, supportive comments while helping the patient out of bed.

Research demonstrates that empathetic intuitions are generally accurate if there are shared backgrounds and experiences, or in the case of nurses, if they have learned vicariously through study. As with other intuitive inferences, empathetic intuitions are used as hypotheses to guide assessment, not as facts. Empathy probably occurs in conjunction with perception and reasoning or has a cognitive dimension. It is difficult to imagine "standing in the shoes" of another without any information about the current context of the other's life. Many times the cues used are nonverbal, such as observing another person's face, tilt of the head, body posture, and movements of arms or legs.

The use of empathy is similar to sharing the perspective or taking the viewpoint of another person that is usually discussed in regard to moral reasoning. Empathetic intuitions lie somewhere between analytical and nonanalytical reasoning and are usually classified as social perception or person perception.

Affective reactions, or feelings and preferences, also denote the apprehension of a whole; in this case the whole personality of another. They are "gut reactions" perceived as feelings, the source of which is difficult to communicate verbally. One author[42] surmises that feelings are learned as a child in the prelinguistic stage of development and therefore there are no extensive and precise words that can be used to communicate feelings.

Nurses are sometimes told to "deal with their feelings" toward clients, not to "jump to conclusions," and to avoid stereotypes in their first impressions. From a more positive viewpoint, be aware that usually it is the lack of information that encourages completing the picture with one's own ideas and assumptions. Assess client's health patterns carefully and reflect on any negative feelings toward and stereotypical impressions of their clients, which might interfere with their nursing care. Nursing research is just beginning to demonstrate that "knowing the patient" is a factor in intervention.[43,44]

INTUITION, ANALYTICAL THINKING, OR BOTH?

There is discussion in the literature about whether analytical or nonanalytical (intuitive) modes best describe human beings' judgments and decisions. There has been a deeply embedded traditional dualism in the way people think: women are supposed to use intuition and men are supposed to use logical, analytical reasoning. Whereas Descartes said, "I think, therefore I am," today many say, "I feel, therefore I am." Implied in the latter is the complete rejection of reasoning; there is no room for open discussion because intuition cannot be challenged—its basis cannot be explained and its validity is based on the authority of the person. It "requires the linear mode to clarify and communicate that which is understood."[45]

In nursing practice both analytical and intuitive inferences are probably used. In general, most thinking in complex situations is neither purely intuitive nor purely analytical.[20] Hammond's cognitive continuum theory[46,47] suggests that some types of clinical judgments may induce either analytical or intuitive thinking. He maintains it is the task or problem that determines the type of thinking that predominates. Human beings adapt to the demands of the judgment situation. The box on the right illustrates three features of judgment tasks that can influence the type of thinking: the complexity of the task, the ambiguity of the cues, and the way information is accessed. If task factors influence thinking, this explains why experts think differently in different clinical judgment situations.[46] The same expert might use an analytical process to identify high risk for pressure ulcer and a combination of intuitive grasp and reasoning when diagnosing hopelessness.

It is not only task factors but also contextual factors that influence thinking. For example, if colleagues or teachers expect every thought and action to be justified logically, intuitions may not be revealed. If the practice setting specifies that a nurse must see one patient every 15 to 20 minutes, as is the case in some health maintenance organizations, or if a shortage of staff in a hospital does not permit time for reasoning, a quick intuitive hunch without benefit of reflection may be the base for judgment. In these situations it is unlikely that any deep knowledge of the person or family could be used in diagnosis and intervention. A student who does not know the generally accepted procedure or rule for diagnosing a particular condition is not likely to use analytical reasoning. If students try using intuitive hunches before they gain the expertise to judge the importance of cues and cue clusters, inaccuracies may result.

The novice and expert

What is expertise and how does it influence thinking? As discussed above, some argue that the characteristics of the judgment task influence the type

---

FACTORS INFLUENCING THE USE OF DIFFERENT MODES OF THINKING

I. COMPLEXITY OF THE TASK
   A. If the number of cues is sufficient and they are relevant and pertinent to the judgment, it is more likely that intuition will be used.
   B. The more cues can be predicted from each other (redundancy), the more likely intuition will be used.
   C. The more likely it is that the cues in a task "add up to" a diagnosis (versus the complicated process of combining and weighting cues), the more likely intuition will be used.

II. AMBIGUITY OF THE TASK (may be interpreted in more than one way)
   A. If interrelations among cues are known, the more likely an analytical approach will be used.
   B. The more familiar the cues and their interrelationships, the more analytical the approach.
   C. The greater the possibility of high accuracy, the more likely that analytical thinking will predominate.

III. FORM OF TASK PRESENTATION
   A. A situation that is a series of small subtasks is likely to induce analytical thinking.
   B. Pictorial information induces intuition, but if the cues are presented numerically or quantitatively, analytical thinking is induced.
   C. If time is short with each patient, intuition is induced.

Modified from Hamm R: Clinical expertise and the cognitive continuum. In Dowie J, Elstein AS, editors: *Professional judgment: a reader in clinical decision making,* New York, 1988, Cambridge University Press.

---

of reasoning a person uses. Others argue that the influencing factor is the level of experience of the diagnostician, that as expertise is gained thinking changes from the analytic to the intuitive mode, and that knowledge and experience are much more powerful influences on the type of reasoning used.

The novice in a domain engages in analytical thinking during the learning phase, whereas the expert reports much more intuitive thinking and the recognition of similarities to past situations and solutions. This is reasonable; the novice does not have a large treasure of past experiences.

The period since the 1960s has been marked by developments in cognitive psychology and artificial intelligence. These developments have generated a great deal of interest in identifying the expert and studying the expert's judgment and decision processes. Studies of chess masters, physicists, doctors, nurses, and other experts suggest that the expert recognizes familiar patterns (pattern similarity recognition rather than individual cues or behaviors). Patterns are clusters or chunks of cues, probably constructed during many years of experience.

The terms *clusters, chunks, patterns, constellations,* and *configurations* are used to describe the possible knowledge structures in the memory stores of experts. Whereas novices seem to go about the process of identification using single pieces of data that they cluster together based on a rule, experts transform the pieces into a pattern or configuration of cues. They have subsumed the rules within the construction of the wholistic pattern.[19] Differences between the expert and novice seem to lie in the way knowledge is structured in memory and the interaction of knowledge structures with processes of reasoning and problem solving.[48] It is also proposed that this structure accounts for the reports that experts make more intuitive judgments than do novices.

The following are excerpts from a summary by Chi and his colleagues[48] of studies in this area (comments in brackets are this author's):

1. *Experts perceive large meaningful patterns in their domain* [patterns may refer to "the picture"]. "For example, chemists solved political science problems much like novices, describing the causes for the problem at a very concrete and specific level, whereas domain experts described more abstract causal categories. This ability to see meaningful patterns does not reflect a generally superior perceptual ability; rather it reflects an organization of the knowledge base."
2. *Experts excel mainly in their own domain* [e.g., a nursing domain]. The obvious reason for the excellence of experts is that they have a good deal of domain knowledge. There is little evidence that a person highly skilled in one domain can transfer the skill to another domain.
3. *Experts are fast: they are faster than novices at performing the skills of their domain and they quickly solve problems with little error.* There are at least two ways to explain experts' speed for simple tasks. . . . (1) The speed that experts have acquired comes with many hours of practice, which makes the skill more automatic and frees up memory capacity for processing other aspects of the task. . . . A further possible explanation for experts' speed in solving problems rests on the idea that (2) experts can often arrive at a solution without conducting extensive search. . . . They have stored straightforward condition-action rules in which a specific pattern will trigger a stereotypic sequence of moves. [One example is the speed of the experienced typist.]
4. *Experts have superior short-term and long-term memory.* With recently presented materials, experts' recall seems to exceed the limits of short-term memory (seven unrelated bits, plus or minus one). This is not because their short-term memory is larger than other humans but because the automaticity of many portions of their skills frees up resources for greater storage. [Possibly stored as "pictures" or patterns rather than as all the elements.] Experts seem to excel in long-term recall as well.
5. *Experts see and represent a problem in their domain at a deeper level (principles; advanced organizing structures) than novices; novices tend to represent a problem at a superficial level (literal objects stated in the problem).* Both experts and novices have conceptual categories, but the expert's categories are semantically or principle-based, whereas the categories of the novices are syntactically or surface feature-oriented.
6. *Experts spend a great deal of time analyzing a problem qualitatively.* At the beginning of a problem-solving episode, experts typically try to "understand" the problem, whereas novices plunge immediately into attempting to apply equations and to solve for an unknown. What do the experts do when they qualitatively solve a problem? Basically they build a mental representation [conceptual interrelations of the whole image] from which they can infer relations that can define the situation, and they add constraints [factors influencing] to the problem. [They create structure in an ill-structured problem.]
7. *Experts have strong self-monitoring skills.* Experts seem to be more aware than novices of when they make errors, why they fail to comprehend, and

when they need to check their solutions. . . . The superior monitoring skills and self-knowledge of experts reflect their greater domain knowledge as well as a different representation of that knowledge.[48]

What can we draw from the review by Chi and colleagues? The implications are different for the nursing student and the expert, or near-expert, nurse; therefore, each will be considered separately.

Transition from novice to expert performance

Dreyfus and Dreyfus[34] have suggested that there is a progression in the performance of skills from novice to expert behavior. Benner[36] has used their model in her study of expert performance in nurs-

ing. The progression with experience is depicted in the box above. A reasonable speculation is that a change in practice area (e.g., psychiatric nursing to adult health nursing) or a change in practice perspective (e.g., a shift from a medical to a nursing model of practice) would require the expert nurse to return to the rule-based performance of the novice or another level.

The transition from novice to expert requires a number of things. The first is long and steady practice; this is the essential ingredient of expertise. Master chess players have spent 10,000 to 20,000 hours staring at chess positions,[48] (p. xxxi) the equivalent to at least 5 to 10 years of nursing practice in direct care. Even with this impressive comparison, the chess players are studying only *one* subject, while in nursing there are over 100 diagnoses. For example, studying the textbook description of a diagnosis and its treatment is probably step one. Then clinical practice with its many variations and interrelationships seen in people and their individual experiences serve to build the "picture" that is stored in memory.[49] That seems to be basic for the intuitive understanding of the expert in nursing. Next, sustained motivation is needed to acquire expert knowledge through practice. Last, the efficiency of the strategies that experts employ is based on learning how to organize, store, and use knowledge effectively and efficiently.[48] (p. 125)

It appears that experience requires the nurse to reflect on his or her practice for learning to occur. Also, it seems that experience in a situation where a model of professional practice predominates facilitates the transition from novice to expert nursing performance.

Expert performance

Rew[35] and Benner[36] suggest that a large portion of the clinical judgments made by expert nurses are based on intuition; that is, an understanding without a rationale. The expert demonstrates a "fine-tuned response to events based upon the lessons of concrete experience"[34] (p. 40) amassed during many years. "When things are proceeding normally, experts don't solve problems and don't make decisions, they do what normally works."[34] (p. 30) Additionally, they are sensitive to when a particular interpretation of information or a particular intervention is "working" and when it is not.

According to Benner,[36] (pp. 24-29) there is a combination of six key conditions for expert intuitive judgment.

1. *Pattern recognition.* This is the perceptual ability to recognize configurations and relationships without prespecifying the components of the situation.
2. *Similarity recognition.* The recognition of a "fuzzy" resemblance despite marked differences in the objective features of past and current situations.
3. *Commonsense understanding.* This involves a deep grasp of the culture and language so that a flexible understanding of persons in diverse situations is possible.
4. *Skilled know-how.* This is based on embodied intelligence (the body takes over a skill).

5. *Sense of salience.* Knowing the importance of observations and events.
6. *Deliberative rationality.* Deliberation occurs when things do not "fit the picture," a perspective on the situation does not seem to be working, or a better idea arises than what experience brings to mind.[36] (pp. 24-29) "Maintaining a perspective in the face of persistent and disquieting evidence is called tunnel vision. Tunnel vision is failing to recognize a potential new perspective that better explains the situation or better dictates future actions."[34] (p. 31) Dreyfus and Dreyfus[34] maintain that these deliberations are not based on rules or principles such as is seen in novices' behavior.[34] (p. 40)

Deliberation is important. Although a judgment may seem plausible based on past experience, yet, as Dreyfus and Dreyfus[34] remark, "The situation may not be *exactly* the same," or not everything "fits the picture." "At this point the expert examines the differences, trying to reduce a sense of uneasiness and may modify the idea which was intuitively suggested. The organizing perspective, or structure, gleaned from intuition is tested in a deliberative way and may improve whole intuitions." [34] (p. 42) Does the expert ever think? As these authors note:

In the idealized picture of the skillfully coping expert . . . it might seem that experts never think and are always right. Of course in reality things are otherwise. While most expert performance is ongoing and nonreflective, when time permits and outcomes are crucial, an expert will deliberate before acting. But . . . this deliberation does not require calculative problem solving but rather involves critically reflecting on one's intuitions.[34] (pp. 30-31)

There must be continual self-monitoring and validation with the client. What can occur with the expert is clearly stated by Schon[50] (p. 73):

Further, as a practice becomes more repetitive and routine, and as knowing-in-practice becomes increasingly tacit and spontaneous, the practitioner may miss important opportunities to think about what he is doing. He may find that he is drawn into patterns of error which he cannot correct. And if he learns, as often happens, to be selectively inattentive to phenomena that do not fit the categories of his knowing-in-action, then he may suffer from boredom or "burn-out" and afflict his clients with the consequences of his narrowness and rigidity.

When this happens, the practitioner has "over-learned" what he knows.

To prevent errors in diagnosis and treatment the expert uses intuitions as possibilities and verifies the insights drawn from this cognitive process. All clinical knowledge is tentative, including that arrived at by intuition. This mode of cognition is just as probable and uncertainty-geared as the cues derived from perception and used in analytical reasoning.

SUMMARY

In this chapter the most critical component of the diagnostic process—information collection—was explored. Unless valid and reliable information is used as a base, health problems may be ideas constructed by the diagnostician rather than descriptions of the client's real signs or symptoms. To avoid having imagination take over, final diagnoses must be firmly based on clinical data.

In the first section of this chapter assessment was defined as health evaluation based on the collection of information (data). It was emphasized that this component of the diagnostic process is continuous during all nurse-client interactions. Four types of assessment situations were identified. First was the initial assessment at admission—a nursing history and examination. The purpose of the initial assessment is to establish diagnoses (if health problems are present) that can direct care planning. Second, the problem-focused assessment has as its purpose the daily or periodic evaluation of the status of a diagnosis. Third, in some situations, such as residential or long-term care, the time lapse between health status assessments (time-lapse reassessment) may be long. A complete history and examination are recommended; yet problem-focused assessment and time-lapse reassessment are designed as follow-ups to previous assessment data. Fourth, the emergency assessment differs from the three other types of assessment in the level of problem formulation and the immediacy of intervention. The differences in the scope of the data, context, and purpose of these four types of assessment were discussed.

The discussion of clinical cues provided an introduction to the nature of the clinical information used in assessment and diagnosis. Four important types of clinical cues to the health status of the client were identified. These cues indicated:

1. A change in a functional pattern
2. A deviation from pattern norms
3. Dysfunctional patterns
4. Pattern development

The uncertain, or probabilistic, nature of clinical data was described. Because of the human capacity for variability in behavioral expression, signs and symptoms predict with less than perfect certainty. Nurses must learn to deal with this uncertain environment. It was emphasized that the most valid and reliable information is most useful. Additionally, the nurse must recognize that judgments based on uncertain data are subject to error. A continual openness to new contradictory or supporting information increases accuracy.

Clinical data can be relevant or irrelevant to the purpose of assessment or to a particular diagnostic hypothesis. Knowing what data are needed prevents the nurse's cognitive processes from being overwhelmed by irrelevant information. Information that does not increase the reliability or validity of judgment is irrelevant. The focus in data collection is on the cues that "pay off" in terms of health status evaluation.

It was suggested that when a nursing framework is used, both subjective and objective data provide important cues. Nurses are equally concerned with the so-called objective observation of the client situation and with the client's subjective perceptions, responses, beliefs, and attitudes. The client's perspective on his or her situation is considered as important in assessment as the nurse's perspective. Rather than discount clients' subjective, personal biases and feelings, nurses use these data in diagnosis.

Historical, current, contextual, and state-of-the-client cues were related to functional health pattern assessment. To understand a pattern, both types of data are necessary. This is why assessment consists of both history taking and examination. The errors and decreased efficiency resulting from an overemphasis on either historical or current data were pointed out. The section may be summarized by saying *important* cues are relevant; they may be historical or current, subjective or objective, and related to the client's state or situational context. Last, important cues are those that represent the most reliable and valid data available.

Two other influential factors were examined. One is the nature of clinical information and its influence on data collection. The probabilistic, or uncertain, nature of clinical data influences a clinician's subjective confidence in diagnoses. In an uncertain situation, collecting more and more data is not the answer; rather, the most valid and reliable predictors should be sought. Important cues were described as those that contribute to evaluative judgments. These cues may be of various types: subjective, objective, historical, and current. Important cues are relevant to health status evaluation and permit reliable and valid judgments.

The last section focused on the diagnostician's capabilities and the judgment task. The diagnostician was viewed as a creative, sensitive measuring device. An examination of perceptual recognition and perceptual sensitivity to cues emphasized the importance of clinical knowledge. It is on the basis of knowing what to expect that sensory input is coded, cues are anticipated, and attention is directed. Examination of short- and long-term memory storage resulted in suggestions for collecting information and for organizing the clinical knowledge necessary for assessment.

Information is also generated by analytical inference and intuition. These two modes of cognition were examined. It is important to pay attention to clinical intuition. Some recent views on intuition and expertise were reviewed.

This chapter and the one preceding it emphasized one component of the diagnostic process, information collection. Information is continually collected throughout all nurse-client interactions. At certain points, when the data indicate, diagnoses are formulated. Information collection is not a random process. Professionals know why information is needed—to reach the long-range goal for which it is collected.

The question at this point is, What do you do with the information collected? Actually, reasoning about the information begins during assessment. A number of thinking processes can be used to derive meaning from the cues and are discussed in Chapter 8. Nursing diagnoses are the judgments that result.

NOTES AND REFERENCES

1. Variation exists in use of the word *assessment* (Bloch, 1974). Some use the term to refer to four activities of the diagnostic process; in this book it means the collection and interpretation of clinical data in any context.
2. Sarbin TR, Taft R, Bailey DE: *Clinical inference and cognitive theory,* New York, 1960, Holt, Rinehart & Winston, pp 144-159.
3. Cardwell JD: *Social psychology,* Philadelphia, 1971, Davis.
4. Herzlich C, Graham D: *Health and illness: a social psychological analysis,* New York, 1973, Academic Press.
5. Koos EL: Illness in Regionville. In Apple D, editor: *Sociological studies of health and sickness,* New York, 1960, McGraw-Hill.
6. Mechanic D, Volkart EH: Stress, illness behavior and the sick role, *Am Sociol Rev* 26:51, 1961.
7. Zola IK: Culture and symptoms: an analysis of patients' presenting complaints. In Spector RE, editor: *Cultural diversity in health and illness,* New York, 1979, Appleton-Century-Crofts.
8. Bruner JS, Goodnow JJ, Austin GA: *A study of thinking,* New York, 1956, Wiley.
9. Functional assessment screening tools have been designed that may be filled out by the patient at home or on admission to a hospital or clinic. The primary nurse reviews the form and completes the nursing components on history and examination. The advantages are twofold: the patient's written response may be different from that given during an interview, and the nurse can focus the assessment based on the screening data, thereby saving time. No reliability measures have been reported.
10. Interaction in the full sense of the word cannot be accomplished when a patient is unconscious, extremely hyperactive, or markedly out of contact with reality. In these instances information is acquired from a knowledgeable person or by examination.
11. Gordon M: *Manual of nursing diagnosis: 1993-1994,* St Louis, 1993, Mosby.
12. Corrigan J: Functional health pattern assessment in the emergency room, *J Emerg Nurs* 12:163, 1986.
13. Cutler P: *Problem solving in clinical medicine: from data to diagnosis,* Baltimore, 1979, Williams & Wilkins.
14. Gordon M: Predictive strategies in diagnostic tasks, *Nurs Res* 29:39, 1980.
15. Gordon M: *Probabilistic concept attainment: a study of nursing diagnosis,* doctoral dissertation, Boston, 1972, Boston College.
16. Hammond K: Clinical inference in nursing: a psychologist's viewpoint, *Nurs Res* 57:27, 1966.
17. Whitehorn JC: Education for uncertainty, *Perspect Biol Med* 7:118, 1963.
18. Kassier JP, Kopelman RL: *Learning clinical reasoning,* Baltimore, 1991, Williams & Wilkins.
19. Brainerd CJ, Reyna VF: Gist is the grist: Fuzzy-trace theory and the new intuitionism, *Dev Rev* 10:3, 1990.
20. Simon HA: The information processing explanation of gestalt phenomena, *Comput Hum Behav* 2:241, 1986.
21. Atkinson RC, Schiffrin RM: The control of short-term memory, *Sci Am* 225:82, 1971.

22. Kassier JP, Kuipers BJ, Gorry A: Toward a theory of clinical expertise *Am J Med* 73:251, 1982.
23. Miller GA: The magical number seven, plus or minus two: some comments on our capacity for processing information, *Psychol Rev* 63:81, 1956.
24. Guyton A: *Textbook of medical physiology,* ed 6, Philadelphia, 1992, Saunders, p 752.
25. Ausabel D: *Educational psychology: a cognitive view,* New York, 1968, Holt, Rinehart & Winston.
26. Devine P, Sherman S: Intuitive versus rational judgment and the role of stereotyping in the human condition: Kirk or Spock? *Psychol Inquiry* 3:153, 1992.
27. Earlier in this book, nursing diagnoses were described as conceptual categories. In this section the focus is on perceptual categories that are the cues or building blocks used in attaining a diagnosis.
28. Rosch E, Lloyd B: *Cognition and categorization,* Hillsdale NJ, 1978, Erlbaum.
29. Categories and relationships might be constructed, but the disposition, curiosity, and time to do this are not always present. Thus there is a tendency to ignore information that cannot be coded.
30. Holt R: Clinical judgment as a disciplined inquiry, *J Nerv Ment Dis* 133:369, 1961.
31. Inductive inferences are general or particular statements representing conclusions drawn from sense data or experience. Conclusions may or may not withstand the test of time, because the next experience may invalidate previous generalizations drawn from experience. One may observe that all swans are white and accept this generalization and then, during a trip to Australia, find that there are black swans. Generalizations can be used to deduce hypotheses. For example, if a high percentage of people with impaired swallowing aspirate, and Mr. James has impaired swallowing after a stroke, the nurse may conclude that he is at high risk for aspiration.
32. Riegel KF: Dialectic operations: the final period of cognitive development, *Hum Dev* 16:346, 1973.
33. Gatens-Robinson E: Clinical judgment and the rationality of the human sciences, *J Med Philos* 11:167, 1988.
34. Dreyfus H, Dreyfus S: *Mind over machine: the power of human intuition and expertise in the era of the computer,* New York, 1984, Free Press.
35. Rew L: Intuition: concept analysis of a group phenomenon, *Adv Nurs Sci* 8:21, 1986.
36. Benner P: From novice to expert, *Am J Nurs* 82:402, 1982. The excerpts from this publication appeared in Benner P, Tanner, C: Clinical judgment: how expert nurses use intuition, *Am J Nurs* 87:23, 1987.
37. Benderly BL: Intuition, *Psychol Today* 35, 1989.
38. Hill OW: Intuition: inferential heuristic or epistemic mode? *Imagination, Cognition, Personality* 7:137, 1987.
39. Wertheimer M: A gestalt perspective on computer simulations of cognitive processes, *Comput Hum Behav* 1:19, 1985.
40. Rew L: Intuition: nursing knowledge and the spiritual dimension of persons, *Holistic Nurs Pract* 3:56, 1989.
41. Leininger M: *Nursing and anthropology: two worlds to blend,* New York, 1970, Wiley.
42. Zajonc RB: Feeling and thinking: preferences need no inferences, *Am J Psychol* 35:151, 1980.
43. Jenny J, Logan J: Knowing the patient: one aspect of clinical knowledge, *Image* 24:254, 1992.
44. Tanner, C: *Image,* 1993 (in press).
45. Gerrity PL: Perception in nursing: the value of intuition, *Holistic Nurs Pract* 1:63, 1987.
46. Hammond KR: *Principles of organization in intuitive and analytical cognition (Report #231),* Boulder, CO, 1981, University of Colorado, Center for Research on Judgment and Policy.
47. Hamm R: Clinical expertise and the cognitive continuum. In Dowie J, Elstein A, editors: *Professional judgment: a reader in clinical decision making,* New York, 1988, Cambridge University Press.
48. Chi M, Glaser R, Farr M: *The nature of expertise,* Hillsdale, NJ, 1988, Erlbaum.
49. Newell A, Simon HA: *Human problem solving,* Englewood Cliffs, NJ, 1972, Prentice-Hall. These authors analyzed previous research on experts in chess and suggested a "perceptual" ability to recognize familiar patterns ("constellations," in their terms) that are clusters of data values stored in long-term memory as a single "symbol" in contrast to storage as separate bits of data, the schemata discussed in theories of perception. Perhaps a pattern is a "set of concepts within a complex, interrelated propositional network that is seen as a whole."[48]
50. Schon DA: From techological rationality to reflection-in-action. In Dowie J, Elstein A, editors: *Professional judgment: a reader in clinical decision making,* New York, 1988, Cambridge University Press.

CHAPTER 8

INFORMATION INTERPRETATION AND CLUSTERING

I n previous discussions information collection was treated independently of the overall diagnostic process. This separation permitted an emphasis on important topics but neglected the fact that information is interpreted and clustered while it is being collected. It may be recalled that interpretation and clustering of cues are two of the continuous components within the diagnostic process:

1. Collecting information (continuous)
2. Interpreting information (continuous)
3. Clustering information (continuous)
4. Naming a cluster or problem formulation (occurs at certain confidence points)

The focus of this chapter is on how to use information.[1] Using information acquired during health status evaluation requires interpretation and clustering of cues on the basis of their meaning. There are various levels at which these aspects of the diagnostic process can be described. At the observable level nurses ask questions and examine a client; then they verbalize and record a diagnosis. How do we explain this behavior, especially when their diagnoses are valid and reliable?

Nonanalytical explanations (involving intuition or pattern recognition) have been proposed to describe expert performance. The use of analytic reasoning and diagnostic strategies during the learning period is thought to be more characteristic of the novice. The emphasis in this discussion will be on the novice and hypothesis generation–hypothesis testing methods—a useful strategy to employ while learning patterns. The selection of information to be collected, the sequence of collection, and the way information is used form a sequence of decisions, which by definition is a *strategy*.[2] Learning how to make a diagnosis requires probing to a deeper level. Exactly what is going on when a diagnostic strategy is employed? Rather, what do we think is going on? From studies of diagnosticians and others, it appears that decisions are based on diagnostic hypotheses that describe the clinician's interpretations of the cues. In fact, over and above routine assessment questions and examination guidelines (Chapter 5), information collection is directed by hypotheses.

Regardless of whether hypotheses are generated by analytical or nonanalytical processes, they have to be subjected to verification. Depending on the diagnostician's level of expertise and familiarity with the situation, hypotheses may be arrived at immediately by matching initial cues to a pattern in memory or by scanning possibilities that are suggested by initial cues.

Hypotheses (possibilities) are alternative interpretations of the data in a functional health pat-

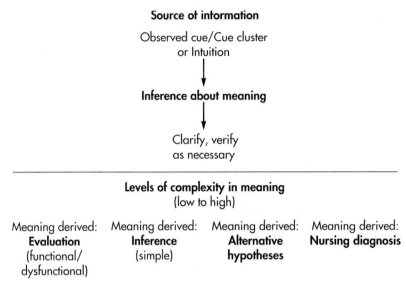

Fig. 8-1   Interpreting the meaning of clinical clues.

tern. Some hypotheses may be discarded, some held, and others revised. Also, new diagnostic hypotheses may be generated as assessment continues. In other words, diagnosticians use their hypotheses about the meaning of the initial data to structure and organize that data. They then shift to a focused search for further information. If the information collected "fits the picture" of a particular diagnosis, then the diagnostician's ideas are made "public." A nursing diagnosis is stated and a treatment plan is developed and recorded. But how do nurses know when the cues "fit the picture"? How do they know what questions to ask and what to observe if the questions and observations are not specified by the standard assessment tool? Where do hypotheses come from?

Answers to these questions lie in the facts and theories of clinical reasoning. Cognitive processes were introduced in Chapter 7 as the diagnostician's basic tools for interpreting and clustering information. They are extremely important in professional nursing because judgments and decisions that result from these processes may affect a client's comfort or life.

In the discussion that follows the interpretation of assessment information is emphasized in the first section and the clustering of information in the second; these processes usually occur together.

In most instances the meaning of a cue depends on the cluster of interrelated cues in which it is embedded. Fig. 8-1 illustrates the process discussed in this section.

INTERPRETATION OF CLINICAL INFORMATION

To be useful, information collected during an assessment must be interpreted. To interpret means to assign meaning to a cue or determine what it signifies. Different levels of meaning can be derived from information. Higher, complex levels require more cognitive skill and ability. For example, interpreting whether a cue indicates a functional or dysfunctional pattern requires less skill than interpreting whether a set of cues mean that a particular diagnosis is present or absent.

Information collected during assessment does not always match the textbook listing of diagnostic signs and symptoms. Thus the diagnostician must be prepared to undertake the following tasks:

1. Clarify and verify cues when necessary before interpreting their meaning
2. Recognize the meaning of direct cues
3. Derive meaning from concealed cues

4. Put initial cues together so that their basic meaning can emerge through first-level inferences[3]

Each of these four elementary processes is considered "the beginning search for meaning" when it is not immediately apparent. The discussion is organized as a series of questions that diagnosticians ask themselves (first consciously and later unconsciously) while interpreting and structuring information early in the diagnostic process:

Is there a need for clarification?

Is there a need for verification?

Is the meaning clear relative to norms for this client and in the context of other cues?

Need for clarification

Before attempting to interpret assessment data, clarification may be necessary. *Clarification* refers to the search for a clearer understanding of the information. Whenever clients use vague, abstract, or ambiguous terms, the data must be clarified; otherwise misperceptions may arise and lead to errors in diagnosis. For example:

What does the client mean by a "poor" marriage?

What are the feelings the client classifies as "anxious"?

What does "I eat good" mean?

Do specific fears underlie a statement such as "I'm afraid of dying"?

What does the client mean by "I feel weak"?

What is the meaning of "I don't know if it is worth going on"?

Without clarification, clinicians tend to place their own meanings on these ambiguous words and statements. They may assume that they know what the client means and later be shocked to find their assumptions totally wrong! For a reliable analysis of information personal meanings should be put aside, especially in the case of important cues; further questions should be asked to clarify what the client means.

Need for verification

Verification of data means double-checking. Verification increases the reliability of information and is necessary when the following situations occur:

1. The diagnostician has doubts about his or her perception.
2. There is a conflict or contradiction among cues.
3. An inference or assumption has been made and is being used as an important piece of data to influence actions.

Verification may be as simple as making sure a client's blood pressure really was 180/80 or as complex as saying to a client after a visitor leaves: "You seem very angry." Verification is also used to validate diagnostic impressions with the client. For example, in the case of health management of medications, the nurse may say to the client: "You seem to be having trouble managing all those medications; I think it might be due to trouble remembering what to take when. Do you think that might be the reason?" Last, when cues appear to be conflicting or contradictory, double-checking can reveal whether assumptions are accurate.

Deriving meaning: evaluation of cues

After clarifying perceptions and understandings (as necessary) and verifying ambiguous information, the diagnostician begins to interpret the meaning of a client's response relative to norms. This process requires evaluation. The purpose of evaluation is to determine if the verbal report or the observation is "normal" or "abnormal," that is, if it is a cue to a functional (healthy behavior) or to a dysfunctional pattern (diagnostic cue). Cue evaluation is an important step because it determines whether the health assessment is to continue or whether a shift to the diagnostic process is necessary, as illustrated in Fig. 8-2. In evaluating a cue or cluster of cues, the diagnostician compares the information obtained from the client with knowledge of norms and criteria retrieved from memory.

Example A

A client's heart rate is measured at 126 beats per minute. To evaluate whether this finding means normal functioning or dysfunction, the nurse considers other information: the measure is from an infant, this infant's baseline heart rate pattern is 120 to 130 beats per minute, and infants have a normal heart rate of 120 to 160 beats per minute. Therefore, a value of 126 beats per minute is evaluated as normal.

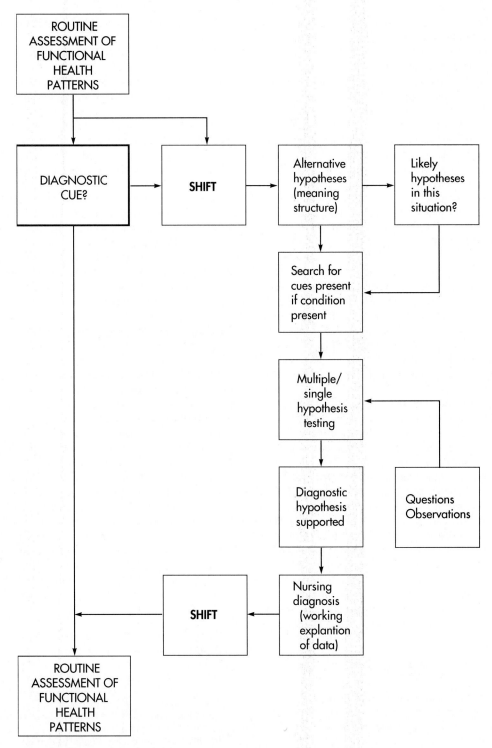

Fig. 8-2 Representation of shifts from routine assessment to the diagnostic process.

The heart rate now begins to take on meaning; it is normal. Evaluation is based on a comparison of a cue with a norm or criterion for health. A problem may be missed if a verbal report or observation is judged to indicate a functional pattern when in fact the health pattern is dysfunctional. The reverse error, an incorrect judgment of a dysfunctional pattern that is actually functional, leads to overdiagnosis. This first level of meaning derived from the data above is limited because the information has not been interpreted in the context of the whole person-situation. To decrease the risk of errors, an evaluation in the context of other cues that are present is necessary; that is, in the context of the whole client-situation complex. Example B is an illustration:

Example B

The nurse inquires about the protein intake of a 22-year-old woman. Her intake is sufficient when evaluated against norms for adult women. Yet when interpreted in the context of other data from the assessment of her reproductive pattern (the woman is 2 months pregnant), the cue takes on a different meaning. In fact, the woman has a potential for protein deficit.

Determining whether an isolated cue is a functional or dysfunctional indicator of a pattern takes the nurse to one level of meaning (Example A). Interpretation of the cues in the context of other data reveals the level of meaning necessary for accurate nursing diagnoses (Example B). These examples illustrate that a reliable estimate of the meaning (functional or dysfunctional) of cues depends on two factors:

1. The use of norms or criteria
2. Other cues that are present

Both single cues and clusters of cues need to be compared with some norms or criteria. At this point consider the knowledge (norms or criteria) stored in memory that is used in the interpretation of data.

Comparison with norms

Evaluating health pattern data involves comparing the observed value with the expected value. Population values (norms) derived from research, individual baselines, or (in some instances) the clinician's past clinical experiences provide the expected values. These are the criteria with which clinical data are compared. The importance of this evaluation must not be underestimated. It is the basis for subsequent diagnostic judgments.

Caution must be exercised in selecting appropriate norms and criteria. *Population norms* specify a range of normal limits for particular groups, frequently age groups. These norms are used as guidelines when physical attributes such as visual acuity, blood pressure, or protein intake are evaluated. For evaluating data such as values, beliefs, self-perceptions, or role relationships, general population norms may be inadequate. Cultural, ethnic, racial, national, and religious patterns as well as clients' baselines need to be considered. For example, the evaluation of data on toilet training practices may be in error if specific cultural norms are ignored. Also, when a social norm is in flux, it may not be useful as a criterion for evaluation. Sexuality patterns are an example; evaluation may have to be based partly or entirely on the client's perception of whether a problem exists.

Individual baselines, if available, are important in evaluating data. *Baseline data* are criteria that permit evaluation on the basis of the client's own functional health patterns. The difficulty arises in obtaining accurate baseline measures. Even during assessment human characteristics may be influenced by the situation and person doing the assessment. An example is "office hypertension" (the client's blood pressure is elevated when it is measured in the doctor's office). The client's previous records may be helpful if functional health pattern assessments have been done. If true baselines are not available, data obtained in the admission history and examination are used as baseline criteria for evaluating change in subsequent assessments.

The critical need for baseline data is the reason many hospitals require a nursing assessment within 6 to 8 hours of admission. Ideally the assessment should be done as soon as a client enters a hospital, clinic, nursing home, or other health care service and has an opportunity to relax and obtain orienting information. The importance of baseline data is the reason the admission assessment should be done with the following goals in mind:

1. The history and examination should be done by a professional nurse.
2. The assessment should be done in an environment conducive to relaxation.
3. An interpersonal situation that facilitates de-

velopment of rapport, trust, and confidence should be established.

4. Privacy, quiet, and adequate lighting to facilitate conversation and examination should be ensured.

Deriving meaning: simple inference

More complex meanings may be derived from assessment information than merely "that's not normal," "wouldn't expect that in this patient," or "that's not usual," as are derived in the levels of interpretation already discussed. When data obtained during an assessment do not meet expected health norms, the diagnostician tries to understand the meaning of the cues and whether or not they "point to" a dysfunctional health pattern. The interpretation of clinical information at this level requires the use of inferential reasoning. That is, an inference or judgment is made about the meaning of a client's verbal report or an observation. *Inferential reasoning is the process by which the unknown meaning is tentatively inferred or predicted from known clinical data.*

As was discussed in Chapter 7, inferences range from simple, immediate judgments, such as "limping gait," to complex chains of reasoning that are deliberate and within conscious awareness. Whether simple or complex, an inference represents a step beyond the information collected to make a judgment and may raise questions such as the following:

1. Why are inferential judgments necessary?
2. Aren't they dangerous?
3. When are inferences rather than observation used?

In answer to the first question, inferences further elaborate the meaning of the information collected. Consider an example of a relatively low level of inference that requires going beyond observations made at 7:00 AM. Note that cues had to be combined in order for an inference to be made and that the inference becomes a diagnostic "cue" that can be termed *restless:*

The patient's bed linen is pulled out from under the mattress and is lying twisted in a wrinkled lump, the blanket is half on the floor, the undersheet is wrinkled, the mattress cover is exposed, and the pillowcase is sliding off the pillow.

INFERENCE: The bed is in disarray.

The patient, a 50-year-old man, sighs and turns first to one side of the bed and then the other. When he notices the nurse, he says he had "quite a night."

INFERENCE: The patient is restless.

This simple example demonstrates the importance of inference in practice. One nurse infers restlessness and investigates the reason for it. Another nurse does not make the inference, as is clear from her comments: "My, you've got your bed in a mess. We'll get it tidied up in a few minutes and make you comfortable." She then hurries out.

As this example shows, an interpretation of the meaning of a set of observations both summarizes the data and provides a selective focus for attention. The expert immediately recognizes restlessness as a deviation from a norm or expected behavior (the restlessness acts as a diagnostic cue). The novice may have to analyze all nine cues (condition of the bed linen, etc., and the patient's actions and comment) before inferring that the data indicate restlessness and then must go on to infer what diagnostic interpretations are suggested by restlessness. The second nurse did not have the time to do so.

Now to the second question: Is it dangerous to make inferences? Inferences may indeed be "dangerous," since inferences or assumptions are created in the mind of the diagnostician. In contrast, observations are open for others to see and validate. On the other hand, as the example illustrates, isolated observations do not have diagnostic meaning unless they are interpretations; thus human beings use inference. *To prevent errors, validate and verify inferences and assumptions. Always remain open to new information and new interpretations of data.*

As we have seen in Fig. 8-1, interpretation occurs at various levels of complexity; one or more levels of interpretation may be required before the diagnostic significance of cues and observations can be inferred. The following process summarizes how to derive meaning from a cue:

1. *Initial interpretation of the meaning and evaluation of cues relative to norms.* First the diagnostician determines whether the information points to a functional or dysfunctional pattern through a comparison with ex-

pected health norms. This is a superficial level of data interpretation.

2. *Interpretation of the meaning of a cue or cue cluster in the context of the available data.* The meaning of a cue may be very different than it seems when considered in the context of the whole person-situation complex.

3. *Interpretation of the meaning of cues to arrive at a simple level of inference,* such as restlessness, anger, or withdrawal. This level of interpretation involves giving some structure to the data and arriving at an inference.

There are two reasons assessment data need interpretation. One is that the human mind cannot manage the large number of isolated bits of information in one pattern area or in the total assessment. (Recall the discussion of "chunking" in Chapter 7.) The other is that interpretations (hypotheses) guide the search for information beyond the routine screening assessment. (Hypotheses are complex inferences about data.)

RECOGNIZING A DIAGNOSTIC CUE

The recognition of a diagnostic cue is extremely important. If a diagnostic cue does not receive attention, the shift from routine assessment to the diagnostic process does not occur. This decision point is depicted as a shift in Fig. 8-2.

A diagnostic cue can be recognized in a number of ways; at least that is what the cognitive theorists propose. (Knowledge of human reasoning is based on indirect measures, verbal reports, and a lot of speculation.) It has been proposed that human beings adjust their cognitive processes to the nature of the judgment task and to their own capabilities. This applies to the recognition of diagnostic cues and the interpretation of their meaning.

Immediate cue recognition and interpretation

In some instances the information collected during assessment may contain client responses or nurse observations that "point directly" to one or more diagnoses. When this occurs, the diagnostic interpretation is simple and routine; that is, there is a similarity to past experiences. The cue, or cluster of cues, corresponds to the characteristics of one or more diagnoses stored in memory. These stored diagnoses are used as hypotheses to be verified by additional data collection. The question, What is the problem in this functional pattern? is quickly narrowed down to one or a few dysfunctional patterns (possible diagnoses). This is the basis for the earlier "intuitive leap" discussed. Immediate recognition occurs through matching a cue or cue cluster to clinical knowledge stored in memory.

It is proposed that the clinical knowledge used in recognizing a cue or situation is stored and can be accessed at at least three levels of complexity. A nurse who is experienced in a particular area should be able to access knowledge for the recognition and interpretation of assessment data at all the following levels:

1. At an elementary level, knowledge is stored as facts, goals, themes, prevalence rates, and generalizations independent of any specific conditions. Connections form a network, and there are rules for using these elements.

2. At a second level, knowledge is "simplified, compressed, and compiled" into prototypes.

3. At a third level are multiple exemplars based on actual experiences with specific patients.[4]

This proposal about how knowledge is stored provides an explanation for the differences in novice and expert performance in various fields.[5] The idea of different storage capabilities also explains why, for some nurses, there is an immediate activation of hypotheses, whereas for another nurse the generation of hypotheses is slower and is done using analytical methods. The sections that follow contain discussions of various ways of generating possibilities to derive meaning from assessment data.

The prototype, or typical case (level 2 above), may be fashioned by experience from the original textbook picture. The cue or cue cluster "fits the picture" or, as some authors say, "fits the problem script."[4 (p. 282); 6 (p. 32)] Comments by nurses such as, "He's our typical cardiac rehab patient, always a little anxious," support the theory of memory stored by prototypes. Another explanation for its recognition and interpretation is that a cue is matched to an exemplar (level 3 in list above). An exemplar has been discussed by Benner[7] as a *specific example of a previous client-situation stored in memory.* Carnavali and Thomas[6] and Kassier and Kopelman [4] (pp. 282-283) refer to these highly specific client-situation complexes as *patient instance scripts.* These scripts contain a story about the context of the problem, its clinical features, causal possibilities, consequences, and other related information. Exemplars may also contain images. These two ways of generating hypotheses depend on abstract (prototype) and concrete exemplars stored in memory as scripts or chunks of information. Diagnosis, according to these theories, involves assessment, the search for an appropriate script by some process of pattern recognition, the selection of the script, and the verification of the script with further clinical data.[4]

As the reader may have anticipated, diagnostic interpretations of the meanings contained in assessment data do not always lend themselves to the simple process of *matching* observed patterns with stored memories. The beginning student and the expert who changes specialties, settings, or frameworks may have to depend more on analytical modes of thinking and methods to generate possible explanations of clinical data.

Data analysis: recognition and interpretation

Some diagnoses describe subjective states that are not visible, whereas others, such as syndromes, describe complex conditions. Before the diagnostic meaning is grasped, it may be necessary to clarify, verify, or determine the basic meaning of some individual cues. Consider an example of pieces of information in the self-perception–self-concept pattern given by two clients scheduled to begin chemotherapy for cancer:

> **Client A:** *I'm so afraid of what will happen to me.*
> **Client B:** *Someone I knew very well had this very same treatment.[8]*

Client A's statement provides a diagnostic cue ("I'm so afraid") that directly suggests the diagnostic hypotheses of fear and anxiety. Neither clarification nor verification of "afraid" is necessary; it is viewed as meaning "feelings of concern about a threatening event," which is a defining characteristic listed in diagnostic manuals for both fear and anxiety. The next step is to determine if the feeling is focused on something specific (fear) or is diffuse (anxiety).[9] In contrast, Client B's statement raises the possibility that "someone's" experience may be used by Client B to predict his own experience. Is this a positive or negative reaction? He "knew" this person—interestingly, he uses the past tense. He might be referring to a memory of events that happened many years ago or that the person is deceased. It may or may not be that Client B views the person's death as related to treatment and it may or may not be that Client B identifies with this person. Before the nurse makes any diagnostic interpretations (for example, fear or anxiety), clarification and verification are necessary.

Selective attention to diagnostic cues

Selective attention is focused attention. It involves "pulling out" a cue or cues from the stream of ongoing assessment and focusing attention (and thinking) on the cue(s). This is not to suggest that attention is not continuous during assessment. Rather, certain cues alert a person's thinking processes more than others. Levine[10] refers to these diagnostic cues or cue clusters as provocative facts; they "provoke" thinking. Others use the term *forceful feature* to refer to data that "force" a response.[11,12] Regardless of the colorful terms used, there are cues that nurses select, attend to, and think about during assessment. They are the diagnostic cues that serve to generate hypotheses. The reader may ask:

1. What is it about information that causes attention to be focused?
2. How does one learn to recognize these cues? During learning, key features of health problems and the meaning of these features are stored in memory. These features include the critical cues of diagnoses that nurses are taught to pay attention to and those they have learned through practice to value as important in a particular group of clients. When these cues are encountered during an assessment, or when other information suggests their presence, the clinician's attention is aroused because the data are seen as having either diagnostic or therapeutic significance. This conclusion motivates the clinician to think about the possible meanings of the data and subsequently to gather more information.

Why is it that some nurses do not recognize and pay attention to important data? First, they may not have learned to recognize a cue and its significance. Second, the way they have organized their knowledge in memory may not permit easy retrieval of possible interpretations when a diagnostic clue is encountered. Third, there may be only subtle manifestations of the behavior; thus the behavior is missed by a novice. Last, clinicians may become distracted by other cues that capture their attention and thinking processes.

Hints for recognizing diagnostic cues

Focusing attention on the cues that have diagnostic significance (those that may signify a problem) is one of the major ways of reducing errors in nursing diagnosis. Of course, the first step in attending to these cues is to learn the defining characteristics of each diagnosis, organize them in some clinically useful way, and use them in practice. For example, NANDA lists about 12 defining characteristics for the diagnosis of Activity Intolerance. They fall into three areas: cardiovascular, respiratory, and subjective report. The critical indicators of the diagnosis are probably one or more of the following:

1. Report of shortness of breath during activity; difficulty observed in breathing during activity
2. Report of fatigue during activity (more than expected)
3. Heart rate changes (increased beyond prescribed level; this indicator also depends on other factors)
4. Failure of heart rate to return to baseline within 3 minutes after activity ceases
5. Report of discomfort and/or pain during activity[13]

Assessment provides information about these characteristics. Of equal importance is "putting things together" during assessment. Previously acquired data may take on significant meaning when combined with other information elicited from the client. Thus a cue may not receive selective attention at the time it is noted but may gain significance and "provoke" thinking after other pattern areas are assessed. To prevent errors, the nurse should always remain open to new information and new interpretations of the data during assessment.

GENERATION OF DIAGNOSTIC HYPOTHESES

When making a nursing diagnosis, attention and thinking are focused on information that has diagnostic and therapeutic significance, which leads to the generation of hypotheses. Diagnostic hypotheses provide further interpretations of the possible meaning of clinical data and serve to structure the diagnostic task. They describe and explain pieces of information. Hypotheses are possibilities. The following list helps clarify this important term:

1. Diagnostic hypotheses are possible interpretations of the meaning of cues (e.g., fatigue may mean activity intolerance).
2. Diagnostic hypotheses are tentative (e.g., possibilities, not certainties; they are "rule-outs").
3. Early diagnostic hypotheses are the basis for a focused cue search to confirm or disconfirm the hypothesis.
4. Diagnostic hypotheses may range from specific to global (e.g., protein deficit to nutritional problem), depending on initial information.

Clinicians go beyond the information contained in cues or cue clusters, first-level inferences, or intuitive inferences to generate a set of diagnostic possibilities. For instance, restlessness may indicate pain, anxiety, fear, anoxia, and a number of other problems because it is usually present in all of these conditions. These possible meanings are diagnostic hypotheses. In a particular client situation, one or all of these hypotheses may be likely enough to warrant investigation. Usually one of the diagnostic hypotheses in the initial pool is found to be the actual diagnosis.

Studies have demonstrated that diagnosticians structure an ill-defined task, such as, Does this client have a health problem? by (1) selectively attending to early diagnostic cue(s), (2) thinking of likely hypotheses that will explain the meaning of the cues, and then (3) testing (or "checking out") their hypotheses by collecting further information.[11,14] There are a number of reasons why this is a useful strategy for managing large amounts of information:

1. The initial cues and those derived from hypothesis testing can be clustered (grouped

into chunks of information) under the related hypotheses. It is easier to think (in working memory) about three or four diagnostic hypotheses than possibly 10 to 20 isolated bits of information.

2. Hypotheses provide some structure for thinking about "what to do next." For example, if cues suggest three possible diagnoses, the task is to check the major critical defining characteristics of the three diagnoses.

3. Diagnostic hypotheses narrow the universe of possibilities. For example, rather than having to hold all the diagnoses describing dysfunctional activity exercise patterns, the universe is narrowed to encompass only the likely diagnoses suggested by the initial data.

In simple terms, hypothesis generation "brings to mind" alternative meanings or explanations for a diagnostic cue or cluster of cues.

Learning how to use knowledge to generate diagnostic hypotheses is not a new behavior for most children and adults.[15] We are all familiar with the "cues" from the *Superman* comic strip:

Distant speck in the sky
Moving toward us.

Three "hypotheses" are generated to explain these "cues":

IT'S A BIRD!
IT'S A PLANE!
IT'S SUPERMAN!

This is a commonplace example of hypothesis generation. Interestingly, this children's comic book expression is consistent with *likelihood estimates.* In real-life experience, birds are the things most frequently seen in the sky. Thus *bird* is a good tentative hypothesis to raise first. A *plane* is the second most frequent explanation of the distant speck in the sky. Estimates of the likelihood of events suggest that the least likely hypothesis (outside the world of fantasy) is *Superman.*

Hypothesis generation is critical to the accuracy of the diagnostic process. If the pool of hypotheses generated to explain diagnostic cues does not contain the actual diagnosis, errors may result and we hear the comment: "I never thought of that." The following example of a set of data and the pool of hypotheses it generates will help clarify the idea of hypothesis generation:

A 50-year-old male client with high blood pressure and mild heart failure is being seen in a clinic. He looks exhausted (dark circles under his eyes, expressionless face, slow gait) and during the assessment of his sleep-rest pattern he reports that he is tired and having trouble sleeping.

This cluster of cues, which contain the diagnostic cue "trouble sleeping," suggests Sleep Pattern Disturbance. Once the cluster of cues has been interpreted in this way, the next thought is: What kind of disturbance? What pool of alternative possibilities might explain the client's appearance and verbal report? The following hypotheses provide alternative structures for this diagnostic problem and some direction for further cue search:

Sleep onset disturbance
Interrupted sleep pattern
Sleep pattern reversal
Early awakening pattern

Further information may reveal that one of these diagnostic hypotheses accounts for the client's "trouble sleeping." If so, the next step is to generates causal hypotheses to explain the problem. Although the data are sketchy at this point, nocturnal dyspnea and fear, anxiety, or depression over deteriorating health should be considered.

The discussion of thinking processes that cannot be seen, heard, or touched is sometimes hard to understand. An idea that may be useful in imagining hypothesis generation is "branching."[16] Branching from a diagnostic cue to generate multiple hypotheses may be compared to the branches on a tree that reach out in various directions. The small twigs coming off a branch represent questions and observations that are used to test hypotheses during a search for further cues. The generation and subsequent testing of hypotheses can be thought of as a decision tree. Consider the following data:

Ms. J. is a 45-year-old white married woman with cancer of the liver and jaundice.[17] She is going home from the hospital in 2 days and is physically able to resume all activities. She states she doesn't know how her friends will react to her color.

Fig. 8-3 depicts three hypotheses, or branches, generated from the cues and pattern areas (role-relationships, self-perception–self-concept, and health perception–health management). All three branches represent viable hypotheses. The reason-

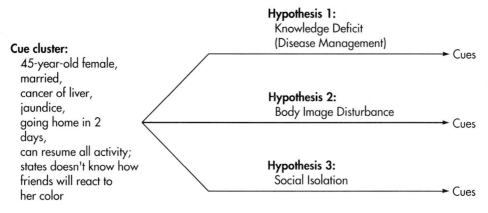

Fig. 8-3 Branching hypotheses that guide cue search.

ing in two of the areas of branching is described below:

1. If jaundice, then abnormality in skin color
2. If abnormality in skin color, then change in outward appearance
3. If change in outward appearance, then feelings of being different
4. If feelings of being different, then negative perception of body or self
5. If feelings of being different, then fewer family and social contacts
6. Check client's perception of self
7. Check for social isolation

The experienced clinician rarely needs to go through this reasoning process. Having cared for many patients with jaundice, he or she probably thinks:

Jaundice → altered body image perception

Jaundice → social isolation

Information is then collected to support or reject the hypotheses. If a clinician were pressed to explain the above reasoning, Goffman's conceptual model of stigma and social identity[18] might be cited.

Consider another example of branching:

In an emergency room a nurse has done a screening of a client for problems in the 11 functional pattern areas. When the role-relationship pattern (work role and relationships) was being assessed, the client said he was a plumber. While dressing the severe laceration of his right hand, the nurse asked him how he would manage at work. This branching question was based on a reasonable inference that the laceration would interfere with the use of the client's right hand. The nurse was checking the inference in a nondirective manner to elicit the client's ideas or plans. The basis for the question was the proposition that plumbers work with their hands, lifting and twisting things. The nurse might also have asked whether the client lived alone. How did he plan to manage his self-care, such as dressing, bathing, and cooking? These questions represent branching from a set of cues, background knowledge, and a sensitivity to human needs for self-care and work. Imagine the branching that would direct the search for cues for a plumber whose work activities became impossible or contraindicated because of neuromuscular, cardiac, respiratory, or psychiatric problems.

To anticipate the possibility of functional problems from a set of situational or contextual cues is an ability whose presence or lack makes care effective or ineffective. This ability requires sensitivity to the likelihood of events. The failure to raise the possibility of a diagnosis is associated with the failure to collect information. If we don't think of a diagnostic possibility, we can't test it. Hypotheses are "theories" about what the cues mean. "Albert Einstein said it best: 'It is the theory which decides what we can observe.' "[4 (p. 70)]

How is this done? Some experienced clinicians say certain cues are "automatically" associated with certain diagnostic hypotheses. Others say the possible hypotheses "just pop up" or "come to mind." Research on experts suggests that their memory stores contain prototypes or patterns, and if a particular cue or cues are representative of a

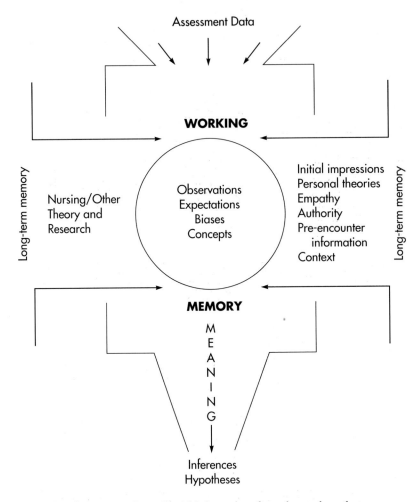

Assessment Data

WORKING

Observations
Expectations
Biases
Concepts

Nursing/Other
Theory and
Research

Initial impressions
Personal theories
Empathy
Authority
Pre-encounter
    information
Context

Long-term memory

Long-term memory

MEMORY

M
E
A
N
I
N
G

Inferences
Hypotheses

Fig. 8-4 Transformation of information: from data to hypotheses.

pattern, it "comes to mind." Similarly, experts have learned what conditions or events occur frequently, and these hypotheses are readily available and activated if the pattern of a set of cues resembles one of them.[19] Experts in an area generate hypotheses effortlessly and ask fewer questions (data collection) than a novice.

These explanations do not help the beginner. When just starting to acquire clinical knowledge for interpreting assessment data, the novice needs to learn how to activate hypotheses stored in memory. This process is depicted in Fig. 8-4. This figure illustrates the use of working and long-term memory. The following discussion suggests some useful ways to "zero in" quickly on likely possibilities by finding the right problem area.

Finding the problem area

The initial information in a pattern may be so specific and diagnostic that it suggests only one problem area. Yet in many instances this is not the case; the actual problem area is not clear. Cognitive "work" must be done to find the most likely area in which the problem lies before a pool of diagnostic hypotheses can be generated. Below are some hints about the use of the assessment framework and other sources of hypotheses.

Pattern areas

The use of the 11 functional pattern areas can facilitate hypothesis generation. Initial hypotheses, such as Sleep Pattern Disturbance or a role-relationship problem, are inadequate as diagnoses, but they serve to structure thinking early in assessment. Newell and Simon[20] are cognitive theorists who propose that the universe of possibilities is narrowed to a limited *problem space* by early information. A problem space can be thought of as an area of clinical knowledge; for example, thinking that a particular set of cues "seems like a nutritional problem." Generally, when a diagnostic cue is observed during assessment in an area, that pattern is the problem space. Each of the 11 pattern areas can narrow the universe of possibilities and focus the clinician's thinking on the diagnoses listed under that pattern area. Use Appendix B or a manual that lists diagnoses under the pattern areas[21] to make the broad hypotheses more specific. For the beginner it may also be useful to think about an admission assessment as a set of questions:

1. Does this client have a health perception–health management problem?
2. A nutritional-metabolic problem?
3. An elimination problem?
4. An activity-exercise problem?
5. A sleep-rest problem?
6. A cognitive-perceptual problem?
7. A self-perception–self-concept problem?
8. A role-relationship problem?
9. A sexuality-reproductive problem?
10. A coping–stress-tolerance problem?
11. A value-belief problem?

If the hypothesis generated is "nutritional problem," the list of diagnoses grouped in that pattern area provides a pool of hypotheses. The following list encompasses currently identified nutritional problems in the adult; eventually the novice will group and store the individual items in memory:

High Risk for Obesity (NANDA: Altered Nutrition: High Risk for More than Body Requirements)
Exogenous Obesity (NANDA: Altered Nutrition: More than Body Requirements)

Nutritional Deficit (Specify) (NANDA: Altered Nutrition: Less than Body Requirements)
High Risk for Nutritional Deficit
Uncompensated Swallowing Impairment
Altered Oral Mucous Membrane
High Risk for Fluid Volume Deficit
Fluid Volume Deficit
Fluid Volume Excess

Let us examine a screening assessment. Try to determine the possible hypotheses and how they may have controlled the cue search.

Assessment

Mr. D. is a healthy-appearing, single 60-year-old salesman with well-controlled high blood pressure.

Health perception–health management pattern. Client views himself as healthy and enjoying life. Takes medications as prescribed.

Nutritional-metabolic pattern. In reviewing his dietary pattern, he states that he avoids meats except for hamburger, doesn't like eggs or fish, and rarely eats raw vegetables or fruits. He comments that he likes everything to be cooked well.

The initial impression, "healthy appearing," indicates that Mr. D.'s body weight, facial expression, speech, skin, and mobility do not *globally* appear to present problems. This tentative impression provides a background for the rest of the assessment. The nurse began assessing the client's nutritional-metabolic pattern by raising the question (broad hypothesis): Does this client have a nutritional problem? The first component reviewed (consistent with the broad hypothesis) was the dietary intake pattern. Note the client's response. It supports the broad hypothesis and indicates the possibility of problems. He eats only soft foods. This kind of diet may be associated with an inadequate nutritional pattern. This report of a soft diet initiated a search for cues guided by less broad hypotheses: Does the client have a nutrient, caloric, fluid, vitamin, or mineral deficit? Inferences from the medical diagnosis—essential hypertension—and the nurse's initial impression suggested a 50:50 chance that any dysfunctional pattern existed. This is typical in the admission assessment, in which there is an equal probability that a problem exists or does not exist. Now data are collected to test the hypotheses generated.

A detailed review of the client's typical daily intake revealed less than minimum requirements for protein and vitamin intake. Intake of other nutrients was sufficient. When asked if this dietary pattern represented a change, Mr. D. replied: "Well . . . yes, I guess in the last year or so."

The nurse's hypothesis, nutritional problem, led to a search for details of the client's daily intake, a comparison with standard requirements, and an evaluative judgment of the data. (Note that some of the original hypotheses were discarded, and the problem narrowed to a protein and vitamin deficit. The next question to the client established that there was a pattern change that evidently occurred over a year ago. At this point the nurse should raise the question of *why the change occurred* and pursue some causal hypotheses. Since a broad question about the reason for the change did not elicit useful information, the questions became more specific:

No indigestion or "stomach trouble" was reported. A question in regard to chewing difficulty produced the report that Mr. D. had had a lot of back teeth pulled as a teenager. Examination revealed many missing back teeth, multiple dental caries, and broken teeth.

Three cue search decisions are evident. The first was to elicit cues in the area of the client's gastrointestinal tolerance for food. The second decision was to seek cues to his chewing difficulties. This cue search led to a third decision, to examine the client's teeth as a possible reason for the soft diet. Two questions were asked, one in the area of gastrointestinal tolerance for food and the other in regard to chewing. The hypothesis of chewing difficulty directed the search for cues by examination of his teeth.

The nurse's inquiry about indigestion was probably based on the proposition that if symptoms or concerns exist about a gastrointestinal problem, then soft foods are eaten. On the basis of this proposition, the hypothesis that the problem was gastrointestinal was tested. The client reported no indigestion or "stomach trouble." This response, plus the absence of any pathological condition noted on medical examination, was sufficient information for discarding this causal hypothesis.

A second causal hypothesis, chewing difficulty and dental problems, was raised. This hypothesis probably rested on the proposition that discomfort in chewing can lead to a change to a diet of soft foods. The age of the client and his verbal report were supporting data. A decision was made to examine the client's teeth, and the data provided support for the hypothesis of dental problems.

The example illustrates hypothesis generation and hypothesis-directed decisions. More information is needed before stating a diagnosis, such as the client's perception of his dental problem, the actions he has taken to deal with the problem, and factors in other pattern areas that may be interacting to produce this problem. The possibility that Mr. D. has a knowledge deficit about minimum daily dietary requirements should also be investigated.

In this example multiple hypotheses were tested simultaneously by asking about dietary pattern (possibilities related to the client's food and fluid intake), quickly narrowing the possibilities. Causal hypotheses about digestive disturbances and dental problems were then pursued one by one. Different hypothesis-testing procedures yield different costs and benefits. For example, one procedure may ensure maximum information but strain memory capabilities (holding and testing multiple hypotheses). Another procedure may control memory strain but may be too time-consuming (hypothesis testing one by one).

When no information is available at the beginning of an assessment, the *first step is to narrow the possibilities*. The list of 11 pattern areas to be assessed is one aspect of a diagnostic strategy that does this. These patterns are the focus of concern in nursing; they circumscribe the important areas of assessment and serve as a problem space structure for retrieving clinical knowledge from memory. Then, as data are collected, broad hypotheses give way to more specific diagnostic hypotheses.

Pattern sequence

The sequence of information collection may facilitate interpretation (hypothesis generation). In addition to suggesting possible diagnostic hypotheses, assessing the health perception–health management pattern first is a good starting point from the client's perspective. It is relevant, regardless of the level of care or the setting. As previously stated, defining the situation and learning how to manage are uppermost in the client's mind when seeking health care.

No research has been done on the relationship between the sequence in which patterns are assessed in the nursing history and the nurse's cognitive processing of information. Therefore it is not known whether or not nurses' use of information is facilitated by the sequence of data collection. As the pattern areas are used more frequently in the nursing specialties, a viable sequence may evolve. Interrelations among patterns may suggest diagnostic and etiological (causal) possibilities. A problem that occurs in one pattern may be caused by a problem(s) in other patterns. For example, the dietary and fluid pattern (nutritional-metabolic) may explain an intermittent constipation pattern (elimination pattern). Excess caloric intake (nutritional-metabolic pattern) and sedentary activity (activity-exercise pattern) may be etiological factors in a pattern of obesity (nutritional-metabolic pattern). Similarly, anxiety (self-perception–self-concept pattern) may be caused by a sleep-pattern disturbance (sleep-rest pattern) or the reverse.

After the health perception–health management pattern has been assessed, a logical sequence from one content area to the next should be followed. For example, it seems logical to assess self-perception–self-concept, then role-relationships, and then the sexuality-reproductive pattern. One flows from the other. Similarly, the nutritional-metabolic and elimination patterns seem logically related. From a psychological perspective, the value-belief pattern (including spirituality) and the sexuality-reproductive pattern may be considered highly personal areas. Most nurses do not assess these areas until rapport has been established and the client is at ease. Hence these patterns should be placed later in the sequence.

The sequence of pattern assessment may be related to individual situations. In a psychiatric setting nurses have found that it facilitates thinking to assess self-perception–self-concept and role-relationship patterns after assessing the client's health perception–health management pattern. In a medical or surgical setting, the nutritional-metabolic pattern might be the second area assessed, followed by the elimination pattern. With experience the clinician can develop an order that

takes the client and the situation into consideration and facilitates information processing during the history. For the first few nursing histories, try this sequence:

1. Health perception–health management pattern
2. Nutritional-metabolic pattern
3. Elimination pattern
4. Activity-exercise pattern
5. Sleep-rest pattern
6. Cognitive-perceptual pattern
7. Self-perception–self-concept pattern
8. Role-relationship pattern
9. Sexuality-reproductive pattern
10. Coping–stress-tolerance pattern
11. Value-belief pattern

SOURCES OF HYPOTHESES (INTERPRETATIONS)

Both the client and the nurse should collaborate in explaining signs and symptoms (hypothesis generation). The person, family, and community may have ideas about their own behavior, and these ideas are also "data." The nurse has the ability to use context, experience, personal theories, authority, and initial impressions to generate hypotheses to explain assessment data (Fig. 8-4). These sources may facilitate reasoning but, without verification, may also be the source of errors in reasoning.

Client's viewpoint

When hypotheses fail to "come to mind," it may be useful to obtain the client's viewpoint. Obtaining the client's viewpoint also involves the client in problem identification and, subsequently, in problem solving. Many nurses take the philosophical position that, as a general rule, clients should be involved. One method of assessing problems from the client's perspective is to use the following set of questions to guide discussion (use a supporting and sincere attitude during questioning, not challenging or interrogational):

1. *Client's definition of the problem* (following a description of the client's signs and symptoms or of a situation): "What do you think that means?" or, "What do you think that is?"

2. *Client's definition of cause:* "Why do you think that occurs (happens)?" or, "I wonder what causes that."
3. *Actions taken in response to the problems:* "What do you do when that happens?" or, "How do you handle that?" or, "How have you managed that?"
4. *Effectiveness of action taken:* "Did (does) that seem to help (work)?"

Clients' descriptions of their problems, their ideas about the causes of problems, and their responses to and evaluations of the actions they have taken provide a wealth of data on health perception, health management, and coping patterns, as well as a measure of personal control and competency.

A philosophy of nurse-client interaction that involves the person, family, or community in problem identification–problem solving always elicits the information described above. Rather than being a way of generating possible interpretations of cues, this method should be an integral part of practice.

Expectancies

Expectancies are ready-made explanations for cues stored in memory. These ready-made explanations are the source of hypotheses that are used to explain cues or predict possibilities; they include the following:

Background knowledge
Contextual information
Generalizations from experience
Personal theories
Generalizations from authority
Generalizations from initial impressions

Background knowledge

Background knowledge and experience stored in memory can be retrieved to predict risk states or derive meaning from assessment data. Stored knowledge can be used as "if-then" propositions or expectancies. An expectancy is a ready-made interpretation derived from memory. Norms are expectancies and can influence the prediction of risk states and nursing diagnoses. For example, most nurses would predict that the skin of an elderly client who is thin, immobile, and incontinent will break down. This expectation suggests the diagnostic hypothesis of High Risk for Impaired Skin

Integrity. Empathetic thinking suggests that the client may be fearful (of hospital procedures) and that the family may be coping ineffectively with the client's illness.

To avoid errors. When generating hypotheses based on past knowledge of "typical" or "similar" client situations (exemplars, prototypes), be aware of the assumptions ("rules of thumb") underlying hypotheses. Examine them for logical error. It might be argued that this is unnecessary because hypotheses are tested by collecting further information. If they are wrong it will become evident in the lack of supporting data. Although this is true, one common diagnostic error is to hold on to hypotheses in the face of disconfirming evidence.

Contextual information

Information available prior to encountering a client may produce expectations and activate memory stores that influence hypothesis generation. This information includes the type of setting, specialty area, medical diagnosis on the admitting sheet, previous records, and colleagues' comments. These historical and current contextual cues, described in Chapter 7, can be powerful influences on perception and diagnostic judgments. For example, the acuteness of the illness and the setting, such as a hospital, long-term care facility, or rehabilitation center, influence the incidence of nursing diagnoses. A knowledge of high-incidence diagnoses can be used in generating hypotheses and anticipating high-risk problems. In a critical care unit a high incidence of Pain, High Risk for Infection, and Fluid Volume Deficit might be expected, but in a rehabilitation nursing setting all the dimensions of Impaired Mobility, Self-Care Deficit, High Risk for Injury, and High Risk for Skin Breakdown should be expected.[22]

In addition to setting and nurse's acuity, specialty areas of practice influence hypotheses. Before seeing clients, a nurse in a cardiac surgical unit expects them to have cardiac problems, to have undergone surgery, and to have nursing diagnoses that are commonly associated with these conditions. The use of expectations increases a nurse's sensitivity to subtle diagnostic cues. For example, in this specialty nurses are sensitive to cues indicating ineffective coping with fear or anxiety regarding surgery and surgical prognosis, knowledge deficits regarding what will happen or how to do breathing exercises postoperatively, ineffective family coping, pain, activity intolerance, and other problems. These hypotheses are generated by cardiac surgical nurses from their knowledge and experience related to the occurrence of medical and nursing diagnoses in the specialty.

In addition to the specialty and the setting, the nurse may draw on information from other sources to generate hypotheses prior to seeing the client. A medical diagnosis of the present illness, records of previous hospitalizations or clinic visits, or referrals from community health nurses may create expectations. Nurses have learned that particular pathologic conditions are associated with changes in certain functional patterns. Some textbooks specify the nursing diagnoses that occur with specific medical diseases. These specifications provide "food for thought" about possible diagnostic hypotheses. There is insufficient research to predict which nursing diagnoses occur with each medical diagnosis. Some have a logical relationship. Nursing and nursing diagnoses focus on the individuality of human responses. Thus the reliability of predicting all nursing diagnoses from medical diagnoses is low.

In wellness clinics, ambulatory health care, and well-child care centers, as well as other community practice areas where persons do not have a disease, preencounter information about a client's age or developmental transitions may suggest hypotheses about his or her health patterns or diagnoses that should be checked.

Other sources of diagnostic hypotheses are the comments and observations of medical or nursing colleagues. A physician calls and says, "I'm sending in a patient; she's been having a hard time with her husband over the surgery." Or a nurse may say, "I just saw him come in on the stretcher; he doesn't look good." Expectations start to form from these comments.

Contextual cues about the client's situation may also be a source of hypotheses. In a research study, nurses used contextual cues to identify the most likely diagnostic hypotheses.[23] When nurses were given the task of determining the presence or absence of a set of surgical complications, the first information they sought concerned the type of surgery performed and the time elapsed since surgery. Even when information was restricted, these were the first data collected, rather than information about clients' surgical complications. In actuality, the nurses' strategy was very efficient; the two contextual cues permitted them to predict the most likely hypotheses and quickly narrow the possibilities. This strategy was labeled *predictive hypothesis testing.*

To avoid errors. Preencounter hypotheses are formed before any interaction with the client and are confirmed or rejected during assessment. Expectancies or predictions may prove true or totally inaccurate. Beware: they may also bias the diagnostician toward a particular hypothesis. Hold them, but not firmly. Wait for the assessment data and make sure the hypotheses are supported by actual data. As reasoning continues in a particular situation, it is not always easy to remember what is observed and what is created from expectancies, but mixing up observations and expectancies increases the possibility of diagnostic errors (of omission and commission).

Generalizations from experience

Hypotheses that structure the data and interpret their possible meaning may be derived from generalizations about experience. These generalizations are based on the recognition of similarities in repeated events. When viewed as similar, repeated events are combined by induction to yield a generalization, rule, or prototype. The generalization may then be used in the next similar situation that occurs. Fig. 8-5 depicts the process and the risk.

In some instances nurses and their colleagues develop maxims. For example, Brykczynski[24] reports maxims used by nurse practitioners, such as "real disease declares itself." This means that, provided a clinician keeps watching a situation in which doubt exists, if the hunch is right and the disease is present, it will eventually declare itself in signs and symptoms. Maxims usually have a link to action. In this case the action is to keep watching if doubt exists.

Various characteristics of client situations are used as a basis for inductive reasoning and generalization. For example, a nurse makes an observation: When one client in a unit becomes very ill or dies, other clients are anxious and upset. Repeated observations of this phenomenon are generalized to: Critical illness or death on a unit produces anxi-

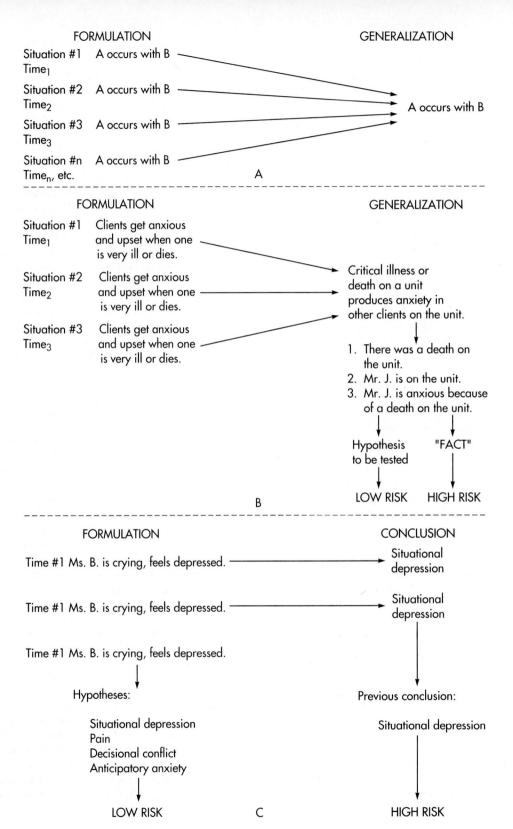

Fig. 8-5 Examples of generalizations from experience (A), across situations (B), or across time (C), and the risk involved in their use.

ety in other clients on the unit. Having acquired this knowledge from practice, the nurse may use it in the next similar situation encountered. Notice that no data are used to indicate whether the clients are also anxious when the situation is absent! Therein lies the risk. If this proposition is treated as a hypothesis to direct cue search, the risk is reduced. If the assumption that "Mr. J. is anxious because of Mr. B.'s cardiac arrest" is acted on without further checking, the risk of error is substantial.

To avoid errors. The key to accuracy when generalizing from experience is not to rush into action before testing the hypothesis. Collecting information will determine the "truth" of the deduction. Unvalidated assumptions are risky; in this example, anxiety regarding Mr. B.'s cardiac arrest may not be the correct or the only hypothesis to explain Mr. J.'s behavior. What explanations might have been proposed if Mr. J. were anxious and no cardiac arrest had occurred? Other hypotheses would have had to be generated.

Nurses can generalize not only from repeated experiences with a particular situational context but also from repeated similar experiences with the same person or persons. For example, the people in a community have been resistant or hostile to developing needed health care services. The nurse infers that today the same reaction will occur (and perhaps responds as if it is occurring). Generalizations from past behavior to expectations of present or future behavior can be risky. When used as rigid assumptions, inferences may close out cues that signal change. On the other hand, generalizations about a person's behavior can sensitize the nurse to important changes from the client's baseline. The key is to be open to cues and remember that most cues have an element of uncertainty.

Consider another example. A clinician, having cared for a number of families in a particular community health nursing district, notices similarities in their knowledge of preventive health measures. He generalizes about the neighborhood: Families in the neighborhood know of the need for immunizations for children. A young family that has lived in this small neighborhood for 10 years encounters some very complex health problems and is added to his caseload. He is very busy. What is the risk of inferring, rather than assessing, family practices regarding their small children's immunizations.

Generalizing from experience is useful if the relevant factors that produce the similar events are identified. A risk is taken if (1) the family that is new to the clinician does not have the same characteristics as the families on which the general proposition was built, (2) important factors producing the relationship are not identified, or (3) overgeneralization occurred initially. Living in the same neighborhood may be totally irrelevant to preventive health measures. On the other hand, it may be relevant because social interactions permit sharing of information about immunizations. The use of induction from experience, as described above, requires that one have a grasp of the likelihood of events. Repeated experiences can suggest to the person making the inference that (1) things are about to change (the gambler's fallacy) or (2) a "run" is occurring; that is, when a relationship between certain events has been observed ten times, it is safe to infer that the same relationship will exist the eleventh time. Both rules may lead to error unless one is sensitive to the risks they entail.

People tend to overestimate the probability of impressive events; they believe more have occurred than has actually been the case.[19] For example, cardiac arrests produce both an emotional and a cognitive impression. As a second example, when students begin the study of pathology, they become impressed by the seriousness of some illnesses and begin to think they and their classmates have the symptoms. These examples describe salient (highly striking) experiences. The nurse in the first example may be more sensitive to cues because of the cardiac arrest experience. The students are sensitive to interpreting symptoms using the new, impressive, readily accessible categories. In both cases there is increased readiness to infer because of experience.

Recall that anticipation facilitated sensitivity to cues and inferences. It can also lead to "systematic and predictable errors."[24] (p. 1131) Past impressive salient events may be highly accessible in memory and because of this may appear to be more likely to recur than they actually do. Generalization from experience (inductive reasoning) is one reference point for hypotheses. Sweeping generalities may be made, or sensitive reflections on multiple experiences during many years of practice may produce clinical wisdom.

Personal theories

In addition to single propositions, complex systems of propositions are sometimes constructed to interpret cues. Health care providers may have their own personal theories of health and disease and even an implicit theory of personality. This is particularly true in areas where science is "fuzzy." These personal theories may reflect reality or contain many illusions. Most contain at least a portion of truth.[25] These so-called theories are constructed during social learning. They are based on experiences in living with other people. Generalizations may be made about human traits, dispositions, and actions. Jones[25] (p. 52) states:

One way to sensitize people to the existence of such beliefs is to pose a question such as "What do you think of a wise, cruel man?"—a jarring inconsistency for most people. For most people, wise men are generally kind, old, and perhaps jaded, but never cruel.

Implicit theories about what people are like, what personality characteristics go together, and what causes behavior may be firmly entrenched. A study in the United States of nurses' inferences of suffering[26] found differences between the inferences of Puerto Rican and other (white or black) nurses. The other nurses inferred that patients experienced less suffering. In general the disease, age, and socioeconomic class of the patients being portrayed influenced the inferences of all the groups of nurses studied. Sociocultural learning was probably influential.

In brief encounters, a person's physical characteristics, a situation, or a patient's disease may be sufficient basis from which to infer traits, dispositions, or secondary health problems; for example, "a high forehead goes with intelligence," "self-confidence predicts a successful and happy person," or "psychiatric patients will be violent."[27] These stored "theories" and related propositional "knowledge" are implicit assumptions whose construction has been worked on since childhood. The tendency to make inferences without factual data is referred to as *bias*.[28] It can influence the interpretation of cues and even perception.

Beliefs about groups of people may be incorporated into implicit theories.[25] The term *stereo-type* describes an inference that all group members are alike. On the basis of one or two cues, a client is classified as a group member and then is assumed to have all the other attributes of the group stereotype. Stereotypic categorization ignores individual differences, as is evident in the group stereotypes about nurses, physicians, various cultures, races, and people of particular religions or nationalities.

Stereotypes are essentially expectations. They are constructed with minimal actual knowledge of the group and sometimes are based on no experience with group members. Stereotypes generally are based on hearsay evidence that is culturally transmitted. Presumably they are not directly related to prejudice (negative attitudes toward a group of persons).[25,29]

A lack of information about, a low degree of interest in, and limited contact with a particular group combine to increase anonymity and subsequent stereotypic classification.[30] This should be kept in mind when decisions are made about having time for an admission assessment. The use of stereotypes based on insufficient information "appears to be a sign of rigidity, occasioned partly by lack of intelligence and insufficient familiarity" with persons.[31] (p. 102)

Biases, errors, and misperceptions result if inferences derived from stereotypes are not subjected to validation. Stated differently, the use of stereotypes or attributions as if they were observed data ignores the uniqueness of the individual. Designating a client as "the gallbladder" encourages anonymity and an extremely broad classification of the client.

When negative stereotypes are used without knowledge or rational thought, they can have unfortunate consequences. Merton[32] defined these consequences as "self-fulfilling prophecy." The false definition of a situation may evoke new client behavior that makes the originally false conception come true. Simply, "if men define situations as real, they are real in their consequences."[33] Extreme caution must be exercised not to draw negative inferences about clients and their behavior from propositions that have no basis in reality.

Consider an example of negative stereotyping (at least negative in terms of its social value): the cancer-patient-as-terminal prophecy. Future-oriented planning by a "terminal" patient is sometimes labeled denial of terminal illness. Considering the great uncertainty in prognosis, many times there is no valid reason for the patient not to expect to survive for months or years. Hypotheses derived from pessimistic propositions or beliefs about death, coping, personal worth, and general ability to control events may be unintentionally communicated to clients during assessment. The potential then exists for the self-fulfilling prophecy to occur.

Empathy is a form of analogy (a correspondence between dissimilar things) and a personal "theory construction" commonly used in nurse-client interactions. The clinician's own feelings and intentions are used to infer the feelings and intentions of a client. In using the self as a theoretical reference point the nurse assumes that all (or many) people share human characteristics and behavior. Therefore the nurse's expectation is that he or she and the client will experience things similarly. The client's behavior is thought to be understood or predicted because it is the way the nurse would feel, behave, or act. Inner experiences of the self plus assumed similarity are the bases for the empathy.[34] In contrast to stereotyping without adequate information, empathy is a form of analogy that is highly valued. In everyday conversation, people understand each other because they share the same meaning of the symbols (words) they use for communication.

Empathy, in contrast, depends on the shared meaning of reactions to human experiences. Empathy is "an attitude of receptiveness, availability, and presence with the whole of one's self."[35] Empathic understanding appears to be an ability closely related to imagination. Sensitivity to the feelings of a person in distress depends heavily on the capacity to imagine how the person feels. Understanding is communicated when a clinician begins to inquire about a client's feeling and intentions. Empathy requires attention to situational cues and the temporary projection of oneself into the situation the client is experiencing. The resulting perceptions are used as hypotheses to direct cue search. Inferences generated by empathic understanding increase sensitivity to cues, particularly cues about feelings and intentions. The use of the self as an analogy is more likely when nurse and client share similar beliefs, attitudes, and personalities; when there is acceptance and liking of

the client; and when they share a similar social status.

Take care that the ability to share empathetic understanding is not influenced by a *set* to interpret events in a particular way. Consider two examples:

Surgical nursing

Sue Jones, a 24-year-old primary nurse, has worked in a gynecological unit for 3 years since her graduation. She was married 2 years ago and has been trying to become pregnant. Today she is caring for Mrs. R., who is a 30-year-old recovering from a hysterectomy (removal of the uterus). Mrs. R. says: "I feel so terrible today." Sue, without hesitation, says: "I know how you must feel, but this hasn't affected your attractiveness and you have two lovely children." With a startled look, Mrs. R. replies: "I mean the pain is terrible. . . ."

Sue learned (the hard way) from this experience. Putting herself in the client's situation caused her to assume that Mrs. R. felt "terrible" because she was unattractive as a woman after the hysterectomy and could not have any more children. Sue *acted* on her feeling of empathy rather than using it to generate hypotheses. Sue decided that in the future she would (1) continue to be empathic but (2) would check her impressions and consider alternative possibilities before she spoke. Sue realized that because *she* thought she would be less attractive to her husband after a hysterectomy and that *she* could not have the children she so desired, she projected these personal feelings onto Mrs. R. She decided that in the future she would keep in mind that the cue "feeling terrible" might mean that any of the following conditions was present:

1. Perceived sexual identity disturbance
2. Grieving (loss of reproductive capacity)
3. Surgical pain
4. Postoperative fatigue

Rehabilitation nursing

John Cari, a 28-year-old primary nurse in a rehabilitation clinic, was seeing Mr. D., who had been in a car accident in which he lost his leg. His wife had been killed in the same accident. Mr. D. was being seen for follow-up on his gait and prosthesis. Initially, Mr. D. had experienced a severe body image disturbance after his amputation. This resolved after he learned to walk with the prosthesis and returned to work. While doing a screening health pattern assessment, John observed that Mr. D. was exhibiting a disinterested manner and that he reported (1) "his computer programming job was very demanding," (2) that all he did was "work and sleep" and "sometimes sleep never comes . . . probably because I'm overtired," (3) that he didn't see that "life is ever going to be more than work and sleep with my job," and (4) that "he didn't have the time to go out and meet new people."

John thought: Is there a reason Mr. D. is choosing to work so much? A body image disturbance might lead to focusing his energy on work if he feels accepted there. His explanation for the sleep-onset disturbance may be correct. If I were in his shoes, with his history, would I throw myself into my work for any other reasons? Maybe he has dysfunctional grieving over the loss of his wife and is using work as an escape from his thoughts. I'll start with the sleep and see if it is more than being tired. Then I'll ask if he had considered changing jobs and why he doesn't get out more.

> **John:** *"You mentioned that the difficulty you have getting to sleep is probably because you are overtired. Is there anything else that could be causing that?"*
> **Mr. D.:** *"No, not that I can think of."*
> **John:** *"All right; it's just that sometimes people start thinking about things and lie awake a long time."*
> **Mr. D.:** *"Yeah, I do that. When I'm overtired I keep reliving the accident and feeling I could have prevented it; I miss Angela so much and just can't seem to get on with my life. The leg isn't a problem now; it's the memories."*

To avoid errors. Personal theories develop as a result of life experiences. At times they are created with only uncertain, ambiguous, or scanty data. Yet they can influence a data base by two routes: information collection and information interpretation. It is essential to be aware that this influence may occur. Although personal theories may lead to sensitivity to cues and the ability to generate hypotheses, a high risk is taken if hypotheses that are based on implicit theories, stereotypes, and empathic reference to the self are not tested and validated by data.

Generalizations from authority

Teachers, textbooks, research journals, and experienced colleagues are frequently used as reference points for inference. The propositions gleaned from these sources may be research conclusions, clinical lore, and experiential wisdom. Inferences drawn from research conclusions are highly valid and useful if clients and situations are similar to the research subjects and settings. Conclusions are probabilistic; that is, they may apply to 95 out of 100 cases. The risk is that a particular client may have a critically dissimilar characteristic or may be within the other 5% rather than the 95% to whom the research findings apply. Again it should be noted that information deduced from any propositions should be treated as constructions of the observer's mind, not as clinical data. Validation in the real world is required if at all possible.

Other nurses also may provide a source of general propositions. Through a process of socialization and instruction, nurses share pooled experiences and probability estimates for certain signs and symptoms. The orientation period for a new clinician provides opportunities for staff to communicate the nature of the client population in both formal and informal ways. New personnel are told—explicitly and implicitly—what cues are important; they are given feedback about their perceptions and are socialized into the norms for assessment and diagnosis.

Socialization into a new role influences expectations. In turn, expectations activate categories and systems of propositions for identifying cues and interpreting data. By activating categories in memory and making them more accessible, socialization increases sensitivity to particular cues.

Bieri and colleagues[36] suggest that the type of setting and type of clients influence perceptual sensitivity and cue search. For example, if a client experienced an increased heart rate and restlessness in a psychiatric nursing setting, there might be a tendency to search for cues to the client's self-concept or role-relationship problems. In contrast, the same signs in a surgical setting might influence the nurse to check the client's temperature, the dressing, and the client's perception of pain or discomfort. Would there not be greater sensitivity to parenting cues in pediatric and obstetrical settings than in medical-surgical nursing settings? Are not intensive care nurses highly sensitive to physiological cues? Indeed they should be, when physiological instability is the major factor required for admission to this type of unit.

Soares[37] has described an aspect of knowledge that is taken for granted in an intensive care unit: that certain norms exist among "inside nurses" (regular staff) and different norms among "outside nurses" (float staff). Inside staff nurses have been exposed to the informal rules of interaction in the particular unit, and they have learned the taken-for-granted meanings that are known to the members of the inside group. Since outside nurses do not appear to understand the meanings conveyed in the unit, as seen by the lack of response to action messages, it seems feasible that these messages and meanings are peculiar to this particular unit.

The degree to which the lore transmitted by nursing and medical colleagues influences an individual's thinking depends in part on that individual's professional confidence and experience. A need to become part of the belief and value system of the group may be expected to facilitate acquisition of group norms. Studies suggest that a person who is uncertain about how to behave in a situation (possibly a new staff member or a new graduate) seeks information that can be used to respond in a "professionally appropriate" manner. Caution must be exercised in accepting statements such as "Oh, yes, all the old people in this community act like that"; "We don't bother with that here; they're only in this unit for 3 days"; or "Just do a quickie assessment; the clients here are pretty healthy and don't have any problems."

To avoid errors. The key is to reflect on the expectancies and probabilities of events communicated by colleagues. Treat the information obtained as hypotheses, not facts. The information may contain gems of wisdom or may lead to the perpetuation of errors. An "anchoring point" in theory, research, and one's own values is the best protection against unwisely adopting others' points of view.

Textbooks and teachers provide the most common anchoring points for generalizations and likelihood estimates about what occurs when and with what. Yet critical, logical examination of any reference point, including self-constructed propositions and ready-made inferences, is always in order.

In this section we have considered research, colleagues, teachers, and books that may be perceived as authoritative. They may be, and generally should be, a source of propositional knowledge to use in deducing the possible meaning of cues. As with all other reference points, caution needs to be exercised. Any hypotheses generated should be tested by collecting further information.

Generalizations from initial impressions

People, including clinicians, seem to need some overall reference point from which to begin to assess what a particular person or group is like. There are two reasons for this phenomenon. The first is idealistic: to be helpful a nurse must know the client as a person (or group) rather than as an object. Objects are observed, but the nurse interacts (or transacts) with people. The interpersonal relationship through which diagnostic information is obtained requires an understanding of people as people, not as an assessment of functional patterns in isolation. The second reason is merely the other side of the coin. Realistically, to perform the clinician's role the nurse must have some understanding of the feelings and intentions of others.

An initial impression of a client and his or her general health and situation is formed early in an interaction.[38] It can influence assessment and diagnosis whether or not the nurse is aware of the influence. Therefore it is important to understand how people form initial impressions of others, what peculiarities of practice influence impressions, and what suggestions can help one get around biased impressions. It should be noted that the following ideas apply particularly to cues about personal attributes and the inferences that result. These form a "backdrop" that can color further assessments, diagnoses, and even intervention.

People learn through experience to make quick inferences about other people's abilities, attitudes, interests, physical features, traits, and behavior. Category labels such as "wholesome," "friendly," "cold," or "hardworking" are used to describe global impressions of people. Value-belief systems "explain" how these personal attributes are related and whether they are to be positively or negatively valued. (What is being described here is a form of implicit theory about personality and social interaction.)

An initial impression is formed when a nurse meets a person or family or enters a community in a professional capacity. Functionally nurses' initial impressions or quick social evaluations permit them to choose their words and behavior in an initial interaction. In addition, but related to the preceding discussion, people may have the general tendency to infer the social characteristics of others. The extremes are the "Pollyanna syndrome" of overoptimism and the negative disposition that "people are no darn good." In general, reports of impressions contain more positive than negative descriptors.[25] The extreme disposition to infer that some people have is usually modified, at least to some extent, by professional education. This tendency to infer does not disappear entirely, as is evident from studies of clinicians' dispositions toward judgments of maladjustment.[39,40]

To avoid errors. Nurses' initial impressions are most likely to be influenced also by the client's health state. If a health problem exists, the medical diagnosis may produce social judgments as well as other impressions. For example, some conditions may be viewed as simply happening to a person (cancer), whereas other conditions may be thought of as the person's or family's fault (obesity or a child's growth delay). Impressions can be useful or lead to erroneous conclusions. If they slip into the data base without validation, diagnostic errors may occur.

Summary: interpretations as a source of hypotheses

To summarize this section on sources of diagnostic hypotheses, it may be said that nurses use their memory stores to generate alternative explanations (hypotheses) for cues. In the previous section retrieval of information from memory was discussed. The stored knowledge, theories, and impressions are used to "fill the gaps" and to interpret ambiguous information. Human beings interpret ambiguous, uncertainty-geared information by using both explicit and implicit generalizations, such as those discussed in the last section. It should be kept in mind that ambiguous information is part of the uncertainty-geared nature of clinical reasoning. Also, inadequate information collection predisposes to ambiguity and the creation of "facts," interpretations, or inferences. Interpretations are

sometimes colored by what care providers "know" is true, or at least is usually true. Ordinarily, people survive quite well on the basis of unexamined and sometimes untested inferences. Perception, as Neisser[41] has said, is self-correcting in the long run. The difficulty in clinical nursing practice is that the "long run" may be too late. Harm or discomfort may result from interventions that are based on unexamined and untested assumptions. Professionals need to set up a system of checks and balances.

Because at times information is ambiguous or insufficient, imagination fills in. The picture is "clarified"; gaps are filled. Inferences based on some data and some imagination are usually the fillers. Checks and balances should be built in to avoid the risk of error; they may be summarized as follows:

1. If at all possible, inferences should be treated as hypotheses to be tested. Inferences should be validated with the client and inferences about the social or physical environment should be rechecked.
2. The roots of inferences (expectations, assumptions, propositions, dispositions, and impressions) should reflect the likelihood of events in the world so that hypotheses are reasonable. Beware of overgeneralizing from experiences that are not representative. Ask for explanations and be curious so that a self-correcting process is established.
3. Inferential or intuitive leaps using minimal data or previous experience should be verified.
4. When inference and imagination are used in diagnosis, get feedback through further observation, follow-up, or colleague review. Always keep in mind the risk of acting with incomplete data. Build in safeguards.
5. Inferences tend to enter the data base used in diagnosis when the data base is incomplete. The more the nurse knows the person or family and their situation, the less need for creating information by inference.

The discussion in this section covered sources of cue interpretation used to generate alternative possibilities (hypotheses) to explain assessment data. The next section focuses on why this is important. Now that the source and importance of hypotheses have been considered, subsequent sections will be concerned with determining likely hypotheses and diagnostic strategies to test the possibilities.

IMPORTANCE OF CONSIDERING ALTERNATIVE HYPOTHESES

Explanations for cues that immediately "come to mind" are useful, but alternative hypotheses to explain the data should be considered, even when everything appears "obvious." Considering multiple hypotheses increases the chance that the correct diagnosis will be in the pool of hypotheses being considered.

One idea for generating multiple diagnostic interpretations of data in a health pattern area is to use knowledge stored in memory by taking a behavioral or environmental cue or set of cues and explaining their meaning using three familiar knowledge frameworks:

1. Physiological framework
2. Psychological framework
3. Sociological framework

For example, consider a client who reports his heart is "jumping." A physiological framework might suggest hypotheses regarding cardiovascular function, such as palpitations associated with excess smoking or caffeine intake. A psychological framework might take into account the possibility of a subjective feeling of fear or anxiety. A sociological framework might suggest that something might have occurred during an interpersonal interaction that generated conflict or anger at a relative. Knowledge stored in memory and available cues lead to inferences; these are converted to hypotheses to guide the search for further cues. The three areas—physiology, psychology, and sociology—are familiar. Many nurses' memory stores of basic knowledge are organized around these three areas. Thus the frameworks are a usable approach for understanding information. *The application of different frameworks to clinical data will help the diagnostician overcome a psychological set to categorize data prematurely.* Alternative viewpoints prevent the distortion of data by the first idea that "comes to mind." The readiness to interpret information in habitual ways may yield one of the following results:

1. Very accurate predictions because the nurse

has learned the real probability of events in practice
2. Errors because the nurse has forgotten that whenever people are involved, cues have a degree of uncertainty and there is always an exception to generalizations. Errors are reduced by always considering alternative explanations.

Studies suggest that with previous education in nursing diagnosis nurses can use diagnostic terms to describe the possibilities they are considering early in the diagnostic process.[42,43] This was observed when only one or two ambiguous diagnostic cues were present. The advantage of this behavior may lie in the subsequent search for cues. For example, if the diagnostician thinks one possible meaning of an initial cue is decreased self-esteem, this hypothesis clearly structures further assessment. The search for cues is focused on the evaluation of self-esteem. In contrast, a vague hypothesis such as "psychological problem" provides no clear focus for further assessment questions or observations.

In one study[43] there was a high percentage of agreement among the nurses that a particular set of diagnostic hypotheses should be investigated further; but the additional hypotheses they generated to explain initial cues showed a great deal of variability. The results were similar to that found in "brainstorming" or divergent thinking exercises. Diagnoses commonly associated with the cues were suggested by a high percentage of the subjects; the variability appeared in the "creative" alternatives that went beyond the diagnostic cues to less obvious possibilities. In this study of 160 baccalaureate staff nurses, the average number of hypotheses generated per task was three.[43]

DETERMINING LIKELY HYPOTHESES

As the determination of likely hypotheses is discussed, we are considering the point in assessment when the diagnostician has only a diagnostic cue or cue cluster in a pattern area (for example, when data indicating only restlessness is present) and three or four likely hypotheses have been generated to explain the meaning of the cue(s).

In the previous sections the reader was encouraged to think about all possible diagnoses that would explain a cue or initial cluster of cues, because studies have shown that if the correct hypothesis is not within the pool of hypotheses, diagnostic errors occur.[11,44] Now the diagnostician must determine the most likely possibilities for the individual client situation.

Why bother estimating which of the alternative hypotheses are most credible? Why not gather assessment data to test them all? The answer lies in efficiency, time conservation, and cognitive strain. It is more efficient and timesaving to eliminate unlikely possibilities. (Of course, if the likely hypotheses must be rejected the more unlikely possibilities should be examined.) Holding both high- and low-probability hypotheses in memory while collecting and interpreting data may strain cognitive capacities, and errors are the result. The reader may be thinking: How do you know which of your hypotheses are the most probable explanations for the data?

The likelihood of a given hypothesis is determined by considering the contextual data and the client situation. These include:

1. Contextual cues such as the client's age or developmental level; gender; culture; previous health history; and medical diagnoses, complications, and treatment. These factors may be used as predictive cues.
2. Functional assessment data already collected. For example, if some patterns have already been assessed, the data base may contain cues that can be used to estimate the likelihood of hypotheses generated to explain the data in subsequent patterns.

As one proceeds through functional pattern assessment gradually a clearer "individualized picture" of the client from a health perspective emerges. This picture may help determine which current diagnostic hypotheses are most probable. The key to estimating the likelihood of hypotheses is to learn the nursing diagnoses that show a high incidence with particular age or developmental levels, medical diagnoses, and the other factors specified above. For example, as nurses use diagnoses and gain experience, they may find a high incidence of social isolation in the frail elderly living alone with no family ties or social support and a high incidence of health management deficit in newly diagnosed diabetic clients with complex medication-exercise-diet regimens. Experts can quickly make

associations between predictive cues and the probability of diagnostic hypotheses. Time and mental energy are not wasted investigating unlikely possibilities.

Predictive hypothesis testing

In some instances early cues point to only one or two hypotheses that can be tested individually. If this is not the case, predictive hypothesis testing may be used to determine the most likely possibilities. Predictive hypothesis testing is defined as *the assessment of factors that establish probabilities.* It involves holding a few possibilities simultaneously while assessing contextual cues. The objectives of the strategy are listed below:

1. To obtain a lot of information quickly
2. To estimate the probability of the hypotheses in the pool
3. To reduce the number of hypotheses to avoid cognitive strain

Frequently the client's medical diagnosis provides a contextual cue to possible dysfunctional patterns. Consider a client who has experienced a cerebrovascular accident (stroke) involving the right side of the brain. Impaired verbal communication related to uncompensated aphasia (difficulty in speaking) is less likely than if the left side of the brain were involved. The presence of a second diagnosis, such as cardiac or respiratory disease, serves as a source of contextual data to increase the probability that self-care deficit, impaired mobility, and impaired home management will be present. The client's age, gender-role responsibilities, and other data may make some hypotheses more credible and others less so.

Although it does not involve nursing diagnoses directly, an example drawn from research findings[22] should further clarify predictive hypothesis testing. Nurses were given the task of determining whether or not a client was developing any postoperative complications (assessment task). All they were told was that they could have any information they wanted by asking for it and stating why it would be useful. The patient had had general surgery; the list of conditions to be assessed (hypotheses) included thrombophlebitis, wound infection, atelectasis, urinary retention, hemorrhagic shock, and no postoperative complications. The nurses were asked which condition(s) they thought were present?

Obviously, if the only initial information given is that the client has had general surgery, one hypothesis is as likely as the other. There are two options: to search for cues to each hypothesis one by one or to pick the most probable and test them first. If the most probable hypotheses can be determined quickly, information collection will be more efficient and less cognitive strain will occur. The information the nurses collected as a result of their first two questions indicated that predictive hypothesis testing was being used (simultaneously assessing multiple hypotheses by collecting contextual data). Their first two questions concerned the time lapse since surgery and the type of surgery performed. These are historical, *contextual cues.* They have nothing to do with the current state of the patient, as would blood pressure or urine output. Even when the nurses were limited to only 12 pieces of information in one of the tasks, these were the first two pieces of information requested. To know whether any surgical complication is present *now,* shouldn't information on the current state of the client be collected? Maybe so, but it may be important to know other information first.

How can we analyze the efficiency of these nurses' approach? In their first two questions they found that the patient had had gallbladder surgery and that it was done at "12 noon today" (in the second task, the time was given as "11 AM yesterday").[45] Using background knowledge and a network of interrelationships stored in memory past events can be restructured or future events predicted. For example, *if* the cues "short time lapse since surgery" and "gallbladder surgery" are present, *then* hemorrhagic shock is probable. Or, in the second case, *if* the cues are 15 to 18 hours postsurgery and gallbladder surgery, *then* atelectasis is highly probable. These are If-then propositions that underlie predictive hypothesis testing using contextual cues.

Is this procedure useful only in the area of identifying surgical complications? Probably not. Logically it would seem to be useful in all anticipatory diagnostic situations. The universe of possibilities cannot be tested, so events must be forecast on the basis of likelihood estimates. Elstein, Schulman, and Sprafka[14] have found that physicians dealing with uncertainty-based medical diagnoses also begin their task with predictive hypothesis testing.

The groupings of currently identified nursing diagnoses within each pattern area in Appendix B may be used as a pool of diagnostic hypotheses. Consider the following example of determining likely hypotheses and then narrowing the possibilities. Before beginning the assessment the nurse obtains the following background information from the client's chart and from observation while entering the client's room.

> Ms. B. is a 40-year-old alert, single executive who looks healthy but slightly overweight. She is sitting quietly near her bed. This is her third admission for gastric ulcer in 2 years.

At this point there are two cues: "slightly overweight" and "third admission in two years for gastric ulcer." The likely hypotheses lie in the nutritional pattern and perhaps also in health management.

The assessment of the likelihood of a diagnosis in the health-management pattern begins with a broad question that provides an introduction to the topic and to the client's view of her health situation. The first question might be: "How has your general health been in the last few years?" Or the nurse might say: "I noticed from the doctor's note that you have been having problems with . . . (insert client's report); how has your general health been in the last few years?" The following information was obtained and documented:

> Ms. B. has always perceived herself as "healthy." No colds or infections. Was thrown off her bicycle six months ago and now rides only on bicycle paths. "I get plenty of exercise and watch my diet. I don't know why the ulcer keeps acting up." In the last 5 months she gained weight from eating ice cream and drinking a lot of milk for an "acidy stomach"; says she looks "terrible" with the extra weight. Severe abdominal pain unrelieved by milk, cream, or antacids in the last week caused her to visit a physician; she was admitted on the same day due to a low hemoglobin level and blood in her stool. She delayed seeking help because of her busy work schedule; she stopped taking pills (name of medication not known) shortly after the last episode of bleeding because she felt better. States she works hard and that "I guess women have to work twice as hard to succeed in some companies."

States the doctor is going to try a regimen of "pills and antacids and see how I do for a few days."

Frequently at the beginning of assessment in a pattern area a broad question will produce considerable information for hypotheses. In this instance the information given decreased the probability of some hypotheses, but the probability is high for a risk for health management deficit (unless the client has a knowledge of medications, symptoms management, and diet). Further information must be collected to test this hypothesis. The client has provided some cues to possible job stress (busy work schedule; working twice as hard), pain management (episodes of severe pain), and body image disturbance (looks "terrible"), but these may be noted and followed up during assessment of self-perception–self-concept and role-relationship patterns. Holding multiple hypotheses in working memory and inferring whether data tend to support or negate each hypothesis may produce cognitive strain, which is usually short-lived. The payoff is that the universe of possibilities has been narrowed. As seen in the next discussion, diagnosticians test the remaining hypotheses one by one, thereby reducing memory and inferential strain to the minimum.

To summarize, when a diagnostic cue suggests a large number of possibilities, simultaneous testing of multiple hypotheses using contextual cues (predictive hypothesis testing) usually helps to determine the most probable hypotheses. Some helpful hints are listed below:

1. Use the routine screening questions suggested in Chapter 5 to investigate a diagnostic cue and consider alternative diagnostic hypotheses to explain the data. Use the diagnoses in the pattern area being assessed. Eliminate those that are unlikely in the particular client-situation; test the most likely possibilities first.
2. During assessment of a pattern area, keep in mind background contextual data related to developmental level or age, gender, medical diagnosis and treatment, and any other data already accumulated.
3. If contextual cues (initial observations of the client situation) predict that a pattern may be dysfunctional, begin assessment in that pattern area with a broad, nondirective question

to elicit maximum information on multiple hypotheses all at once. Sometimes examples of how to ask those questions are helpful; here are a few examples from the health pattern areas:
   "How has your general health been lately?"
   "How has your appetite and food intake been lately?"
   "Do you find your energy level is sufficient for doing what you want or need to do?"
   "How are working relationships in your job?"
   For an elderly person: "As people get older, they sometimes find that their sexual relationships change. How has it been for you and your husband?"
4. Generating, testing, deleting, revising, and adding diagnostic possibilities continue throughout the functional pattern assessment.

As previously discussed, hypotheses may be vague or highly specific depending on the information available. Some refer to such diagnoses as prediagnostic and diagnostic hypotheses. Prediagnostic hypotheses are the vague "educated" or "intuitive" guesses, such as, "I think there is a relationship problem here," or "She's really not managing her disease well." If these early hypotheses survive, they become more specific diagnostic hypotheses that describe the problem and etiological factors: "weak mother-infant attachment related to early separation" or "protein deficit related to scarce financial resources." (The novice who is learning to use diagnostic categories may find a manual helpful for suggesting special ideas and diagnostic terms.)

INVESTIGATING DIAGNOSTIC HYPOTHESES

Discussion in this section centers on strategies for testing hypotheses and the kind of data that increase confidence in diagnostic judgments. Weighting cues and resolving inconsistencies in the data are also important topics considered in this section. This discussion leads to the problem of how to state a nursing diagnosis, which is the subject of the next chapter.

Hypothesis testing takes the diagnostician beyond the routine assessment guidelines discussed in Chapter 5. Now questions and observations are focused on the high-probability diagnostic hypotheses under consideration. This is the point at which the most likely hypotheses for explaining an initial diagnostic cue or cluster of cues have already been identified. Now the important question is: Does sufficient data exist to support the presence of any of the hypotheses being considered?

Which hypothesis offers the best explanation of the cues? (*Best,* of course, means "most useful for thinking about intervention.") The answer is determined by a focused search for critical defining characteristics (diagnostic cues) specific to the diagnostic category represented in each hypothesis. Critical diagnostic cues are the signs or symptoms that are nearly always present if the diagnosis is present.

Moving from vague "hunches" to specific diagnostic hypotheses during the diagnostic process requires a series of decisions about acquiring, retaining, and utilizing assessment information. The sequential set of decisions is called a *strategy.* A diagnostic strategy includes decisions about what information to collect, in what sequence to collect it, and how to use the information.[2]

Various hypothesis-testing strategies may be used to learn which of the possibilities best describes the client's health problem. The overall objectives of any strategy are efficiency, accuracy, and confidence in the diagnosis attained. To meet these objectives, the following are necessary:

1. A knowledge of what cues would be present if the health problem described by a diagnosis were present. These cues will be the focus of the cue search. Learn the critical defining characteristics of the common diagnoses in your practice.
2. A reliance on highly valid and reliable cues so that confidence will be sufficiently high to use the final diagnostic judgment as a basis for planning intervention.
3. Prevention of "thinking errors" by controlling cognitive strain during information collection and processing.

Perhaps the best way to discuss hypothesis testing is through examples. Cues or cue clusters and diagnostic hypotheses will be presented and then the process by which the hypotheses are tested will be examined.

Case 1: initial data

Billy Smith, a premature baby, is 4 weeks old and weighs 6 pounds. He has been transferred to a medical center 10 miles from his home for treatment of a congenital defect in his heart. He has progressed well since birth and does not require an incubator at this time. Billy is the third child of 26-year-old parents; the other two children are 3 and 5 years old. During visiting hours the parents stand viewing their baby at the nursery window. Only after the nurse's aide offers do they say they would like to hold their baby. Mrs. Smith holds the baby on her lap with the child facing Mr. Smith. They continue to talk to each other. No inquiries are made about the baby's condition. During the second visit that day the same behavior is repeated. When the baby cries, Mrs. Smith rocks him on her knee.

Case 1: early hypothesis generation

Observations and background data contained diagnostic cues. These cues suggested hypotheses that could structure the diagnostic task. The following hypotheses were generated in the order of most to least likely (see p. 182 or the *Manual*[21] for defining characteristics):

Weak parent-infant attachment
Early parent-infant separation reaction
Fear (attachment to sick infant)
Reactive situational depression
Knowledge deficit (baby care skills)
Postpartum depression

The initial behavioral cues suggested that the parents' attachment to their baby was weak; early separation may produce this condition. On the other hand, the baby's cardiac condition may be viewed as life threatening, and the parents' reaction may be fear of bonding to an infant they think is going to die. A reactive situational depression is also plausible if they think the baby is going to die. The cues may be explained by postpartum depression, but the frequency of this condition is low. Knowledge Deficit (Baby Care Skills) is possible but unlikely, since the parents have two other children. The major cues of concern are the parents' lack of inquiry regarding the baby's condition and the parent-baby interaction. Lack of inquiry alone may not be significant, as the parents may have consulted with the physician. Yet when this cue is combined with the interaction cues, both gain significance.

Case 1: determining the most likely hypotheses

The nurse in a friendly way introduces herself and asks the parents how they are managing. The response to this broad question should elicit cues to be used in estimating the likelihood of the hypotheses in the set. The cues listed below in column 3 would have to be present if the conditions were present (the defining characteristics of the remaining diagnostic categories may be found in the *Manual*.[21])

Keep the diagnostic hypotheses in mind and use each piece of the case data to estimate their probability (high, medium, low). Consider the response of the parents to the nurse's question and her accepting, attentive manner:

Parents responded (hesitantly at first) that they "have this feeling that this is not our baby but know that it really is"; "It's a strange thing to have these feelings; the baby is cute."

(Estimate the probabilities of the previously listed hypotheses with each piece of data; watch how they change or remain the same.)

The nurse asks why they think these feelings are occurring. (She is thinking about weak parent-infant attachment and fear of attachment. If depression exists it probably is a secondary reaction to the other conditions.) The parents respond that the baby was premature and had a heart condition. They couldn't touch or hold the baby "because of the incubator and tubes." They said it was "so devastating that we began to visit less frequently. We had trouble handling the news about the cardiac condition, but the doctors say the baby will do fine. . . . Don't know why, but sometimes it seems to me (mother) like we are giving our love to our other children and don't seem to have any left for this one. I feel sad about this but really think it will be better now that they let me touch the baby; we really wanted a boy, seeing we had two girls." No mention here of fear of losing the baby (thus fear of attachment is reduced in probability for the moment). During this interaction Mrs. Smith is holding the baby as described above. The nurse asks her if she is comfortable holding the baby this way and if Mr. Smith wants to hold the baby. The mother replies: "I didn't even realize how I was holding him; see—that's an example of my not feeling close; I know how to hold a baby!" Nurse suggests she let Mr. Smith hold Billy and that she guide him in how to hold the baby.

Case 1: formulating a working diagnosis

At this point a diagnostic judgment is to be made. When the problem is this complex, thinking about the diagnostic judgment as a "working diagnosis" may be useful. Which of the hypotheses is supported by the data; that is, which cluster of signs and symptoms listed below or found in the *Manual*[21] most closely corresponds to the cluster

Hypothesis	Focused cue search (assessment)	Cues supporting the diagnosis
Weak parent-infant attachment	Facial expression, talking to baby; eye contact, kissing; holding position, comforting measures used; inquiries regarding baby's feeding, care, physical condition	Minimal smiling, close contact, enfolding, and talking to baby; does not assume "en face" position; little eye-to-eye contact; minimal kissing; continues unsuccessful comforting measures; infrequent inquiries regarding baby's condition
Early parent-infant separation	Time lapse; postpartum parent-baby interaction; frequency of interaction and caring activities	Postpartum separation of baby and parents or low-frequency contact for holding, cuddling, feeding, caring activities
Reactive situational depression	Mood state; degree of hope; current life situation and perception of situation	Expressed feelings of sadness, hopelessness, or despair; crying; feelings of failure or powerlessness; perception of current situation as crisis, stress, unmanageable

of signs and symptoms collected from the nurse's questions and observations thus far? It is a good idea to write down each hypothesis and then list supporting and nonsupporting data beneath each. Then see which hypothesis has sufficient support in the data. State your conclusion: what the problem is and what is contributing to the problem (etiology) that nursing can do something about. Following this, see Note 46 at the end of the chapter. Then consider another example:

Case 2: initial data

> Mr. W. is an alert, 75-year-old retired teacher who was admitted for removal of rectal polyps. A secondary diagnosis was chronic arthritis. Assessment of his cognitive-perceptual patternrevealed: Hearing aid, left ear; perceives whisper with hearing aid. Glasses for reading; checked 1 year ago; reads newsprint. No recent change in memory; keeps pills in kitchen near coffee so he is reminded to take them in the AM. Reports no difficulty in making decisions; balances checkbook for his daughter. No reported sensory changes in extremities. Complains of periodic aching pain in left hip joint, especially in the AM after arising. Arthritis diagnosed 10 years ago. Pain getting progressively worse in last 2 years; takes buffered 1 tab aspirin 4 times per day (not sure of dose). Grimacing noted when Mr. W. rises from sitting to standing position.

Case 2: early hypothesis generation

When assessment revealed a diagnostic cue (pain in hip joint), the nurse switched from the routine assessment format of the nursing history to the diagnostic process. The diagnosis of Pain is clear. The critical diagnostic criterion that must be present is a verbal report of pain or pain descriptors. Pain may signify serious conditions. In this case the order of likelihood is:

Arthritic pain

Post-hip fracture

Other pathological condition of bone

Further checking revealed no history of injury to the hip, and the physician's examination revealed minimal osteoporosis. The nurse concluded that the pain was associated with the documented medical diagnosis, chronic arthritis. The client's report of periodic pain and its character were noted in the chart for the physician. Consultation with the physician is necessary in order to discuss the drug

regimen. Having referred the pain cues to the physician, the nurse began to consider how nursing might be able to help this man. From a nursing perspective, what would be a useful way of thinking about this problem?

The diagnostic hypothesis that guided further data collection was chronic pain and self-management deficit. Cues to chronic pain were present, but was there a self-management deficit? If this condition were present, the following additional cues would also have to be present:

1. Lack of use of pain management techniques appropriate to the type of pain
2. Physical and cognitive ability to self-manage chronic pain

Case 2: hypothesis testing

Further assessment revealed that Mr. W. did not know how to manage arthritic pain. This information, plus the previous data on his cognitive and physical abilities, met the criteria stated above. At this point the nurse had to think about what was contributing to the problem. The etiological factors considered were arthritis and insufficient knowledge (pain-management techniques).

In general, focusing on the medical diagnosis as an etiological factor is not useful. Recall that etiological factors are used to plan the definitive nursing interventions. What definitive treatment can the nurse provide for arthritis, a medical diagnosis? None. The definitive treatment plan for the pathophysiology of arthritis is within the physician's domain of practice. For the time being, the nurse decided to formulate the diagnosis as Chronic Pain Self-Management Deficit/Insufficient Knowledge (Pain Management Techniques). She then continued her admission assessment. When the assessment was completed she began to review the dysfunctional patterns that she had diagnosed. This is a step that must not be missed. During a final review of findings, judgments are made in regard to interrelationships among problems. Earlier in the assessment, the nurse had diagnosed impaired mobility on the basis of Mr. W.'s report:

1. He did not walk much any more (maybe once a week) because of the progressively increasing joint pain
2. The presence of some limitation in range of motion (15 degrees right hip; 25 degrees left hip).

The nurse reasoned that if he could be helped to manage his pain (by drugs and other techniques), his mobility would improve. Then he could be started on an exercise program and daily walks, which would improve his general health and feeling of well-being. These thoughts led her to revise her diagnosis. The nursing diagnoses were:

1. Impaired Ambulation (Level II)/Chronic Pain/Self-Management Deficit
2. At Risk for Health Management Deficit (Arthritis)

The treatment plan was focused on the chronic pain/self-management deficit. The daily evaluation focused on the problem of impaired mobility. Two additional points need to be discussed in regard to the formulation of this problem. First, the nurse might have missed the interrelationship between the activity-exercise and cognitive-perceptual dysfunctional patterns if the final review of data and diagnoses had not been done. Second, two of the diagnostic categories listed in Appendix B were used to describe the problem. A second diagnosis was made in consultation with the clinical nurse specialist regarding Mr. W.'s management of his arthritis. There were a number of things he could be taught to do that would facilitate this area of his health management. Why is it formulated as a risk state? This formulation was made because if the problem was not addressed by the nurse he would be at risk for this condition. One of the cues supporting this formulation was the client's knowledge deficit regarding the management of this chronic condition.

Having discussed hypothesis generation and testing as the "route" to formulating nursing diagnoses, we now consider two strategies that were mentioned during the discussion: simultaneous and successive scanning. The terms mean that either a single diagnostic hypothesis is tested, such as sleep onset disturbance, or multiple hypotheses are tested simultaneously, such as sleep onset disturbance, early awakening pattern, sleep pattern reversal, and other disturbances. These two major hypothesis testing strategies, identified originally by Bruner and his colleagues,[2] influence other areas, such as:

1. *Information intake.* This refers to the amount of information obtained from a question or observation. If three hypotheses are being tested simultaneously and the diagnostician uses the assessment information in evaluating the hypotheses, the information value is tripled. If only one hypothesis is being tested, the information intake is one bit. (This would not apply if the clinician were reasoning on the basis of exemplars.)
2. *Cognitive strain.* The major cognitive processes involved in diagnosis are memory and inference (retrieval of knowledge from memory, holding new and retrieved information in working memory, and deductive and inductive inference). Memory and inference requirements are greater when multiple hypotheses are tested with each question or observation. Thus the cognitive strain is greater.
3. *Risk regulation.* Strategies can control the risk of (a) not getting sufficient information to make a diagnosis with confidence and (b) errors in processing because the cognitive capacity of the diagnostician is overwhelmed.

The simultaneous hypothesis-testing strategy is useful early in pattern assessment when the universe of possibilities must be narrowed. It is also useful when two diagnoses share the same cue but each has a different value. Successive scanning or single-hypothesis testing involves assessing a client or situation to test one diagnostic hypothesis at a time. This is a reasonable approach when critical, differentiating cues apply to only one diagnosis. Moreover if, after predicting likely hypotheses, only one or two hypotheses remain, they can be tested one by one. Further discussion and examples of these strategies are contained in Appendix K.

Weighting cues in judgment

Weighting refers to the power of a cue to influence judgment. The respective weight given a cue by a diagnostician influences which information gets clustered under a diagnostic hypothesis and which information is discounted as not useful.

Much research and rhetoric have taken place in order to explain how clinicians put information together. Do they add one cue to another, or are cues weighted? Some resolve this controversy by demonstrating that clinicians may do either.[47,48] When cues are added together to make a diagnostic judgment (Dx) the procedure is merely $a + b + c + d = Dx$. The whole (Dx) is merely a sum. For example, the following cues might be added together:

1. A 2-cm-wide break in the skin over the coccyx
2. Demarcated border
3. White and glossy lesion
4. Minimal depth
5. Redness at borders and in adjacent skin
6. History of long periods of lying on (his/her) back
7. Verbalized pain and discomfort
8. Left-sided paralysis

The problem would be decubitus ulcer. Should all pieces of information be weighted exactly the same? Are some cues in the list above not as important an influence on the diagnosis as others? The highest weighting would be given to the 2-cm-wide break in the skin over the coccyx. This is an ulcer. The term *decubitus* refers to lying down; the cue "history of long periods of lying on (his/her) back" should be given weight equal to the skin break in the diagnosis of a decubitus ulcer. "White and glossy lesion," "minimal depth," and "redness at borders and in adjacent skin" are cues to the severity (the grading) of the lesion. They permit a finer discrimination and are of equal value in judging severity. The cue "demarcated border" would be weighted and valued lower; it is not as influential in judging the presence of the condition. "Verbalized pain and discomfort" is of low diagnostic value; it supports the observation, but the diagnostic judgment can be made without it. The verbal cue would not be available if the patient was comatose. (Actually, this cue points to another problem, that of pain management.)

Consider another example in which the judgment is not as clear. The setting is a community clinic. The client is being treated for hypertension. These cues are present:

1. Tense posture
2. Flat, low tone; slowed speech; dull, depressed facial expression
3. Client has lost his job (company closed plant)
4. Depressed thoughts, but no thought of suicide
5. Perceived himself as self-made success in past
6. Perceives himself as self-made failure now
7. Wife has diabetes that is poorly controlled
8. Cannot discuss problems with friends: "They would think I was a failure."

9. Does not know what to do: "The job market is so bad"; "I just sit all day"; "This never happened to me before."

Considering these cues, which of the following is the best diagnostic judgment? (A slash separates problem and etiology.)

☐ Self-Concept Disturbance/Role Change
☐ Ineffective Coping/Role Change
☐ High Risk for Suicide
☐ Situational Depression/Role Change

The selection of Self-Concept Disturbance/Role Change suggests that cues 5 and 6 were weighted most heavily in the judgment. Cues 8 and 9 may be most impressive to some readers, who might then choose Ineffective Coping/Role Change. Cues 2, 4, 7, and 9 may have been most influential, thus leading to the conclusion that Situational Depression/Role Change was present. Selecting High Risk for Suicide suggests that the cue "but no thought of suicide" was discounted; this verbal report must have been weighted very low or considered unreliable as a predictor. Now let us see whether adding two other cues can influence judgment. One is a situational cue and the other is historical information. The clinic is a community mental health clinic and the client has a history of suicide attempts. Did these additional cues influence your weighting of the previous cues?

The example suggests that pieces of information are not always judged independently of one another. One cue may influence the weighting of another. Also, the example demonstrates that different people may be influenced differently by information. This is especially true when data are uncertain, as some clinical data are. Weighting and clustering information differently are probably the reasons experts sometimes differ in their diagnoses.

A third point demonstrated in this example is that information may be discounted in making a diagnostic judgment. Care providers make an estimate of the quality of information. Their estimates can be affected by other information or inferences about the client and situation.

Resolving inconsistencies

Previous information, regardless of its source, sets up expectations of new information. New information that conflicts with expectations constitutes an inconsistency. To inquisitive clinicians such inconsistency creates a dilemma. They know that ignoring inconsistencies increases the risk of diagnostic error and may also result in harm to the client. The dilemma must be resolved. Through expectations we "know" how things *should* appear, come about, or be related. Inconsistencies represent an inability to fit data together.

To recognize inconsistencies, first a comparison is made between what was expected and what has been observed. Then the nurse reasons deductively, using "If-then" statements. For example, if a client reports not eating much, then obesity should not be present. When "things don't turn out as they should," the question of "why" arises. Resolution of inconsistencies must take into account possible sources for the apparent conflict:

Measurement error

Expectations

Conflicting or unreliable reports

Inconsistencies caused by measurement error

When inconsistencies arise, a measurement error should be considered. During a nursing history, verbal reports by the client may be misunderstood. At times this happens because the nurse is listening inattentively. Misunderstanding may also result from a lack of clarity in a client's communication. If there is any doubt as to whether a client's statement was heard correctly, the client should be asked to validate or repeat the information. Care must be exercised to explain the reason for the repetition, because rephrasing or requesting repetition is also a technique for confronting a person or focusing attention on statements. During examination of a client, measurement errors may produce apparent inconsistencies. Observations should be repeated if doubt exists. Instruments—for example, sphygmomanometers—should be checked, as well as the technique used to obtain the blood pressure measurement.

Inconsistencies caused by expectations

What appear to be inconsistencies in data may be merely a nurse's incorrect expectations. Inadequate knowledge or inexperience can produce faulty expectations. In addition, expectations are based on interpretations; thus errors in previous or current reasoning may be the basis for apparent inconsistencies. Sometimes an understanding of the client's personal intentions, values, or beliefs provides a logical interpretation of the client's behavior and resolves what had seemed to be inconsistencies in the data. This situation is different from viewing behavioral data using one's own inferences and perspective.

Inconsistencies caused by conflicting reports

Clients' and families' verbal reports may conflict, producing apparent inconsistencies among their reports. Or the same person may give inconsistent reports at different times.

It is not uncommon for conflicting or contradictory reports to be given by a client and family member, by different members of a family, or by different groups within a community. The question arises: Whose information is to be taken into account and whose discounted? A number of hypotheses may be formulated. Do biases or cognitive deficits explain the conflicting reports? Is it a matter of different perspectives, such as objective (others') versus subjective (client's) points of view?

Resolving conflicting reports requires caution and tact. The strategy should be well thought through. Direct confrontation may serve only to induce guilt or defensiveness in the client. If conflicting reports are discussed only with one party, interpersonal conflict between two parties involved might arise later when they become aware of their differing reports. In some instances it may be wise to discuss the differences in perceptions with both parties together. A major factor in the decision is the current mental or physical health of the people involved.

Conflicts may also be apparent when a client's previous and current verbal reports differ. For example, a client may report an event or set of symptoms that is not consistent with the report the client had given to another health care provider or at another time. Temporary memory lapse, an interpersonal milieu in which the client felt the need to report things differently, or the way questions were formulated may explain the conflict in data. The client may be asked in a gentle manner about the apparent inconsistency.

Inconsistencies caused by unreliable reports

A client's verbal reports during a nursing history may be judged unreliable. Extreme caution must be exercised in making this judgment if errors are to be avoided, because information considered to be unreliable will be discounted and therefore given minimal weight in diagnostic judgments. Also, making this judgment may have ethical implications regarding the person's ability to make his or her own decisions. Assumed incompetency is one reason verbal reports are judged unreliable. The presence of cognitive or sensory deficits in a client may suggest to the care provider that the client's verbal reports should be used cautiously. Yet errors may result if a client's reliability has been incorrectly assessed. For example, many times elderly clients are stereotyped as incompetent or cognitively deficient because they "look old," whereas in fact no deficit may exist.

A well-publicized case of psychiatric stereotyping was reported[49]; it dealt with "being sane in insane places." The behavior of a group of persons was interpreted as manifesting psychosis because psychotic behavior was what was expected in the setting, which was a psychiatric hospital.

Concluding that information is biased is a second reason for discounting it as unreliable. Situations occur wherein clients or family members consciously or unconsciously provide biased reports. For example, a strong motivation, and perhaps a realistic need, to leave the hospital may influence a client to bias reports of his or her health state. Moreover, family members may overemphasize or underemphasize certain symptoms because of their basic anxieties or needs. These situations are usually easily recognized, because the reported information is inconsistent with other observations. The nurse needs to focus on discovering the underlying problem and why the conflicting reports have been given.

A third reason some observers discount information as unreliable is their prior classification of the character, or personality type, of a client or relative. Consider the following client classifications: drug addict, alcoholic, hospitalized prisoner, hypochondriac, malingerer, sociopath, murderer. When admitted to an in-patient facility, these negatively valued clients may predispose health care providers to question their verbal reports, which might lead to very serious error.

Reasonable and respectful consideration should be given to any client report without discrimination based on character stereotypes. Health care providers may infer that five instances of complaint that have no basis are predictors that the sixth complaint will be of the same type. Sometimes this is the instance when the appendix actually ruptures or the client does perform some act in desperation. Resolving, as opposed to ignoring, inconsistencies decreases the risk of error. An awareness of inconsistencies prevents fitting the data to hypotheses. Rather, hypotheses should be generated to fit the data actually present.

SUMMARY: INTERPRETATION OF CLINICAL INFORMATION

This section was concerned with the interpretation of clinical information. It stressed that meaning does not come with clinical data but must be derived through analysis and interpretation of the data by a clinician. After any needed clarification and verification, the diagnostic work begins. Cues are evaluated against norms, simple inferences are made, and selective, focused attention is given to diagnostic cues. Sometimes a diagnostic cue is clear and points to only one or two health problems (nursing diagnoses). At other times deriving the possible diagnostic meaning (hypotheses) of a cue requires cognitive work. Some helpful hints were given for generating possible diagnostic hypotheses that might explain the initial cues and give some structure to the diagnostic task. These hints included the use of pattern areas, pattern assessment sequence, client's viewpoint, expectancies derived from contextual information, and related knowledge stored in memory.

In a typical admission history and examination the nurse is presented with many discrete cues. It is impossible for any human being to process this amount of information at one time. The objective is to reduce the information by combining interrelated cues in a cluster (chunking) under a set of tentative hypotheses that gives them meaning. After considering a client's background data and initial data, some diagnostic hypotheses will be eliminated from the mental list of possibilities. This further reduces the information that must be held in working memory while hypotheses are tested.

Only a few initial cues are necessary to generate patterns that are described by the tentative diagnostic hypotheses. Hypotheses about the diagnostic meaning of cues are created in the mind of the clinician to structure the search for cues. It is only when they are tested by further information collection and analysis that their validity is revealed. Always be conscious of the fact that diagnostic hypotheses and, subsequently, nursing diagnoses are created; only the human behaviors upon which they are based are close to reality. Keeping this in mind increases the probability that unsupported hypotheses or diagnoses will be modified or discarded.

Going from no information to a well-supported diagnosis is not always a smooth process. Inconsistencies and conflicts in the data are sometimes observed. One topic discussed was how to resolve these inconsistencies. During hypothesis testing, cues are clustered together. To do this, the nurse must make decisions about how information is to be combined. Does this cue support a possible diagnosis? Does that cue suggest the problem is not present? Frequently these judgments are not easy to make. Inconsistencies among cues must be resolved. In the discussion of information clustering it was seen that one cue can influence the interpretation of other cues in the cluster and that some cues influence judgment more than others. Collecting, interpreting, and naming information is continuous throughout the process of nursing diagnosis. Conflicts and inconsistencies may arise as the data accumulate.

In the following case example a client-situation is analyzed. This analysis affords a total picture of how information is interpreted and integrated to yield a holistic picture of a person-family complex. The case illustrates topics in this chapter and the diagnostic process. Readers will be better able to evaluate their grasp of diagnostic reasoning by completing the case in Appendix I before reading the interpretation below. The setting is a hospital. While reading the nursing assessment, take notes and attempt to cluster the cues that signify actual or potential health problems. Readers should use the *Manual of Nursing Diagnosis*[21] to be able to apply some of the ideas that have been discussed. Then return to this discussion of the case to evaluate your reasoning and diagnostic judgment. Also,

> ## CHECKPOINTS FOR HYPOTHESIS GENERATION AND TESTING*
>
> At this point have I, the nurse,
> 1. Clarified and verified information as necessary so that I understand the client's reports and have confidence in my observations?
> 2. Paid attention to diagnostic cues in the data?
> 3. Interpreted what the client's verbal reports mean or signify? Used norms in the context of other data?
> 4. Considered alternative explanations for the cues? Eliminated those not applicable in this client situation?
> 5. Recalled all the critical diagnostic characteristics for the diagnoses I am testing and assessed for these characteristics? (See *Manual of Nursing Diagnosis.*[21])
> 6. In my best (unbiased) judgment, have sufficient data to confirm the diagnostic hypothesis? Can I justify my diagnostic judgments (nursing diagnoses) to others? Can I be accountable for the outcomes of my diagnoses (e.g., are they nursing diagnoses)?
>
> *Specific guidelines are found in the discussion.[50]

the following checkpoints can be used for self-evaluation. Learn to evaluate your clinical practice using these checkpoints (number 1 cannot be applied in this example, since the assessment data are given).

CASE EXAMPLE

Before making this assessment the nurse had received background information from the physician's history and physical examination. The client, Mr. K., had a 5-year history of "slightly elevated blood pressure." One year ago he had experienced an episode of dizziness for 12 hours. At that time he started taking medication for his blood pressure. Six months ago he had discontinued the medication, since he felt better. In the last 6 months before his admission, two other episodes of dizziness occurred, which lasted 1 to 2 hours and were relieved by rest. Frequent headaches were also reported.

Mr. K's father, now deceased, had had diabetes and hypertension. The client's mother, who died 1 year ago of a stroke, had also had hypertension. His wife and two children (14 and 10 years old) are well. An episode of dizziness and numbness of his left arm brought Mr. K. to the emergency room. The physician described him as a 55-year-old obese Caucasian male who was head of a Spanish center in a large southern city. The medical diagnosis at admission was hypertension and transient ischemic attack. This diagnosis and his family history placed Mr. K. at risk for a stroke.

When the nurse began the nursing history and assessment, Mr. K.'s dizziness and numbness had gone. The background information suggested the possibility of problems in his health perception–health management pattern. The following assessment data were collected; the main diagnostic hypotheses the nurse raised during the assessment are added in italics.

Nursing history and examination

First hospital admission of 55-year-old married, obese, white male administrator of a Spanish center. Sitting upright in bed, tense posture and expression *(fear; obesity)*.

Health perception–health management pattern
Viewed health as good until 1 year ago when diagnosed as "having high blood pressure." States job as "stressful . . . but the people need me" *(job stress)*. Had headaches for last 6 months and two episodes of dizziness (one at work and one at home) each lasting about 2 hours. Rested and symptoms went away. Delayed seeking care because was "too busy" *(job stress)*. Thought dizziness was caused by "overwork," not blood pressure *(job stress)*. Discontinued blood pressure medication and M.D. visits about 6 months ago "when blood pressure came down and I felt better"; states medicine caused impotence *(risk for noncompliance/disease management)*. To emergency room today because of left arm numbness and fear of stroke. Mother died of "stroke" 15 months ago. Concerned that he hasn't been taking care of himself; states, "I need to learn about what to do." Wants to know "everything" *(fear of stroke or death)*. Asked if OK to do some job-related paperwork if someone brought it in *(job stress)*. Takes no medicines currently except Alka-Seltzer and laxative; doesn't smoke; social drinking.

During introductions and while stating the purpose of the interview, the nurse's first impression was of a person in fear. Mr. K. was sitting upright in bed; his posture and facial expression were tense. It was inferred that he had been very frightened by the loss of feeling in his arm. Was he interpreting his symptoms in the context of his past experience (mother's stroke and death)? The hypothesis of fear influenced the conduct of the interview. It was important to establish the client's trust in care providers and to provide some reassurance.

The hypothesis of *obesity* was also generated from the initial impression. The nurse planned to follow up this topic when nutritional and activity patterns were assessed.

Review of the client's health perception pattern indicated a change. He had thought his health was good until 1 year ago, when high blood pressure was diagnosed. Although his blood pressure had been "slightly elevated" for 5 years, the change in health perception probably occurred with the first episode of dizziness and start of medication. This was also about the time of his mother's death.

Six months after beginning treatment, Mr. K. perceived that his "blood pressure came down" and he "felt better." Sexual impotence had occurred (impotence is common with certain blood pressure medications) and he discontinued medication and medical care. Further symptoms occurred and the client's action was to rest. This action was consistent with his previous interpretation of the cause of symptoms, "overwork" and being "too busy." There seems to have been delay in seeking health care, but today the loss of sensation in his arm could not be ignored.

Previously there may have been denial of change in health state or vulnerability. In addition the client may not have had knowledge to interpret the physical signs. What should the present data suggest to a nurse? One, the present symptoms have had an impact. Two, the client wants to "learn what to do." Yet knowledge deficit may not be the only reason for his past behavior.

The tentative diagnostic hypothesis, *risk for noncompliance,* served to cluster early cues and inferences—past history of not attending to symptoms, discontinuation of medication and care, misinterpretation of symptoms, and possible conflict between his health management and work-related activities. *Knowledge deficit* may be one risk factor, but the cue of "too busy" suggests motivational or time-management factors. The need to "learn what to do" is suggestive; yet readiness for learning and actual knowledge deficiencies need further assessment. Moreover, the client does not yet have medical recommendations for future care, so teaching about self-care in compliance with the medical regimen will have to be deferred.

Mr. K.'s asking whether he might do job-related paperwork might have meaning. Does he need to take his mind off his concerns, need diversion, have guilt about being away from his responsibilities, or need to maintain the self-perception of being well enough to do work?

"Wants to know everything" was tentatively interpreted as either fear, need for control, or motivation toward better health management. This and the cues to dysfunctional patterns cited previously were underlined during note taking for follow-up as other patterns were assessed.

The nurse suggested to Mr. K. that he seemed to want and need more information to help him plan how he could take care of himself. Then a smooth transition was made to the next area discussed, which was his nutritional-metabolic pattern.

Nutritional-metabolic pattern
Mr. K.'s diet history revealed adequate protein, excess carbohydrate and fat, minimal high-roughage foods (fruits and vegetables), approximately 3 cups of coffee per day, but a fluid intake of 700 to 800 mL/day *(constipation pattern)*. No history of lesions in mouth corners or mucous membranes. Has gained weight gradually last 15 years *(exogenous obesity)*; dieting unsuccessful; problem is "probably the stress of my job; I get home and eat a big supper and snacks in the evening"; no food dislikes *(caloric excess)*. Takes lunch (sandwich and cake) to work and eats at desk. Restaurants in area not good. Some indigestion and heartburn after lunch attributed to days with multiple stressors *(job stress)*; takes Alka-Seltzer.

At this point the nurse reevaluated Mr. K.'s emotional state. He had begun to relax his body and facial muscles.

Unsuccessful dieting, excessive intake of carbohydrate and fat, "big supper and snacks," minimal high-roughage foods, report of gradual weight gain last 15 years, and the absence of an endocrine disease (medical assessment data) suggested that the probable cause of obesity was caloric intake. Intake of both fluid and high-roughage food was low. These cues will have to be followed up when Mr. K.'s elimination pattern is assessed. The cues "days with multiple problems" and "stress of job" supported the previous hypothesis of job stress. This stress will have to be further assessed; it is influencing hypertension management and the client's nutritional pattern. The nurse then assessed the elimination pattern.

Elimination pattern
Daily bowel movement pattern with 2 or 3 episodes per month of constipation (hard stools and straining) lasting 2 days; laxatives used when constipation occurs *(intermittent constipation pattern/dietary habits)*. Attributes constipation to his diet; knows he should eat better.

The data about this pattern supported the hypothesis of intermittent constipation pattern. Was the constipation related to dietary habits (low fluid intake, minimal high-roughage foods) previously reported? Job stress may be a contributing factor. In this pattern there is again evidence of Health-Management Deficit. A picture of conflict between health practices and work "responsibilities" seems to be emerging.

Activity-exercise pattern
Spectator sports, uses car, minimal walking due to time schedule, sedentary job, considers self too old for exercise. Increasing fatigue last few weeks, less energy during the 2 months before admission; no self-care deficit *(decreased activity tolerance* and *knowledge deficit: age-exercise)*. Recreation consists of reading novels, watching TV, dining with other couples. Lives in first-floor apartment in city and drives ¾ mile to work *(exogenous obesity/caloric intake–energy expenditure imbalance)*.

Activities (work and leisure) suggested a sedentary pattern with minimal exercise. The perception of having less energy was not attributable to anemia (laboratory tests) or heart failure (physician's examination). Yet the perceptions of fatigue and less energy were real; the hypothesis was descriptive of the functional problem, decreased activity tolerance. Again, there was further indication that a busy schedule was conflicting with health management. Knowledge Deficit existed regarding age and exercise. Also, note the revision of the hypothesis about obesity; information from two pattern areas was clustered and exogenous obesity/caloric intake–energy-expenditure imbalance was formulated.

Sleep-rest pattern
Averages 4 to 6 hours of sleep per night, quiet atmosphere, own room with wife, double bed, uses bed board. Presleep activities include watching TV or completing paperwork from job; difficulty with sleep onset 1 month; awakens many mornings thinking about job-related problems *(sleep pattern disturbance/presleep activities; job stress)*.

A Sleep Pattern Disturbance existed. This may have been contributing to the increasing fatigue. A probable cause lay in the presleep activity (paperwork from job). Comments about awakening with thoughts of job-related problems supported the nurse's supposition that job stress was an influential factor for this client. Cues were clustered under this etiological hypothesis.

Cognitive-perceptual pattern
Sight corrected with glasses, changed 1 year ago; no change in hearing, taste, smell. No perceived change in memory; "I couldn't take it if I started losing my mind, like with a stroke" *(fear of stroke)*. Learning ability: sees self as somewhat slower than in college, alert manner, grasps questions easily. Takes no sedatives, tranquilizers, other drugs. No headache at present.

Again during discussion of this pattern there was mention of stroke. Fear (Stroke) was further supported.

Self-perception–self-concept pattern
Sees self as needing to do things well (job, father role, husband role); "Sometimes I don't think I'm doing well with my family, having them live in this area, but in my job you have to be near when people need help" *(role conflict)*. "It will be just great [sarcasm] if I get sick and they have to take care of me instead of me taking care of them" *(fear of dependency)*.

Conflict between the sense of responsibility to family and to job seemed to be present. Now he will have three responsibilities to balance: family, job, and responsibility to self (health). Fear (Stroke) was changed to Fear (Dependency). The cue "just great if I get sick and they have to take care of me . . ." influenced this modification.

Role-relationship pattern
Describes family as happy and understanding of his job commitments; wife former social worker; "kids good." "But I know we'll have trouble as Joe [10 years old] gets older"; "Maybe I should move out of [lower socioeconomic neighborhood]"; 10-year-old assaulted 4 months ago; 14-year-old boy interested in sports and "keeps out of trouble, so far" *(family concerns)*. Family usually "sits down together" to handle problems. Social relationships confined to "a few other couples"; finds this sufficient. Job demanding 9 to 10 hours per day; "always trying to get money to keep the center solvent" *(job stress)*. Assistant taking over while in hospital. Enjoys job and helping people; co-workers are "good to work with." Wife states the two of them are close; worried about husband's health; states he is more concerned with other people than himself; she admires him for this. Wife able to handle home responsibilities during hospitalization. States she and children had physical exams recently; no health problems; no elevation in blood pressure.

The family relationships elicited were positive and supportive. Concern and indecision were voiced regarding the environment (assault on son, "know we'll have trouble," and "maybe I should move"). The neighborhood environment could be a source of worry and stress in addition to the job problems (center's financial solvency).

A picture of his work was emerging: indigestion and heartburn on "days with multiple problems"; "stress of job"; "job was cause of high blood pressure"; "too busy"; "overwork"; wants to do job-related paperwork in hospital; sedentary job; awakens thinking of job-related problems; financial solvency; presleep activities sometimes job-related; and job demands 9 to 10 hours per day. These data were clustered as job stress. Is he saying that although his work is stressful he enjoys it and his co-workers?

Concern expressed by Mr. K.'s wife was expected under the circumstances. She and the children were managing, so at present there was no evidence of family coping problems. How did her comment about the client's concern for others fit into the picture? Is this a value that the client and his wife hold?

Sexual-reproductive pattern
Two children; states impotent when on BP medication. When BP "went down," stopped meds;

potency returned *(risk for noncompliance)*. No problems perceived in sexual relationship.

These data generated no new hypotheses. The information about impotency related to blood pressure medication would be a useful aid to the physician in his or her choice of medication.

Coping–stress-tolerance pattern
Feels tense at work *(job stress);* has tried relaxation exercises with some alleviation; doesn't always have time. States the best way to deal with problems is to "attack them." Afraid of having a stroke and being dependent: "This thing today has really scared me" *(fear of dependency)*. "I have too many things to think about at work and at home, and now this blood pressure thing" *(role conflict)*. Life changes: father died 3 years ago; mother died of stroke 15 months ago; took job at Spanish center 2 years ago to be near mother who "was getting old." Pleased he did this and feels good about it.

The previous mention of job and family stressors led naturally to a discussion of the coping–stress-tolerance pattern. "Attacking" problems seemed to be the predominant coping pattern expressed. The continuing theme of job stress was evident. Job stress was not interpreted as the factor receiving the "blame" for his state of affairs.

Further support for the Fear (Dependency) hypothesis was found in the cue "This thing . . . really scared me. The tentative hypothesis of conflict received support from the cue, "Too many things to think about, and now this. . . ." Questions regarding his mother's death elicited no verbal or nonverbal cues to unresolved grieving.

The life changes as well as the assault on his child placed considerable strain on coping patterns. Yet there were indications of support (family relationships) and a disposition toward finding a solution for present problems.

Value-belief pattern
"Life has been good to me"; feels deeply about "injustices in society" and wants to do something about them *(value conflict)*. States family is important to him. Religion (Catholic) important to him; would like to be active in church affairs.

In response to a question about things important to him, "injustices" and family were mentioned. These data prompted a change in the earlier hypothesis of role conflict. A value conflict is more likely present. This hypothesis revision was supported by cues about (1) family concerns and

perceived responsibilities, (2) the valuing of the needs of others, and (3) time available.

The nurse performed an examination following the history. The above hypotheses were kept in mind. There was also an openness to further cues.

Examination
Vital signs: BP 205/118; T 37.6° C (99.8° F); P 80, regular and strong; R 18.

Nutritional-metabolic pattern:

Skin: No redness over bony prominences; no lesions. Dryness, calluses on feet with discomfort when touched.

Oral mucous membranes: Moist, no lesions.

Height and weight: 180 cm (5 ft 11 in); 104 kg (230 lb) actual weight; 99.8 kg (220 lb) reported weight.

Activity-exercise pattern:

Gait: Steady.

Posture: Well balanced.

Muscle tone, strength, and coordination: Hand grip firm left and right; lifts legs; can pick up pencil; tenseness in neck and shoulder muscles.

Range of motion (joints): Within normal limits.

Prosthesis and assistive devices: None.

Absence of body part: No.

Cognitive-perceptual pattern:

Perception: Hears whisper; reads newsprint with glasses.

Cognition: Language: English; grasps ideas, both abstract and concrete; speech clear; attention span good.

Self-perception–self-concept pattern:

General appearance: Well-groomed, evidences good hygiene.

Nervous or relaxed: Tense; some relaxation during history taking.

Eye contact: Yes.

Attention span: Good.

Role-relationship pattern:

Interactions: Communications with wife supportive, both somewhat tense; children not present.

Obesity was further confirmed by the client's height and weight measurements. Tenseness of neck muscles was clustered with other cues to Fear (Dependency). Numbness had disappeared. Calluses are relevant to his exercise pattern.

The nursing history and examination provide a

beginning understanding of the client's health patterns. The history and examination also demonstrate the individuality of clients and show how assessment can identify clients' problems. Diagnostic hypotheses in Mr. K.'s situation were added, deleted, and revised as follows:

Fear → Fear (Stroke; Death) → Fear (Stroke) → Fear (Dependency)

Obesity → Exogenous Obesity → Exogenous Obesity/Caloric Intake–Energy Expenditure Imbalance

Job Stress → (delete; incorporated under Value Conflict and Responsibilities)

High Risk for Noncompliance (Health Management)

Constipation → Intermittent Constipation Pattern/Dietary Pattern → Intermittent Constipation Pattern/Dietary and Exercise Pattern

Caloric Excess → (delete; incorporated as etiology of Obesity)

Decreased Activity Tolerance (to be evaluated further after medical treatment)

Knowledge Deficit (Age and Exercise) → (incorporated under Health Management)

Sleep Pattern Disturbance/Presleep Activity, Job Stress

Family Concerns → (delete; incorporated under Value Conflict and Responsibilities)

Role Conflict → (delete; incorporated under Value Conflict and Responsibilities)

Value Conflict → Value Conflict/Perceived Job and Family Responsibilities

A final review of findings produced further revision. The following nursing diagnoses, supported by data, were recorded (a slash separates the problem and the etiological factors):

Exogenous Obesity/Caloric Intake–Energy Expenditure Imbalance

Intermittent Constipation Pattern/Dietary and Exercise Pattern

Sleep Pattern Disturbance/Presleep Activity, Perceived Responsibilities

Fear (Dependency)/Perceived Risk of Stroke

High Risk for Health Management Deficit

Value Conflict/Perceived Job and Family Responsibilities

The diagnoses related to obesity, sleep, and constipation became more specific as data accumulated. It can be noted that these represent a problem in one pattern area and etiological factors in other pattern areas.

Fear (Dependency) was probably related to the perceived risk of a stroke. A care plan that emphasized developing a feeling of personal control through reduction of risk factors might help this client.

High Risk for Health Management Deficit was used to describe the history of noncompliance with medication and follow-up care and the client's general neglect of health. The diagnosis High Risk for Noncompliance might have been used. Yet no evidence was present to suggest there was previous intention to comply.[51] In addition, there were data to support an interest in learning "what to do." The care plan would emphasize teaching and counseling for general health promotion. Special emphasis would be given to correcting misinformation about age and exercise. A podiatry referral was recommended to Mr. K. to relieve his calluses, which may cause sufficient discomfort to prevent walking and other forms of exercise. Specific teaching would be provided about hypertension and other areas of risk factor management.

A conflict in values existed. Mr. K.'s family was important to him. Also important was his contribution to resolving "injustices" through his work. A sense of responsibility "to do things well" in both areas produced conflict. The cues were: "need to be near when people need help," "maybe I should move . . . ," "sometimes I don't think I'm doing well with my family . . . ," more concerned with others than himself, enjoys job and helping people, and multiple references to demanding responsibilities in his job. The cues were clustered and described as Value Conflict Related to Perceived Job and Family Responsibilities.

From the nurse's perspective, the problem is more complex. The client's value system (hence his conflict) should also include responsibility to himself, to protect his own health. A serious illness would not permit Mr. K. to realize either set of values or carry out the responsibilities he has chosen to assume. Yet at this time there are few cues that his conflict includes health-maintenance responsibilities to self. The nursing diagnosis must describe the conflict that exists, not the conflict that *should* exist.

Nursing care should focus first on helping the client to examine the possibility of balancing his life. First, things important to him will be discussed, that is, his perceived job and family responsibilities. It is expected that current health concerns will come to be perceived as a third area of conflict. This insight can then lead to an examination of how a balance of responsibilities may be attained. The nurse must exercise caution during these explorations of Mr. K.'s personal values and lifestyle, since clients have a right to choose how to conduct their lives. The nursing responsibility is to help them look at alternatives that include health promotion. In the end, the client chooses.

The case of Mr. K. illustrates the broad life pattern that was previously discussed as an overriding pattern that encompasses all diagnoses. For example, *all* of Mr. K.'s health problems seem to be related to the choices he has made and the responsibilities he has chosen, or not chosen, to assume. In fact, a nursing diagnosis might be stated as: Health Management Deficit Related to Value-Choice Pattern. Currently some nurses intuitively grasp clients' life pattern problems and intervene at this broad level. But questions remain. Is this level of problem identification useful for planning intervention? Are both broad and specific levels of diagnosis needed? Can this broad pattern be identified without going through the step of identifying specific diagnoses, such as Exogenous Obesity and Sleep Pattern Disturbance? Probably not.

The first step toward answering these questions is to have nursing diagnosis an integral part of nursing practice. Then it will be possible to see at what level diagnoses should be formulated. Facilitation of care planning will always be an important criterion by which nursing diagnosis is further developed, and decisions about levels of diagnosis will be made in accordance with that criterion.

SUMMARY

Discussion in this chapter focused on how to analyze and interpret diagnostic cues during assessment. As previously summarized, first the clarity of the data is evaluated. Following this, the meaning of cues is interpreted and structured by hypotheses (possibilities). The most likely alternative hypotheses provide a focused search for cues. Data that should be present if the condition is present are collected, evaluated, and clustered under the appropriate hypothesis. When psychological confidence in the "best" working hypothesis is present, a nursing diagnosis is stated. This nursing diagnosis provides a focus for projecting outcomes and planning treatment until a "better" hypothesis is generated. Note that this last statement suggests an attitude toward diagnosis that will prevent some of the errors to be discussed in Chapter 9.

NOTES AND REFERENCES

1. The initial assessment will be used in examples. Various other types of assessments are discussed in Chapter 7.
2. Bruner JS, Goodnow JJ, Austin GA: *A study of thinking,* New York, 1956, Wiley, p 51.
3. First-level inferences are concrete impressions arrived at by combining observations. *Cyanosis* is an example; it describes a bluish tinge to the skin in several parts of the body. *Restlessness* is a first-level inference derived from body movements over a short period of time and sometimes from disarray of the bed.
4. Kassier JP, Kopelman RL: *Learning clinical reasoning,* Baltimore, 1991, Williams & Wilkins, p 282.
5. Larkin J et al: Expert and novice performance in solving physics problems, *Science* 208:1335, 1980.
6. Carnevali DL, Thomas MD: *Diagnostic reasoning and treatment decision making in nursing,* Philadelphia, 1993, Lippincott, p 32.
7. Benner P: *From novice to expert: excellence and power in clinical nursing practice,* Menlo Park, CA, 1984, Addison-Wesley.
8. Does Client A fear the chemotherapy? That is a good example of an inference. Putting together "afraid" and "chemotherapy" creates the inference that they are related. Next this "creation" must be validated.
9. The differential diagnosis of fear versus anxiety depends on the client's focus of concern. If the client reports a specific focus of concern, the condition is called fear; if the focus is diffuse, it is anxiety.
10. Levine ME: *Introduction to clinical nursing,* ed 2, Philadelphia, 1973, Davis.
11. Gale J, Marsden P: *Medical diagnosis: from student to clinician,* New York, 1983, Oxford University Press.
12. Thyne JM: *Psychology of learning and techniques of teaching,* London, 1966, University of London Press.
13. These characteristics were rated as nearly always or frequently present (very/quite characteristic) with activity intolerance by more than 50% of 212 critical care nurses in a national study. Gordon M: *Critical characteristics of high-frequency nursing diagnoses in critical care,* manuscript submitted for publication, 1993. The first three characteristics were viewed as nearly always or frequently present by 70% or more of the nurses. These characteristics are also included in American Association of Critical Care Nurses: *Outcome standards for nursing care of the critically ill,* Laguna Niguel, CA, 1990, The Association. In addition, these are the signs and symptoms listed in most textbooks.
14. Elstein AS, Schulman LS, Sprafka SA: *Medical problem solving: an analysis of clinical reasoning,* Cambridge, MA, 1978, Harvard University Press.

15. Levine M: *A cognitive theory of learning,* Hillsdale, NJ, 1975, Erlbaum.
16. Aspinall MJ: Use of a decision tree to improve accuracy of diagnosis, *Nurs Res* 28:182, 1979. The results of this study suggest that performance in the diagnostic process improved when there was conscious awareness of the idea of branching.
17. Jaundice is a yellow coloring of the skin and whites of the eyes associated with bile pigment in the blood, in this case due to changes in liver cells and obstruction.
18. Goffman E: *Stigma: notes on the management of spoiled identity,* Englewood Cliffs, NJ, 1965, Prentice-Hall.
19. These are the representativeness and availability heuristics identified in the early 1970s by Tversky A, Kahneman D: Judgment under uncertainty: heuristics and biases, *Science* 185:1124, 1974.
20. Newell A, Simon H: *Human problem solving,* Englewood Cliffs, NJ, 1972, Prentice-Hall.
21. Gordon M: *Manual of nursing diagnosis,* St Louis, 1993, Mosby.
22. Gordon M: High-frequency–high-treatment priority nursing diagnoses in critical care and rehabilitation nursing practice. Study in progress. Boston College School of Nursing, Chestnut Hill, MA 02167.
23. Gordon M: Predictive strategies in diagnostic tasks, *Nurs Res* 29:39, 1980.
24. Brykczynski KA: An interpretive study describing the clinical judgment of nurse practitioners, *Scholarly Inquiry for Nursing Practice: An International Journal* 3:75, 1989.
25. Jones RA: *Self-fulfilling prophecies: social, psychological and physiological effects of expectancies,* Hillsdale, NJ, 1977, Erlbaum, p 52.
26. Davitz L, Davitz J: *Inference of patient's pain and psychological distress,* New York, 1980, Springer.
27. Dion K, Berscheid E, Walster E: What is beautiful is good, *J Pers Soc Psychol* 24:285, 1972.
28. Kaplan MF: Stimulus inconsistency and response dispositions in forming judgments of other persons, *J Pers Soc Psychol* 25:58, 1973.
29. Young L, Powell B: Effects of obesity on the clinical judgment of mental health professionals, *J Health Soc Behav* 26:233, 1985.
30. Berger PL, Luckmann T: *The social construction of reality,* Garden City, NY, 1966, Anchor, p 33.
31. Sarbin TR, Taft R, Bailey DE: *Clinical inference and cognitive theory,* New York, 1960, Holt, Rinehart & Winston.
32. Merton RK: *Social theory and social structure,* rev ed, New York, 1957, Free Press.
33. Thomas WO, Thomas DS: *The child in America,* New York, 1928, Knopf.
34. Morse JM, et al: Exploring empathy: a conceptual fit for nursing practice? *Image,* 24:273, 1993.
35. Zderad L: Empathetic nursing: realization of a human capacity, *Nurs Clin North Am* 4:655, 1969.
36. Bieri J, et al: *Clinical and social judgment,* New York, 1966, Wiley.
37. Soares C: Low verbal usage and status maintenance among intensive care nurses. In Chaska NL, editor: *The nursing profession: views through the mist,* New York, 1978, McGraw-Hill.
38. The client is probably also picking up an initial impression of the nurse. Frequently this impression is generalized to all the staff and the agency. Clients, like nurses, go beyond the information given to reach inferential conclusions: "She's nice"; "He's a considerate nurse"; "She'll know what to do if something happens."
39. Weiss JH: Effect of professional training and amount of accuracy of information on behavioral prediction, *J Consult Psychol* 27:257, 1963.
40. Schmidt HO, Fonda CP: Reliability of psychiatric diagnosis: a new look, *J Abnorm Soc Psychol* 52:262, 1956.
41. Neisser U: Perceiving, anticipating, imagining. In Savage GW, editor: *Minnesota studies in the philosophy of science,* vol 9, *Perception and cognition,* Minneapolis, 1978, University of Minnesota Press.
42. Craig J: Types of statements made by nurses as first impressions of patient problems. In Hurley M, editor: *Classification of nursing diagnoses: proceedings of the sixth conference,* St Louis, 1986, Mosby.
43. Gordon M: Strategies for teaching diagnostic reasoning. In Carroll-Johnson R, editor: *Classification of nursing diagnoses: proceedings of the eighth conference,* St Louis, 1990, Mosby.
44. Ciafrani KL: The influence of amounts and relevance of data on identifying health problems. In Kim MJ, McFarland G, McLane A, editors: *Classification of nursing diagnoses: proceedings of the fifth national conference,* St Louis, 1984, Mosby.
45. Accuracy was very high when the information was limited and the correct judgment was hemorrhagic shock. When the information was unlimited and the correct judgment was atelectasis, 52% of the judgments were inaccurate; errors were attributed to information overload and other aspects of the nurses' strategy. The current time they "did the assessment" was known to be between 2 and 5 PM. The nurses could have used simple subtraction to find how many hours had elapsed since surgery.
46. The nurse believed she had sufficient data to support the diagnosis of Weak Parent-Infant Attachment/Early Parent-Infant Separation.
47. Anderson NH: Looking for configurality in clinical judgment, *Psychol Bull* 78:93, 1972.
48. Elstein AS: Clinical judgment: psychological research and medical practice, *Science* 194:696, 1976.
49. Rosenhan DL: On being sane in insane places, *Science* 179:250, 1973.
50. Nurses just beginning to learn nursing diagnosis may wish to photocopy these checkpoints and refer to them before recording their nursing diagnoses on the chart/Kardex/computer.
51. Noncompliance is defined as a client's failure to participate in carrying out the plan of care after indicating an initial intention to comply. Some prefer the diagnosis Health Management Deficit (Specify). Ineffective Management of Therapeutic Regimen is also suggested. The author prefers Health Management Deficit with the specification of the area (e.g., Activity, Medication Regimen).

CHAPTER 9

DIAGNOSTIC STATEMENTS AND DIAGNOSTIC ERRORS

It will be recalled from Chapter 1 that nursing diagnosis is defined as a process of reasoning and judgment and as a category used to label the judgment that results. Diagnostic categories describe dysfunctional or potentially dysfunctional patterns. This chapter is about diagnostic judgments that result from the process and their description using diagnostic category labels.

At the point a diagnosis is stated confidence exists in the diagnostic judgment. The diagnostician is ready to make the judgment public (charting) and to use the diagnostic statement (problem and etiological or related factors) to design a treatment plan. To facilitate the use of nursing diagnosis in nursing process the diagnostic statement has to be precise, clear, and sufficiently supported by critical defining characteristics.

Stating the diagnosis is the end point in the process of problem formulation. Actually, problem formulation began when the first diagnostic cue was noticed. This is an important point to remember. Errors can result if one thinks information collection and diagnosis can be separated in time (diagnosing the problem after all information is collected) and space (back at the desk or community agency office) and person (one person collects the information and another makes the diagnosis).

This chapter emphasizes how to state a precise nursing diagnosis and how to deal with the uncertainty and dilemmas inherent in making clinical judgments. Continued validation of the diagnosis during treatment will be considered as well as ways to avoid the major diagnostic errors that can occur.

REVIEW OF ASSESSMENT FINDINGS

When learning nursing diagnosis, it is difficult to follow the advice in Chapter 7; that is, to review the health problems identified with the client at the end of the assessment. (This was demonstrated in Chapter 8 with Mr. K.) Sometimes time to think is needed and all that can be expected is a vague statement, such as "I think while you're here, I can help you with some of the things you have mentioned . . ." (insert: things that seemed important to the client, such as how to take medications, helping to relax, information about the surgery). For the novice diagnostician this is better than leaping in and stating health problems that one later regrets. In fact, in some cases guiding *clients* to identify the problem would increase their learning and thus their independence in monitoring their own health. This is also a more advanced behavior for the clinician.

Kelly[1] makes an important point in regard to reviewing findings with the client. She points out that the medical diagnosis of disease does not require involvement of the client except as a reporter of symptoms. Nursing diagnoses focus on human responses and require inclusion of the client and his or her subjective perspective. The nurse's interpretation of the significance of behavior may change when the client's view of a situation is obtained, and the client's understanding may shift when the nurse's professional knowledge and experience are shared.

The client's situation as a whole as well as the individual patterns are observed during history and examination. The skill to move back and forth between a holistic and an analytic perspective in order to gain understanding is a skill that develops. Health pattern areas are only a way of organizing data and coping with the complexity of the human situation. In addition to alternating between abstract judgments and concrete cues during an assessment, a final review of the assessment data is necessary. This will ensure that diagnostic judgments are not made in isolation. Patterns are *interactive and interdependent;* thus each problem has to be reviewed in the context of the whole client situation.

Formulating the diagnostic statement

As the reader will already have learned, a diagnostic statement consists of a problem and etiological or related factors. In this section some guidelines will be offered about how to state a problem, the probable cause(s), and the relationship between the problem and the probable cause(s). Included also will be the formulation of high-risk diagnoses, syndromes, and how to describe the conclusions of an admission assessment when there are no problems, high-risk states, or syndromes—truly a healthy state.

PROBLEM STATEMENTS

The problem describes the state of the client at the time the diagnosis is made. If the critical diagnostic criteria for a category match the cluster of cues observed, then the category name is applied. It has to be kept in mind that the nurse will use the problem statement to project outcomes that describe the desired state the client or someone acting on behalf of the client wishes to attain. The following are characteristics of useful problem statements:

1. It is a phenomenon of concern to nurses.
2. It is a condition that the client, nurse, or both agree requires changing.[2] It is a problem, a high-risk problem, or a condition where

there is potential for growth in a health-related area.
3. The name given to the cluster of observed signs and symptoms is an accepted diagnostic label (unless none of the current labels apply). This applies mostly to the learner; others may wish to experiment with new diagnostic category labels.
4. The diagnostic category label is clear and concise.
5. A sufficient cluster of signs and/or symptoms can be documented to justify the diagnosis. Critical diagnostic criteria are included in the cluster.

Precision in diagnostic judgment

Precision refers to specificity. If a problem statement is to be used to project outcomes and measure the effectiveness of nursing care, it must be fairly specific. (As will be seen in the next chapter, diagnoses are also being used for staffing, reimbursement, and health statistics.) For example, Alterations in Parenting is not specific; Total Self-Care Deficit is specific. When considering alterations in parenting, the question arises: What type of alteration? In contrast, by definition total self-care deficit means feeding, bathing, toileting, dressing, and grooming.[3]

Specific focus or level

A second factor that increases precision is the term *specify,* which follows certain diagnostic categories (Appendix A). This requires that the diagnostician include the focus or level of the problem. For example, Fear and Noncompliance are nonspecific. Fear (Anesthesia), Noncompliance (Follow-Up Care), Skill Deficit (Insulin Administration), Activity Intolerance (Level I), Total Self-Care Deficit (Level IV) are specific. In the case of Self-Care Deficit, diagnosing the level provides a very useful specification. The definition of Level IV is: "dependent and does not participate in self-care." When a diagnostic category requires specification, assessment has to continue until the focus or level is determined.

Specific modifiers

Some diagnostic categories require that the level of acuity be determined. This specification clarifies the description of the problem; in some instances acuity can be used to prioritize diagnoses. Anxiety is not a specific formulation; mild anxiety is. Grieving is nonspecific but acute dysfunctional grieving is a useful formulation.

Further refinement of diagnostic categories will establish the cluster of cues that represents each specific acuity or risk level. Until this occurs try to identify levels that influence treatment decisions and continue assessment until the level can be specified.

The following are clear, concise problem statements:

Column 1	Column 2	Column 3
Caregiver Role Strain	Moderate Anxiety	Delayed Pattern Onset
Constipation	Preoperative Fear (Pain)	Pressure Ulcer (Specify Stage 1 or 2)
Ineffective Airway Clearance	Impaired Bed Mobility	Support System Deficit

Column 1 contains NANDA-accepted diagnoses. These are what the American Nurses' Association refers to as standardized terms in the developing Uniform Nursing Language System. Column 2 contains clinical modifications of the standard terminology that increase the precision of the diagnoses. Column 3 contains diagnoses that are clinically useful but have not been submitted to the NANDA review process. Notice the similarity in structure among the three columns. This is important when creating new terms to describe diagnostic judgments. The following are two "creations" and one NANDA-accepted diagnosis observed in manuals, textbooks, and client records:

1. Altered Respiratory Status	No clue to how it is altered, nonspecific, and are nurses responsible for the treatment plan? See discussion below on collaborative problems.
2. Impaired Adaptation	Too global. This is a conceptual framework for all the diagnoses—all could be viewed as impaired adaptations.
3. Altered Protection	Much too global. Includes characteristics from itching to altered clotting. (NANDA-accepted but there are other diagnoses listed that describe its characteristics.)

Tentative diagnostic hypotheses

In some instances the cluster of cues is insufficient for identifying a problem. The data suggest only tentative diagnostic hypotheses. Further data collection is not possible at the time. As will be discussed in the next chapter, this situation requires a diagnostic plan and further assessment. Some authors[4,5] suggest describing the cluster of cues as a "possible problem," such as "possible body image disturbance." This would communicate that some diagnostic cues are present but they are not sufficient to justify a diagnosis. Presumably this means that the most likely hypothesis is chosen to be labeled "possible." From a clinical reasoning perspective, does this encourage premature closure on the diagnosis as opposed to recording the cluster of cues? In medicine the concept of rule out (R/O) is used but usually includes more than one condition. As will be recommended in Chapter 10, a cluster of cues requiring further investigation is included in the diagnostic plan.

JUDGMENTS ABOUT CAUSAL FACTORS

Any discussion of causal (related) factors cannot begin without calling the readers' attention to the importance of formulating these factors in a clear, clinically useful way. Etiological or related factors are the basis for nursing intervention.

Dysfunctional patterns described by diagnostic categories in Appendix B can be interrelated in a causal manner. This can happen in at least three ways:

1. One dysfunctional pattern can contribute to the development and maintenance of another dysfunctional pattern. For example, Activity Intolerance can lead to Social Isolation in an elderly person.
2. Two conditions within the same pattern can

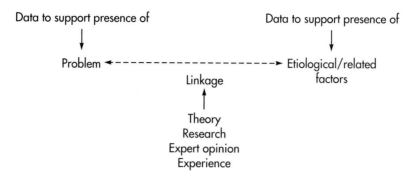

Fig. 9-1   Formulation of problem-etiological factors linkage.

be related. For example, Activity Intolerance can be a causal factor in Self-Care Deficit, and the major reason for Weak Mother-Infant Attachment may be Mother-Infant Separation. (This may be a result of surgery on the newborn or the need for constant observation in the neonatal intensive care unit.)

3. Risk factors for a potential problem (high-risk state) can be in a number of patterns and can be described by current diagnostic categories in Appendix B. For example, impaired bed mobility is a factor in the diagnosis High Risk for Pressure Ulcer.

Probable causes of a problem are referred to as contributing factors, etiological factors, or, in the case of NANDA, related factors. There has been controversy over which terms should be used and the possible legal implications. (These are causal factors and nurses intervene on the probable causes of health problems, *but* this label would be even more controversial!) None of these terms as currently used in health care circles contradict the belief that the causes of a health problem are multiple and based on uncertainty-geared judgments.

How do you know a problem is an etiological or related factor? The question is very important because in an initial assessment a few problems or dysfunctional patterns may be identified. Assessment data support the judgment that a dysfunctional pattern exists; that is, the judgment is substantiated by the critical, diagnostic cues. This is the first judgment made by the diagnostician: a dysfunctional pattern exists.

It is a second-level diagnostic judgment to say that one dysfunctional pattern is the problem and

another is a probable cause of the problem. This requires application of theory, research findings, experience, or a combination of these. The problem-etiology link is an inference that is not observable. The clinician makes the linkage—creates it. For example, can you observe that a particular client's Activity Intolerance is the major factor causing Self-Care Deficit (Level II)? No, you cannot; but you can provide observational data that support the presence of Activity Intolerance *and* Self-Care Deficit (Level II). Further, you can argue from observations and theory that Activity Intolerance is more likely producing the Self-Care Deficit than incontinence! Fig. 9-1 illustrates the linkage of two dysfunctional patterns. This linkage can be logically argued from theory, research, expert opinion, and experience.

At the present time the problem-etiology linkages for most nursing diagnoses have to be based on subjective probabilities and clinical judgment. Recognize this when you use the "related to" statement and the problem/etiology format. Think through and be able to justify the "causal" reasoning that underlies the problem-etiology linkage you propose. As a helpful hint: Many times the extra effort of thinking through causal connections for problems that occur frequently "pays off"; the next time the same problems occur you will have already built the knowledge. It is useful because common problems occur frequently.

Try to learn the cause-and-effect relationships between health-related events. Nursing intervention seeks to modify the chain of events that leads to or maintains a problem. Fig. 9-2 illustrates the relationships among inferences about problems/

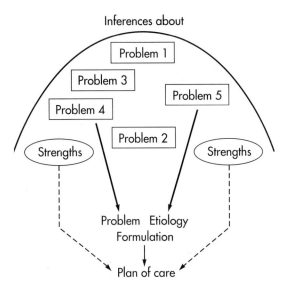

Inferences about

Problem 1

Problem 3

Problem 5

Problem 4

Problem 2

Strengths   Strengths

Problem Etiology
Formulation

Plan of care

Fig. 9-2   Relationships among problems/strengths, problem/etiology formulation, and plan of care.

strengths–problem/etiology formulation and a plan of care. Because of their importance to intervention, etiological or related factors should meet the same requirements for precision as discussed above in regard to problems. Characteristics of the dysfunctional patterns designated as etiological factors in a client-situation are:

1. Nursing treatment can usually resolve the pattern or factor; thus a nurse can assume responsibility for the outcomes.
2. It is a pattern or factor that the client, nurse, or both agree(s) could be one reason for the problem.
3. The name given to the pattern or factor is clear and concise. (Diagnostic categories in Appendix B are used to describe etiological factors when possible; e.g., Sleep-Onset Disturbance Related to Anxiety.)
4. A sufficient cluster of signs and/or symptoms including critical diagnostic criteria can be documented to justify the presence of the pattern or factor.

It is recognized that at this time most of the etiological factors listed in manuals or by NANDA are not defined, nor do they list diagnostic criteria. The exceptions are when *other* diagnostic cat-

egories listed in Appendix A are used to describe etiological factors. A number of views have been expressed regarding the concept of etiology, and the reader may wish to review these.[6-11] The following are clear, concise, etiological factors; note, nurses intervene to help clients modify these factors:

Column 1	Column 2
Activity Intolerance	Job stress
Knowledge Deficit (Specify)	Ineffective chronic pain self-management
Fear (Specify)	Parent-infant separation anxiety
Hopelessness	Reactive situational depression
Impaired Mobility (Specify Type and Level)	Weak parent-infant attachment

Diagnoses in Column 1 are "problems" that are the focus for nursing interventions. Note that they are from the listing of NANDA-accepted diagnoses in Appendix A. In Column 2 are some etiological factors that nurses can treat; they need to be developed and added to our "dictionary" of diagnostic terms used in describing clinical judgments (Appendix A).

JUDGMENTS ABOUT HIGH-RISK PROBLEMS

As discussed in Chapter 6, potential problems or high-risk states alert the nurse to the need for preventive intervention. Preventive intervention for high-risk conditions has always been a priority in nursing. Unlike other taxonomies, the nursing taxonomy is replete with at-risk categories. This focus of nursing practice was supported in a study in critical care and rehabilitation nursing diagnoses.[12] In both areas a high percentage of nurses rated potential problems as high frequency and high treatment priority.

In 1992 NANDA replaced the term *potential* with *high risk problems*. (This is a format first used by the American Nurses Association–American Association of Neuroscience Nurses in their nursing standards.)[13]

More specificity can be achieved by modifiers. Specifying High Risk for Infection as High Risk for Wound Infection would be an example. It was interesting to note in a study of the NANDA defining characteristics of the diagnosis High Risk for Infection there were four nested diagnoses.[12]

High Risk for Respiratory Infection
High Risk for Skin Infection
High Risk for Wound Infection
High Risk for Urinary Tract Infection
High Risk for Puerperal Infection

One defining characteristic, rupture of amniotic membrane, suggested High Risk for Puerperal Infection. The question for clinicians is: Do we need this degree of specificity or is it of mere academic interest? Would you do anything different or would assessment and teaching be any different if the person were at risk for respiratory infection rather than urinary tract infection? If so, then we need the specificity for clinical practice. The broad category will still be useful for describing the state of immunosuppressed persons who are susceptible to all types of infections.

It is useful to note that if etiological factors contribute to the development and maintenance of an actual problem, then logically they are major risk factors for a potential problem. For example, when a person has one or more of the following, he or she is usually unable to manage independently the treatment for a complex disease or his or her health promotion activities (health management deficit):

Activity intolerance (Level IV)
Uncompensated cognitive impairment
Uncompensated visual or hearing loss
Impaired reality testing
Depression

These conditions are major reasons for a health management deficit. Now shift thinking. If you had a client with one or more of the conditions above, wouldn't the client be at risk for a health management deficit? When the need to state a high-risk problem exists and no labels are available, review the etiological factors for the actual problem.

Even with all the guidelines that books offer for formulating the diagnostic statement, difficulties will arise. In the next section we will try to anticipate some of the dilemmas.

JUDGMENTS ABOUT SYNDROMES

Syndromes in nursing were not discussed in the literature until a decade after the work on diagnostic language began. The first, Rape Trauma Syndrome, was submitted to NANDA in the 1980s. It described a biopsychosocial cluster of problems associated with rape and its aftermath. Rather than a cluster of signs and symptoms as in a diagnosis, a syndrome represents a cluster of interrelated problems, usually with biopsychosocial dimensions.

The central causative factor for the cluster of problems is incorporated in the title. In other health care professions syndromes are defined as a cluster or group of signs and symptoms that almost always occur together. Together these clusters represent a distinct clinical picture.[14] McCourt suggests that the common characteristics of NANDA-accepted syndromes are:

1. Syndromes represent a cluster of nursing diagnoses.
2. Their labels give cues to the cause.
3. Syndromes have initial and long-term phases.
4. Syndromes have emotional, social, and physical components.
5. Syndromes represent complex clinical conditions requiring expert nursing assessment and expert nursing interventions.[14]

The current NANDA-accepted syndromes are Rape Trauma Syndrome, Relocation Stress Syndrome, and Disuse Syndrome. It would be interesting to investigate if there is a theoretically related cluster of problems occurring with some cases of activity intolerance and chronic pain. Also perhaps instead of the diagnosis Fatigue being defined simply as overwhelming exhaustion, the diagnosis should be developed to describe a chronic fatigue syndrome.[15] A syndrome is not a typology of problems under a broad category. This is suggested when Self-Care Deficit is converted to a syndrome.[16] When diagnosing a syndrome it is important to:

1. Identify the central etiological factor in the syndrome (e.g., rape, disuse, relocation, etc.).
2. Assess that all the nursing diagnoses/problems described by the syndrome are present.
3. Include all the problems in the development of a plan of care.

Perhaps the key to clinical recognition of a syndrome is the single etiological factor. In addition, this type of diagnosis involves more complex, integrated treatment planning to address multiple, interrelated problems.

DIAGNOSTIC STATEMENTS

At this point some guidelines that summarize the final formulation of the diagnostic statement will be helpful. Most guidelines identified by Iyer and her colleagues[17] and other authors are included or adapted in the following; these structural and functional guidelines can be reviewed prior to entering a diagnosis on the client's record.

1. *The nursing diagnosis describes a dysfunctional or potentially dysfunctional pattern using accepted diagnostic category labels.* This applies particularly to the novice, who needs some standard language to practice the diagnostic process; others may wish to test refinements or new diagnoses in their practice prior to submission to NANDA. The diagnosis does not describe or include in the statement a therapeutic need, medical diagnosis, treatments, staff problems, and other clinical terms discussed in Chapter 2. (Some would include a life process formulated as a "health diagnosis" or "potential for enhancement of . . ." as a nursing diagnosis.) Appendix B has terms that can be used to label judgments.

2. *The relationship between the diagnostic categories describing the problem and etiological factors is indicated by a "/" or "R/T" or the words, "related to."* Some authors refer to the problem and etiology as the "two part" statement or the "two clauses." It is preferable to use the terms *problem* and *related factors;* "parts" and "clauses" do not remind diagnosticians of what they are stating—a causal relationship. Avoidance of "caused by" or "due to" and use of "related to" seems to be the prevailing opinion in the nursing diagnosis literature.

3. *Both the problem and etiology refer to distinct clusters of signs and symptoms. The observed signs and symptoms contain the critical defining characteristics for the problem and etiological factors.* As Iyer and others[17] (p. 101) caution, the problem and etiology should not describe (a) *the same condition or whole-part relations* (alteration in bowel elimination related to constipation) or (b) *the condition and a defining characteristic of the same condition* (body image disturbance related to "can't look at colostomy" or "fear related to nervousness about threatening event").

Definitely avoid the routine use of diagnostic categories, such as Ineffective Coping and Self-Care Deficit, as umbrellas for specific diagnoses or as a "routine label" that fits every ill client or distressed family. Alterations in Health Maintenance also is not an "umbrella" for the medical diagnoses of a client. "Altered (broad category . . .)" is not a clinically useful statement to use as a base for intervention. It is too broad. Alteration in parenting is an example. What are the alterations of concern to nurses? NANDA[3] has identified Parental Role Conflict; Gordon[7] has identified Weak Parent-Infant Attachment and a number of altered growth and development areas; and Herdman[8] has identified Parental Fear of Attachment, Parent-Infant Separation, and High Risk for Developmental Delay (Specify).

4. *Structure of the problem and etiological factors are concise, clear, and include the recommended specifications (e.g., levels, acuity, etc.).* Precision will facilitate treatment planning. This guideline refers to categories that require a specification, such as fear (specify focus). Avoid stating the focus as the etiology (fear related to surgery or dysfunctional grieving related to loss of spouse). In neither case can the nurse change these etiological factors (surgery, death). It could be sleep deprivation related to fear (surgical prognosis) or dysfunctional grieving (loss of spouse) related to social isolation. Note in the last item that loss of spouse does not suggest the reason the grieving is *dysfunctional;* one might suspect that the nurse should intervene to help the person with the grieving process, thus treating *this* problem as the etiology! Thinking this way would suggest a little deeper review of findings to identify other problems that dysfunctional grieving is probably causing. Fear in the second example may also be the treatment focus (etiology) because it is contributing to sleep deprivation. Recall the suggestion to be conscious of what you are inclined to treat; consider the idea that that condition may very well be the etiological factor.

5. *(a) The etiological factors or critical risk factors for a potential problem can be predicted to change with nursing intervention, and (b) the change can be predicted to resolve the problem.* The author realizes that nursing does not have the research base for the types of predictions in (b); thus consider this an ideal to think about but not a reason for discarding a diagnosis. A second but related idea is that the etiological factors and risk factors should include conditions that are usually resolved by nursing intervention. For example, Chronic Pain Related to Arthritis requires medical planning and intervention. If this condition were viewed as a problem in the client's management of pain (viewed as the probable cause), the nurse would intervene on the self-management of the pain, not the Arthritis (inflammation of the joint). Also rather than trying to find a nursing intervention for Decreased Cardiac Output, Excess Fluid Volume Deficit, Fluid Volume Deficit (at least the levels requiring intravenous therapy), Impaired Gas Exchange, and Altered Tissue Perfusion, consider these collaborative treatment problems. In many instances these conditions occur with nursing diagnoses. For example, persons with Decreased Cardiac Output (Congestive Heart Failure) usually have Decreased Activity Tolerance.

6. *The problem and etiological factors are written without ambiguous or highly value-laden words and in legally advisable terms.* Nursing diagnoses are value concepts; that is, they express what the profession or society deem as "unhealthy" or as a problem. Going further to say "inadequate parenting" or "poor sleep patterns" is both ambiguous and laden with personal values and criteria.

Don't imply malpractice, as in "pressure ulcer related to inadequate turning." Nursing diagnoses are not used to discipline nursing, medical, or other care providers; if there is malpractice or ethical misconduct, report it to the proper agency person or legal or professional authorities.

Many of the topics discussed in this chapter thus far can be reasons for structural errors, such as can occur in stating a diagnosis, and procedural errors, such as those related to some of the "dilemmas in the following section." Let us now consider the difficulties that students and staff nurses report when using nursing diagnoses.

POSTASSESSMENT DILEMMAS

Any of the following prediagnostic situations or combinations of situations may exist at the end of an admission assessment for both the novice and expert:

No diagnostic cues
Cluster of cues; no idea of the problem
Nothing fits the cues
A lot of problems formulated
Imprecise problem formulation
Problem formulated; is it a nursing diagnosis?

Let us consider the way out of each of these wicked dilemmas.

No diagnostic cues

After a functional pattern assessment, it is difficult to face the fact that there are no cues or cue clusters that point to a diagnosis. This can be a dilemma for a student who believes the instructor assigned the patient so that diagnostic judgment could be practiced or for the staff nurse who believes the client must have one.

Possibility 1

There are no nursing diagnoses; the client is healthy and even with a disease is managing well.

Action. Provide feedback to ensure that the client realizes that health practices being employed are beneficial. If the setting is appropriate, see if there is potential for growth to higher levels of functional well-being.

Possibility 2

The assessment was superficial; therefore cues were missed.

Action. Check the screening assessment in Appendix H. Were the items assessed and attention paid to client reports and observations? See Chapters 5 to 7.

Possibility 3

The assessment was adequate but the diagnostic meaning of cues was not derived. Hypotheses were not generated to guide branching questions and observations.

Action. See Chapter 8.

Cluster of cues; no idea of problem

A dilemma exists if assessment resulted in a set of cues and there is no idea of how to formulate the problem. Yet this is more positive than the situation above where information collection and first-level interpretation skills may be missing. Having cues without a problem formulated is usually expressed as "I didn't know what to call it!"

Possibility 1

Knowledge of diagnostic categories, labels, and critical cues (diagnostic criteria) is insufficient. This is an example:

> States he becomes fatigued about midday after minimal activity; feels heart thumping and some shortness of breath after "getting breakfast and doing the morning dishes." Medical diagnosis: Congestive heart failure, arteriosclerosis.

If it can be assumed that cue evaluation was correct and diagnostic cues *are* present (as in the example above), the difficulty lies in placing the appropriate diagnostic label on the cluster.

Action. In a clinical situation think why even a broad dysfunctional pattern was not identified, such as activity problem. To solve the immediate need on the clinical unit, look up the diagnoses grouped under Exercise-Activity Pattern in *Manual of Nursing Diagnosis*[17] (for now look at Appendix B) and see if a few category labels seem applicable. Go to the pages in the *Manual* listing applicable diagnoses and read the defining characteristics. Do any match the assessment data? In the future modify the information collection procedure by collecting and organizing data under each pattern area. Diagnostic cues will then be within a pattern and will indicate the *general area* of a problem. Then look at the diagnoses under the pattern in your *Manual*. See if the cluster of cues matches any of the diagnostic categories within the pattern area and their defining characteristics. The data above should have suggested activity intolerance.

Possibility 2

The cluster of cues under consideration includes more than one set of diagnostic cues. The difficulty lies in trying to make one diagnosis when more than one is possible. For example:

> Thin, lanky 16-year-old during check of an arm cast states: "Those guys (parents) are always making me feel like a kid; come in by 10, clean my room, get better grades; wish they'd leave me alone. I can't wait till I finish school and can live on my own." States mother checks cast every day but "now she's working and is never home when I get home from school like she used to be." Reports he comes home after school and gets "some junk food out of the refrigerator" and then doesn't eat supper. States he doesn't prepare a lunch for school, gets food out of the machines. "She yells at me for that too."

Action. Recognize that the nurse, not the client, organizes the information into clusters of cues; the nurse has to be sensitive to the different meanings in a communication and must organize the data under the patterns. This will help in processing the data. The client has a nutritional deficit and also may be having a developmental independence/dependence conflict that requires more investigation.

Nothing fits the cues

A dilemma exists when none of the current diagnostic categories can be applied and a diagnosis needs to be made to guide care planning. A number of explanations exist.

Possibility 1

There is a cluster of cues but none show the critical defining characteristics. This is associated with lack of confidence in applying *any* diagnostic category.

Action. Try focusing on hypothesis generation during assessment. Diagnostic hypotheses direct you beyond the routine questions to the assessment of critical cues (see Chapter 7). Also learn the critical cues for common diagnoses.

Possibility 2

The cues signify a disease, complication of a disease, or adverse effect of medical therapy. For example, a client with bladder cancer may report blood in the urine.

Action. This is an important cue to be reported to the physician if the condition is not already documented on the chart. Avoid creating a label such as "alteration in urinary elimination: bleeding" when you record this observation. The physician will never find the data recorded under this label; document under the medical diagnosis to which the data apply.

Possibility 3

There is no current diagnostic category that describes the information collected.

Action. After checking the current listing carefully, try to come up with a concise category label and check it out with an instructor/clinical specialist. Chapter 12 provides some guidelines for creating new diagnostic category labels. Never use a category that does not fit the clinical "picture" described by the data. That would be a forced classification.

A lot of problems formulated

This situation is typical of the *advanced* beginner, who can derive meaning from cues, cluster the data, and identify dysfunctional patterns (perhaps a list of six to ten) but has difficulty in knowing what goes with what. When this happens, frequently the difficulty may be expressed as "Today, I really don't feel like working up more than three or four (student who has to chart and also write lengthy recordings or staff nurse who has two other admission assessments to do)."

Possibility 1

The client-environment situation is complex and there *are* a lot of problems and etiological factors. This can occur in long-term care or with multi-problem families.

Action. Check to see if some problems do not require immediate treatment. Are they low priority today (e.g., discharge preparation in a pre-operative client)? Record them; do the treatment plan tomorrow. Make sure good judgment is exercised (e.g., that client is not going home tomorrow).

Possibility 2

The six to ten "problems" are dysfunctional patterns, but a final synthesis of the assessment data

was not done. If the causal links or relationships among problems was determined, there may only be three or four.

Action. Always remember to do a final review of the findings; this provides a holistic look at the client's health. Learn to "put things together" as you move from assessment of one pattern to another by thinking while assessing. Possibility 2 is a typical difficulty; the following is a list of problems that were not linked at the end of the assessment (75-year-old female, 2 days after fractured hip and concussion):

1. Sleep Onset Disturbance
2. Self-Care Deficit (Level II)
3. High Risk for Impaired Home Maintenance Management
4. Ineffective Airway Clearance
5. Anticipatory Fear (Future Loss of Independence)
6. Impaired Bed Mobility (Level II)
7. Viscous secretions, pain in hip with cough

Reviewing the findings made it clear that relationships existed among these problems. Rather than trying to do a care plan for each, the dysfunctional patterns were examined for causal links. Some were seen as the problem and others as the probable cause; the problem/etiology format was used, thereby reducing the number of diagnoses and providing a useful focus for treatment planning:

1. Sleep Onset Disturbance/Anticipatory Fear (Loss of Independence)
2. Self-Care Deficit (Level II)/Impaired Bed Mobility (Level II)
3. Ineffective Airway Clearance/Viscous Secretions, Pain in Hip with Cough
4. High Risk for Impaired Home Maintenance Management

Imprecise problem formulation

At times novice diagnosticians get feedback that their diagnoses are vague and imprecise. It is a dilemma when the reason cannot be found. Precise diagnoses are important because they facilitate treatment planning and communication among care providers.

Possibility 1

Insufficient assessment. The diagnosis is made but lacks specificity. Certain diagnoses require specification of the acuity, level, or focus. Examples are:

Self-Care Deficit (Specify Level)
Pain (Acute, Chronic)
Knowledge Deficit (Specify)
Health Management Deficit (Specify)

Action. Continue assessment after the problem is identified. Include specifications as in the examples that follow:
Self-Care Deficit (Level III)
Knowledge Deficit (Medication Regimen)
Acute Pain
Health Management Deficit (Follow-up care)

Possibility 2

Affirming a causal relationship between the whole and component parts. A diagnosis is imprecise when the problem-etiology merely communicates the relationship between the whole and its parts or divisions. Imprecise diagnoses would be Alterations in Parenting Related to Weak Parent-Infant Attachment or Self-Care Deficit Related to Bathing Deficit. Self-Care Deficit represents the "whole" diagnostic class and has components: feeding, bathing, dressing, and toileting. Thus bathing deficit is not a contributing or etiological factor but rather a component. Treatment is directed toward factors contributing to the problem; thus whole-part formulations are not useful clinically. It would be comparable to the physician writing a medical diagnosis such as: "cardiac disease related to rheumatic fever."

Action. Use the specific, not the general, classification category. Try to determine the major contributing factors. For example:
Self-Bathing Deficit (Level III) Related to Uncompensated Hemiplegia
Weak Parent-Infant Attachment Related to Parent-Infant Separation Anxiety

When terms such as "alterations in . . ." or "impairment of . . ." come to mind, assess further to determine the *specific* alteration or impairment and the etiological factors.

Possibility 3

The diagnostic category requires refinement. The novice cannot be blamed for using "accepted" nursing diagnoses that are imprecise (see Appendix A). Diagnostic categories are in the process of

development by staff nurses, specialists, faculty, researchers, and theoreticians. All agree that the classifications will be much more precise 50 years from now.

Action. Learn what precision means (see section above) and obtain help when you are tempted to use broad categories. As diagnostic abilities increase
1. Think of all the types of "alterations in . . ." that are encountered.
2. Refine the diagnostic category and clinically test the specific categories.
3. Submit to NANDA for review and listing.

Problem formulated—is it a nursing diagnosis?

The way a diagnostic statement is structured can be elegant, but it may not represent a condition amenable to nursing intervention. A dilemma exists if the condition is recorded as a nursing diagnosis and it is not. The primary nurse may not be able to assume accountability for the outcomes.

Possibility 1

There is unclear understanding of the nursing diagnosis-treatment realm of practice as opposed to the collaborative practice domain. The possibility exists that the "obvious" is focused on and problem formulation is superficial. For example, the medical diagnosis is very "obvious" in acute care settings. Some may assume that everything has to be tied to the medical diagnosis or it will "get lost." The following incorrect diagnoses result (problem/etiology format): Activity Intolerance/Chronic Obstructive Pulmonary Disease (COPD) or Body Image Disturbance/Hysterectomy. Etiological factors are used to focus the nursing treatment plan; but nurses do not assume independent responsibility for treating diseases (COPD) or surgical procedures. Thus chronic obstructive pulmonary disease and hysterectomy are not useful as etiological factors. A more useful formulation would be Situational Depression/Body Image Disturbance.

A second reason given for the possible "loss" of the medical diagnosis in the suggested format is that nurses treating Situational Depression/Body

Image Disturbance will not realize that the client had a hysterectomy. How could this occur? Surgical procedures and medical diagnoses have high clinical visibility. Errors result if *any* diagnosis is treated out of context—the whole client-environment situation.

Action. When you are inclined to view the medical diagnosis as the etiology of a problem, (1) consider looking deeper into the situation, (2) assess for etiological or related factors that will respond to nursing treatment, and (3) formulate the diagnosis in nursing terms. As one author frequently states, Florence Nightingale cautioned that we should not mix nursing and medicine; it confuses them both.[19] Understand the independent and interdependent (collaborative) areas of nursing practice; this leads to a clear view of responsibility and accountability in each area of clinical judgment.

Also always consider the possibility that the "problem" you have identified may in fact be the etiology. Consider activity intolerance/COPD. Now ask the question: If a person had activity intolerance, what problems might this produce? The diagnosis, from a nursing perspective, may be Impaired Home Maintenance Management/Activity Intolerance or Self-Care Deficit (Level III)/Activity Intolerance.

Possibility 2

The nursing diagnosis is defined by the diagnostician as *both* independent and interdependent (collaborative) practice. Not all nurses agree that nursing diagnosis should only describe conditions within the independent area of nursing practice. They suggest, for example, that Activity Intolerance/Decreased Cardiac Output is a nursing diagnosis. Some accept Body Image Disturbance/Hysterectomy as a diagnosis.

Action. Consider the pro and con arguments (Chapters 1, 5, and 9), take a position, and test its clinical usefulness in practice and in your work with physicians or other care providers.

CONSISTENCY AMONG CARE PROVIDERS' DIAGNOSES

Some would argue that nursing diagnoses should be consistent with medical diagnoses or those of other care providers. Consistency by definition means compatible, noncontradictory, or conforming to some principle or course of action. This is unattainable for the following reasons.

There may be no medical diagnosis and thus the requirement is impossible. Second, problems diagnosed by nurses, physicians, and social workers are in three different domains: functional patterns, disease, and personal social matters. Clients can have various problems in each area and in many combinations. Is a nursing diagnosis of unresolved grieving consistent with the medical diagnosis of Appendicitis? A client could have both of these diagnoses, yet neither consistently predicts the other.

Apparent inconsistencies may arise in regard to assessment data collected by different professionals. Although used in different ways, many of the same data are gathered by the various health care providers. If the data are inconsistent, discussion among the professionals and reassessment can usually resolve any contradictions. If an apparent inconsistency occurs at the level of diagnosis, disagreement on a diagnosis that is well supported by data is also resolved by discussion. The opinion of the care provider who is expert in the problem area and most knowledgeable about the client should be weighed most heavily.

AVOIDING ERRORS IN REASONING AND JUDGMENT

The reader will recall from Chapters 7 and 8, in which the diagnostic process was outlined, that there are four critical components: collecting, interpreting, clustering, and labeling judgments. Each component is a potential source of error. In reading this section try to reflect on those components as they are pointed out. Suggestions for avoiding errors will draw heavily on the content from those chapters. It will be noted by the repetition that a particular type of error can occur for many reasons. For example, errors of omission can be attributed to (1) not viewing information as relevant to nursing diagnosis and therefore not assessing the pattern indicator, (2) assessing but not "seeing" the relevance of a cue, or (3) lacking knowledge that the cue should influence judgment in a particular direction.

Data collection errors

The information collected during assessment influences the *entire* diagnostic process. If data are omitted, diagnoses can be missed. If large amounts of data are collected in an unorganized manner, cognitive processes can be overwhelmed. Irrelevant data can produce the same effect. Thoroughness is important. Yet data must be relevant to areas of nursing concern.

Interviewing and examination skills are critical factors in perceptual accuracy. These activities include inquiries, supportive replies, silence, touching, and examination. Characteristics such as physical attributes of the head, face, shoulders, arms and posture of a client in bed are observable. Actions are required to elicit data about less readily apparent characteristics. If these actions are not taken, not chosen wisely, or not performed correctly, the nurse's perceptual accuracy suffers.

To maintain a low rate of error in data collection, think of what the data collection process involves: (1) perceptual accuracy, (2) organization, and (3) interviewing and examination skills. First, consider *perceptual accuracy*. What may influence this? Clinical knowledge is one factor. People may at times observe without perceiving. Many errors in perception result from not having available categories for classifying sensory information. These categories are based on clinical knowledge. The nurse must be curious and question what is observed; this is how knowledge develops and errors are avoided for both the novice and expert diagnostician.

Perception is a neuropsychological phenomenon. Thus it is influenced by health states, fatigue, and boredom or routine. It is particularly important for perceptual alertness that nurses maintain their own functional health patterns, particularly sleep and rest. One could surmise that extended work shifts may tax perceptual-cognitive processes, perhaps especially in settings where continuous alertness is critical.

Neglecting to collect critical data is another source of potential error. The nurse may overlook critical cues because of distraction, lack of organization, or inadequate clinical knowledge. For example, lack of knowledge about coping deficits or about risk factors in skin breakdown can lead one to miss cues. Too narrow a concept of nursing may cause one to exclude some material for assessment (for example, coping patterns).

Failure to obtain client reports in areas about which the client's subjective information is critical is another source of inaccuracies. Similarly, relying on only predictive (contextual) data and inferences increases the rate of error; current data about the state of the client are also needed. Sometimes data are collected but not considered in analysis. Ignoring a critical cue that should have been pursued leads to errors of omission.

Overload of data can also lead the diagnostician astray. When large quantities of irrelevant data are collected, cognitive capacities for processing information can be overloaded. For example, questions may be irrelevant or clients may ramble.

Methodological errors can be caused by inaccuracies in measurement of a client characteristic. Questions asked during history taking may lead the client to say what seems to be expected. Or the nurse may not listen attentively. Perceptual errors, such as underestimating the depth of respirations, or faulty equipment can also be a source of measurement error.

A second factor related to data collection errors is *organization*. There are two aspects: (1) preorganization and (2) organization during assessment. *Preassessment organization* has been emphasized in previous discussions. Briefly, one must know one's conceptual focus and the pattern areas. The critical areas for data collection within patterns should be listed. In addition, one must decide how to begin and select a possible sequence.

As data collection begins, *concurrent organization* is needed: that is, as the assessment proceeds the nurse has to organize the data by generating diagnostic hypotheses that permit clustering of data and by also recording the data under the functional health pattern areas. The human mind cannot handle large amounts of unorganized data. Some method of keeping track of what has gone before is needed because previous data and hypotheses influence what questions are asked in branching. One of the major reasons for missing critical cues is lack of concurrent organization of data during history taking and examination.

Data interpretation errors

If the meaning of cues is inaccurately interpreted, diagnostic errors result. Cues signifying a dysfunctional pattern may not be interpreted as dysfunctional; an error of omission will result. Overdiagnosing occurs when a functional pattern is interpreted as dysfunctional. Usually the diagnostic errors occur because of inadequate clinical knowledge. Not taking developmental or individual norms into account also contributes to errors of interpretation.

Another source of error in data interpretation is overgeneralizing from one observation of client behavior. The behavioral sample can be inadequate (too few observations, or atypical ones) or interpreted outside the context of the situation in which the behavior took place. One episode of hostility does not mean the client is a hostile person. Remember that assessment relies on patterns of behavior, not isolated events.

To maintain a low rate of error the nurse must validate his or her inferences. Errors occur if hypotheses are not treated as tentative and subject to revision. Furthermore, generating hypotheses early does not mean that early ideas are the only ones considered. Additional data may require additional hypotheses.

When judgments have an element of uncertainty, probabilities have to be taken into account. Errors can result from incorrect notions about the likelihood of diagnoses. As described, an element of forecasting or prediction enters into diagnosis. Adequate testing of hypotheses helps to control errors in prediction.

One technique for examining interpretations of data is *reframing*.[21] This is a process of shifting perspectives. A familiar example is looking at the sky and deciding the day is partly cloudy; from another perspective the day is partly sunny. Reframing can be applied to one or two cues, a tentative hypothesis, or a cluster of cues in a diagnosis. Try to reframe the following cues:

This behavior is familiar to nurses who work in pediatric, public health, or school settings with "shy" children. A child who clings to his mother, withdraws, and does not play with other children is apt to make a lasting impression on a nurse. There is a tendency to call this "separation anxiety."[20] (p. 840)

After attempting to look at these cues in a different way, read the following. Note that Clark reinterprets data from the perspective of the child's thinking:

Reframing will enable the nurse to pick out the adaptive portions of the child's behavior from his point of view. The child does not know what the new experience holds. He only knows he has been taken to a strange place for some unclear purpose. He is actually to be commended for sticking close to the one familiar object in the environment, his mother, until he can figure out what is happening. In this sense, the child's behavior is quite adaptive, since it allows for some stability through closeness to mother until information can be gathered on what action is appropriate.[20] (p. 840)

The earlier interpretation of separation anxiety may be realistic if the behavior continues. If separation anxiety is ultimately diagnosed, having considered adaptation as an alternative should increase the nurse's confidence that error has been avoided.

Try another example adapted from Clark.[21] For medical reasons a client requires complete bed rest. He is not to get out of bed. This activity restriction has been discussed with him and he acknowledges the need for it. Repeatedly the nurse observes the client out of bed. Obviously, the problem is noncompliance with activity prescription! What might be the reasons for this behavior? Is there a deeper problem? Here is how Clark reframed this data:

To reframe the patients' behavior from his point of view, staying in bed may seem like an attempt to force him into a dependent, helpless position, and getting out of bed may be an adaptive maneuver. A patient who refuses to accept the "sick role" may harm himself physically in the short term, but he may be taking steps to preserve his long-term self-image. In other words, refusing to accept the "sick role" can be adaptive.[20] (p. 840)

Reframing is similar to branching. It is an important concept in reducing errors. Try to see the world from the client's eyes when interpreting cues. Also, as previously recommended, obtain the client's perception of the health problem, its probable cause, and any action that has been taken to remedy the problem. A total reformulation or rejection of a hypothesis may result.

Data clustering errors

Clustering, it may be recalled, is the combination of cues. Three kinds of errors can occur in clustering: A nursing diagnosis may be made prematurely, incorrectly, or not at all.

Premature closure is a common error. A diagnostic judgment is reached before all critical information has been considered or even before all information has been collected. The observations that have been made are inadequate supporting data.

One of the reasons the problem-oriented method for charting was introduced in hospitals around the country was to prevent premature closure. Problem-oriented recording requires the diagnostician to list the subjective and objective data for each problem. Clearly this form of charting forces the clinician to specify the data base for each diagnostic judgment. Having recorded the cues used in making each judgment, the clinician can examine whether or not sufficient supporting evidence is available. More will be said about this charting system in the next chapter.

Incorrect clustering of cues can occur in formulating the problem, in identifying the etiology, or in combining the problem and etiology. The result of incorrect clustering is that data supposedly supporting the diagnosis clearly contradict it.[21] This error is usually related to inadequate knowledge of critical signs and symptoms. It is similar to labeling a chair as a table. The rules for using any language apply also to diagnostic "language."

Lack of standardization of diagnostic categories used in nursing diagnosis contributes to this type of error. If the difference between a chair and table was not specified in dictionaries, errors in use of the terms would occur. The situation is similar in nursing diagnosis. Try to use currently identified signs, symptoms, and category definitions. The potential for errors will be reduced but probably not eliminated until precise definitions and critical characteristics are standardized.

Not *synthesizing* (not combining cues) obviously leads to errors of omission. Whereas some nurses tend to close prematurely, others delay diagnostic judgment. This delay may represent an attempt to reach absolute certainty when in reality the situation is inevitably based on some degree of uncertainty. Think of a nursing diagnosis as the best hypothesis of the moment; be open to new information that can reject or further confirm judgments: These are the keys to working with uncertainty-based data and judgments.

Attribution errors

Errors can occur if the reasons (etiological factors) for a problem are attributed to the client's behavior, when in fact the reason lies in the situation or in client-environment interaction. This type of error has a direct effect on intervention because a treatment plan is based on etiological factors. Obtain the client's viewpoint regarding probable causes of the problem and consider these in formulating etiological factors. Always keep in mind that usually there are multiple causes for problems. Focus on helping clients change their behavior or change the sources of a problem in their situation or environment.[22]

IMPLICIT RULES

In an interesting article about unwritten rules for making decisions, Scheff[23] examined differences in tolerance for certain errors of judgment. The following synopsis of his ideas will serve as a basis for considering what implicit rules might influence nursing diagnosis.

In a court of law a person is innocent until proven guilty. The rule is "when in doubt, acquit." Underlying this rule are the assumptions that (1) conviction will do irreversible harm to a person's reputation, (2) the person is weak and defenseless relative to society, and (3) society can sustain some errors without serious consequences.

Note the dilemma. A legal judgment of guilty when innocent has serious consequences for the individual. Yet a judgment of innocent when the person is guilty can have serious consequences for society. An acquitted offender may commit further crimes. Western society resolves the dilemma in favor of the individual; in fact the assumption of innocence is stated in legal codes and accepted by jurists.

What is actually occurring? There are two types of errors a jury could make:

Type I error. The accused is *actually guilty,* but the hypothesis of *not guilty* is accepted.

Type II error. The accused is *actually innocent,* but the hypothesis of *guilty* is accepted.

Before receiving data from witnesses and the interpretations of lawyers, juries are instructed to avoid a type II error. Society does not tolerate convicting the innocent; if doubt exists, acquit.

In the profession of medicine, the same types of errors are possible when clinical data are ambiguous:

Type I error. The client *actually has a disease,* but the hypothesis of *no disease* is accepted.
Type II error. The client is *actually disease-free,* but the hypothesis of *disease* is accepted.

Colleagues, clients, and the general society generally do not tolerate a type I error. What implicit rule is followed by practitioners of medicine?

According to Scheff,[23] the rule is not always explicitly stated or as rigid in medicine as in law. Yet it does exist: "When in doubt, diagnose disease." This bias can influence medical assessment. It encourages the physician to consider symptoms as possibly signifying illness until disease is ruled out. When in doubt, it is far more important to continue to suspect illness than to suspect health.

The assumptions that underlie this implicit rule are: (1) undetected disease will have serious consequences, (2) diagnoses are reversible, and (3) society expects disease, if present, to be diagnosed. Physicians are aware that a malpractice legal decision can result from a type I error. That is, a client may sue if dismissed as healthy when in fact disease was present and subsequently produced harm. Furthermore, if a client remains in society with untreated infectious disease or behavior harmful to others, there may be serious consequences.

A dilemma accompanies the rule "When in doubt diagnose or suspect illness." Calling clients' attention to their bodily state can produce physiologic and psychologic changes. The client may alter many aspects of life and assume the sick role in work, family, and social situations.[24] Furthermore, psychiatric as well as some medical disease labels carry social stigma. Type II errors are costly to individuals or society, and many people question whether unnecessary surgical and psychiatric treatment is occurring. Yet the implicit rule of "Better safe than sorry" prevails.[23] (p. 100)

Scheff suggests that personal biases toward type I or type II errors are influenced by the disease characteristics, the physician, the client, and the

health care setting in which diagnoses are made. He raises a number of possibilities that are relevant to nursing as well as medical diagnosis:

Physicians who generally *favor active intervention* probably make more type II errors than physicians who view their treatments only as assistance for natural bodily reactions to disease. The physician's *perception of the personality of the patient* may also be relevant; type II errors are less likely if the physician defines the patient as a "crock," than a person who ignores or denies disease.

The organizational setting is relevant to the extent that it influences the relationship between the doctor and the patient. In some contexts, as in medical practice in organizations such as the military or industrial setting, the physician is not as likely to feel *personal responsibility* for the patient as he would in others, such as private practice. This may be due in part to the conditions of financial remuneration and perhaps equally important, the sheer volume of patients dependent on the doctor's time. Cultural or class differences may also affect the amount of social distance between doctor and patient, and therefore the amount of responsibility which the doctor feels for the patient. Whatever the sources, the more the physician feels personally responsible for the patient, the more likely he is to make a type II error.[23] (p. 104)

It is also interesting to think about whether nurses are influenced by their perception of the personality of the client; for example, in the initial impression. Does perception of personal responsibility for a client versus perception of team responsibility influence diagnostic errors? Do nurses who view nursing as assisting the client make fewer type II errors than nurses who view nursing as doing things for the client? Answers are not available, but the questions provoke thought.

No research has been published about nursing diagnostic errors. One could imagine that there are rules that bias practitioners toward either of the following errors:

Type I error. The client actually has a *functional health problem,* but the hypothesis of *no problem* is accepted.
Type II error. The client is *actually problem-free,* but the hypothesis of *functional problem* is accepted.

In doubtful situations are the rules in nursing similar to those of the courtroom? When in doubt, assume health. Or are nurses' implicit rules and assumptions similar to those of their colleagues in medicine? When in doubt, diagnose a problem (or continue to suspect a problem).

Many comments are heard admonishing nurses *not* to be problem-focused. It is said that the client's strengths, not problems, should be emphasized. This is quite true in *treatment.* Focusing on strength—areas of wellness and capabilities—is an approach that mobilizes the client's resources. In *diagnosis,* a bias toward recognition of health rather than of problematic states can result in diagnostic errors of omission, type I errors. If symptoms signifying a nursing diagnosis are not investigated, problems can be missed.

With regard to observing signs and symptoms of disease, nurses are told that when in doubt they should assume these signify complications and call a physician. As Hammond[25] (p. 29) has suggested, nurses have to think for themselves as well as think "as" the doctor thinks; when observing disease states and carrying out medical treatment the nurse is under the "cognitive control of the doctor." Within this cognitive set may be the rule "When in doubt, diagnose or suspect disease complications." Is it difficult to shift to an opposite rule in nursing diagnosis? This question would make an interesting clinical study.

Legal as well as moral responsibilities argue for avoiding errors of omission. It is understandable that one may not wish to diagnose potential for injury or trauma when cues are uncertain. This diagnosis, for example, might necessitate cautioning the truck driver with uncontrolled seizures not to drive although his employment would be interrupted by following that recommendation. Values enter into any judgment. The best thing is to be aware of the potential consequences of diagnosis and treatment when symptoms are doubtful.

Also be aware of the consequences of delay in diagnosis and treatment. If delay is the action of choice, continue to collect data and attempt to resolve ambiguities. Learn the technique of discussing observations with clients in a nonthreatening, nonanxiety-producing manner. It is important not to reinforce the sick role but instead help clients to *feel capable* of handling any health problems diagnosed.

In addition to errors of omission (type I) and errors of commission (type II) there is an "error of the third kind," solving the *wrong* problem.[26] Pre- paring a care plan for the wrong problem wastes nursing time. Most important, the real problem can cause client discomfort if allowed to progress.

Diagnosing and treating the wrong problem can usually be avoided if the meaning of client behavior is explored. The only way to understand the behavior of the client is to ask. It is as simple as that. Inferences made without checking the client's viewpoint can lead to completely erroneous problem formulations and ineffective care plans.

RETROSPECTIVE EVALUATION OF DIAGNOSES

When uncertainty in diagnosis can be reduced but not eliminated, it is helpful to have ways of checking judgments. Checking that critical defining cues are present is one way of validating a diagnosis before intervention begins. A second way is to evaluate change in signs and symptoms of the problem after problem-specific intervention has been initiated. This second check involves retrospective evaluation of a diagnostic judgment.

Nursing care is directed at the probable cause of a problem and effectiveness of care is measured by client outcomes. The outcome of nursing care is a positive change in the status of the problem, therefore the nurse may assume that the previously identified factors were at least one probable cause. This procedure of evaluating the correctness of causal factors by observing the effectiveness of the intervention is a *retrospective* test of the cause of a problem.

Consider an example. If (1) knowledge deficit is *correctly* viewed as the predominant factor causing noncompliance and (2) the intervention is designed to increase the client's knowledge, then (3) the outcome assessment should indicate a change from noncompliance to compliance. What if this expected outcome does not occur, as shown in Table 9-1?

As seen in Table 9-1, one cannot make clearcut assumptions about etiological factors from outcome data. If there is no change in signs and symptoms, several possible reasons have to be considered. Returning to the example about knowledge deficit, let us assume the intervention was the best possible for the diagnosis. Four questions can then be raised. Was knowledge deficit the correct etiology? Could there have been other, unidentified factors? Were some events or situational factors overlooked? Was noncompliance just a sign of another problem? These are possible reasons why nursing care did not produce a change.

Now let us assume that the etiology is correct but the intervention was ineffective. As can be seen in Table 9-1, either the choice of intervention or its implementation (or both) may not have been correct. Knowledge deficit may indeed have been the predominant factor, but teaching methods may have been ineffective—maybe the client's readiness for learning new information was not considered. It is useful to think about intervention as a test of the accuracy of problem formulation.

The questions for consideration when the expected outcomes *are* attained (again see Table 9-1)

Table 9-1 Outcome Evaluation of the Problem— Etiological Factors Identified

Outcome evaluation	Considerations
I Change in problem status not as predicted (e.g., signs and symptoms of problem still present)	1. Were the assumed etiological factors (cause) not correct? 2. Were other unidentified factors, etiological or otherwise, operating? 3. Was the intervention inadequate to produce change in the problem? 4. Were the intervention methods applied correctly?
II Change in problem state as predicted (e.g., signs and symptoms of problem not present)	1. Are there any other explanations for the change in the problem? 2. Was the intervention influencing only the assumed etiological factors or others also?

will benefit future clients. Asking these questions enables the nurse to learn from practice experiences. For example, was knowledge deficit the predominate cause of the client's noncompliance? Could it be that the human concern and rapport established during teaching influenced the client's *motivation,* and that motivation, rather than learning, produced change? Perhaps the intervention influenced other unspecified factors as well and the combined effect produced the result.

Unless these questions are considered, the previously effective combination of problem, etiological factor, and intervention, when applied in a future situation, may not produce the outcome. Why? Mainly because a *group* of factors may be operating, not just the one or more that have been identified (in the present example, knowledge deficit). By chance, the intervention dealt with these unrecognized factors and hence produced the desired outcome.

Conclusions from unexamined judgments cannot be applied to future clients' problems. The kind of reflection just discussed is necessary. Essentially, this is called "learning from practice." Future clients benefit from the nurse's past experience. (This is probably why employment advertisements specify "experience required"; the implicit assumption is that past experience has been used to increase clinical judgment and skill.)

SUMMARY

The focus of this chapter was on formulating nursing diagnoses. It was pointed out that diagnoses begin to be formulated when attention is paid to a diagnostic cue. Guidelines were provided for stating problems, etiological factors, and potential problems. Precision in stating the diagnosis was stressed in the discussion because the nursing diagnosis is used to project outcomes, design a treatment plan, and evaluate outcomes. A number of postassessment dilemmas reported by learners were discussed and suggested actions were outlined. It was pointed out that the criterion of logical consistency among care providers' diagnoses was probably not relevant. Different domains of diagnostic focus will result in unrelated diagnoses in most instances.

Sources of diagnostic error were considered, as were some implicit rules that may apply. The potential for errors in nursing diagnosis lies in data collection, interpretation, clustering, and the attribution of cause. Retrospective tests of diagnostic formulations were suggested. It was seen that if anticipated outcomes do not occur, both diagnoses and interventions should be examined for error. Perhaps the most important way of self-monitoring diagnostic accuracy is to be open to new information, to recognize that biases can enter the diagnostic thinking process, and to treat nursing diagnoses as tentative judgments.

NOTES AND REFERENCES

1. Kelly MA: *Nursing diagnosis source book,* Norwalk, CT, 1985, Appleton-Century-Crofts.
2. Ideally, because most diagnoses require "work" on the part of the client, both should agree that the problem exists and needs to changed.
3. North American Nursing Diagnosis Association: *NANDA Taxonomy I,* Rev, Philadelphia, 1992, The Association.
4. Carpenito LJ: *Nursing diagnosis: application to clinical practice,* New York, 1993, Lippincott.
5. Iyer P, Taptich B, Bernocchi-Losey D: *Nursing process and nursing diagnosis,* Philadelphia, 1986, Saunders.
6. Forsythe G: Etiology: in what sense and of what value? In Kim MJ, McLane A, McFarland G, editors: *Classification of nursing diagnoses: proceedings of the fifth conference,* St Louis, 1984 Mosby, pp 63-72.
7. Halfman TM, Pigg JS: Nurses' perceptions of rheumatic disease patient problems as evidenced in nursing diagnoses, etiologies, defining characteristics, expected outcomes and interventions. In Kim MJ, McLane A, McFarland G, editors: *Classification of nursing diagnoses: proceedings of the fifth conference,* St Louis, 1984, Mosby, pp 216-223.
8. Ziegler SM: Nursing diagnosis: the state of the art as reflected in graduate students' work. In Kim MJ, McLane A, McFarland G, editors: *Classification of nursing diagnoses: proceedings of the fifth conference,* St Louis, 1984, Mosby, pp 19-208.
9. McLane A, Fehring RJ: Nursing diagnosis: a review of the literature. In Kim MJ, McLane A, McFarland G, editors: *Classification of nursing diagnoses: proceedings of the fifth conference,* St Louis, 1984, Mosby, pp 526-527.
10. Dederian A: Etiology: practical relevance. In McLane A, editor: *Classification of nursing diagnoses: proceedings of the seventh conference,* St Louis, 1987, Mosby, pp 65-77.
11. Fitzpatrick J: Etiology: conceptual concerns. In McLane A, editor: *Classification of nursing diagnoses: proceedings of the seventh conference,* St Louis, 1987, Mosby, pp 61-64.
12. Gordon M: Identification of critical defining characteristics of high frequency–high treatment priority diagnoses in critical care. Study in progress. Boston College School of Nursing, Chestnut Hill, MA 02167.
13. American Nurses Association–American Association of Neuroscience Nurses: *Standards for neuroscience nursing practice,* Washington, DC, 1985, Author.
14. McCourt AE: Syndromes in nursing: a continuing concern. In Carroll-Johnson R, editor: *Classification of nursing diagnoses: proceedings of the ninth conference,* Philadelphia, 1991, Lippincott, pp 79-82.
15. This condition is discussed in medicine from a physiological grouping. It may very well be better conceptualized as a biopsychosocial problem.
16. Carpenito LJ: *Handbook of nursing diagnosis,* ed 5, Philadelphia, 1993, Lippincott.
17. Gordon M: *Manual of nursing diagnosis,* St Louis, 1993, Mosby.
18. Herdman TH: Critical defining characteristics of high frequency–high treatment priority diagnoses in neonatal intensive care. In progress. Boston College School of Nursing, Chestnut Hill, MA 02647.
19. Halloran E: Nursing complexity, the DRG, and length of stay. In McLane A, editor: *Classification of nursing diagnoses: proceedings of the seventh conference,* St Louis, 1986, Mosby, pp 391-398.
20. Clark N: Reframing, *Am J Nurs,* 77:840, 1977.
21. Voytovich A, Rippey R, Suffredini A: Premature conclusions in diagnostic reasoning, *J Med Educ* 60:302, 1985.
22. Abraham I: Causal analysis in clinical inference of depression: influence of general cognition on causality, *J Human Behav Learn* 4:61, 1987.
23. Scheff TJ: Decision rules, types of error, and their consequences in medical diagnosis, *Behav Sci,* 8:97, 1963.
24. Haynes RB et al: Increased absenteeism from work after detection and labeling of hypertensive patients, *N Engl J Med,* 299:741, 1978.
25. Hammond KR: Clinical inference in nursing: a psychologist's viewpoint, *Nurs Res* 15:27, 1966.
26. Mitroff I, Featheringham T: On systematic problem solving and the error of the third kind, *Behav Sci,* 19:383, 1974.

CHAPTER 10

USE OF NURSING DIAGNOSIS IN DIRECT CARE ACTIVITIES

T he previous chapters have defined nursing diagnosis and attempted to lay before the reader the process of diagnostic judgment. This earlier discussion had one end: the application of diagnosis to client care.

In a profession with a social responsibility, thinking and reasoning skills must be applied, not learned just for abstract, theoretical purposes. In fact, it is questionable whether true learning about concepts like diagnosis can occur without application in the real world. The test of an idea is its usefulness in practice: Does nursing diagnosis facilitate direct client care activities? If nursing diagnosis is merely an intellectual exercise, a status symbol, or an ivory tower idea, why learn it?

The reader would not have been led through the preceding chapters if nursing diagnosis had no clinical relevance. In this chapter it will become clear that the effort spent in formulating diagnoses greatly facilitates the planning of effective nursing care. First we shall consider the rightful place of diagnosis, that is, within the nursing process. It will be demonstrated that diagnosis is used as a focus for decisions about the care that is needed to attain the desired outcomes.

Verbal and written communications are an inte-gral part of direct care activities. How nursing diagnoses enhance the transfer of information about a client's condition and nursing care needs is a second topic. Examples will demonstrate that diagnoses organize thoughts for purposes of communication.

A third topic, discharge planning, builds on the understanding of nursing diagnosis in nursing process and in communication. The process of care planning is taken beyond a daily activity to a continuity of planning between settings and care providers. Again, examples will illustrate how nursing diagnoses are the basis for making and communicating discharge plans. A fourth topic, resource allocation, includes a consideration of the cost of nursing process and how a nurse's time is allocated on the basis of the decisions made about client's diagnoses and their treatment.

Diagnosis and the nurse's legal responsibilities and risks are interrelated. We shall consider a way in which diagnostic judgments might enter into cases of alleged professional negligence. By a case example it will be made clear that diagnostic judgments are a "duty" in the legal sense; not diagnosing can be as serious as misdiagnosing. This will lead us to the last topic of this chapter, who should diagnose.

NURSING DIAGNOSIS IN NURSING PROCESS

As currently conceived, nursing process is a problem identification and problem-solving approach to client care. It is the way in which a helping relationship, characterized by knowledge, reason, and caring, is established. The art of caring for human beings involves the application of clinical judgment, nursing science, intuition, empathy, and technical skills. Structurally, the nursing process is adapted from the scientific approach to solving problems; the knowledge and judgment used identifies the process as nursing.

Previous chapters have emphasized the problem identification phase of clinical thinking. We have seen that the diagnostic process is used in this phase to identify and label problems and strengths. When sufficient understanding of the client's health problem and contributing factors is gained, the nurse shifts from a diagnostic to a problem-solving process. At least, that is what many say. Actually, during the problem identification phase the nurse begins to consider what actions might be taken. Any one phase may contain activities found in other phases. Thinking is not in a straight line—a linear process. Yet it makes sense to describe the nursing process as a set of steps similar to those shown in the box on the right, because in a superficial sense one phase follows another. For example, it would be difficult to solve a problem that had not been assessed. Within the problem identification phase are "background" operations related to nursing actions and outcomes.

The elegance of this approach lies in its broad applicability to reasoning in any domain. Yet clearly the skeletal structure needs to be clothed. Nursing process becomes a process of nursing when the above components are attired in *values, concepts,* and *standards* of nursing.

Guiding values

The way problem identification and problem solving are carried out depends on a nurse's values and beliefs about human nature and helping. Some nurses believe that clients should diagnose their own problems. Others advocate having the nurse act as diagnostician and expert decision maker. Neither approach is applicable to *all* nursing situ-

---

> ## TWO MAJOR PHASES OF NURSING PROCESS
>
> I. *Problem identification using diagnostic process*
>   A. Data collection
>   B. Diagnostic judgment
>   C. Diagnostic labeling of actual and potential problems
> II. *Problem solving using problem-solving process*
>   A. Outcome projection
>   B. Care planning
>   C. Intervention
>   D. Outcome evaluation

---

ations. This will become evident as we examine two extremes.

At one extreme a nurse may believe that a client comes to a health care provider for help. What is sought is clinical expertise in the identification and solution of health problems or potential problems the client alone cannot identify and solve. The nurse serves the client as resource and expert. Strategies for implementing nursing process require that the nurse collect data, diagnose, and intervene. The client provides information, and then steps are taken to improve his or her health.

This belief system and strategy for using nursing process are useful if the client is unconscious or feels too weak to participate; but if applied to all clients and situations, it becomes an authoritarian approach.

At the opposite extreme is the position that all nurse-client interactions should promote growth toward the realization of human potential. The nursing role is "helper, assistant, and colleague in a cooperative search" for health.[1] (p. 214)

The second philosophy leads to a strategy in which the client is considered the expert in assessing situations, diagnosing problems, and arriving at effective solutions. Nurses operating under this philosophy accept responsibility for creating conditions in which the client carries out these activities, not for identifying problems and solutions. This procedure is similar to the problem-solving method of social work practice discussed earlier.

This approach to nursing process requires that the client have both the energy and the inclination to develop insight into problems and to engage in problem solving. It is applicable in situations in which change in the client's perceptions and behavior must occur in order to facilitate healthy functional patterns. The nurse retains responsibility for labeling any health problems the client identifies. The strategy associated with this form of helping requires expert diagnostic and problem-solving skills because conditions must be created in which the client develops insight, considers options, and makes choices.

Values that guide nurses' decisions and actions within nursing process are derived from their philosophical beliefs about human beings and human interaction. One particular set of professional values is in the area of ethics. These values, as described in the section on standards, are expressed in a code of ethics that guide professional conduct.

Guiding concepts and theory

Problem identification and problem solving are guided by a set of *abstract concepts* and *practice theory*. The abstract concepts provide a way of thinking about the following:

1. The health problems that are of concern to nurses
2. The kinds of solutions (outcomes) sought
3. The types of interventions to be used to attain outcomes

This triad, as discussed in Chapter 4, is a framework for nursing. Suppose, for instance, that actual and potential self-care deficits were the focus of concern. The diagnosis Nutritional Deficit/Food Selection would be thought of as a discrepancy between self-care agency and self-care demand. An educative and supportive system of care would be designed to assist the client in learning about food selection.[2]

A conceptual framework is necessary to guide thinking. Within the self-care agency framework a nurse thinks of problem identification as identification of self-care agency deficits. Problem solving focuses on the design of a nursing system of care. Goals, or outcomes, are expressed in terms of independent self-care management. Other frameworks, such as the adaptation, life process, or behavioral systems previously discussed, provide different concepts to guide nursing process.

Practice theories, facts, and principles are the body of knowledge within nursing science. Recall the discussion of deriving meaning from cues in Chapter 8 (simple, inferential, and diagnostic meaning) and the discussion of etiological factors that describe the probable causes of a problem. The knowledge used to derive meaning from cues, make diagnoses, and identify probable causes rests on practice theory learned in the classroom, from books, and from experience. Similarly the knowledge to predict that certain nursing actions will resolve certain nursing diagnoses is based on practice theories. For example, does providing information about what is going to happen during the surgical experience reduce a client's fear of the experience? Practice theory suggests it does (if fear is due to insufficient information), and this theory is the basis for nursing intervention. Why would taking in insufficient fluids and a low-roughage diet contribute to constipation? What are the arguments for a causal relationship between fluids, diet, and constipation? You have just stated a practice theory!

Guiding standards

A profession derives its authority to practice from society. In return it has a responsibility to be mindful of the public trust. Standards and practice guidelines are developed by a profession to guide and evaluate practice and demonstrate accountability to society. They describe an acceptable level of care. There are two types

Standards of care

Standards of professional performance

Standards are broad statements that apply to the care of *all* clients, to the professional behavior of *all* nurses, and to the full scope of professional nursing practice. Standards of care for specialty practice (e.g., neonatal nurses or neuroscience nurses) are developed by the specialty organizations using national standards as a generic guide.[3] Standards are important when legal actions are taken by clients' families against care providers, as will be seen later in the chapter.

The box on p. 218 contains the standards of care for nursing. Note the reference to nursing diagnosis. Based on these national standards, consumers

STANDARDS OF CARE

Standard I. Assessment

The nurse collects client health data.

Measurement criteria

1. The priority of data collection is determined by the client's immediate condition or needs.
2. Pertinent data are collected using appropriate assessment techniques.
3. Data collection involves the client, significant others, and health care providers when appropriate.
4. The data collection process is systematic and ongoing.
5. Relevant data are documented in a retrievable form.

Standard II. Diagnosis

The nurse analyzes the assessment data in determining diagnoses.

Measurement criteria

1. Diagnoses are derived from the assessment data.
2. Diagnoses are validated with the client, significant others, and health care providers, when possible.
3. Diagnoses are documented in a manner that facilitates the determination of expected outcomes and plan of care.

Standard III. Outcome identification

The nurse identifies expected outcomes individualized to the client.

Measurement criteria

1. Outcomes are derived from the diagnoses.
2. Outcomes are documented on measurable goals.
3. Outcomes are mutually formulated with the client and health care providers, when possible.
4. Outcomes are realistic in relation to the client's present and potential capabilities.
5. Outcomes are attainable in relation to resources available to the client.
6. Outcomes include a time estimate for attainment.
7. Outcomes provide direction for continuity of care.

Standard IV. Planning

The nurse develops a plan of care that prescribes interventions to attain expected outcomes.

Measurement criteria

1. The plan is individualized to the client's condition or needs.
2. The plan is developed with the client, significant others, and health care providers, when appropriate.
3. The plan reflects current nursing practice.
4. The plan is documented.
5. The plan provides for continuity of care.

Standard V. Implementation

The nurse implements the interventions identified in the plan of care.

Measurement criteria

1. Interventions are consistent with the established plan of care.
2. Interventions are implemented in a safe and appropriate manner.
3. Interventions are documented.

Standard VI. Evaluation

The nurse evaluates the client's progress toward attainment of outcomes.

Measurement criteria

1. Evaluation is systematic and ongoing.
2. The client's responses to interventions are documented.
3. The effectiveness of interventions is evaluated in relation to outcomes.
4. Ongoing assessment data are used to revise diagnoses, outcomes, and the plan of care, as needed.
5. Revisions in diagnoses, outcomes, and the plan of care are documented.
6. The client, significant others, and health care providers are involved in the evaluation process, when appropriate.

From American Nurses Association: *Standards of clinical nursing practice,* Washington, DC, 1991, The Association.

Table 10-1 Comparison of Nursing Standards, Nursing Process, and the Problem-Solving Model

Nursing standards*	Nursing process	Problem-solving model
Assessment (I)	Assessment	Observation, data collection
Diagnosis (II)	Diagnosis	Problem identification
Outcome identification (III)	Outcome projection	Problem solving
Planning (IV)	Planning	(methods, goals, outcomes)
Implementation (V)	Implementation	Problem-solving actions (intervention)
Evaluation (VI)	Evaluation	Evaluation

*Roman numerals refer to particular standards listed in full in the box on p. 218.

can expect that nursing diagnoses will be derived from their health assessments. Standards represent a consensus of the profession and are published by the American Nurses Association (ANA). Practice standards and the assurance of quality care are relatively new; standards for conduct expressed in a code of ethics are not.

Standards of care

Traditionally the quality of practice has been monitored by colleagues and state licensing boards. In recent years public pressure for assurance that quality care is being delivered has prompted the development of practice standards. In 1991 the Congress of Nursing Practice of the ANA published the standards of care for professional nursing practice in any setting.[4] Why are standards important and what do they have to do with nursing diagnosis?

Standards are valued and achievable criteria for nursing performance against which actual performance can be judged. For example, suppose a registered nurse wishes to know whether the way he or she practices is satisfactory. A comparison between personal practice and the national standards of care could be made. Or suppose a nursing student wants to evaluate the progress he or she is making toward professionally accepted nursing standards. The student could make the same comparison, knowing that by the time of graduation the standards should be met.

Standard II is of particular interest in this discussion. It states that diagnoses are derived from assessment data. The fact that this standard exists

means that nurses have stated a criterion for satisfactory professional practice in the area of nursing diagnosis. Thus consumers can expect nursing diagnoses to be made if they are getting an acceptable quality of care. *Professional nurses have a responsibility to ensure that standards of care are met for clients, since many cannot ensure this for themselves.*

Problem identification and problem solving, nursing process, and standards of care have many similarities. The resemblance is evident in the comparisons presented in Table 10-1. The 1991 Standards of Care are more consistent with the categories of nursing process than the previous eight standards. One change in Standards is the deletion of "nursing" as a modifier of diagnosis. This deletion broadens the concept of diagnosis in nursing, perhaps allowing for nurse practitioners' practice. Criterion 2, Standard II, page 218, states "diagnoses are validated with health care providers when possible." This is unclear, an unusual practice in health care, and may be unrealistic.

Clearly both the standards and nursing process are similar and both are based on problem identification and problem solving. It is well to appreciate these similarities and not to think three different things are being referred to when the different labels are encountered.

To supplement the general process standards, the ANA councils and the specialty organizations, such as the American Association of Critical Care Nurses,[5] are currently writing standards for nursing diagnoses. Discussion and examples of these specific standards are included in Chapter 11 in the section on assurance of quality care.

Practice guidelines

"Guidelines are systematically developed statements to assist nurse and patient decisions about appropriate health care for specific clinical conditions."[6 (p. ii)] They may be developed locally by a unit or a health care agency for in-house use, by a professional nursing organization and nursing specialty organizations, or by a national task force. For example, the first national guidelines from the Agency for Health Care Policy and Research (AHCPR) of the U.S. Department of Health and Human Services were published in the early 1990s. The guidelines are for three nursing diagnoses: Pain, Pressure Ulcer, and Incontinence, but can also be used by other disciplines. During their development nurses and physicians chaired panels related to their practice areas, and a pharmacist, psychologist, physical therapist, patient/consumer, and ethicist collaborated on the development of some of the guidelines. All the available research has been reviewed and evaluated, making these guidelines highly relevant for nursing practice. Each treatment recommendation is accompanied by a "strength of evidence" rating from A to C.

Acute pain is one of the foci for guideline development. It is a condition in which "as necessary" orders are written for its control with drugs. Problems in undermedication have been reported and attributed to the choice of drugs, dosage, inadequate assessment, or a combination of these. There is much variation in practice. It is pointed out that "health care is both a technical and ethical enterprise. The ethical obligation to manage pain and relieve the patient's suffering is at the core of a health care professional's commitment."[6 (p. 4)]

The pressure ulcer national guideline is listed in Appendix M. This guideline is badly needed, as the condition causes clients much pain and discomfort. As is the case with pain, there is much variation in treatment, and the cost of care is tremendous. The box on the right contains a summary of the recommendations from this national guideline. Guidelines should soon become available for HIV/AIDS, smoking cessation, general anxiety/panic disorders, and prenatal care. The concern about variations in medical practice across the country was one of the motivators for developing practice

---

CLINICAL PRACTICE GUIDELINE 3. PRESSURE ULCERS IN ADULTS: PREDICTION AND PREVENTION

Clinical Practice Guideline: A Summary of Recommendations for Pressure Ulcer

1. Assess patients with regard to the risk factors for developing pressure ulcers using the Braden Scale and monitor daily.
2. Ensure that skin is kept clean, warm, well moisturized, and free of wetness.
3. Avoid massage over bony prominences.
4. Encourage patient mobility if possible.
5. Protect against pressure, friction, and shear.
6. Ensure good nutrition.
7. Educate all relevant health care providers and the patient on pressure ulcer risk, prevention, detection, and management.[6]

---

guidelines for specific situations. There are probably also variations in practice patterns in nursing, and these guidelines may address that issue.

The following criteria for selecting nursing diagnoses/clinical conditions as a basis for guideline development are suggested by the ANA:

Variation in practice (the way the condition is treated)
Costly; high economic impact
High prevalence (high volume)
Variation in outcome (i.e., outcomes attained)
Improved methods of prevention, diagnosis, prescription, and clinical management
High-risk potential
Amenable to nursing intervention[7]

Diagnoses such as High Risk for Infection, Impaired Mobility, High Risk for Injury (e.g., falls), and Nutritional Deficits or Obesity meet many of these criteria.

Ethical standards

Standards for ethical conduct are presented in the box on p. 221; they are called the Code of Ethics for professional practice. They represent areas of moral accountability to the consumer of nursing. Standards of this type are monitored by colleagues and professional organizations. State

NURSING CODE OF ETHICS

1. The nurse provides services with respect for human dignity and the uniqueness of the client, unrestricted by considerations of social or economic status, personal attributes, or the nature of health problems.
2. The nurse safeguards the client's right to privacy by judiciously protecting information of a confidential nature.
3. The nurse acts to safeguard the client and the public when health care and safety are affected by the incompetent, unethical, or illegal practice of any person.
4. The nurse assumes responsibility and accountability for individual nursing judgments and actions.
5. The nurse maintains competence in nursing.
6. The nurse exercises informed judgment and uses individual competence and qualifications as criteria in seeking consultation, accepting responsibilities, and delegating nursing activities to others.
7. The nurse participates in activities that contribute to the ongoing development of the profession's body of knowledge.
8. The nurse participates in the profession's efforts to implement and improve standards of nursing.
9. The nurse participates in the profession's efforts to establish and maintain conditions of employment conducive to high quality nursing care.
10. The nurse participates in the profession's effort to protect the public from misinformation and misrepresentation and to maintain the integrity of nursing.
11. The nurse collaborates with members of the health professions and other citizens in promoting community and national efforts to meet the health needs of the public.

From *Code for nurses with interpretive statements,* 1985, American Nurses Association.

nurses' associations are the bodies that discipline members who violate the code.

The interpretive statements that accompany the ANA code of ethics[8] are quite explicit in items 4 and 6, which relate to nursing diagnosis. The major points regarding ethical/moral responsibility are excerpted in the following (italics are the author's):

1. *The regulation and control of nursing practice by nurses* demand that individual practitioners of professional nursing must bear primary *responsibility* for the nursing care clients receive and must be *individually accountable for their own practice.*
2. Nursing obligations are reflected in the ANA publications *Nursing: A Social Policy Statement*[9] and *Standards of Clinical Nursing Practice*[4] (see also the box on p. 218).
3. In order to be *accountable,* nurses act under a code of ethical conduct that is grounded in the moral *principles of fidelity and respect for the dignity, worth, and self-determination of clients.*
4. Nurses are *accountable for judgments made and actions* taken in the course of nursing practice. *Neither physician's orders nor the employing agency's policies relieve the nurse of accountability for actions taken and judgments made.*
5. Inasmuch as the nurse is responsible for the continuous care of patients in health care settings, the nurse is frequently called on to carry out components of care delegated by other health professionals as part of the client's treatment regimen. The nurse *should not accept these interdependent functions if they are so extensive as to prevent the nurse from fulfilling the responsibility to provide appropriate nursing care to clients.*[8]

Beliefs about helping relationships, concepts, theories, and standards guide the use of nursing process and its component, nursing diagnosis. Previous chapters demonstrated how diagnostic categories are used in problem identification. In the following sections the relevance of nursing diagnoses to care delivery will become clear. The objective is not an in-depth discussion of problem-solving activities; rather, the emphasis is on how to use nursing diagnoses in these activities.

NURSING DIAGNOSIS IN CARE PLANNING

The nurse's desire to change the course of events gives nursing care planning its momentum. A health problem may have dire consequences if left to run its course. It also may cause the client great discomfort even if it resolves naturally. Nurses attempt to alter these possibilities by thinking ahead, making decisions, and formulating nursing care plans. This involves therapeutic reasoning.

Once the client's health problems and contributing factors are recognized and labeled as nursing diagnoses, responsibility for treatment arises and decisions are required. The decisions to be made in the treatment of any nursing diagnosis are:

1. What are the desired outcomes?
2. What plan of nursing care is needed to reach the outcomes?
3. After implementation of nursing care, were the desired outcomes actually reached?

Nursing diagnosis is merely an intellectual exercise unless it is used in making these therapeutic judgments.

Let us consider the way nursing diagnoses can help in decision making. During the discussion the nurse is the decision maker. If the process is understood and practiced, the important ideas can then be modified for application to situations in which clients are guided to do their own decision making and planning. The first step is to decide what health outcome is desired and attainable.

Projected outcomes

Suppose you wish to be in San Francisco on Tuesday to meet a friend. Deciding this before starting a trip increases the probability that you will get there. Otherwise on Tuesday you may be in Louisiana. This failure to specify what outcome is desired may produce inconvenience, additional cost, distress, and delay.

The reasoning is similar in nursing. Being in San Francisco on Tuesday would be called the desired outcome. In health care an *outcome* is a valued health state, condition, or behavior exhibited by a client. It may be, for example, a client's verbalized intention to take some particular health-promoting action, or it may be a behavior or condition observed by a nurse.

Other similar terms are in use, such as *objectives* and *goals*. *Outcome* is synonymous with *behavioral objective;* both specify observable behaviors of the client. *Goals* are usually broader statements that require further specification. Measurable outcomes that indicate goal attainment must be identified.

Adding the term *projected*—projected outcome—means that a prediction or forecast of a future behavior has been made. Outcomes are projected in order to guide decisions about care; later they are measured to evaluate the effectiveness of the care that has been given. *Projecting outcomes permits the nurse to know when the problem is resolved.*

Outcomes are projected before nursing actions are planned or carried out. There are two reasons for this:

1. The health problem describes the present health state of the client; the projected outcome describes the desired health state. When the discrepancy between present and desired state is consciously examined, the treatment focus becomes evident and nursing actions can be considered. The actions most likely to lead to desired outcomes are selected and implemented.
2. Outcomes precede plans and actions because they are the basis for deciding when actions should cease. When outcomes are attained the client is discharged from care. During implementation of the nursing plan, projected outcomes are used to evaluate daily progress toward their attainment.

Of what relevance to outcome projection is a nursing diagnosis? Without a diagnosis that describes the health problem it is difficult even to attempt to specify outcomes. Projected outcomes describe the state of a client after, or at some stage of, problem resolution. Thus the health problem is the basis for outcome projection.

Consider an example of a hospitalized client:

Mr. Jones is a 25-year-old with paralysis of the lower half of his body as a result of a car accident in which his spinal cord was severely damaged. A number of risk factors predispose him to reduced circulation to tissues over the bony prominences of his body. The nursing diagnosis was High Risk for Skin Breakdown.

Given this diagnosis, what nursing care outcome would be desirable at the time of the client's discharge from the acute care setting? Obviously the valued outcome is *skin intact at discharge*. Notice what has occurred. The diagnosis of High Risk for Skin Breakdown was made, and then the reverse of breakdown, intact skin, was stated as the desired outcome of nursing care.

Converting the diagnosis into a desired health state is a quick method for projecting outcomes. The critical signs and symptoms that define a diagnosis are useful in the transformation. Logically their opposites define the resolution of the problem. Even positive changes in symptoms indicate progress toward problem resolution. The "rule" to remember is: Outcomes are derived from the problem, which is a part of the problem-etiology statement.

Consider another problem. A client with heart failure is unable to bathe; whenever she tries, shortness of breath and fatigue occur. The nursing diagnosis is Self-Bathing/Hygiene Deficit (Level II, requires assistance), and the probable cause is Decreased Activity Tolerance. Mentally transforming the problem into a desired functional state permits outcome projection. In this case the outcome would be self-bathing.[10]

Notice that outcomes in the previous examples are stated concisely and definitely. Specificity is necessary to guide planning; vague words and statements make it difficult to know exactly where one is going. Furthermore, only with specific outcomes does one know when the nursing goal has been reached. For example, "good skin color" or "good knowledge of . . ." are difficult to measure. How is "good" to be recognized?

Consider the following diagnoses and outcomes; which of these are useful for planning care and evaluating progress (diagnoses are written in the problem/etiological factor format)?

1. Exogenous Obesity/Caloric Intake–Energy Expenditure Imbalance
   Outcome: weight loss 10 pounds; 5-week visit
2. Ineffective Airway Clearance/Decreased Energy
   Outcome: breath (lung) sounds clear, day 2
3. Weak Mother-Infant Bonding/Separation
   Outcome: parental attachment behaviors present; 3-week visit

Examples 1 and 2 are measurable outcomes that can be used in planning care and evaluating the effectiveness of nursing intervention. The third statement is too broad. What attachment behaviors are to be present? What should be expected in 3 weeks?

Value-laden decisions

Outcomes are value decisions. In the example above it may be inferred that having intact skin and bathing independently are highly valued by most people. The arguments are numerous: (1) bathing removes dirt, dead skin, and secretions; (2) intact skin prevents infection; and (3) independence is "better" than dependence. Most adults probably would agree. Yet in essence, writing an outcome is stating a personal value—the profession's value or a social value. The desirability of intact skin raises little if any controversy, but with many other diagnoses the situation is not as clear.

The client has the right to choose outcomes. In their enthusiasm to promote health, nurses may easily unconsciously impose their own personal or social values on others. Outcomes for problems related to cognition, beliefs, self-perception, or relationships require choices that are best made by the client or in collaboration with the client. *Philosophically, if the nurse believes clients should participate in actions to solve their problems, it follows that clients must be involved in deciding outcomes. From a practical perspective, participation in setting outcomes increases motivation toward achieving those outcomes.*

In many instances the client says what he or she wishes remedied; listening enables the nurse to know what that is. On the other hand, clients may not know what outcomes are possible. Additionally they may have difficulty coping with an event or may be in conflict about making a choice; their ability to use their problem-solving capacities may be lowered. In these situations a nurse may suggest alternatives and act in the client's best interest.

A 65-year-old woman had a nursing diagnosis of Social Isolation Related to Body Image Disturbance and Fear of Rejection. After having a leg amputation and being fitted with an artificial limb, she stayed in her apartment. She told most close friends that she was unable to have visitors and avoided other tenants. The desired outcome for the health problem was: Resumes previous level of social relationships.

The nurse took an indirect approach because of the high degree of stress the woman was experiencing. Yet the client was given an opportunity to reject the outcome. In essence, here is how the diagnosis and projected outcome were translated to the client: "You mentioned before that you are trying to avoid your friends because you think they would be disgusted by someone with a leg missing. Can we think about how they would react and how you could handle this if you decided to invite them?" The nurse paused for the client's reactions to the subtly introduced outcome of inviting friends to her apartment. The client looked down and said, "I do miss having people in." The nurse interpreted the statement as a wish to resume previous social contacts. At that time the client was unable to agree to the outcome more directly because of her fear of rejection by friends.

Some have advocated written, signed contracts for outcomes. It has been demonstrated that such contracts with clients have some effect on compliance with needed behavior changes, such as dieting. But contracts produce a formalism in the nurse-client relationship that many nurses reject.

To introduce the idea of projecting outcomes by using nursing diagnoses, the concept of problem resolution has been somewhat oversimplified. Transforming indicators of a problem (signs and symptoms) to positive health behaviors is easier to do "in the head" than "in the world of reality." The final resolution of a client's health problem may require several steps rather than one leap.

If short-term resolution of a diagnosis is not possible, outcomes representing progress toward resolution are stated. For example, outcomes may be projected for accomplishment by the date of hospital discharge *and* for 3 months, 6 months, or longer if the client is under continuing care.

Time, resources, and costs are factors to be considered in projecting outcomes. Before individualized outcomes can be specified within a realistic time frame for outcome attainment, the nurse must know what interventions will be used. What is done (nursing and client actions) influences the client's progress toward resolution of the health problem. Yet what is done is influenced by clients' choices, capabilities, and resources.

Importance of outcomes

With soaring health care costs has come an emphasis on the achievement of outcomes. Governments, private insurers, state funders, corporations paying employee health care premiums, and consumers are paying high costs. They want to make sure that projected outcomes are achieved. This goal has generated many models of care delivery that emphasize outcomes. Faster achievement of outcomes and nursing methods that guarantee outcome achievement are valued. The expression "outcome-driven care" embodies the emphasis in today's health care delivery system.

Even in short-stay acute care settings, nurses now use intermediate outcomes in addition to discharge outcomes to evaluate the care they provide. The idea behind this method is not to wait until discharge to measure outcomes but rather to check whether progress is being made at an intermediate point as measured by previously stated intermediate outcomes. In other models particular days or weeks are designated as goals for measuring outcomes, indicating progress toward discharge, or progress toward a long-term outcome in a managed care program, which is discussed in Chapter 11.

Interventions

Thinking of ideal outcomes such as being in San Francisco on Tuesday motivates a person to find a way of getting there. Realistically, the traveler must consider wardrobe, packing, transportation schedules, and finances. With these considerations in mind, outcome attainment may be set for a Tuesday 3 years hence! Similarly, in care planning the current state of the client and the highly valued outcome are considered first, then the way of getting "from here to there."

Interventions are the actions taken to help the client move from a present state to the state described in the projected outcomes. They may involve doing for, doing with, or enabling a client to do something to influence or resolve the health problem. The type of intervention selected depends on the nursing diagnosis and outcomes. As Fig. 10-1 shows, specific interventions for individual clients depend on the choices, capabilities, and resources of the client; the creativity of the nurse; and research findings.

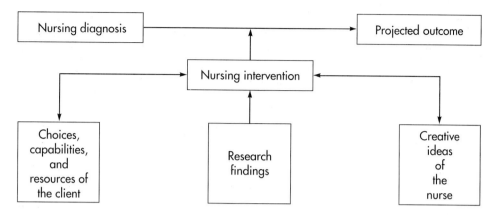

Fig. 10-1 From diagnosis to outcome.

Nursing intervention research in the 1980s, prior to the classification of nursing interventions published in 1992, was disorganized. This situation was similar to that of research on client conditions prior to the development of a nursing diagnosis language system. A uniform language for nursing interventions allows access to literature and improved communication among clinicians and researchers. Egan and colleagues[11] point out the importance of a clear definition of an intervention when studying its effect. It is clear from nursing care plans in clinical settings and in many educational settings that the language of interventions is fuzzy, to say the least.

As a result of a large, federally funded, continuing project at the University of Iowa, McCloskey and Bulechek,[12] have defined nursing intervention and developed a nursing intervention classification (NIC). Their definition follows:

A nursing intervention is any direct care treatment that a nurse performs on behalf of a client. These treatments include nurse-initiated treatments resulting from nursing diagnoses, physician-initiated treatments resulting from medical diagnoses, and performance of the daily essential functions for the client [who] cannot do these.[12] (p. 21)

Interventions "are at the conceptual level and require a series of actions or activities to carry them out."[13] Note that *intervention* means "direct care treatment"; that is, direct care of the client. Two types of nursing intervention with examples are defined in Appendix N. As specified in the NIC, one type of intervention is "nurse initiated," which is based on nursing diagnoses; a second is "physician initiated," which is based on medical diagnoses but done by a nurse until clients can do it for themselves. (A third is daily essential functions—which nurses do if assistants are not available—such as finding supplies, cleaning equipment, and picking up meal trays.) Each nursing intervention has a definition in the NIC.[12]

Interventions are action concepts. (In contrast, nursing diagnoses are descriptive concepts.) Each intervention has a list of activities that are defined as the specific things to be done when the intervention is implemented.[12] What defining characteristics are to nursing diagnoses, activities are to interventions. They illustrate the meaning of the concept. Recall that in the case of nursing diagnoses not all the listed characteristics need to be present; similarly, not all the activities listed under an intervention need to be used in a particular client situation. Further study may indicate which activities are critical to the meaning of the intervention and thus must be implemented; the number of critical interventions will probably be few.

An example may clarify the concept of intervention. For the diagnosis of Ineffective Airway Clearance related to thick, viscous secretions, the interventions of airway management, fluid therapy, and their related nursing activities may be the treatments a nurse will order.

From reviews of the literature and research studies approximately 400 intervention concepts (word labels) and their associated activities have been identified. These terms are listed in Appendix N. The interventions have been incorporated into the National Library of Medicine System so they can be accessed by computer, libraries, or individuals. This listing might be used for the documentation of services provided and converted into a format for reimbursement and a minimum data set. This list would be similar to the *Physicians' Current Procedural Terminology,* published by the American Medical Association,[14] which is used for coding services performed by physicians. Further validation of the intervention concepts is in progress. Research needs to be directed to the diagnosis-intervention linkages; at present these links are based on clinical judgment. A number of other intervention classifications in nursing are also evolving.[15-19]

Focus for interventions

A nursing diagnosis provides a focus for thinking about what interventions may resolve a problem. The alternative approach is to treat isolated or unorganized signs and symptoms such as frequent crying spells, difficulty in breathing, or inability to bathe self. Interventions based on these symptoms may help for the moment but rarely resolve the underlying problem. If the truth of this last statement is not apparent, try to identify interventions by using the above signs and symptoms as a focus. Contrast these interventions with those you would use for the diagnoses stated in the following paragraph.

Using a diagnosis and projected outcome as a focus increases the probability of selecting effective nursing interventions. For example, each of the previously listed signs (crying spells, difficult breathing, and inability to bathe) was investigated and clustered with other signs and symptoms. The problem and etiology were formulated in each case and labeled as follows: (1) the crying client's diagnosis was Ineffective Coping/Perceived Incompetence (Parenting); (2) Ineffective Airway Clearance/Thick Secretions was the statement formulated for the client with dyspnea; and (3) Self-Bathing Deficit (Level III)/Activity Intolerance suggested many more specific interventions than did the sign *inability to bathe self.* In the third situation, bathing the client might solve the immediate need, but helping the client to increase his or her activity tolerance gets at the essence of the problem.

Trial and error is a common approach if isolated signs and symptoms are used as a focus for care planning. This method is wasteful of nursing time. It also may prolong the client's discomfort, allow problems to become more severe, and lead to adverse effects. The trial-and-error method is used either because no meaning has been derived from the unclustered signs and symptoms or because possible meanings have not been validated. Think of the multiple meanings of the sign *crying.* Each is associated with a different intervention.

Diagnoses are concepts from which a knowledgeable nurse can derive meaning. Consider the diagnosis Ineffective Airway Clearance/Thick Secretions. Biopsychosocial theories and research about airway obstruction, secretions, and client responses may be used as a framework to determine an approach to care. Specifically, theories provide help in understanding a problem, designing possible interventions, and calculating when intervention may be effective. Thus identifying problems facilitates the retrieval of related theory from memory or a textbook. This in turn provides meaning and ideas that guide care-planning decisions.

Focusing on the nursing diagnosis and on the available theoretical knowledge is similar to what occurred in the generation of diagnostic hypotheses during problem identification. Selecting the right problem area opened up multiple possibilities. In problem solving, this occurs when a problem area in memory or a textbook index is searched for alternative interventions.

Although on the surface a routine intervention may appear sufficient, clients deserve thoughtful planning of their care. This requires *thinking of alternative methods, their consequences, and the probability that they will be effective* for the particular client and situation.

Generating interventions based on probable cause(s)

When searching textbooks or memory stores for possible interventions, the nurse should keep the problem in mind but *focus on the etiological or related factors.* If the probable cause can be influenced, the health problem should change.

Consider first a basic example: E (etiological factor) is the probable reason the P (problem) exists. If E is removed, the prediction is that P will be resolved. Intervention is directed primarily at E.

This abstract reasoning is applicable to clinical situations. Recall the 65-year-old woman whose diagnosis was Social Isolation/Body Image Disturbance. After her leg amputation she learned to use an artificial limb but continued to stay in her apartment and allowed no friends to visit. Before the amputation she went shopping, had friends in for coffee, and was socially active in her church. The outcome desired by the client and nurse was "resumes previous level of social relationships." What should be the focus of intervention for the visiting nurse?

Just recommending that the client socialize has a low probability of success. The problem alone does not offer a focus for generating interventions. If Body Image Disturbance is a major contributing factor, influencing the client's body image may increase socialization. *Etiological factors identified in the diagnosis are the focus of intervention.* If these factors can be changed, the problem should begin to resolve.

Another example should help clarify the need to *focus on etiological factors in generating alternative interventions.* A second client also had Social Isolation, but the etiological factor was Impaired Mobility. This 65-year-old woman had been, as she described it, "a social butterfly"; staying in the house was "confining", and she was becoming despondent. Visiting friends and going to holiday celebrations and the theater were important to her, yet the permanent peripheral vascular changes caused by her diabetes impaired her mobility for climbing stairs and walking distances.

The intervention for this client was entirely different, *although the problem specified in the nursing diagnosis was the same.* The focus for thinking about a solution was the etiological factor Impaired Mobility. The nurse generated alternative interventions. Keeping these in the back of her mind, she encouraged the client to think of ways to circumvent the mobility impairment. The choice was to rent a wheelchair for steps (ramps) and distances; friends gladly helped. The visiting nurse arranged for the chair, and the client was delighted that they had found a way for her to resume social activities.

In these examples the alternatives for intervention were clear-cut. When more complex situations are encountered, the nurse must stop and think through the situation. The first step in deciding on an intervention is to answer the question, What is the therapeutic problem?

A therapeutic problem exists if interventions to attain outcomes have a low degree of success; are unknown; or, while known, have been unsuccessful in the client's particular situation. Aptly named, this is the *wicked decision problem.*

The nurse must define the therapeutic problem: Is a behavioral change needed? Is it conflict resolution? Are there other ways of looking at the therapeutic problem? The nurse should keep etiological factor(s) and outcome in mind and then think of offbeat or "far-out" ideas—methods that will increase creative thinking. Logical analysis is applied only *after* the ideas are generated.

Individualizing interventions

During the process of generating alternative interventions, the nurse thinks about the contributing factors and the particular client and situation. Consideration of these factors individualizes interventions. *Individualizing interventions increases treatment success rate.*

The following are the areas of information in which data are needed to individualize care:

1. *Personal client factors:* The client, whether an individual, family, or community, has unique characteristics that influence intervention. If interventions are being considered for an individual, then age, developmental stage, gender, culture, religion, family structure, and other personal characteristics are considered. Some of these considerations are equally applicable in family or community intervention. In some instances further data collection may be necessary.

2. *Client's perception:* The client may associate various causal factors with his or her problem even though objectively they are unrelated. Unless the correction of misperceptions and faulty associations about the cause of a problem is built into the intervention plan, intervention may fail because the client considers it unrelated and therefore meaningless.

3. *Current level of compensation:* The client may have mobilized some strengths, defenses, or resources to compensate for the problem. Data about this compensation help the nurse decide about the degree of nursing assistance required and also allow recogni-

tion of the client's strengths. Diagnoses may be classified as compensated (monitoring only is necessary), partially compensated (some nursing assistance is needed), or uncompensated (the client requires full nursing assistance).

4. *Problem magnitude and urgency:* The acuity or severity of a problem influences the type and timing of intervention. Certain conditions are urgent, and intervention must be immediate. These are health problems that may result in harm to the client or others.

   As an example, a client who is having surgery in 24 hours and who is near panic and not coping effectively requires immediate intervention. Either the surgery should be cancelled or the anxiety should be reduced quickly. With diagnoses such as High Risk for Injury or High Risk for Violence, the immediate reduction of risk factors is needed.

5. *Extended effects:* Interventions have the potential for extended effects. Indirectly or directly they can influence members of the client's family, work group, or social circle. For example, what effects will a major diet change have on the other household members? Forethought is needed when interventions are planned, so that no additional problems are created by their extended effects.

   Interactions among nursing diagnoses should also be considered in planning intervention. If treatment for one problem is planned in isolation, there may be extended effects on coexisting problems. As an example, the usual treatment for one diagnosis may be contraindicated when another nursing diagnosis is present. Similarly the treatment for a nursing diagnosis may negatively or positively influence a disease or a medical treatment; the reverse may also occur. *Interactions among all diagnoses and all treatments must be taken into account in decision making.*

6. *Cost-benefit factors:* The consequences of treatments are a consideration in decision making. Each intervention has a "price." The costs may be financial, social, or psychological. *Benefits* are the advantages that accompany (or are expected to result from) the outcomes of treatment in terms of (1) optimum

health and well-being or (2) an immediate or long-term life goal of the client. The possible benefits of the results of various interventions being considered are weighed against their possible costs.

One dimension of cost-benefit considerations is the psychological or social cost related to the functional benefit. Before recommending or guiding clients to change their behavior patterns, nurses should consider the payoff. They should be knowledgeable about the predicted benefits of change so that clients can weigh alternatives and make informed choices. Changing behavioral patterns is one of the most difficult things for people to do, especially during adulthood.

A client may value the expected outcome as a benefit but feel the cost (e.g., stopping smoking or giving up desired foods) is too high. In this situation the nurse and client should try to find a way to reduce the cost of the intervention. Perhaps a less valued outcome (e.g., switching to low-tar cigarettes) is all that can be accomplished at present. It may also be possible to increase the client's value of the beneficial outcome enough to make the client willing to pay the price.

A second dimension of the cost-benefit factor is financial cost related to the functional benefit of the expected outcome. Given today's soaring health care costs, if two alternative interventions for a diagnosis result in the same beneficial effect, the less expensive one should be chosen. Referral of nursing problems to other disciplines also increases costs. *Before consultations, equipment, or services for the treatment of the problem are ordered, consider whether the benefit is worth the cost.* Consumers are currently demanding that cost-benefit ratios be considered in treatment planning.

Predicting effectiveness of interventions

Consideration of the six factors just discussed should narrow down the treatment alternatives for a particular client's nursing diagnosis. The remaining alternatives are subjected to final scrutiny. The one with the greatest probability of being effective is chosen.

The *predicted effectiveness* of an intervention is the probability that it will lead to the projected outcome. For example, suppose the probability that intervention A will lead to outcome C is 60 percent, whereas the probability that intervention B will produce outcome C is 90 percent. If A and B "cost" the same, B should be chosen.

Predicted effectiveness takes into account all six factors above relevant to the diagnosis. Thus the predicted effectiveness is a prediction about individualized interventions for a particular client and situation. Obviously the intervention with the highest probability of being effective is chosen and implemented.

Priority setting

A client may have multiple diagnoses, not all of which can or should be treated at the time they are identified. Priorities for treatment depend on (1) the urgency of the problem, (2) the nature of the treatment indicated, and (3) the interactions among diagnoses.

Nursing diagnoses that, if untreated, could result in harm to the client or others have the highest priority for treatment. Examples include High Risk for Violence, High Risk for Trauma, and Ineffective Airway Clearance. In these examples the priority is clear. In many other instances thorough knowledge of the client and situation is necessary before the nurse can be sure what patient conditions are urgent.

The type of treatment indicated also helps determine priorities in particular cases. If a client is physiologically unstable, as might commonly be the situation in an intensive care unit, treatment of diagnosed conditions that requires learning behavioral changes should not be given a high priority. Intensive care units are not designed for treating knowledge deficits about postdischarge health management; nor is an emergency room designed for the treatment of noncompliance with a weight reduction program. *The cost of keeping a client in an expensive nursing care setting for a problem that can be treated in a less expensive setting* must be considered.

Another factor that influences priority setting is the possibility of interactions among diagnoses. Suppose a 10-year-old client has the following problems: Chronic Exogenous Obesity/Caloric Intake-Activity Imbalance; Dysfunctional Grieving/(Loss of Parent); and Compromised Family Coping. Should priorities be set, and if so, how?

Although the coping and grieving problems are not judged to be probable causes of obesity, they are problems that potentially can interact. Improved family coping may provide greater support to the child and assist in resolving the grief process. When these problems begin to improve, the child may be helped to lose weight, ideally with family support. Priority setting enhances treatment when the client has multiple problems. *Yet priority setting would be impossible without clearly identified nursing diagnoses.*

When considering treatment priorities, it is important to have a grasp of the broad types of activities nurses perform. McCloskey and Bulechek[12] (p. 20) list seven:

1. Assessment behaviors to make a nursing diagnosis.
2. Assessment behaviors to gather information for a physician to make a medical diagnosis.
3. Nurse-initiated treatment behaviors in response to nursing diagnoses.
4. Physician-initiated treatment behaviors in response to medical diagnoses.
5. Daily essential function behaviors that may not relate to either medical or nursing diagnoses but are done by the nurse for patients who cannot do these things for themselves.
6. Behaviors to evaluate the effects of nursing and medical treatments. These are also assessment behaviors, but they are done for purposes of evaluation, not diagnosis.
7. Administrative and indirect-care behaviors that support interventions.

Notice how the activities relate to nursing process. Items 1 and 2 are related to assessment; 3, 4, and 5 are related to intervention; and 6 is related to outcome evaluation. The authors state that activities 5 and 7 may overlap.

When a nurse in acute, critical, or community care working with any age group observes that nearly all of his or her time is spent in activities 2, 4, and 6, there is cause for serious concern. The nurse should examine exactly what role he or she was assuming. A professional model of nursing practice (in contrast to a model of physician assistants' practice) should encompass all seven activities. Factors contributing to this situation need to be examined, such as the nurse's role perception and the staffing patterns or caseload.

Treatment priorities are influenced by the setting and the level of patient acuity implied by the setting. For example, the treatment priorities in

Table 10–2 High–Treatment Priority Nursing Diagnoses in Two Nursing Specialties*

Nursing diagnoses	
Critical care nursing	Rehabilitation nursing
1. Pain	1. Impaired Physical Mobility (Transfer, Locomotion, Ambulation, and Bed Mobility)
2. High Risk for Infection	2. Knowledge Deficit
3. Ineffective Airway Clearance	3. Self-Care Deficit (Bathing, Hygiene, Dressing, Grooming, Toileting, and Feeding)
4. Anxiety	4. Activity Intolerance
5. High Risk for Impaired Skin Integrity	5. High Risk for Impaired Skin Integrity

*Based on a national stratified sample of 616 critical care nurses and 730 rehabilitation nurses who rated each condition as nearly, always, or frequently a treatment priority in their practice. Diagnoses are consistent with those identified by specialty organizations.

critical care are different from those of rehabilitation nursing. Table 10-2 contains those diagnoses rated by more than 75% of the nurses in two studies as nearly always or frequently a treatment priority.[20] These diagnoses were also rated as highly prevalent in these national studies. This type of information is useful in different areas of practice. It not only sensitizes nurses to possibilities but also help students to prioritize treatments.

Implementation and evaluation

After decisions about interventions and priorities are made, the treatment plan is begun. During implementation of the plan, continued assessment provides feedback that is used to evaluate prior diagnostic judgments and treatment decisions. Assessing the client's progress toward the projected outcomes enables the nurse to evaluate the effectiveness of the interventions. Progress toward out-

comes is evaluated during the course of nursing intervention by *problem-focused assessment* as described in Chapter 7. Data collected about the status of the problem are the basis for evaluative judgments. If the intervention is effective, the signs and symptoms used to diagnose the problem should be changing.

At this point we may summarize the use of diagnoses in problem identification and problem solving. The first concern is to identify the client's health problems and apply diagnostic labels to these judgments. Then the use of a systematic problem-solving process takes precedence. During this problem-solving phase of the nursing process, diagnoses are the bases for projecting desired outcomes, deciding on interventions by which to attain the outcomes, using judgments about the probable cause(s), implementing interventions, and evaluating the attainment of diagnosis-specific outcomes.

After this process of problem identification and problem solving has been completed, it appears in retrospect to have been a sequence of steps. In actuality, the entire set of activities is always kept in mind. Each decision influences other decisions. It is a matter of greatest importance to maintain an open mind about observations and new data that are collected during all phases of nursing process. Never hesitate to consider new data and revise judgments; continued assessment and open-mindedness are the keys to handling uncertainties in clinical information.

When a hypothesis about disease progression or complications is supported, judgments are made to verbally inform the physician, note the information in the client's record, carry out or withhold treatments designated by existing physician's orders or nursing protocols, carry out palliative treatments based on nursing judgment, or execute a combination of these actions. In contrast, the main responsibility after nursing diagnosis is to plan and execute treatment and to facilitate treatment coordination by communication with other health care professionals.

Treatment coordination

When a client has both nursing and medical diagnoses, treatment must be coordinated. Otherwise interventions may conflict and outcomes may not be attained. Ideally, the professionals involved should have regularly scheduled time for sharing information. Regular communication promotes an understanding of each care provider's diagnostic judgments and treatment decisions. It also increases the probability of integrated care and promotes working relationships.

It is easy to understand the need for coordination. Yet implementation in certain settings requires ingenuity and initiative. Who shall take the initiative? In acute care settings, such as hospitals, nurses have 24-hour responsibility for implementing client's medical and nursing treatments and for seeing their families. Accordingly, nurses need to be aware of the total care plan. To gain this overview, nursing staff may need to take the initiative to institute changes in communication patterns; for example, care conferences between the client's primary nurse and physician might be scheduled.

Change takes time and is sometimes accomplished by small steps. Minimally, a front sheet on the client's chart might be used for the care providers from all professions to record their diagnoses. A perceived need for scheduled joint conferences might evolve from this beginning. Physicians and nurses who have separate rounds on all clients should combine them. The methods employed to promote change must be specific to a particular institution.

NURSING PROCESS IN DISEASE-RELATED CARE

Nursing process is a problem identification–problem-solving process. As such, it is adaptable to domains of problems other than nursing diagnoses; one domain is that described by medical diagnoses. Although the subject of this book is nursing diagnoses, some consideration should be given to nurses' disease-related care activities and the clinical judgments on which care is based.

The first judgment made after a client is admitted is based on the quick-scan emergency assessment described in Chapter 7. This assessment differentiates between emergency and nonemergency situations. For example:

> Mr. F. was brought to the emergency room by ambulance after a fall. Head injury was obvious from his bleeding laceration, minimal spontaneous

activity, and sluggish response to verbal communications. The situation was judged to be a medical emergency and a physician was immediately summoned.

Judgments about emergencies and the need for a particular health professional's services are continually made in nursing. Although the need for medical evaluation was quite obvious in this case, frequently judgments are uncertain when clinical signs are ambiguous:

> Further physical assessment of Mr. F., a 45-year-old man in previous good health, involved the search for cues to his neurological status. The most likely possibility was intracranial bleeding from trauma. Signs observed signified moderate head injury (concussion).

A client with a history such as Mr. F.'s requires immediate assessment and continued close observation upon admission to an acute care unit. Judgments about the level of nursing care required are based on a nurse's medical knowledge. Regardless of whether or not physician's orders were written, Mr. F. should have been observed for increased intracranial pressure, intracranial bleeding, associated spinal cord injury, other undetected injuries, and infection of his head laceration. These hypotheses are generated from the cues present on admission and the medical diagnosis. Hypothesis testing involves a search for cues that define these conditions:

> Two hours after admission, Mr. F. showed changes from baseline data collected at admission (decreased level of consciousness, no spontaneous motor activity, reaction only to strong stimuli, increased dilation and fixation of right pupil, and changes in vital signs).

The observed physical signs suggested the hypothesis of further intracranial bleeding and a subdural hematoma. Having generated this hypothesis, the nurse caring for Mr. F. immediately called the physician and anticipated surgical intervention. Mr. F.'s physiological problems and the nurse's responses demonstrate the similarities and differences between nursing diagnoses and disease-related nursing judgments:

1. *Similarities:* Assessment or information collection, hypothesis generation, and hypothesis testing. (Only one set of cognitive behaviors need be learned.)

2. *Differences:* The kind of information collected and processed and the actions taken. (A body of knowledge in medical science and experience in its application are required.) The problem is then referred.

Carpenito's Bifocal Clinical Practice Model[21] offers a way of thinking about nursing practice that includes nursing diagnoses and collaborative problems. "Collaborative problems are certain physiological complications that nurses monitor to detect onset or change in status. Nurses manage collaborative problems using physician-prescribed and nurse-prescribed interventions to minimize the complications of the events."[21 (p. 30)] This model provides a way of thinking about the medical diagnosis and complications that have been traditionally addressed by nurses in various ways. Actions and judgments include the following:

1. Carrying out or assisting clients to carry out the physician-prescribed treatments for diseases or mental disorders until clients can do these tasks for themselves (medications, treatments, dressings, etc.)
2. Clinical judgments for purposes of referral to another care provider (assessing and recognizing complications of disease/mental disorder/treatment that are outside the domain of nursing)
3. Clinical judgments about whether or not to institute medical treatment protocols (interventions for medical problems/diseases/disorders)
4. Clinical judgments about the supplementation and/or individualization of physician-prescribed treatments carried out by nurses (adapting a treatment order without changing any factors that would influence the efficacy or intention of the treatment)

The list above includes the areas defined by Carpenito in slightly different terms and with some additions.[1 (pp. 28-36)]

She suggests a format for documenting collaborative problems. The following are some examples from her discussion:

Potential complication: increased intracranial pressure

Potential complication: dysrhythmia

Potential complication: asthma[21 (p. 30)]

Under each would be listed the observations to be made and reported and the nurse-initiated interventions. Nurses find this method useful for thinking about and documenting problems in this domain.

Why not just use the medical disease terminology to trigger thinking about nurse-initiated treatments for these conditions and for documenting? This approach is certainly feasible: It would be easier for the physician to find the documentation. Many nurses are reluctant to do this. It may be that for the last few decades nurses have been educated in the problem curriculum, in which the stress is on problems (e.g., increased intracranial pressure, decreased cardiac output, impaired gas exchange, or impaired glucose metabolism) rather than on diseases (e.g., Congestive Heart Failure, Chronic Obstructive Pulmonary Disease, Diabetes Mellitus). The problem-focused curriculum organizes diseases around common problems. Thus thinking is about problems that cut across diseases, and knowledge structures in memory may be organized in this way. Carpenito's[21] bifocal model fits well with this memory structure. The focus on potential complications is also well placed, since most clinical judgments about interventions in this domain are "clinical judgments for purposes of referral." *Potential complications* implies "watch for," "check for," and other terms that nurses use to direct observation and "watchful vigilance."

High touch and high tech in nursing intervention

Health care has become very technologically oriented with machines that substitute for organs and the monitoring of body functions by machine-generated information. What were once technological options in selected cases have become mandates for routine practice. This change is apparent in prenatal and genetic testing, electronic fetal monitoring, and postoperative pulmonary care.[21] It is important that nurses "counter the magnetic quality of monitors that tends to draw attention to the machines themselves and away from patients."[22 (p. 37)] Machines can redefine a situation, as in the intensive care unit where the emphasis is on machine technology rather than on nurses' "watchful vigilance."[23 (p. 56)] Not much has been said about the nurse-client interaction that is the basis for nursing process because there are many good books on the subject. Yet it is the nurse's interaction and caring that many times leads to the success of interventions.

NURSING DIAGNOSIS AND COMMUNICATION

When more than one person is responsible for the health care of a client, communication is necessary. Actually, even in private practice, records of diagnoses and treatments must be kept. In this section the relevance of nursing diagnoses to various types of written and verbal communication within and among professions is examined. The problem-oriented permanent record and the nursing care plan are important methods of communication and are discussed in detail. Nursing diagnoses provide a concise and organized means of communication.

Communicating diagnoses and interventions in writing has benefits, yet it is difficult to get health professionals to "do their charting." Perhaps an awareness of the benefits would increase the motivation to document data. Documenting accomplishes the following goals:

1. Prevents memory strain and errors due to memory lapses
2. Encourages health professionals to organize their data, diagnostic judgments, and treatment decisions
3. Facilitates continuity and coordination of care when two or more health professionals provide care
4. Provides a record in the event of alleged harm to a client
5. Permits research and reviews of care (quality assurance) that can lead to the improvement of care
6. Provides data for staffing, cost reimbursement, and health statistics

The costs in time and effort are minimal when compared with these benefits and the legal protection documentation provides.

Verbal communication

Nurses use verbal communication with other nurses in shift reports, informal discussions of clients' health problems, formal case conferences, nursing rounds, and reports to supervisors. During nurse-physician communication, a physician may inquire about a client's sleep pattern or nutritional pattern during hospitalization, or the nurse may initiate a verbal communication about a nursing diagnosis that might have an impact on medical treatment.

In all these kinds of communications, nursing diagnosis provides a succinct and clear mode of communication. Consider the following examples:

1. *Shift report:* "Ms. K. is ineffectively coping with the threat of impending surgery. I have . . ." [night nurse lists interventions and outcomes].
2. *During coffee break:* "I'm really having trouble coming up with a way of dealing with Mr. G. He is at risk for fluid volume deficit and I can't get him to drink anything. I hate to see him have an intravenous infusion. Can you think of anything?"
3. *Case conference:* "I've picked Mr. L. because his major problem is common to so many of our clients. His diagnosis is self-care deficit due to left-sided neglect. We aren't treating this effectively, and so I have done a review of the literature and I've come up with an idea that may suggest some additional possibilities."
4. *Nursing rounds:* "Mr. F. is a 45-year-old construction worker; his medical problem is uncomplicated myocardial infarct. Currently he has an independence-dependence conflict. The probable cause is the restriction of his activity and self-care. I am . . ." (states intervention).
5. *Report to supervisor (service director):* "I have one client with impaired home maintenance management/decreased activity tolerance. I taught her energy conservation techniques, but I've decided she also needs a homemaker 2 days a week. Tomorrow I'll orient the homemaker. I also have two clients for whom the referral states alterations in parenting. I'll see them tomorrow. The home health aide is implementing my plan for Ms. S. Her mobility has decreased and . . ."
6. *Nurse-physician:* "I finally found out that Jamie's passive dependence is not due to fear but to parental overprotection. I'm helping his parents develop a plan for allowing him more independence. When you talk to the parents . . ."

The preceding communications are concise and to the point. Hesitation and confusion over a multiplicity of signs and symptoms are avoided. Data have been organized by the use of nursing diagnoses.

Written communication

In contrast to verbal communication, which relies on human recall and human interaction, written information takes on a quality of permanence. In the developed nations, important observations and decisions are nearly always recorded. Others can read how an event was seen and interpreted 1 hour, 1 day, or years later.

In health care situations written communications provide a sequential record of the client's health status as well as care providers' diagnostic judgments, treatment plans, and actions. These records provide the means for continuity and coordination of plans across settings, care providers, and time. Written records not only preserve data; certain methods of recording also provide a means for checking thought processes.

Nurses and other care providers use various modes of written communication. Some are permanent records of the client's progress; others are working records that are summarized and discarded at intervals.

A permanent record, commonly referred to as the medical record or client's chart, is used in private, institutional, and community practice. Its main purpose is to provide continuity of care, but it also is used for research and teaching purposes. In addition, this record is used as evidence in legal proceedings. State laws require that a record of care provided to an individual or family be kept for a number of years.

Different chart formats are in use, particularly for nursing recordings. Some institutions separate medical and nursing notes within a chart. Others use one section for all health care providers' histories, examinations, progress notes, and treatment orders.

Historically, nurses communicated important observations and actions in long paragraphs. Additions to the record were made at least three times a day, once on each work shift. Communications of certain observations were required: clients' sleeping, eating, comfort, and doctors' visits. Some-

times long dissertations were critically important and sometimes not. Little evidence existed that physicians or supervisors read nurses' notes, and after the client's discharge they were discarded. Understandably, this type of nurse's note has become nearly extinct. In addition, the nurse's judgments had to be carefully worded in the written record. Every student learned the cautious, conservative phrase "appears to be" in the first nursing course. These words were modestly applied to nurses' judgments—"appears to be bleeding," "appears to be uncomfortable," or even "appears to have expired."

In recent years judgment has been emphasized in nursing. Most important, nurses themselves are beginning to believe their observations, diagnostic judgments, and treatment decisions are important. They diagnose and treat health problems within their scope of practice and communicate these via a permanent record.

Computer-based communication

It is predicted that most health care agencies will be using computer-based clinical records by the mid-1990s. Already a number of hospitals and community agencies have discarded paper records, and all charting is entered into a computerized system. Printouts provide the nursing care and medical care plans for daily care; laboratory and other data are also entered into the computerized record. The computer provides a readily accessible system of information to guide daily care activities. When an entire hospital uses computerized records, the term *hospital information system* is used. The nursing portion of the system is called the *nursing information system.* More will be said about computerized systems in the next chapter. For now it suffices to say that this type of clinical record permits documentation and access to the following:

1. Current nursing diagnoses and supporting data
2. Projected outcomes
3. Treatment orders and progress notes
4. Personal data about the client (age, next of kin, etc.)
5. Current medical diagnoses, treatment orders, lab tests, progress notes, and other health care professionals' treatment plans and notes

Table 10-3   Admission Problem List for One Client

Problem number	Active problems	Date entered	Date problem inactive
1.	Diabetes mellitus	5/20	
2.	Hyperglycemia; acidosis	5/20	
3.	Exogenous obesity/activity-caloric intake imbalance	5/20	
4.	High risk for injury	5/20	
5.	Four-day history of not taking insulin	5/20	

6. History of dysfunctional patterns and illnesses
7. Name of primary nurse and physician

A computerized system of clinical data recording produces a printout of a client's current nursing and medical plan of care to guide daily activities. Appendix I lists suggested components of a practice-based computerized system for nursing care delivery.

FORMATS FOR DOCUMENTATION

Each health care agency develops a specific format for documentation that is useful for their client population and setting. This section reviews general formats that are in wide use; these include problem-oriented recording (POR) and Kardex. The sections of the POR and Kardexes organized by nursing diagnosis-outcome-intervention contain elements similar to those used in a computerized system. Also, consideration will be given to the documentation of disease-related care in this section.

Problem-oriented recording

In 1969 Lawrence Weed, a physician concerned about the poor quality of records, designed a format that organizes and indexes information around client problems. This format has been implemented in many care delivery settings. Interestingly, it was about the same time that many nurses began to think about their practice in terms of nursing diagnoses. Merging the two ideas permitted nurses to move easily into the new charting system, which is designed to facilitate care, teaching, and research. The structure has four parts:

1. *A problem list:* This is a cumulative listing of client problems and potential problems providing a continually updated indexing system. All health care professionals list their diagnoses on the master problem list using a number, date of diagnosis, and date when resolved. This list is found at the front of the chart. Each nursing diagnosis (problem/etiological factors) is recorded on the master problem list and assigned the next consecutive number. (If other professionals do not wish to use this listing, nursing diagnoses only may appear on the list, or it may be agreed that nurses copy the medical diagnosis from the progress sheets so that they may index their charting.) Problems that are of a very transitory nature should not be listed on the master problem list. An example of a problem list from a chart is contained in the box above.

2. *A defined data base:* The term *data base* refers to all the information about the client's health. The nursing component includes the nursing history and examination, incorporating supporting data for nursing diagnoses.

3. *Initial and revised plans:* This component includes all professionals' treatment plans, revisions in plans, and discharge plans.

4. *Progress notes:* All professionals caring for the client chart their observations about the client's progress or lack of progress on sheets called *progress notes.* Each entry is labeled with the number of the diagnosis being addressed. Thus to review the progress of problem resolution, it is easy to go through the notes and read about the particular numbered problem.

Documentation: admission assessment

The nursing history and examination are documented on progress sheets in the form illustrated in Appendix I. The process of recording data in this manner helps the clinician think through the problems that have been identified. The objective is to be clear, concise, and complete. The documentation of an admission assessment has two purposes: (1) It provides a baseline with which changes may be compared, and (2) it is a record of the health status of the client when admitted to the nurse's caseload. The latter is important from a legal perspective in the event of a malpractice suit against the health care agency or the nurse.

Conciseness and clarity in documentation are important. First, others may want to review the nursing assessment, and second, a nurse's time should not be wasted with wordy descriptions. Note how extraneous words are deleted in the examples of admission assessments in this text and in Appendix I. For example:

1. *Not concise:* The patient says he has a dull, aching pain in his right knee when he walks to the bathroom or around the house.
2. *Concise:* Patient reports dull aching pain in right knee when ambulating.

To assure clarity in documentation, use quotation marks to signify client's words. This distinguishes verbal reports from a nurse's observation or inference:

1. *Concise but not clear:* Husband gets angry and beats the children when he gets drunk. Has essential hypertension, diagnosed in 1982. Work is stressful for him.
2. *Concise and clear:* Client states "husband gets angry and beats the kids when he gets drunk." Reports husband has "essential hypertension, diagnosed in 1982." States husband's work is "stressful."

Documentation of the nursing history and examination must be complete. First, data on each functional pattern should be documented even if there are no problems. *If assessment in a pattern area is deferred, the reason should be stated concisely.* Second, it is not advisable to record only conclusions about important data; rather, all data should be documented. For example:

1. *Incomplete:* Seems anxious about surgery.

2. *Complete:* Restless, in and out of bed five times this morning; eyes darting about; startled response to noises; reports feeling "anxious" about the outcome of surgery and whether he "will ever go back to work."

Documentation: nursing diagnoses/treatment plans

The problem-oriented recording system has a particular format for documenting diagnoses and treatments. The format is concise and permits organization of the products of clinical reasoning. The components are:

1. *The health problem (P):* As defined in Chapter 6.
2. *Subjective clinical data (S):* Client reports, as described in Chapter 7.
3. *Objective clinical data (O):* Nurse observations, as described in Chapter 7.
4. *Assessment (A):* Analysis and interpretation of reasons for the problem (etiological or related factors, as described in Chapter 6) and any factors related to the prognosis of the problem. Also include strengths of the client situation that would influence treatment plans.
5. *Plan (P):* The desired outcomes and the treatments to be carried out. (Some authors suggest adding a sixth component *[O]* for outcomes to the list; it seems useful to include all elements of nursing process and adapt the format to *SOAOP*.)

The formulation of nursing diagnoses was discussed in other chapters. Below is an example of documentation of one of the problems listed in the box on p. 235.

> Problem 4. High Risk for Injury (Table 10-3)
> S: Reports reduced touch sensation in legs; minimizes bruise and scratches on legs; can't recall trauma; "they're nothing"; uses scatter rugs without nonskid padding; "At times I hate to wear my glasses around the house"; does not put on lights to cross hall to bathroom during the night; hates to arouse her dog.
> O: 3-cm bruise on left leg; scratches on both lower legs; diabetic neuropathy (see physician's notes); decreased sensitivity to touch.

What outcome(s) would be projected? What would be the treatment plan for this diagnosis?

In thinking about these questions, it is important to note that a treatment plan is written for each diagnosis. Plans always include items 1 and 2 below; depending on the diagnosis, item 3 may be included. If the diagnosis is not completely formulated, item 4 would be expected to appear on a care plan:

1. Projected outcomes
2. Treatment orders
3. Patient education orders when indicated by the diagnosis
4. Collection of further diagnostic information

Projected outcomes clarify the behavior that indicates the resolution of the risk state (or in the case of actual problems, the resolution of the problem). These outcomes are the criteria for judging the quality of care delivered. Thus it is important that outcomes are realistic, clear, and concise and that they emphasize critical indicators of problem resolution. Below are the outcomes and treatment plan stated at admission for the client with High Risk for Injury:

O: Outcome: Absence of leg injuries; states plans for implementing measures in home to prevent injury.

P: P_{Dx}: Observe degree of caution exercised when ambulating.

P_{Tx}: Environmental management: Room check for jutting objects, slippery floors; eyeglasses worn during ambulation; adequate lighting at all times when ambulating.

P_{Ed}: High Risk for Injury with sensory deficit to be explained. Teach precautions regarding ambulation, adequate vision, lighting, scatter rugs, slippery floors, jutting objects, ill-fitting shoes or boots, nail cutting.

The diagnostic plan (Dx) at admission was to collect further information about the degree of caution exercised by the client when ambulating in the hospital. Plans for further data collection should always be included when the problem list includes uncategorized but potentially important signs, for example, problem 5 in the box on p. 235 (4-day history of not taking insulin). Admission data may not be sufficient to specify etiological factors; this situation also necessitates a plan for data collection.

The treatment plan (Tx) was designed to ensure the client's safety during ambulation in the hospi-

tal and to attain the stated outcome, absence of leg injury. While these interventions were being implemented, incidental teaching might be done. Yet to attain the outcome "States plans for implementing measures in home to prevent injury," an *educational plan* (Ed) was needed.

The P-SOAP (or SOAOP) format provides immediate feedback on cognitive processes. Contradictions can be seen. For example, it is possible to check whether the subjective (S) and objective (O) data are sufficient to support the recorded problem and etiology. First, a cross-check using a manual of diagnostic category definitions may help. Second, the nurse can check to be certain that the projected outcome (O) is consistent with the problem and that the treatment plan is consistent with the etiological factors identified (or with the risk factors of a potential problem). The checkpoints in the box on p. 238 may be useful. Consider the checkpoints and use these to identify errors in the following examples. Errors occurred as nurses were learning to use nursing diagnoses and problem-oriented recording. Try to pick out the inconsistencies found in these three charts:

Example 1

1. Self-Bathing Deficit (Level II)/Extreme Obesity-Fear of Falling

   S: Fears falling in shower; bathes self at sink daily but has difficulty reaching all body parts due to extreme obesity.

   A: Has plans to lose weight.

   O: Personal hygiene poor; body odor and urine odor detected; hair unwashed; skin unclean on admission.

   P: 1. Obtain long-handled sponge and tub chair.
      2. Arrange for equipment to be used in shower at home after practice in hospital.
      3. Teach 1000-calorie diet.

Example 2

1. Sleep Pattern Disturbance

   S: "I am unable to fall asleep at least three or four times a week; I awaken easily and have nightmares when I take Valium."

   A: Job stress; family stress.

   P_{Dx}: Observe and record sleep pattern in hospital.

   P_{Tx}: Back massage at bedtime; check comfort level.

PROBLEM-ORIENTED RECORDING: GUIDELINES AND CHECKPOINTS

No.___: Problem number and label

State clear, concise diagnostic label for the problem.
1. Check below to ensure that S and O contain sufficient supporting data (diagnostic criteria) for the problem.
2. If insufficient information available to label the problem, record the possible diagnoses being considered or major signs/symptoms; continue assessment.

S: Subjective data*

List pertinent diagnostic indicators from verbal reports by individual or family.
1. Record quotes when applicable.
2. Check for consistency with objective data. Attempt to resolve incongruities or inconsistencies in data before recording.

O: Objective data*

List pertinent diagnostic indicators from direct observation and examination of individual or family; observations of context or milieu; and observational reports of other care providers, if pertinent.
1. Check for measurement error, observer bias, and consistency with subjective data. Attempt to resolve incongruities or inconsistencies in data before recording.

A: Assessment

State etiological or related factors contributing to the problem in No.___.
1. Use clear, concise terms.
2. Check that S and O data provide diagnostic criteria for etiological factor(s).
3. If insufficient information available to label etiological factors, record possible etiologies being considered; continue assessment.
4. Include functional strengths pertinent to resolution of the problem and any relevant prognostic statements.
5. Potential problems have risk factors recorded in S and O. These are the factors contributing to the high-risk state.

P: Plan

State projected outcome(s) and interventions.

Projected Outcome(s): State concise, explicit, measurable, critical, attainable outcome(s) for the problem. State time of outcome attainment (e.g., discharge, 3 days; 4-week visit). If applicable, state a sequential set of outcomes and time frame.
1. Check that outcomes are specific to problem in No.___.
2. Check that date of outcome attainment is realistic. Consider etiological factors that may influence time for outcome attainment.

Interventions: State intervention goal (optional). List concise nursing treatment orders. Include specific actions (time and amount, if applicable).
1. Check that treatment orders are consistent with etiological factors stated in A and are specific to the individual client. If potential problem, check that treatment orders will reduce risk factors specified under S and O.
2. Check that treatment orders have a high possibility for attaining outcome(s).
3. If useful, classify plan by treatment orders (P_{RX}), diagnostic orders (P_{DX}), and teaching orders (P_{ED}).
4. Check that treatment plan includes strengths that can be mobilized by the client/family situation to help resolve the problem or risk state. After the format is learned, errors in documentation are usually attributable to errors in clinical reasoning.

*S and O data must provide sufficient diagnostic criteria to support problem and etiology. Use a manual to check defining characteristics of a diagnostic category.

Example 3

1. Impaired Verbal Communication
    S: States husband died 8 months ago; 4 days ago was told she has extensive cancer of abdominal organs.
    O: Weak, halting speech; uses short sentences; no apparent shortness of breath.
    A: Decreased strength.
    P: 1. Facilitate verbalization of feelings.
    2. Provide encouragement, support, and motivation.
    3. Work with family.

In Example 1 a question may be raised about plan 3: Is "Teach 1000-calorie diet" an intervention for Self-Bathing Deficit/Extreme Obesity-Fear of Falling? Fear of falling is the reason for the client not taking a shower (see data). Difficulty reaching body parts is a second reason for the problem. Obesity, especially the exogenous type, due to a caloric-intake–energy-expenditure imbalance, is a second diagnosis. It should be recorded separately as problem number 2. Further, the plan is inadequate for the diagnosis of obesity.

Example 2 illustrates a common error of the novice. The data base is inadequate for the diagnosis. The recorded data do not support the etiological factors stated in "A," work and family stress. Actually the nurse had data to support this diagnosis in the role-relationship pattern recorded in the history. In addition, the plan is inadequate for the diagnosis. Palliative treatment is prescribed, but no interventions are directed toward the stress factors.

Obviously the nurse who recorded Example 3 did not appreciate how problem-oriented recording provides a check on clinical reasoning. The data do not support the diagnosis. It appears that objective data were heavily weighted in the nurse's diagnostic judgment. Do the subjective data support the diagnosis? Absolutely not. Furthermore there is no data base to support "decreased strength," the etiology recorded under "A."

In Example 3, if the nurse had reread and examined the consistency among problem, etiology, and plan, the errors would have become obvious. Facilitating verbalization, providing support, and working with a family are not the treatments for impaired verbal communication. Second, the plan, even if appropriate, is too vague. What does support entail? Work with the family toward what objective?

Rather than cross-checking judgments and decisions in memory, the written SOAP format should be used. Instructors or clinical specialists can provide feedback, but it is important to learn how to pick up contradictions oneself.

Now consider some reasonably good examples of problem-oriented recording in the box on p. 238. Try to discover the one element of the POR format (or of nursing process) that is missing.

Did you find difficulty in evaluating the treatment plan? That is because no outcomes are stated. In the box on p. 240, noncompliance with activity prescription was a problem of a 35-year-old construction worker in an intensive care unit for treatment of myocardial infarction (heart attack). In this case the nurse did not have sufficient data to determine the etiological factors. Thus the tentative hypotheses and the etiological factors that were ruled out (Knowledge Deficit) were recorded under assessment. An assessment of activity tolerance was included. High Risk for Skin Breakdown was diagnosed for another client during a home visit by a community health nurse. The wife was taking care of her husband, who had had a transection of the spinal cord at the level of the third lumbar vertebra. The third example was written in a psychiatric setting; the diagnosis was Impaired Socialization/Inability to Trust. Probably some further questions can be raised at this point that might be answered by considering ongoing documentation during care delivery. Questions might include: How do I document what I do? and, How do I know when to stop treatment?

Documentation: progress notes

Progress toward outcomes is charted on each problem by number on sheets called *progress notes*. Theoretically, progress notes are written only when a change is observed in the status of the problem or when there is no response or an unexpected response to treatment. In actuality, if treatment is aggressive, daily changes in hospital settings or at each visit in private practice settings, clinics or at community nursing home visits should be observed and documented. Not all components of

---

RECORDED NURSING DIAGNOSES

Intensive care unit

1. Noncompliance with activity prescription
   S: States feels better: "heart OK now," and "able to do my own bath." Told M.D. that he understood the need for rest and wanted to "do everything to get it healed."
   O: Out of bed × 3; stays at bedside; heart rate increased 5 beats per minute with no arrhythmias when out of bed; restless when in bed; activity prescription is complete bed rest.
   A: Possible postmyocardial infarction denial or independence-dependence conflict; no knowledge deficit regarding activity limits; heart rate response to being out of bed suggests tolerance.
   P_{Dx}: Reasons for noncompliance; assess denial or conflict over required dependence.
   P_{Tx}: Anticipate needs; discuss activity orders and patient's tolerance limits with M.D.; may need activity tolerance evaluation.
   P_{Ed}: Problem solve with client regarding activity restriction if prescription is not changed.

Community: home-care

2. High Risk for Skin Breakdown
   S: States likes to lie on left side to look out bedroom window; has no discomfort at site of redness.
   O: 3-cm reddened area over left greater trochanter; no ulceration; decreased pain perception below L3.
   A: Wife competent and will be able to carry out plan with neighbor's help.
   P_{Ed}: Discuss with wife: (1) relocation of bed, OOB as tolerated when assistance available; (2) 1½-hour position change and functional positioning; (3) signs of impending skin breakdown; (4) care of potential pressure sites; (5) adequate nutritional intake, especially protein.

Psychiatric unit

3. Impaired Social Integration
   S: States he doesn't want to sit with or talk to others; they "frighten" him.
   O: Single; no family in this part of country; no group involvement; at times appears to be listening to group conversations from a distance but does not interact.
   A: Inability to trust.
   P: a. Milieu (social environment) activities with staff person he relates to.
   b. Explore these difficulties with patient when he is observed to be listening to conversations.
   c. Assist patient to develop plans for joining activities.
   d. Provide support from trusted staff person when he agrees to join in activities.

---

the P-SOAP format need be included in each progress note. If initial plans have not changed, no entry is made under plan (P). A progress note on the client with high risk for injury (pages 236-237) might be:

Problem 4. High Risk for Injury
S/O: No further trauma to extremities. Keeps eyeglasses on top of bedside stand; uses when ambulating. Twenty-minute teaching session on sensory deficit and risk for trauma; client suggested she use a night-light in the hall and dog would accommodate; plans to talk to daughter re: scatter rugs and waxed floors.
P: Other risk factors to be discussed tomorrow.

Note that it was difficult to separate objective and subjective observations. In this author's opinion, this may not be as crucial in nursing as in medicine. It is clear from this progress note that treatment is leading to risk-factor reduction. The most important cue for future health management is the client's intention to use a night-light and plan to talk to her daughter. One senses that the nurse engaged the client in solving her problem, rather than "telling" her what to do!

To return to the second question posed: *When should treatment cease?* The answer is simply, When the projected outcomes are reached. One outcome was *Absence of leg injuries*. This is a discharge outcome; therefore "room check" and observation for leg trauma should continue until discharge. As a method of teaching and evaluation, the nurse might observe the client's assumption of responsibility for room check and whether any risk factors are identified. The second outcome was, *States plans for implementing measures in home to prevent injury.* When the client and her daughter outline plans for correcting the risk factors in the home environment, treatment may be discontinued. If this client was receiving home visits, the community nurse would have described the outcome as, *Implements measures in home to prevent injury* and would observe for corrective actions. When the client names a podiatrist who will cut her nails and check her shoes/boots, this outcome will be reached. To evaluate teaching, the client might be asked to write her plan for preventing injury to her legs. She would then have a written plan to take home. When outcomes are reached, the client may be discharged from the primary nurse's caseload. At that point a discharge summary is written.

Documentation: discharge summary/referrals

Nursing discharge summaries are similar to medical summaries. A note is written about the progress, or lack of progress, toward outcomes for each nursing diagnosis. Other care-related information that should be summarized for future care providers is included. In some agencies the nursing diagnoses on the discharge summary are coded so that the client's record can be retrieved easily for purposes of research or health statistics. Consider the discharge summary for the nursing diagnosis High Risk for Injury:

> Problem 4. High Risk for Injury (pp. 236-237)
> Stated plan for implementing measures in home to prevent injury to legs (sensory loss-diabetic neuropathy). Observed caution in hospital and demonstrated understanding by writing plan for a nightlight, padding for scatter rugs, and nonskid wax on floors. Wore glasses when ambulating and stated name of podiatrist who would check shoes/boots, cut toe nails and corns. No trauma to legs at discharge.

Documentation: disease-related care

The emphasis in this chapter has been on nursing diagnosis and treatment. Yet, as pointed out in Chapter 1, nursing practice also includes carrying out aspects of medical therapy that clients cannot manage for themselves. These aspects of nursing care are determined by physicians' orders or established protocols for medical treatment.

Disease-related observations and treatments must be recorded. Presumably, if a disease or symptom has been identified, the physician will have recorded it on the problem list. In the sample problem list in Table 10-3, the physician made two entries: (1) diabetes mellitus and hypoglycemia; and (2) acidosis. In charting observations or treatments related to the disease process, the nurse can use the SOAP format previously described. The differences from that format are listed below:

1. The plan (P) is not used unless supplementary *nursing* orders are required; these may include "observe for . . . ," "watch for . . . ," or other monitoring orders and any individualized adaptations of the physician's order that do not alter the intention of therapy, such as "give with orange juice," "notify M.D. if systolic above 170," or other orders relative to equipment used in treatment.

2. The medical diagnosis and its number (from the master problem list or medical notes) are the title for charting the nurse's observations and actions relative to the disease. For example, if symptoms of thirst or frequent urination were observed, the nurse would record them using the heading: #1 Diabetes Mellitus, or High Risk for Complications: Diabetes Mellitus.

As with nursing diagnoses, one must be aware of contradictions in the charting of disease-related information. For example, recording "able to administer own insulin injection effectively" under diabetes mellitus is a contradiction. The client's ability has no *direct* relationship to the pathophysiology of diabetes. This observation may indicate that a nursing diagnosis of Knowledge Deficit (Insulin Administration) was present but not diagnosed. *Beware of placing observations related to nursing diagnoses under medical problems.*

There is no need to create new terms for diseases or pathophysiological processes in order to chart disease-related observations and treatments. The medical diagnoses provide terminology. Use of those terms does not constitute medical diagnosis, provided that the physician has already identified and recorded them as his or her diagnostic judgment. If the medical diagnoses have not been recorded, either the symptoms were overlooked or new problems have occurred. In either case, notification of the physician is appropriate.

KARDEX CARE PLANS: NURSING AND MEDICAL DIAGNOSES

In addition to recording diagnoses and plans on the client's chart, many nurses use a Kardex, a flip-card tool that has sections for recording information about each client. Usually the following information is recorded: name, age, room number, religion, admission date, medical diagnoses, scheduled medical tests (e.g., cardiac catheterization) and medical treatments, nursing diagnoses, nursing treatments, and nursing outcomes.

The main advantage of the Kardex is that it provides rapid access to the client's overall plan of care. It is used in shift reports, in planning staff assignments, and as a quick reference about all the clients on the hospital unit. The alternative way to acquire information is to leaf through each client's chart or problem list. Proponents of the Kardex system extol its merits. Some nurses decry the Kardex's usefulness. They claim the Kardex duplicates information on the chart, is usually not up to date, and is rarely used by the professional staff.

If a Kardex is used, nursing diagnoses provide a method of organizing treatment plans. The diagnoses are stated in the problem/etiological factor format, and the interventions and outcomes are then listed. The data base for a diagnosis is not included, as may be seen in the following example of one nursing diagnosis of a client who has pneumonia and chronic lung disease (the data for diagnoses is on the chart):

Problem: Fear (Inability to Breathe)/Pain on Inspiration and Cough.
Intervention: 1. Discuss with M.D. need for a liquefying cough medicine and humidifier.

2. Repeatedly reassure client (regarding breathing problem) that nurses are present; provide call system that does not require verbalization (client is concerned that he will not be able to speak into intercom if respiratory problems occur).
3. Monitor breathing difficulty every half hour.
4. Teach relaxation techniques.
5. Ensure adequate fluid intake to assist in liquefying secretions.
Outcomes: 1. Verbalizes perception of ability to breathe adequately.
2. Verbalizes comfort on inspiration.

In some institutions a nurse's order sheet specifying interventions is used as a supplement to the client's chart. Orders—for example, "teach relaxation techniques"—are transferred directly from the chart to the order book.

Disease-related interventions

Nurses write nursing orders for treating nursing diagnoses. In addition, they write orders related to a client's disease, possible complications, or adaptations of medical treatments. For example, a client may require observation for heart failure, bleeding, or a change in neurological signs. Or observations and adaptations (e.g., "give with orange juice") may be necessary while the nurse is carrying out medical orders for administering drugs and other aspects of medical treatment.

In ordering or recording nursing interventions related to diseases, it is not necessary to label disease-related care with nursing diagnoses. One simply records on the Kardex or in the order book the interventions required. The same format as that for recording nursing diagnoses may be used, except that the medical diagnosis is listed as the problem. For example:

Problem: Diabetes mellitus.
Intervention: Observe for irritability as sign of impending ketoacidosis. See that daily blood samples are drawn *before* breakfast.
Problem: Right Hip Fracture.
Intervention: Obtain fracture pan; maintain functional alignment of right leg.

It is not necessary to change a diagnosis of "diabetes mellitus" to "alterations in glucose metabolism" in order to write interventions or make observations. Nor is it necessary to change "myocardial infarction" or "congestive heart failure" to "alterations in cardiac output" in order to observe for arrhythmias or pulmonary edema. It is expected that *after* a medical diagnosis is made, nurses will make pertinent observations and carry out appropriate treatments. Communications about these conditions are organized under disease labels, not nursing diagnoses. An alternative, *Potential Complications*, was discussed on p. 232.

In summary, nursing diagnoses organize written and verbal communications. They provide a concise label for a health problem and thereby increase the speed and clarity of communication. Use of the problem-oriented clinical information system is facilitated by nursing diagnoses. In fact, without diagnostic labels the system is difficult to use. In addition, if a nursing Kardex or nursing order book is employed, diagnoses organize the recording of nursing care plans. In the near future recording will be on computerized systems.

NURSING DIAGNOSIS AND DISCHARGE PLANNING

The high cost of health care requires that needs and resources be correctly matched. Clients should receive a level of care and the technology appropriate to the severity of their health problems. To match needs and resources may require that clients be transferred through many levels of care within a few months. The following are two typical examples:

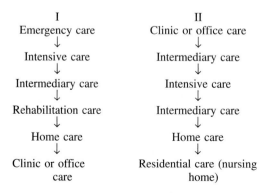

I	II
Emergency care	Clinic or office care
↓	↓
Intensive care	Intermediary care
↓	↓
Intermediary care	Intensive care
↓	↓
Rehabilitation care	Intermediary care
↓	↓
Home care	Home care
↓	↓
Clinic or office care	Residential care (nursing home)

These transfers offer the appropriate level of care for different phases of an illness; but from the client's perspective the repeated changes in care providers, routines, and the environment may be additional sources of stress. By planning for continuity of care between levels, the nurse can decrease the impact of change.

Ensuring continuity of nursing care between acute care hospitals and the community has been a problem. In response to this difficulty, many hospitals have established continuing care programs to assist in coordinating clients' needs and available community resources. Even with these programs, continuity may be jeopardized. If needs are not clearly evaluated and communicated from one care setting to another, fragmented care results.

The requirements for continued medical care as the client moves from one setting to another can be clearly specified. Plans are organized and communicated from physician to physician by using the medical diagnosis. In contrast, nursing has not agreed on the focus for the predischarge evaluation or postdischarge communication of treatment plans. Additionally, many times medical and nursing plans for the client's continuing care have not been coordinated.

The set of decisions and activities involved in providing continuity and coordination of care after hospitalization is called *discharge planning*. In many instances it is required by federal or state law[23] or by hospital policy.

In the following sections it will be seen that nursing diagnoses provide an excellent focus for discharge planning. Communicating a client's care requirements to nurses in community agencies and coordinating resources for continuing care are also facilitated. In fact, a nurse would not know that a client *needed* continued nursing care unless unresolved nursing diagnoses had been identified. A brief consideration of predischarge planning, referral decisions, and communication of nursing plans illustrates how diagnoses facilitate these activities.

Predischarge planning

Discharge planning begins when diagnoses are made. Outcomes that can and should be attained before discharge are projected. These discharge outcomes specify the level of problem resolution and probable time required before a client can (1) undertake independent health management at home or (2) manage with less than 24-hour acute hospital care.

Many conditions currently identified by nursing diagnoses may be treated with less expense to the consumer in nursing homes, rehabilitation centers, home care programs, or office and clinics than in hospitals. Thus a patient's discharge is seldom delayed because of nursing diagnoses.

The time of discharge is a combined decision of all health professionals who treat the patient. Sometimes nurses and social workers leave this decision to the physician if it is assumed that the nursing and social work diagnoses (1) will be resolved before the physician is ready to discharge the client or (2) can and should be treated in another setting. In other instances coordinated discharge planning is necessary. No one professional should be expected to make decisions in isolation without information about the client's overall program of care. Too-early discharge may result in harm, and delayed discharge adds to financial costs.

Most problems arise because of inadequate communication and delayed planning and intervention. The solution to these problems is (1) early discharge planning, (2) an established structure for multidisciplinary discharge planning, and (3) discharge nursing assessment.

Nursing activities in discharge planning

The structure and implementation of multidisciplinary discharge planning has been described by McKeehan.[24] In order to participate in multidisciplinary planning, the nurse must do the following:

1. Assess the level of problem resolution as discharge approaches. Review the status of each current nursing diagnosis. If there is doubt that all nursing problems have been diagnosed, a functional health pattern assessment is done.
2. By reviewing nursing treatment orders, decide what continuing care is needed.
3. Assess the client's capabilities as well as available family and community assistance. The client's (or responsible family member's or guardian's) understanding and plans for personal management of the medically prescribed treatment are also evaluated. (New

---

POSTHOSPITAL RESOURCES AND FACILITIES FOR CONTINUED NURSING CARE

Hospital clinics
Private office practice
Health maintenance organizations
Neighborhood health centers
Rehabilitation centers
Hospital home care programs
Home health care agencies (visiting nurse or public health agencies)
Hospices
Residential centers (long-term care)
Nursing homes
Long-term care hospitals

---

nursing diagnoses may arise when medical discharge plans are formulated. They may include knowledge or planning deficits in the management of symptoms, medication, diet, or activity.)

Discrepancies between the nurse's and the client's (or family member's) assessments of the client's capabilities for managing outside the hospital also need to be identified. For example, if a client does not feel capable of carrying out a health care recommendation, support services will have to be arranged until the client develops confidence.

4. Assess the client's need for referral for continued care. When the nurse knows the current diagnoses, the posthospital nursing care that will be required, and the client's capabilities and environmental resources, the next questions are: What care will not be handled adequately by the client, family, or friends? What home or environmental adaptations that are necessary for optimal (or at least acceptable) health promotion cannot be handled by the client, family, or friends? The answers to these questions provide the basis for matching the client's needs for continued nursing care, the available community resources, and the client's preferences about continuing care.

Referral decisions

The last step in planning for a client's discharge is to determine what type of referral to make. Some options for postacute nursing care are listed in the box on p. 244. Clinics, nurses in private practice, health maintenance organizations, and neighborhood health centers provide periodic nursing care. The emphasis is on health maintenance and promotion. Clients with nursing diagnoses requiring follow-up care on an ambulatory basis are referred to nursing services such as these.

With certain nursing diagnoses a long period of time and highly skilled nursing care are required to reach optimal outcomes. In these situations, plans may be initiated to refer clients to rehabilitation centers or rehabilitation units in acute care hospitals. Specialized services may be considered with diagnoses such as Impaired Mobility, Self-Care Deficit, Perceptual Deficit, or Chronic Pain Self-Management Deficit. Referrals for rehabilitation are appropriate only for clients who have the potential for improvement of their functional patterns. Reliable predictions of potential are important.

Both hospital-managed home care programs and community nursing agencies provide family-centered care and help with the adaptation from hospital to home. Clients with nursing diagnoses requiring continued home care or supervision are referred to visiting nurses in these agencies. Examples of such diagnoses are High Risk for Noncompliance (Disease Management), Self-Care Deficit Due to Short-Term Memory Loss, High Risk for Injury, and Unresolved Grieving. Actual or potential family problems in coping, interaction, or home maintenance may also require home visits for evaluation and treatment. The availability of professional visiting nurses, homemakers, and home health aides varies from 24 hours a day in some communities to 8 or fewer in others; thus client and family capabilities must be carefully determined.

Residential and hospice centers provide living environments for clients who cannot manage in their homes. Conditions such as profound mental retardation or severe cerebral palsy may require long-term residential care in a sheltered environment. A hospice is both a living environment and a philosophy of care for terminally ill clients. Resi-dential care and hospice centers are, respectively, options for clients with nursing diagnoses related to permanent cognitive or motor impairments and terminal illness.

Depending on the resources available and the person's choice, a diagnosis such as Chronic Mobility Impairment may be treated in the home or may require long-term institutional care. If continuous 24-hour nursing care is required over a period of time, nursing homes or long-term care hospitals may be chosen. The period of care may be weeks, months, or years, depending on the client's progress toward independence in decision making, mobility, and self-care.

The nurse discusses with clients and their families the type of care required and the options available, or clients and their families may attend multidisciplinary planning conferences. These conferences include all health team members involved in the client's care and discharge planning.

Two or more clients may have the same nursing diagnosis but different discharge plans. This is to be expected because interventions are always individualized. Consider the example of two clients with total self-care deficit (level III) due to sensorimotor loss (spinal cord transection). After rehabilitation, both were able to manage self-care with the assistance of one person and assistive devices. One client was referred to the visiting nurse service for home care. The other was discharged to a long-term care facility. Why the difference? The first client's spouse and neighbors valued home care and were able to adapt the home setting and provide care with the assistance of the visiting nurse. The second client had no family and lived alone, although he liked social contact. Twenty-four-hour home services were not available; even if they had been they would probably have been too costly and would not have provided sufficient social interaction. A nursing home was chosen where he could be near his friends.

Before discussing the writing of referrals, it is important to examine why discharge planning begins when nursing diagnoses are made and outcomes projected. If referral for continuing care is necessary, information will be needed for making decisions about the referral. A great deal of information can be collected and charted while daily care is being given. Without this ongoing information gathering, discharge planning may be very time consuming—it is rushed and ineffectively done.

Discharge planning judgments are critically important both for the client's safety and for the quality of the person's life. Diagnoses must be made accurately. If the capabilities of the client or situation are overestimated, further problems may arise; if they are underestimated, the client is subjected to unwarranted financial expense. The best data available should be obtained.

Communication of plans

The communication of plans is as important as planning. Clear and concise treatment orders and the bases for orders should be communicated to the next care providers. Good communication increases the probability that nursing care will proceed without interruption.

Nursing diagnoses organize communications and clarify the rationale for nursing orders. Problem-oriented recording of the diagnoses (P-SOAP format) further facilitates concise communication of critical information.

Standardized forms are used in most hospitals for client referrals to frequently used community agencies; visiting nurse referral forms are an example. Discharge summaries may also be used by nurses to refer clients with unresolved diagnoses. A discharge summary referral is sent to nurses in clinics, private practice, and other ambulatory care settings. When some problem or aspect of follow-up care needs particular attention, a telephone call may be the quickest, most efficient means.

The following two examples of the use of nursing diagnoses in writing referrals demonstrate the clarity and conciseness of communication which results. The first client was a 12-year-old intelligent, sports-loving boy referred for periodic nursing care at a hematology (blood) clinic. His medical diagnosis was hemophilia. The following two nursing diagnoses and SOAP notes were recorded on the nursing section of a referral:

ND$_x$:[1]   1.   High Risk for Injury (Bleeding)
   S: Likes sports, especially football; active child; states he thinks he can still play on team if he plays a different position.

O: Factor VIII deficiency, 1% plasma factor activity; recent football injury.
A: Moderately severe risk for hemorrhage; knows about bleeding problem and that he will not be able to play football but can attend games; overheard telling mother he could play.
P$_{Dx}$:   Assess whether client has resigned from Little League team.
P$_{Ed}$:   Repeat instructions regarding caution in avoiding trauma. If trauma occurs, mother is to bring child to emergency room.

ND$_x$:   2.   High Risk for Parental Overprotection.
   S: Mother states, "I feel so guilty, but I'll be sure he doesn't get hurt"; father says he will buy books and child can come home and read after school; asks if they should get rid of dog.
O: Both parents express concern and nervousness whenever child's activity discussed.
A: Parents understand tendency for overprotection and say they will try to avoid it; plan to contact National Hemophilia Foundation and join parent support group.
P$_{Dx}$:   Assess for restrictions placed on child by parents; check to see whether they have joined parent support group.
P$_{Tx}$:   Continue to reassure parents that guilt is a normal reaction; assist them in identifying their strengths as parents; child to hospital for plasma factor VIII if trauma and bleeding occur.

Another example is that of a referral to a visiting nurse. The client's medical diagnosis was Adult Onset Diabetes Mellitus. She was a 65-year-old retired secretary. In the nursing section of the visiting nurse referral the following appeared:

ND$_x$ 1.   Dysfunctional Grieving
   S: States lost her father 1 year ago; cared for him at home before he died of cancer; verbal expression of distress, sadness; states she has no one now and doesn't know what to do.

O: Altered sleeping, eating, and dream patterns in hospital; mild inability to concentrate; crying spells.

A: Loss; possible fear of newly acquired independence. States will try to become involved in community activities after discharge.

P_{Dx}: Evaluate state of grieving after return home.

P_{Tx}: Grief Work Facilitation: Encourage contact with son and his family for support. Encourage joining voluntary community group; client expressed interest in this.

ND_x 2. Disease Management Deficit (Insulin Administration)[25]

S: "I don't know if I can do this injection adequately. I could never give my father injections." States knows importance of insulin administration.

O: Has successfully administered morning insulin twice. Hand shakes; dexterity is fair. Client has asked to practice on an orange. Able to draw up dose accurately.

A: Fear (perceived incompetency and error). Motivated but still needs supervision. Supervision and experience increase confidence.

P: Supervise insulin administration in home ×2 (likes to eat breakfast at 9 AM). Reevaluate competency.

ND_x 3. Disease Management Deficit (Compensated)

S: Reassured by plans for nurse's home visit.

O: Verbalizes correct dietary and activity plans. States principles of skin care, urine testing, and signs of complications to be reported; skills demonstrated.

P: Review management during home visit. To be seen in doctor's office in 1 month.

Nursing referrals about unresolved diagnoses help community agencies provide continuity of care. Referrals should also be sent from these agencies when their clients are treated in hospitals.

In summary, nursing diagnoses facilitate continuity of care in different care settings. Diagnoses provide a focus for early evaluation of continuing care needs, and suggested plans can be communicated in a concise, organized manner. Most important, individualized interventions can be written and communicated for each problem. Good communication between care providers decreases the client's stress in adjusting to different health care providers, routines, and environments.

NURSING DIAGNOSIS AND THE LAW

From the perspective of many nurses, nursing diagnosis merely recognizes what nurses have always done. This was not the view of hospital administrators, lawyers, or physicians in the 1970s. For many the term *nursing diagnosis,* when heard for the first time, set red lights flashing. The lights usually change to green when the concept is explained. Today this reaction is rare.

Even nursing colleagues were heard to say to each other, "Legally, you can't do that," or, "You'll put your license in jeopardy." Another often-heard comment by nurses was, "Our hospital hasn't accepted nursing diagnosis." The purpose of the discussion in this section is to explore whether the first statements are true or false and to see whether the latter has any relevance. The concepts of duty, cause, and harm, as they relate to negligence, will first be examined in order to provide a basis for judging the truth of the above or similar statements encountered in practice. It will be seen that *formulating and documenting nursing diagnoses can help nurses and institutions avoid negligence claims.*

Negligent conduct on the part of a nurse is a basis for malpractice litigation. The client, relative, or other must provide evidence about four issues: (1) duty, (2) breach of duty, (3) cause and effect, and (4) personal or economic harm.[26]

As a good example, a nurse, hospital, and physician were sued by the wife of a client. Her husband fell in the hospital and fractured his femur. She maintained that his care was negligent. The facts of the situation were as follows:

On December 1 the patient, an athletic-appearing sociable 30-year-old male was admitted to a hospital because of slight muscle weakness. The chart stated that tests for multiple sclerosis were to be done. According to the wife, she told the admitting nurse that her husband had fallen twice at home. The physician's ambulation order was

"Out of bed as desired." On the morning of December 2, the nurse told the client he could wash in the bathroom and then left to care for others. The client fell while going to the bathroom. X-ray films revealed a fractured femur. The client was unable to reach the call light; the private room door was shut, and it was claimed that he lay in pain for half an hour before the nurse returned.

Element of duty

The first element to be established when the possibility of negligence is being assessed is duty to the client. Basically the nurse must protect the client against unreasonable risks by adhering to a certain standard of conduct. How is a nurse to know what the standard of conduct is?

In response to this question, the ANA standards of care or the ANA code of nursing ethics may come to mind. These nationally accepted professional guidelines for the conduct of nursing practice can be used by a trial lawyer. The situation is similar to obtaining a nurse expert witness. A lawyer might ask, "Would this [citing alleged negligence] be common practice by a nurse?"

As previously discussed, the *Standards of Clinical Nursing Practice*[4] states that nurses do assessments and that nursing diagnoses are derived from health status data. In this case, there was no indication in the client's chart that the nurse had assessed mobility or gross muscle strength even though they were the reason for admission.

A nurse expert witness would probably testify that it was reasonable to expect that the risk factors (history of falls, muscle weakness, and possible multiple sclerosis) would suggest the diagnostic judgment of High Risk for Injury. The recognition of High Risk for Injury should be followed by supervision while ambulating and other preventive measures. Although this diagnosis was within the domain of nursing practice (Appendix A), there was no evidence that the diagnosis was made and supervision instituted.

Before resorting to the standards or nursing textbooks, the client's attorney should check the state nurse practice act. The incident occurred in one of the states whose nurse practice law includes the term *diagnosis* or *judgment.*

Lawyers also examine rules and regulations promulgated by state boards of nursing; some states specify the nursing process components as functions of the registered nurse. State practice acts and board of nursing rules and regulations are the legal basis for nursing; standards are professional, not legal, guidelines.

Breach of duty

The second element that must be present in negligence is breach of duty to a client. The chart in this man's case was evidence that the nurse did not conform to the state practice act: No diagnostic judgment was on record about the High Risk for Injury. Most important, there was no indication that the client's ambulation was being supervised by nurses.

Cause and effect

A relationship between the nurse's conduct and an alleged injury is the third element necessary for demonstrating negligence. In the case cited, a reasonably close relationship had to be demonstrated between the fracture and the nurse's lack of client supervision. *Why* the nurse did not supervise the client's ambulation is irrelevant from the legal perspective. The court is interested only in the fact that there was negligent supervision. Nurses and hospital administrators ask for the reason in order to prevent future occurrences; for example, why was a nursing history and examination not done at admission?

Nursing diagnosis represents a synthesis of clinical data and a judgment about whether or not a health problem is present. Once this synthesis and problem identification take place, it is difficult to ignore the state of the client. The nurse becomes motivated to act. This is how diagnosis helps prevent a breach of duty that results in harm to the client.

Harm or injury

The fourth element to be proven in a negligence case is actual injury (physical, psychological, or both) and loss, including economic loss. In the case illustrated, x-ray reports demonstrated a fractured femur. Because of the long period required for healing, economic loss as well as injury was claimed.

The main point to be understood from this discussion is that the law is concerned with diagnosis in only one respect. That is, the court wishes to establish what the state of the client is. Once this is established, the law is primarily concerned with nursing actions appropriate to the client's state. An act that is *committed* or *omitted* in regard to that state *and* results in harm is a basis for a malpractice determination. As Fortin and Rabinow state, "The law is primarily concerned with diagnosis-related action."[27] (p. 553)

Legal decisions

No cases have been found in which the court cited nursing diagnosis, although "judgment" increasingly appears to be something nurses are expected to exercise.

Can nurses make medical diagnoses? This is not the most fruitful way of framing the question. Rather, the question should be: What judgments are nurses expected to make? Two cases cited by Fortin and Rabinow[27] show that judgment beyond the domain of nursing diagnoses is expected.

In the first case, a company nurse was considered negligent for not recognizing a basal cell carcinoma and referring the employee who had developed it. As cited, the court said that "a nurse . . . should be able to diagnose . . . sufficiently to know whether it is a condition within her authority to treat as a first-aid case or whether it bears danger signs that should warn her to send the patient to a physician."[27] (p. 560) In the second case, nurses judged that a child's fever was not serious. No physician was called. The child died of congestive heart failure after an attack of rheumatic fever.[27] (p. 560) In both cases, the courts required the nurses to make tentative medical diagnoses to some degree. In many states the extent of a nurse's responsibility for making medical diagnoses is unclear.

Interpreting signs and symptoms and judging how to treat them (nursing diagnoses) or making referrals (tentative medical diagnoses) are nursing responsibilities. In both instances the nurse has the legal responsibility to use the diagnostic process skillfully. Otherwise diagnostic judgments may lead to injury and the risk of malpractice.

One additional point should be made. There are reasons some physicians pale when they encounter nursing diagnoses. They may believe they are legally responsible for *all* care. What needs to be clarified for such physicians is that a nurse practices under his or her own license, not the physician's. Second, it should be made clear to physicians that the law requires nurses to make diagnostic judgments; the previously mentioned court cases might be cited. Third, the nurse can find out whether the state practice acts or rules and regulations specify "diagnosis," "diagnostic judgments," or merely "judgment." If "diagnosis" is specified, physicians might be given copies of such state acts or rules. They may not have had the opportunity to learn the legal scope of nursing. In many medical schools little is taught about nursing practice.

DIAGNOSTIC RESPONSIBILITY

Who should diagnose? The answer is usually a classification, such as clinical specialist or professional, technical, or practical nurse. At times the question is abstract; at other times it is highly pragmatic and is posed for legal, administrative, or educational purposes. It may also be reworded: Who *can* diagnose? This wording introduces the idea of ability.

The answer is important when staffing and nursing care delivery are being examined. It is also important in decisions about delegating care to nonprofessionals when the nurse assumes managerial responsibility for groups of clients.

What the answer is depends on multiple factors. An exploration of these factors and the "state of art" of nursing diagnosis suggests that diagnosing is a professional activity influenced by the situation in which the professional is practicing. Bruce and Snyder[28] provide an excellent review of rights and responsibilities in diagnosis.

Legal considerations

Laws regulating nursing practice are not worded consistently from one state to another. In some states, practice acts specify diagnosis as a function of the registered nurse (baccalaureate, associate degree, and diploma graduates). The question is sometimes asked whether initial assessment and diagnosis can be delegated to practical nurses. Practice acts controlling practical nursing usually state that the practical nurse must have the *direction and supervision* of a registered nurse, physician, or dentist. Diagnostic judgment cannot be directed; thus it cannot be delegated. Moreover, supervision during assessment would require presence of a registered nurse as data are being collected; thus there is no point in delegating assessment.

Direction and supervision usually refers to the activities of observation and treatment. These can be clearly directed *after* diagnoses are made. Non-complex judgments related to observation and treatment are within practical nurses' scope of practice, but the complex diagnostic judgment is not.

The delegation of nursing diagnosis to practical nurses places an unwarranted burden on them. If harm occurs, it can easily be established that the practical nurse is not educated to diagnose and should not have accepted this responsibility. A comparable situation would exist if a physician delegated a liver biopsy to a registered nurse. Both risk malpractice claims if harm occurs.

This argument does not negate the fact that practical nurses contribute observations of importance to nursing diagnosis. Neither does it detract from their contribution to treatment, once the treatment plan has been specified.

Professional considerations

Registered nurses consider assessment, diagnosis, care planning, and evaluation to be professional—as well as legal—duties to their clients. Standards of practice, nursing textbooks, and journal articles specify diagnosis as a professional function. In addition, standards of the Joint Commission on Accreditation of Hospitals state that a registered nurse assesses clients and plans their care.[29] Clearly, consumers deserve professional nursing care.

NANDA supports the concept that only registered professional nurses are responsible and accountable for identifying nursing diagnoses for their patient population.[30] One argument for this statement rests within the educational curricula of nursing programs, as discussed in the next section.

Educational considerations

Another way of answering the question of who should diagnose is to examine the curricula of nursing programs. Such an examination reveals that diagnostic judgment is seldom if ever taught in practical nursing programs. In baccalaureate and master's degree programs, nursing diagnoses and the judgment skills used in making diagnoses are usually integrated into nursing courses.[31] In diploma and associate degree programs it may be expected that at least an introduction to nursing diagnosis is given when nursing process is taught. Currently diploma and associate degree graduates are prepared for registered nurse functions.

When competency statements for professional and technical practice (and thus education) are discussed, professional competency includes formulating nursing diagnoses. Technical nurses' competencies are usually viewed as the ability to contribute observations to the formulation of diagnoses and to understand relationships between diagnoses and care planning.

Process considerations

From earlier chapters it should be clear that the diagnostic process is not a task to be undertaken by nonprofessional nurses. Diagnosing requires a good clinical knowledge base, training in inferential and analytical skills, and the ability to conceptualize a client's condition for purposes of intervention. Nevertheless, it is not uncommon to hear that initial assessment or diagnosis may be delegated to nonprofessionals.

A distinct problem arises if one person collects clinical data (for example, taking the health history) and another tries to formulate diagnoses. A critical step is missed: branching on the basis of clinical knowledge and hypotheses. In earlier chapters, it was pointed out that assessment and diagnosis are not separate activities. *The diagnostic process begins after the first few pieces of information signifying a possible problem are collected.*

Furthermore, a diagnosis dictates care. It is impossible to separate the components of nursing process into an assembly-line activity. The nursing process is just that—a process—not independent steps.

A second major argument for diagnosis as a

professional activity is the clinical knowledge base required. If all nurses had equally good diagnostic process skills, the successful and unsuccessful diagnosticians could probably be separated on the basis of their theoretical knowledge, suggesting that the best diagnosticians would probably be at the clinical specialist level. These are the nurses who should be used as consultants to those less knowledgeable and experienced.

As an example, consider what many think is an "easy" diagnosis to make: High Risk for Skin Breakdown. Anyone can recognize reddened skin if motivated to do so. Yet to make an early diagnosis and institute preventive care, a multiplicity of factors in judgment must be weighed. It is not enough that a client is on bed rest; age, nutrition, current pathophysiology, motivation, and emotional state are also factors that determine the risk state. The weight of each factor must be considered in making the judgment that the client is at risk for skin breakdown.

The currently accepted diagnoses (Appendix A) may appear very basic. In fact, from a cognitive perspective, they require more complex judgments than do many medical diagnoses.

A third major argument for restricting diagnostic responsibility to professional nurses is the state of the art in nursing diagnosis. Professional nurses at this time are just learning how to formulate clients' actual and potential problems in diagnostic terms. Equally true, the diagnostic nomenclature is still evolving. When ambiguity exists, professionals are required. This is exemplified in the levels of certainty discussed in Chapter 3.

In other professions, it takes many years of training to be considered a good diagnostician by one's colleagues. Perhaps in the future, new nursing graduates, like medical interns, will routinely have the opportunity for a year of supervised practice. The value of postgraduate supervision of diagnosis and treatment is already recognized in psychiatric–mental-health nursing. Most people presumably agree that clients with other types of conditions also deserve this quality control.

Situational considerations

The reality is that not all clients who need nursing care have access to professional nurses. In some settings, such as primary care, the shortage of professional nurses may be related to insufficient reimbursement for nursing, a topic to be considered later. The lack of sufficient professional staff in nursing home settings is widely recognized, but barriers to change exist.

Why is there a shortage of professional staff? Conditions of employment have been implicated. Nursing as a profession has not articulated the client problems requiring professional care; in the absence of this information, staffing has been based on the only available data, the medical diagnosis and its severity. Yet no administrator would be able to refute the need for staff if there is documentation to show that nursing diagnoses are going untreated. It takes time to collect data on staffing needs in relation to the problems nurses treat, but such data may prove exceedingly useful in the long run to justify whether professional staff are needed.

In response to shortages, busy nurses too often delegate the history, examination, diagnosis, or care planning at admission to a nonprofessional person. In actuality, it would be safer to turn over technical or administrative duties to the nonprofessional. Professional care planning makes a difference; more specifically, diagnosis-based treatment makes a difference. Many will attest to this.

Experiential considerations

Among professional nurses there are both experienced and inexperienced diagnosticians. Some nurses may not have had the opportunity to learn diagnostic skills in basic or continuing education programs. In-service programs or self-study groups can remedy this.

As a nurse attains competency, whether a student or graduate, it is important that she or he recognizes the need for consultation. No one is an expert on everything. Legal and ethical considerations suggest that assistance should be sought from colleagues or specialists in the problem area. As in medicine, general practitioners in nursing seek specialist consultation for complex diagnostic problems. Thus the practitioner learns and the client receives quality care.

In summary, registered nurses have the responsibility for diagnosis. Within this category there may be varying levels of expertise. This variety is the result of the nature of educational programs as well as of continuing education opportunities.

Projections about the future indicate that clinical specialists will be the expert diagnosticians of the profession. Baccalaureate graduates will be competent in diagnosis and, through experience, will build on these competencies. The shorter programs cannot be expected to develop more than an introduction to the concept of diagnosis and diagnostic skills used in nurse referrals. Practical nurses will become aware of diagnosis and of the relevant data to be documented. Projections are always tentative, especially when a profession is in the process of change, as is currently the state in nursing. Furthermore, projections are not based on research in diagnostic competencies but rather on opinion derived from the legal, educational, and process considerations just discussed.

SUMMARY

In this chapter the use of nursing diagnoses in direct client care was discussed. Nursing process was described as the method nurses use to deliver care and to implement the concepts, values, and standards of nursing.

Two phases of the nursing process were delineated: problem identification and the focus of problem solving.

Nursing process involves an interrelated set of decisions. The discussion in the chapter covered how, in the problem-solving phase, a nursing diagnosis, describing the client's present state, is used as a focus for projecting health outcomes. The diagnosis and the desired outcomes are used in combination as a basis for decisions about nursing intervention.

One of the values held by the profession and expressed in its *Standards of Clinical Nursing Practice*[4] is individualized nursing care. Accordingly, although clients may have the same diagnosis and desired outcomes, *their individuality is considered in care planning.* Personal factors, the client's perceptions about the problem, its severity, the level of compensation, situational effects, and cost-benefit factors were discussed as considerations in care-planning decisions that individualize care.

To ensure *coordination of care,* and for legal reasons, communication of nursing process decisions is necessary. Both *written records* and *verbal communications* are enhanced by using nursing diagnoses to organize clinical data. The problem-oriented method of recording provides clarity of communication as well as an important cross-check of cognitive processes.

Using nursing diagnoses increases the clarity and conciseness of verbal and written communications. One result is improved coordination of care. Examples of communication in discharge planning demonstrated how diagnoses can be used to facilitate continuity of care.

In an examination of *nursing diagnosis and the law,* negligence was defined. In malpractice suits involving negligence, one criterion to be demonstrated is duty to the client. According to the professional standards of practice, duty includes diagnostic judgments. Some state nurse practice acts or board of nursing rules and regulations for practice also specify nursing diagnosis as within the scope of generic (general) registered-nurse practice. From a legal perspective, must the nurse diagnose? The law is concerned with whether harm and injury might have been prevented if a diagnostic judgment had been made and whether standards, acts, or rules and regulations were violated. Nursing diagnosis is a cognitive tool that directs conscious attention to the meaning of a set of cues. Attention to a client's need for care usually results in nursing action. This is how nursing diagnosis, as opposed to isolated and sometimes meaningless cues, protects a nurse against negligence litigation and a client against harm.

Who should diagnose? Standards and laws clearly dictate that diagnosis is a professional activity. Nonprofessionals contribute data as diagnoses are made. Can diagnosis be delegated to nonprofessionals? Certainly, just as cardiac surgery may be delegated to a registered nurse. However, no nurse would accept this delegation because none is prepared and licensed to practice medicine. The situation is similar where nursing diagnosis is involved. *Delegation* is associated with *legal risk,* both for the person delegating and for the one accepting. Nonprofessional activities, not assessment and diagnosis, are appropriately assigned to nonprofessional personnel. Professional authority should not be used to subject others to situations they are unprepared to handle.

NOTES AND REFERENCES

1. Combs AW, Avila DL, Purkey WW: *Helping relationships*, Boston, 1971, Allyn & Bacon.
2. Orem D: *Nursing: concepts of practice*, St Louis, 1985, Mosby.
3. There are many recognized specialty organizations in nursing. The American Association of Critical Care Nurses and the American Association of Neuroscience Nurses are examples. Most of these organizations publish their specialty standards of care with the ANA. Several of these organizations have published their core curricula, which contain specialty knowledge and standards. One example is *Core curriculum in rehabilitation nursing*, McCourt A, editor, Skokie, IL, 1993, American Association of Rehabilitation Nurses.
4. American Nurses Association: *Standards of clinical nursing practice*, Washington, DC, 1991, The Association.
5. American Association of Critical Care Nurses: *AACN outcome standards for nursing care of the critically ill*, Laguna Nigel, CA, 1990, The Association.
6. AHCPR: *Clinical practice guideline: acute pain management and pressure ulcers in adults: prediction and prevention*, Rockville, MD, 1992, US Department of Health and Human Services.
7. Committee on Nursing Practice Standards and Guidelines: *Guideline Panels Memo 3/2/92*, Washington, DC, 1992, American Nurses Association.
8. American Nurses Association: *Code for nurses with interpretative statements*, Washington, DC, 1985, The Association, pp 7-11.
9. American Nurses Association: *Nursing: a social policy statement*, Washington, DC, 1980, The Association.
10. The diagnostic category Self-Bathing/Hygiene Deficit has four levels. These levels of dependency (Chapter 6) may be used to state progress toward a client's independence.
11. Egan E, Snyder M, Burns K: Intervention studies in nursing: is the effect due to the independent variable? *Nurs Outlook* 40:187, 1992.
12. McCloskey J, Bulechek G: *Nursing intervention classification (NIC)*, St Louis, 1992, Mosby.
13. Bulechek G, McCloskey J: *Nursing interventions: essential nursing treatments*, Philadelphia, 1992, Saunders.
14. American Medical Association: *Physicians' current procedures terminology*, ed 4, Chicago, 1986, The Association.
15. Verran J: Delineation of ambulatory care nursing practice, *J Ambul Care Manage* 4:1, 1981.
16. Saba VK: A nursing intervention taxonomy for home health care, *Nurs Health Care* 12:296, 1991.
17. Martin KS, Sheet NJ: *The Omaha system: applications for community health nursing*, Philadelphia, 1992, Saunders.
18. Benner P: *From novice to expert: excellence and power in clinical nursing practice*, Menlo Park, CA, 1987, Addison-Wesley.
19. Kane M et al: *A study of nursing practice, role delineation and job analysis of entry-level performance of registered nurses*, Chicago, 1986, National Council of State Boards.
20. Gordon M: *Identification of high frequency–high treatment priority nursing diagnoses in critical care and rehabilitation nursing*, study in progress, 1993, and Herdman HT: *High frequency-high treatment priority nursing diagnoses in neonatal intensive care*, study in progress, 1993, Boston College School of Nursing, Chestnut Hill, MA 02617.
21. Carpenito LJ: *Nursing diagnosis: application to clinical practice*, Philadelphia, 1993, Lippincott, pp 28-36.
22. Sandelowski M: Toward a theory of technology dependency, *Nurs Outlook* 41:36, 1993.
23. Fairman J: Watchful vigilance: nursing care, technology, and the development of intensive care units, *Nurs Res* 41:56, 1992.
24. McKeehan KM: Nursing diagnosis in a discharge planning program, *Nurs Clin North Am* 14:517, 1979.
25. Note: The problem label heads the referral. Etiological factors are under assessment.
26. Mancini M: Proving negligence in nursing practice, *Am J Nurs* 79:337, 1979.
27. Fortin JD, Rabinow J: Legal implications of nursing diagnosis, *Nurs Clin North Am* 14:553, 1979.
28. Bruce JA, Snyder ME: Right and responsibility to diagnose, *Am J Nurs* 82:645, 1982.
29. Joint Commission on Accreditation: *Accreditation manual*, Chicago, 1993, The Commission.
30. McLane A: General assembly minutes. In Kim MJ, Moritz D, editors: *Classification of nursing diagnoses: proceedings of the third and fourth national conferences*, New York, 1987, McGraw-Hill.
31. McLane A: Nursing diagnosis in baccalaureate and graduate education. In Kim MJ, Moritz DA, editors: *Classification of nursing diagnoses: proceedings of the third and fourth national conferences*, New York, 1981, McGraw-Hill.

CHAPTER 11

RELEVANCE OF NURSING DIAGNOSIS TO PRACTICE ISSUES

In this chapter the relevance of nursing diagnosis to issues slightly removed from direct care is considered. The *assurance of quality care* for populations of clients is one issue. This area is examined in order to understand how diagnoses can be the focus for nursing quality assurance programs. Ideas in this section will be familiar because quality care review is a review of nursing process components and the outcomes of the process discussed previously. It will become evident that nursing diagnoses must be recorded during direct care in order for the required review to take place.

One factor that may influence quality care is the client's access to professional nurses. The section on *staffing patterns* demonstrates that current methods of allocating staff leave much to be desired in the opinion of institutional administrators. Staffing patterns are unsatisfactory partly because nursing has not sufficiently described client needs from a nursing perspective. Studies are in progress to design staffing patterns that are based on clients' nursing diagnoses. The essential understanding to be gained from the discussion is that each nurse must record clients' diagnoses and related interventions in order to help institutions plan professional staff allocations.

Access to professional nursing in the community is also a problem. The issue has some similarities to staffing problems in institutional care. In both settings the rationale for reimbursement for nursing care is either vague or lacking. An understanding of *third-party payment* for the treatment of nursing diagnoses may lead to a clearer articulation of what should be reimbursed.

Nursing diagnoses are relevant in determining the *scope of nursing practice*. Nurses need to communicate to consumers, legislators, and administrators specifically what health conditions they treat. In this chapter it is argued that the scope of practice becomes much clearer when nursing diagnoses are identified. Of course, not everything about nursing can be captured by nursing diagnoses; for instance, the personal intention and philosophy of a nurse as expressed in his or her caring interactions or transactions with clients.

Issues such as how to describe the domain of nursing practice will lead us to consider the development of nursing science. Nursing diagnosis is particularly relevant to this subject. Diagnoses may offer a focus for the development of *nursing practice theory,* which will eventually provide scientific knowledge to be used in direct care activities.

Identifying health conditions that concern practicing nurses will have an impact on the issues already discussed. Thus we come full circle: As nursing diagnoses are identified a focus is provided for measuring quality client care, for allocation of professional staff, and for third-party reimbursement.

NURSING DIAGNOSIS AND QUALITY CARE REVIEW

As costs rise, consumers demand quality goods and services. People have long been concerned about the cost and quality of toasters, automobiles, and plumbers' services. Since more public funds have been funneled into government-sponsored health programs, demands for assurance of quality care have grown.

External review

In 1972 the Congress of the United States mandated professional review of health care services, particularly emphasizing medical services. Since that time, care delivered to recipients of Medicare (people over 65 years of age), Medicaid (low-income populations), and maternal and child health programs must be reviewed. A national and state-wide system of professional review was created. This system is responsible for ensuring that all health care whose costs are reimbursed from federal funds is *necessary*. In addition, care must (1) meet professional standards and (2) be provided economically in an appropriate setting (Public Law 92-603).

The federal legislation just described was based on the concept of *peer review*. This concept means that members of a profession develop the bases for evaluation of their care. They also carry out the evaluation process. Care may be reviewed (evaluated) while it is being given or retrospectively. In the latter case charts are examined after the clients are discharged. The purpose of peer review is to identify less-than-acceptable care delivery. Once problems are identified, remedial action can be taken. Through educational programs, administrators and practitioners may be helped to bring care to an accepted level.

In addition to the required review of hospital and long-term care, many institutions voluntarily submit to another type of care review carried out periodically by the national Joint Commission on Accreditation of Healthcare Organizations (JCAHO). The focus of the commission's review

is on the individual health care organization's plan for quality improvement, rather than on traditional quality assurance. One of the standards for accreditation that went into effect in 1992 is described below:

> Nursing care data related to patient assessment, nursing diagnoses and/or patient needs, the nursing interventions, and patient outcomes are permanently integrated into the clinical information system (for example, the medical record).[1]

This statement is consistent with the professional standards discussed in Chapter 10. When this JCAHO standard was instituted, there was much discussion regarding the deletion of the care plan requirement. A care plan for every patient had been a traditional requirement. Deletion of this requirement permitted the use of any documentation system that met the standard above, such as a computerized information system. Rather than deleting nursing diagnosis, treatment, and outcome, it makes these components much more visible than the "care plan" had done.

As discussed previously, there is an emphasis on outcomes of care in any quality care review. Outcomes indicate resolution of the nursing diagnosis or progress toward resolution. The accrediting body is interested in a well-defined program of quality assessment, correction of problems, and following this reassessment. Most important, reviewers are interested in the results of actions that were taken for improvement in the quality of care. This goal requires changes based on an ongoing internal review of the quality of the care delivered.

Internal review

In the discussions that follow, concepts of quality assurance are reviewed. This review provides a basis for understanding how nursing diagnosis may be used in care review, problem identification, and remedial actions. It is also important to understand the concept of accountability to consumers that underlies quality assurance.

Assuring quality care for large groups of clients is sometimes thought of as a responsibility only of administrators. Actually, *concepts of quality assurance must be integrated into every nurse's practice*. Regardless of whether they are directly or indirectly involved in quality assurance, nurses should clearly understand issues such as this that affect their professional practice. Understanding is facilitated when each nurse becomes involved in developing standards, reviewing care, or planning for care improvement. As professionals, all nurses are responsible and accountable for the standards that are set for their practice and the level of care delivered to consumers.

Overview of concepts

What are measures of quality nursing care? This is the first question to be answered when a department of nursing begins quality care review. Various options exist. The competence of nurses certainly influences quality care, as do the resources they have available. Also, what nurses do for clients has an impact on care and can be measured. Finally, it is argued that the outcome of care, that is, the health state of the client, is one of the best measures of quality care delivery.

The areas just discussed represent three traditional components of care delivery that can be evaluated within a health care organization:

Structure

Process

Outcome

In each of these components, standards and guidelines can be developed using sources such as research literature and expert opinion. The three components are defined below (*standards* is used as a generic term):

1. *Structural standards* are statements describing valued characteristics of the care delivery setting. These characteristics indirectly influence care. Some examples are the number and preparation of nurses, physical facilities, equipment availability, in-service education, policies, and procedures.
2. *Process standards* are statements describing valued characterisitics of care delivery. They describe what consumers can expect from nurses (assessment, diagnosis, planning, and so forth). Standards of care are process standards. Treatment guidelines for the management of nursing diagnoses contain specific process standards.
3. *Outcome standards* are statements describing the health characteristics, behavior, or

state of the client. Descriptions of a client's mobility and of a client's knowledge about medications are examples of the focus of these standards. Outcomes are presumed to result from nursing intervention (although cause-and-effect relationships are hard to establish).

Theoretically structural, process, and outcome components are interrelated as are links in a chain. Structural resources are needed to carry out the processes of care delivery; in turn, processes (interventions) influence client health outcomes. Yet many other factors operating in either the client or the environment may influence outcomes.

The focus of *standards* has been changed in recent years in order to be consistent with terms used by the U.S. Department of Health and Human Services and its Agency for Health Care Policy and Research.[2] Standards are statements that describe the professional behavior of all nurses. In contrast, a *guideline* contains recommendations for care management that pertain to particular populations. (A *population* is a classification or grouping of clients who have some characteristic in common. A diagnosis may be a characteristic used as a basis for grouping.) The term *guideline* is probably more neutral from a legal standpoint than is the term *treatment standard*. In addition, guidelines serve as criteria for judgments about quality care. The following definitions will be used in the discussion on quality assurance: *Guidelines* are recommendations to assist nurses in making decisions about therapeutic management with specific nursing diagnoses or clinical conditions. *Criteria* are guideline statements used as a basis for measuring quality of care.

Setting standards for client populations is an activity of great importance. Once set, they cannot be ignored. In a sense they are a commitment to certain health care values. Suppose, for example, a standard is set in a hospital for clients with high risk for fluid volume deficit; ethically, the standard should then be met for every patient with that diagnosis. Standards should be based on the best scientific and clinical knowledge available. They must be realistic and attainable in all situations unless there are extenuating circumstances.

To understand the issue, imagine for a moment that your colleagues are going to use a set of criteria to grade (evaluate) your nursing care or your clients' health outcomes. Imagine further that outsiders are going to know what grade you receive. Are you concerned about *what* is evaluated and *how* the evaluation is done? For example, do you want your colleagues to measure *what patient education you provided?* Or instead, should they evaluate *your clients' health knowledge and skills?* Suppose you taught a client how to take his medications, but when your care was evaluated the client stated incorrect information. Does that mean you gave poor quality care?

There is a second important issue with which nurses must be concerned. Full accountability may be assumed only for the health problems nurses diagnose and treat. This statement may seem so logical that it need not be said. As quality assurance began, however, criteria sets were developed according to medical conditions such as Myocardial Infarction and Appendectomy. This gave the impression that nurses were assuming accountability for quality of care not within their control. Actually, the criteria sets were mislabeled; many sets contained processes and outcomes of unlabeled *nursing* diagnoses.

Nursing diagnoses describe the independent domain of nursing practice. Thus nurses assume accountability for health problems described by these diagnostic labels. It follows logically that nursing diagnoses should be used to define client populations for care review[3-5] and that diagnoses provide the ideal tool for writing guidelines, identifying care delivery problems and planning remedial actions.

The use of nursing diagnoses as a framework for care review brings some uniformity to quality assurance activities in different health care settings. Criteria based on diagnoses rather than on unique features of one setting or another may be shared and consequently decrease the cost of implementing review programs.

Selecting populations

The national guidelines cited in Chapter 10 and Appendix M were based on populations (e.g., clients with pressure ulcer, incontinence, or pain) that generated high health care costs. Health care agencies planning to develop guidelines may want to focus on high-volume, high-cost conditions. In a health care setting a small, representative group of nurses usually undertakes the task of developing

> ## USEFUL QUESTIONS FOR IDENTIFYING TRACERS OF QUALITY NURSING CARE
>
> 1. Does the tracer diagnosis have a definite functional impact on clients?
> 2. Is the tracer diagnosis relatively well defined and easy to diagnose?
> 3. Is the incidence of the tracer diagnosis high enough for adequate data to be collected?
> 4. Does the quality of nursing care influence the progression of the tracer diagnosis?
> 5. Is the prevention or treatment of the tracer diagnosis sufficiently well defined?
> 6. Are the effects of nonnursing (environmental) factors on the tracer diagnosis sufficiently understood?
>
> Adapted from Kessner DM, Kalk CE, Singer J: Assessing health quality: the case for tracers, *N Engl J Med* 288:189-194, 1973.

guidelines. This task requires a set of decisions. Because of time and costs, it is seldom possible to review all care given to all patients; therefore the first decision is to designate several diagnostic populations. Later the number of populations may be increased. To decide which patient populations will be studied, high-incidence nursing diagnoses must be identified by staff familiar with the setting. A listing such as that in Appendix A or data in Table 10-2 can facilitate the process of selection.

Tracer methodology is a systematic way of making final decisions about populations.[5] The common nursing diagnoses identified by staff may be narrowed by use of this technique. A tracer is a nursing diagnosis that can reflect the quality of care being delivered. For example, High Risk for Skin Breakdown may be one good tracer for long-term institutional care. A tracer such as Noncompliance or Health Management Deficit (Specify) may reflect an aspect of ambulatory care quality.

The questions in the box above may be applied to a list of diagnoses that are common in the particular setting. Those nursing diagnoses that have most of the characteristics are probably good tracers, and the clients who have those diagnoses become the tracer populations. Problems in selecting the focal population for the guideline will arise. For example, if a high-volume, high-treatment priority nursing diagnosis in a particular service is Self-Care Deficit Related to Activity Intolerance, it seems logical that a treatment guideline be based on Activity Intolerance. The guideline would address diagnosis, treatment, and prevention, as do the national guidelines.[2] As work begins, the developers will have to see if Self-Care Deficit is only relevant to outcome, not treatment, guidelines. Are guidelines written only for conditions nurses treat, that is, for etiological or related factors? (Many conditions in Appendixes A and B are the focus of treatment.) This approach sounds reasonable, but only experience will determine the best method.

Writing guidelines

Sufficient nursing literature exists to enable nurses to begin to delineate processes and outcomes for currently approved nursing diagnoses. As clinical research on these conditions grows, guidelines will have a more substantial research base. Until then theory, the available research, and expert opinion will prevail.

The box on the right illustrates a commonly used model for writing guidelines. When treatment guidelines are written, both the problem and the etiological factors must be considered. Look at the differences in the standards in Table 11-1. Although the problem in the two diagnoses is the same, the criteria are different because the etiological factor differs. The probable cause of a condition directly influences what is done to treat it; thus the acceptable criteria for what is done changes with the etiological factors. Table 11-2 contains another example of process criteria.

Outcome standards are characteristics of the client that describe a desired health state; they describe only the state of the client, not how it came about. If the health problem improves or disappears, the assumption is that quality care was delivered. Outcome standards and their measurement were important when determinations were made about the appropriateness and effectiveness of care. As McCourt[4] reports, they are extremely important today:

Consideration is now being given to the feasibility of using outcomes as indicators for reimbursement, for de-

---

MODEL FOR WRITING STANDARDS/CRITERIA FOR NURSING DIAGNOSES

1. Diagnostic category (from NANDA-approved list).
2. Specific nursing diagnosis (related to category).
3. Assessment criteria (defining characteristics of nursing diagnosis).
4. Etiologies or risk factors (major causes of health problems).
5. Process criteria (interventions)(statements to guide nursing care of groups of patients).
6. Outcome criteria (projected goals) (changes in health status resulting from nursing interventions).
7. Review of literature (significant references).
8. Standards Committee, New England Sinai Hospital (date)

From McCourt A: Nursing diagnosis: key to quality assurance. In Hurley M, editor: *Classification of nursing diagnoses: proceedings of the sixth conference,* St Louis, 1986, Mosby.

---

termining level of nursing home placement, and even for licensure of long-term care facilities. This thinking reflects the rapidly changing climate of professional accountability.[4 (p. 137)]

When outcomes are being written, the definition and defining characteristics of the problem statement are helpful; for accepted diagnoses they may be found in manuals.[7,8] When defining characteristics are converted to positive health behaviors, they provide the content for outcomes. For example, the outcome indicating resolution of Impaired Home Maintenance Management might be one of those listed in Table 11-3. They are the opposite of the critical defining characteristics of the diagnosis. Similarly, converting the characteristics of a diagnosis such as Ineffective Coping to the signs of effective coping results in measurable outcomes. In most instances, irrespective of the probable cause (etiology), with quality care the outcome should be attained. Therefore, etiological factors are not as influential when outcome stan-

Table 11-1   Diagnosis-Specific Process Criteria

Diagnosis:	Impaired Home Maintenance Management/ Decreased Activity Tolerance (Level 2)
Process standards:	1. Energy conservation techniques for cleaning, cooking, lifting, pushing, etc., are taught.
	2. Assistance is given in planning home management activities and rest periods.
Diagnosis:	Impaired Home Maintenance Management/ Knowledge Deficit (hygiene practices)
Process standards:	1. Relationships between the lack of hygienic home practices (cleanliness, food storage), the spread of harmful microorganisms, and human infections are explained.
	2. Assistance is given in planning home maintenance responsibilities with family.
	3. Information is given about methods and resources to prevent vermin.

Table 11-2   Diagnosis-Specific Process Criteria*

Diagnosis	High risk for pressure ulcer
Process criteria:	1. Systematic skin inspection once a day with attention to bony prominences.
	2. Skin cleansing at time of soiling and (specify times). Tepid water and mild cleansing agent applied with minimal force and friction.
	3. Maintain room humidity at 40% or higher; for dry skin, apply a dry-skin moisturizer.
	4. No massage over bony prominences.
	5. Avoid shear during positioning, transfer, and turning; reduce friction by use of lubricants, protective films, protective dressings, and protective padding.
	6. Inadequate protein and caloric intake corrected by support with eating, supplements, or enteral/ parental feeding.
	7. Current activity level, mobility, and range of motion maintained or improved if compatible with goals of therapy and potential.
	8. Interventions and outcomes monitored and documented.[6]

*See Appendix M.

dards for populations are written. Notice that in Table 11-1 the probable causes of the two diagnoses were Decreased Activity Tolerance and Knowledge Deficit (Hygienic Practices). Clients with Impaired Home Maintenance Management from *either* cause should reach the same accepted outcome.

Although not influencing the *content* of outcomes, etiological factors influence the length of time to their attainment. Outcomes must be realistic (attainable); hence the time frame may be different when etiological factors require complex, extended interventions.

The time by which the outcome must be reached is specified. For a population with Impaired Home Maintenance Management, food stored safely (1 week) would be an example. Some outcome standards also require consistency of client behavior across time; for example, food found stored safely at three visits (3 weeks). Thus the client's progress would be assessed, but outcome attainment would not be evaluated against the criteria until after 3 weeks and three visits.

In addition to nursing diagnoses, nurses assume accountability for assisting clients in carrying out therapy ordered by physicians. Although no data exist, it may be estimated that nursing judgment is involved in nearly 50% of the disease-related acute care clients receive. This percentage in-

Table 11-3 Diagnosis-Specific Outcome Criteria

Diagnosis:	Impaired Home Maintenance Management
Outcome standards*:	1. Food stored safely
	2. Wastes disposed of safely
	3. Vermin absent
	4. Surroundings generally clean

*Time and methods of measurement are not specified.

cludes making and reporting clinical observations and judgments about complications, administering "as necessary" medications, and carrying out protocols. How is this aspect of nursing care reviewed?

The quality assurance review of medical-diagnosis–specific nursing care requires only process standards. Nurses do not assume accountability for medical, or disease-related, outcomes.[9]

Process standards can be developed for complications, actions based on assessments, and actions based on physician orders or hospital protocols. Caution must be exercised in writing these standards. Expectations cannot go beyond the knowledge commonly acquired in professional education, and processes for the treatment of nursing diagnoses must not be mislabeled under medical diagnostic population groups.

Information retrieval

After criteria (guidelines) are written, the quality of care is evaluated. Clients' permanent records are reviewed to see whether (1) admission was necessary (facility utilization review); (2) care being delivered is at an acceptable standard (concurrent review or retrospective review); and (3) outcome standards are reached (retrospective review). The time expenditures and other costs make it necessary for most monitoring to be done by reviewing clients' records. Thus it is extremely important that daily recordings be clear, concise, and complete.

There are difficulties, but not unsolvable ones, in grouping clients and writing criteria according to nursing diagnoses. In most health care settings clients' records can be retrieved (selected for inclusion in the audit) only on the basis of medical diagnoses. This chart retrieval system exists because hospital statistical reports are based on medical diagnoses. Unless provision has been made to also record nursing diagnoses in the call-up system, record retrieval is difficult. For example, 100 charts of clients with ineffective coping patterns or impaired home maintenance management cannot be easily retrieved from among 10,000 records.

The mechanical problem of retrieval does not have to dictate the way criteria are written. Nurses are working toward placing nursing diagnoses in computerized or other information systems. Until this occurs other methods of record retrieval must be used.

One method is to use medical diagnoses for retrieval and nursing diagnoses as a focus for writing standards.[2] (pp. 85-86) A second method of retrieval is to write discharge notes containing both resolved and current (unresolved) nursing diagnoses. This kind of discharge note makes it easier for record librarians to code and retrieve records according to nursing diagnoses.

Interdisciplinary reviews

Some institutions combine nursing, medical, and other health professionals' quality care reviews into one program.[4] Again, because of the retrieval process, medical diagnosis is usually the main client classification. Nursing diagnoses may be a subset.

Interpretation of care reviews

If standards are not reached by the specified time, two alternative interpretations are possible. One possibility is that quality care was delivered but client or situational factors interfered with the expected outcome. If clients with Noncompliance/Knowledge Deficit become disoriented, it is understandable that they might not attain the expected knowledge level. This kind of situation constitutes an exception to the standard, but information about the client's disorientation would have to be found in the client's chart.

Not reaching an outcome may also mean that treatment of a particular nursing diagnosis was not at an acceptable level. This finding leads to the identification of care delivery problems.

Identifying problems

The use of nursing diagnoses in population monitoring facilitates identification of care delivery problems. The group of clients who are receiving less than quality care is clearly specified, and the reasons for the inadequate care can be determined.

Problems in care delivery are identified by raising questions. For example: Why did 30% of the client population with the diagnosis of High Risk for Fluid Volume Deficit develop dehydration? Why did 10% of the population with High Risk for Skin Breakdown develop pressure ulcers (bedsores)?

Where do auditors find the answers to these questions? The nurse who thinks that possible answers lie in the processes of care (nursing interventions) or in the structural resources of the setting has grasped a major concept in quality care assessment. That is exactly where nurses look for the reasons why client outcomes are below standard. Charts that do not pass the outcome screening standard are examined. Guidelines that have been developed for relevant diagnoses (for example, High Risk for Fluid Volume Deficit and High Risk for Skin Breakdown) are compared to the actual care documented in the chart. It may be found that treatments for these diagnoses were not consistent with accepted standards of treatment. Why?

For answers, structural factors in the setting are examined. Was there sufficient staff competent in treating clients with these diagnoses? Did they have the necessary equipment and materials, such as special mattresses to prevent pressure ulcerations? Does the method of nursing care delivery or philosophy of care promote individual accountability for the treatment of diagnosed problems? These searching questions are asked by both practitioners and administrators.

It is advisable to begin a quality care assurance program with a concurrent audit of all (or a sample of) charts, using the ANA standards (p. 218). This preliminary audit may be done while committees are preparing diagnostic population standards. The major elements for this general audit are identified in the box on the right. Included in the general process audit are assessment, diagnosis, outcomes, in-

---

GENERAL PROCESS AUDIT

1. Assessment contains information relevant to Health perception–health management
   Nutritional-metabolic
   Elimination
   Activity exercise
   Sleep-rest
   Cognitive-perceptual
   Self-perception–self-concept
   Role-relationship
   Sexuality-reproductive
   Coping–stress-tolerance
   Value-belief
2. Nursing diagnoses are supported by and consistent with history and assessment data.
3. Unstable or potentially unstable physical parameters are identified for observation; for example:
   Blood pressure
   Pulse
   Level of consciousness
4. Outcomes for diagnoses are stated.
5. Diagnosis-specific nursing activities are listed in the plan of care.
6. Progress notes are written about each diagnosis.
7. Information relevant to progress toward outcomes is documented.

---

terventions, and evaluation of progress toward discharge outcomes. At this early point in the audit only the presence or absence of these elements is the objective of the audit.

An audit of this type identifies gross deficiencies. If nursing diagnoses, plans of care, progress notes, and discharge assessments of care outcomes are not recorded, diagnostic populations cannot be monitored economically. Thus the first step is to determine whether broad standards are being met. If not, why not? After remedial actions are taken by nurses to correct these charting deficiencies, the previously described tracer population audits can be done from records.

When quality care assurance programs are built on nursing diagnoses, periodic review of the validity of diagnoses may be necessary. Nurses may not be making valid assessments or correct diagnostic judgments; these errors affect audits that are based on recorded diagnoses. Periodic review of items 1 and 2 in the box on p. 261 would reveal these diagnostic errors. An actual reassessment of some clients might be done to check diagnostic accuracy, but this procedure involves added time and expense. The same problem occurs in medicine. An elevated blood pressure may have been overlooked, but this lack of diagnosis and treatment would not be revealed in a process or outcome audit of a fractured-femur population.

Taking remedial actions

Using nursing diagnoses for developing guidelines and identifying problems facilitates the next step in quality assurance. That is the step of nurses taking remedial actions. Let us suppose that both the resources and the care provided are problems found in certain diagnostic populations. As an example, consider the situation in which the incidence of skin breakdown is too high. Nurses and administrators determine the problem is twofold: inadequate professional staff and inadequate methods of prevention used by current staff.

The ultimate purpose of quality care review is to offer opportunities for institutional administrators and care providers to improve care. In the skin breakdown example, reasonable actions would include (1) obtaining more professional staff and (2) increasing staff education programs. The nursing diagnosis and management of High Risk for Skin Breakdown would be an excellent topic for inservice education programs in this setting. Early diagnosis, judgments about risk factors, and prevention need to be emphasized. If the problem was correctly identified and addressed, it should now be found that standards indicating quality care are being reached.

In summary, accountability to the consumer underlies quality assurance programs. Individual nurses of course evaluate the effectiveness of the care they give to individual clients; quality assurance evaluates the nursing care delivered to groups of clients. In essence, care review requires that nurses decide in what areas of health care their accountability lies. Clearly, nurses' accountability, first and foremost, is to the health problems described by nursing diagnoses. Just as physicians as-

sume accountability for quality treatment of diseases described by medical diagnoses, nurses assume accountability for recognizing and intervening in the dysfunctional health patterns described by nursing diagnoses.

Writing standards, identifying problems that exist, and taking remedial actions are made easier when nursing diagnoses are used. Diagnoses impart clear direction to these activities. The result is that nursing assures quality of care within its own domain of practice. When each profession achieves this, overall health care quality is assured.

Future directions

Two issues are clearly important to the future of quality assurance. One is the need for a scientific base for nursing care evaluation. The second is the identification of care delivery problems and creative solutions that have immediate payoff in terms of quality.

Writing standards of care makes it clear to all involved that "mature knowledge" (replicated studies) in nursing is sparse. There is a great diversity of opinion when a group of nurses try to state what nurses should do for a particular nursing diagnosis and what health results are expected. Even if the matter of quality assurance is put aside, research is needed to determine effective treatments and related outcomes as a basis for everyday practice.

The second major issue for the next few years is the cost-benefit aspect of quality assurance. In simplest terms, activities have to pay off; thus problems in care delivery must be prioritized. The highest priority must be given to those care delivery problems that have a significant impact on illness, death rates, and actual financial costs.

Inadequate preventive care is one example of a care delivery problem that, when remedied, can lower health care costs. If potential problems were diagnosed and preventive care instituted, many dollars and days of disability could be saved. It is estimated that the treatment of a decubitus ulcer costs thousands of dollars, but preventive nursing care of 2 hours daily costs less than $20 a day. As a second example, imagine the reduction in cost, disability, and mortality if people were helped to improve their functional health patterns. Merely reducing the speed limit on highways has enormously lowered the number of automobile accidents, one of the leading causes of death and disability.

One hospital, by focusing nurses' attention on the nursing diagnosis High Risk for Injury, substantially reduced clients' falls.[10] Imagine the savings in money and days of disability and discomfort if even 10 fractures of the hip were prevented. This is an example of identifying care delivery problems that have immediate payoff in monetary and human costs. Containing these costs will be the major emphasis in future quality assurance activities.

A number of factors should facilitate the development of quality assessment and quality assurance programs. As discussed in Chapter 10, McCloskey and Bulechuk's study[11] begins to identify, label, and classify nursing interventions. Work is also beginning on identifying, labeling, and classifying outcomes.[12] And, as will be seen below, a national data base for nursing is already a reality.

NURSING DIAGNOSIS AND NATIONAL DATA BASES

A *data base* is a collection of information on particular elements or things. For example, all the courses in a college and all the students registered for each of those courses in an academic year constitutes a data base in the university information system. To continue the analogy, a national data base in the U.S. Department of Education may include the percentage of students in U.S. colleges and universities who are majoring in nursing or in the health-related disciplines. The latter might provide interesting statistics about the size of the future work force in these disciplines.

Statistics on the conditions of therapeutic concern that are described by nursing diagnoses will never be available without a national data base. Such a data base requires a uniform nursing language system.[13,14] Four evolving nursing classification systems were recently placed in the National Library of Medicine Metathesaurus of the Unified Medical Language System[13,15]:

1. Taxonomy I, developed by the members of the North American Nursing Diagnosis Association[7]
2. Classification of Nursing Interventions, developed as part of the University of Iowa Intervention Project[11]

3. Client Management Information System for Community Health Nursing Agencies, developed by the Omaha Visiting Nurse Association[16]
4. SABA Home Health Care Classification, developed at Georgetown University[17]

Readers should be familiar with the concept of a thesaurus, which provides synonyms for words. A metathesaurus provides a structure for cross-indexing similar words.

The advantage of a metathesaurus in the health care field is that all nursing and medical data bases may be cross-indexed. A second advantage is that the computer can generate information on how much overlap exists in classifications 1, 3, and 4 in the list above and how much overlap there is in classifications 2, 3, and 4. Also, the thesaurus will enable developers to access the words that are available to describe a particular phenomenon so that developers need not create their own. The thesaurus will also enable developers of information systems in health care organizations to access terminology. The distinct advantage to people who have been wedded to a particular system is that such a thesaurus allows them to access all studies on a particular NANDA diagnosis, as well as studies on synonyms in another system, such as the Omaha and SABA. As the head of the national task force, Norma Lang, recently said:

> Ultimately, we envision the nurse in clinical practice—who may need information on an intervention—having direct computer access to such a system.[13]

In addition, a uniform nursing language for diagnoses, interventions, and outcomes will facilitate billing for services and analyzing the cost of nursing care.

NURSING DIAGNOSES AND THIRD-PARTY PAYERS

At what stage health care reform will be when this book is published is anyone's guess. Will it be a single-payer system, a pay-or-play system, an incremental reform of the present system, or "business as usual"? Whatever the stage of health care reform, it is predicted that nursing will have a greater role than before. Let us consider where we are as a basis for examining the evolving reform.

A large proportion of U.S. citizens pay for nursing care through a third party, commonly an insurance company. In fact, as will be discussed, a fourth party—the physician or hospital—enters into the payment for nursing care. A brief overview of the current system of paying for care will demonstrate that some people have minimal access to nursing care and some have little choice. The historical development of the situation is interestingly portrayed by Welch[18]; changes in the current situation may be facilitated by nursing diagnosis.

Rather than paying for health services at the time of care delivery, people pay monthly premiums to nonprofit (for example, Blue Cross and Blue Shield) or profit-making (Mutual of Omaha, Aetna, etc.) companies. Also, government funds are available for care of the elderly (Medicare) or medically indigent (Medicaid). Insurance companies and the government are referred to as *third-party payers,* and their process of payment is called *reimbursement.*

Treatment of a nursing diagnosis, except in a few instances, is not reimbursed. This means that consumers do not have direct access to nursing unless they are willing to pay the fees themselves. It means, furthermore, that the poor and medically indigent have no choice in the type of care provider they can choose. Yet there are loopholes whereby payment for nursing can be obtained.

A client who wants nursing care may be admitted to a hospital or clinic; the nursing is included in the reimbursable bed-and-board charges or clinic fees. But to get into a hospital, the client must have a disease or possible disease. Another route is to convince a physician that nursing care is needed. If a physician certifies the need, a client can obtain home nursing, private duty nursing, or community-based care by a nurse in private practice. As Jennings[19] points out, although consumers are paying high premiums, in the current system a consumer is not entitled to receive any health care unless it is directed or executed by a physician.

Under the current system, many functional health problems are not diagnosed early or are not diagnosed until disease is present. Many cases could be cited: the untreated Body Image Disturbance that must progress to Severe Depression; the potential shoulder contracture that, when fully developed a year after mastectomy, requires surgery; and the Ineffective Coping pattern that is not di-

agnosed until child abuse results. As many have said, the current health care system is disease oriented rather than preventive care oriented.

What can be done? Groups are currently working with legislators and insurance companies to determine reimbursement plans. This, of course, is a threat to the current system. Counteracting proposals, such as reimbursement for health education when ordered by the physician, continue to be offered.

Consumers need to be informed about the controls the present system imposes on access to care. Public education requires clear communication about what is to be reimbursed. Communication should be focused on the actual and potential health problems nurses diagnose and treat, rather than on tasks nurses do. Competency and quality care can be assured to consumers and third-party payers if the reasons (nursing diagnoses) for actions are specified.

In addition to these efforts to obtain reimbursement for community-based care, work is underway to study the use of nursing diagnoses to determine costs of hospital nursing. This work involves the concept of client classification for staff allocation, which is discussed later in this chapter.

Prospective payment programs

Prospective payment to hospitals for persons covered by the federal Medicare program was introduced in 1982. This means that hospitals know prior to care delivery what payment will be received for particular diseases. Previously, costs were established after services were delivered. This is similar to your employer (or school) telling you prior to a trip to Boston how much money you will receive to finance your trip, instead of you submitting your actual costs after your return. Think of how these two different situations might influence your behavior and you will appreciate the magnitude of change that has occurred in health care reimbursement. Thompson and Diers[20] described the reasons the federal government changed from retrospective to prospective payment:

1. Spiraling health care costs
2. Increasing use of hospital services
3. Wide variation in care costs among hospitals

A method of payment based on a standard cost for

specific disease groupings was instituted in the early 1980s. These standard costs are based on resources consumed. Payment remains the same regardless of the length of hospital stay or the number of tests given. Clients with (1) similar conditions who supposedly use (2) similar resources which cost (3) a similar amount are grouped together. The 468 disease groupings are called diagnostic-related groups (DRGs). Hospitals classify individual clients into the DRG group that includes their disease/surgery/complications. There is a *standard payment for each DRG and a standard room and board for the length of stay* permitted under the DRG. Similar to the "prospective payment" for the trip to Boston, hospitals keep the extra money they will receive if they can decrease the costs and length of stay below the DRG allowance. They absorb the extra cost if there are more services and a longer stay. Hospitals, as well as the traveler to Boston, have to pay attention to cost control.

The DRG prospective payment system is saving money, but the results of these changes are: a strain on home health care agencies; people going home earlier and sicker; people in hospitals more acutely ill; and many procedures and surgery, formerly done in the hospital, being done in clinics and health maintenance organizations. For example, Medicare paid hospitals $1200 to $1500 for placing an artificial lens in a patient's eye on an in-patient basis but paid hospitals or physicians up to $2800 for this procedure if done on an outpatient basis[19]; this type of inequity encourages the extension of cost controls. After this introduction to prospective payment, the question arises: *What is the relevance of nursing diagnosis?* Nursing diagnosis accounts for a substantial portion of the costs of care and influences discharge from hospital settings.

DRGs AND NURSING DIAGNOSIS

A DRG refers only to medical diagnoses, not nursing diagnoses. This is because DRGs (1) take into account only the therapeutic services the client receives and (2) assume that all care is disease-related.[21] This is a shocking situation. Traditionally, nursing has been part of the "bed and board" charges. It is covered under the per diem rate for a particular DRG, along with housekeeping and

meal services. A number of researchers have pointed out the problems.[22-24] For instance, not all clients within a DRG require a similar intensity of nursing care; individual clients have different nursing diagnoses. Also, nursing diagnoses are one reason the length of stay in a hospital varies. This suggests that nursing diagnosis is extremely important in any cost containment program and raises more questions: *What increases resource consumption and costs? What increases length of stay in the hospital?* The consumption of resources in-creases above the average for the DRG if complications result or if the length of stay is exceeded. Also, too early discharge may result in readmission, complications, and death. Below are some important points in delivering care:

1. If High Risk for Injury, Skin Breakdown, or Infection is not diagnosed and treated, costs can increase. In general, risk-factor control is important both for cost containment and for preventing client discomfort.

2. Inattention to *early discharge planning,* especially for clients who have High Risk for Impaired Mobility, Pain Management Deficits, Self-Care Deficits, or Impaired Home Maintenance Management, which can prolong the length of stay. Discharge planning should begin when the diagnosis is made and outcomes projected.

3. Delays in diagnosis and ineffective treatment plans can prolong hospitalization. In some instances the lack of recognition of clients' High Risk for Anxiety, Ineffective Coping, Situational Depression, or Body Image Disturbances can influence the course of convalescence and produce complications. *Precision in diagnosis and effective and efficient treatment methods* are important.

4. *Quality care review and monitoring of attained outcomes* at discharge are necessary to prevent discharge before the client is ready and when community or family resources are absent.

Most nurses are employed by hospitals; if a hospital loses money, the impact will be felt in salaries, reduced staffing, or layoffs. Nurses also appreciate the escalating costs of health care when they pay their own hospital insurance premiums. They have always tried to prevent unnecessary hospital admissions and maintained that most clients do better at home. Thus nurses are motivated to control costs, length of stay, and quality of care. A number of authors predict changes in the DRG system that will produce a more sensitive measure of the actual amount of resources consumed. It is likely that in the future DRGs will be supplemented with an acuteness-of-illness factor and nursing diagnoses. As will be discussed in Chapter 12, prospective payment systems and other health care issues increase the need for clinical studies to refine nursing diagnoses and link diagnoses/outcomes/interventions to cost. Nursing is definitely a therapeutic service, and nursing services have a definite impact on the cost and quality of care; it is important that this be demonstrated.

Halloran and colleagues[23] have implemented a nursing diagnosis classification system for determining staffing (Appendix O) that has yielded other interesting data. "The nursing diagnosis–based patient classification scheme supports the resource allocation decisions made by bedside nurses."[25 (p. 224)] For each client, nurses fill out a daily checklist of the nursing diagnoses of the clients they are treating. The use of this classification has revealed the following:

1. Having a greater percentage of registered nurses on a unit decreased the cost of care delivery.[26]
2. Nursing diagnoses predict the client's nursing care requirements with 50% more precision than do medical diagnoses.[22,23]
3. Nursing diagnoses predict 20% more of the variation in the patient's length of stay in an acute care setting than does the DRG.[27]
4. Nursing care is provided on the basis of the nurse's judgment about the level of patient need, *not on the basis of the medical diagnosis.*[25]

NURSING DIAGNOSIS AND STAFFING PATTERNS

Previously, the *number* of professional staff was used as an example of a structural characteristic of a care delivery setting that influences the quality of care. *Staffing pattern* refers to the allocation and utilization of nurses. An ideal pattern exists when the number and competency of the nurses who work in a setting match the nursing care requirements of the clients.

The degree of control a nurse has over the num-

ber of clients in his or her caseload varies with the institution. Whether or not involved in this determination, each nurse should have some understanding of how staffing is done and how daily assignments are made. If fewer staff are available than are needed, quality care or dedicated nurses suffer; if staffing is excessive, the cost to consumers and taxpayers rises.

This section includes a brief overview of how staffing patterns are determined and how nursing diagnoses can facilitate these decisions. The influence of nursing care requirements and budgetary allocations will be examined.

Current systems of classifying clients' care requirements receive much criticism. It is equally true that the way hospitals are currently reimbursed for care does not allow for variability in nursing care requirements. This in turn has an effect on staffing, as is illustrated in two projects that involve studies of nursing diagnosis as a basis for determining clients' use of nursing services.

The discussions that follow emphasize that (1) both internal and external factors influence staffing on a unit, (2) nurses need to find ways of describing their practice more accurately so that staffing patterns support quality care, and (3) nurses must incorporate diagnosis into their practice so that they can study the potential uses of nursing diagnosis.

Determination of staffing patterns

Nurses can set standards of quality care, but these standards will be difficult to realize if equal consideration is not given to staffing. Many factors influence the number of professional nurses on a hospital unit, in a clinic, or in a visiting nurse district. Two primary factors we shall consider are client care requirements and budgetary allocations.

Classification of care requirements

Client care requirements for a nursing unit may be determined by various means. The purpose is to predict the amount of *nursing time* that clients on a unit require. Quantifying care in terms of nursing time is the usual basis for allocating nurses.

Global approaches for determining nursing time, such as counting the number of clients, have been used. Such approaches are not too successful in predicting staffing needs because clients differ in their care requirements. Recognition of this fact has led to client classification as a basis for allocating nursing staff. *Classification* is the process of categorizing clients according to their nursing care requirements.

Classifications may be based on single or multiple indicators of care needs. For example, acuteness of illness is one gross predictor of required nursing time. It is assumed that critically ill clients need more nursing care time than do convalescent clients. If nurses gave only physical care, the assumption might be true.

What if health counseling and teaching were used as indicators of the nursing time required by clients? Then it might be found that convalescent clients need more or as much nursing time (and staff) as do critically ill clients. Clearly the indicator used for classifying clients ultimately influences decisions about staffing.

Most current systems of classification are based on task-oriented, "doing for" views of nursing. Clients' needs for bathing, feeding, ambulation, and medication are not always valid predictors of the professional nursing time required. These indicators do not take into account the scope of client problems and current standards of nursing care. By maintaining the status quo, classification systems of this type hinder developments in professional practice. In turn, clients are deprived of new developments in practice. A comparable situation would exist if a faculty-student ratio did not permit instructors to institute new methods of teaching or a physician-client ratio did not permit clients to benefit from new medical developments.

If professional staffing is based on poor predictors or poor use of predictors, shortages become the rule, not the exception. Understaffing limits the implementation of current practice standards, including nursing diagnosis. Yet, if instituted, nursing diagnoses may provide a more valid measure of staffing needs.

Simmons[28] recognized the utility of diagnosis as a basis for staffing specifically in relation to community heath nursing. Her comments about the use of nursing diagnoses (nursing problems) apply to other levels of care also:

Problem labels and their signs and symptoms, stated clearly and concisely, can be useful in interpreting community health nursing services to others. A clear interpretation of services can be especially crucial when the agency must compete for funding and justify the need for existing or new programs.

Cost analysis and cost effectiveness can be enhanced by using the problem classification scheme. Nursing activities can be related to specific client problems resulting in cost centers for different client needs. Proficient use of the problem classification scheme will demand less time in recording and allow more nursing time for direct client care.[28 (p. 5)]

Giovanetti[29] notes that classifications are consistent with current ways of thinking about practice and with the nomenclature of the time. When nursing was conceptualized as tasks and procedures, the presently used classification systems were developed. She states:

As the nomenclature changes, so will the basis for classification. Two relatively new nomenclatures to describe nursing process are now beginning to emerge: (1) patient problems and (2) nursing diagnoses. It seems reasonable to expect that as the validity of these descriptions becomes more evident, one or both may well lead to new patient classification systems, which, in turn, may be more responsive to the true nature of the patients' care requirements.[29 (p. 92)]

Budgetary allocations

A second important factor influences the number and competency of the nurses with which the unit is staffed. This factor is the budget allocated for nurses' salaries by the institution. The nursing department budget for salaries is usually about one third of a total hospital budget. To a great extent the hospital budget, and thus the salary budget, is controlled by outside forces.

Hospital income is based on direct client payments and reimbursement by insurance companies and public funds. The external control of reimbursement rates (by state agencies) directly influences nursing department budgets. State rate-setting commissions determine the reimbursement hospitals receive per client (excluding Medicare clients).

It must be recognized that in the majority of institutions the cost of nursing care *is included in the basic daily room charge.* This charge is a flat rate for all clients at particular levels of care (acute, intensive, long-term). As an example, reimbursement is not provided for clinical specialist consultation. In the past, when nursing mainly provided glorified maid service using apprentices, inclusion in the "hotel rate" may have been appropriate.

Today many nurses argue that nursing should be a separate charge, as are physical therapy, radiology, and other hospital services. Would this increase consumers' bills? Perhaps not; rather, there might be more equitable distribution. Those clients requiring minimal care would probably pay less than they now pay. Charging separately for nursing would also pressure the profession to determine a base for fee-for-service charges. Actual and potential problems diagnosed and treated by nurses may be an answer.

In summary, hospital staffing patterns are controlled both from within an institution and by external forces. In institutions, clients are categorized (usually by medical diagnosis and acuteness of illness), and their care requirements are estimated and translated into the nursing time that will be needed to give that care. This process is the basis for staffing patterns. More accurate predictions of nursing time requirements may result from using nursing diagnoses to estimate the care that will be needed.

Externally, the regulation of reimbursement rates by state agencies influences hospital budgets and, therefore, staffing patterns. Charges for nursing care are included in the daily room rate along with the cost of laundry, meals, and housekeeping. Other ways of establishing charges for nursing care are being studied; hospitalized clients of the future may pay a direct fee for nursing services.

As professionals, nurses have an obligation to clients to see that current standards of quality care are not compromised. The responsibility also exists to see that excess costs are not imposed by overstaffing. As employees, nurses seldom have much direct control over caseloads; as professionals, they are responsible for communicating clients' care requirements to enhance staffing pattern decisions.

COST CONTAINMENT AND MODELS OF NURSING CARE DELIVERY

Models of care delivery impact on the cost of care. In addition they may or may not facilitate nurses'

diagnostic and treatment decisions. Two models of care delivery that have appeared on the hospital scene recently are "patient-focused care"[29] and case management. It is important that nurses ensure that the professional aspects of practice are not lost in the restructuring of care delivery to reduce hospital costs. More than 50% of vice presidents in charge of nursing are restructuring nursing care delivery in attempts to cut costs and inefficiency.[30] Perhaps the benefits of primary nursing to clients as well as nurses' central role in diagnosis and treatment can be preserved in the current cost-conscious environment.

Case management

Nursing diagnoses and medical diagnoses are the focus of activities in case management. They describe the health-related, therapeutic concerns that are to be managed in an effective and cost-efficient way. Case management has been defined as a "set of logical steps and a process of interaction with service networks, which assures that a client receives needed services in a supportive, cost-effective, efficient manner."[31] The logical steps are health assessment, planning service procurement, delivery, coordination, and monitoring. *Case management, case coordination, service management,* and *care management* are terms that share many similarities.[32] Community health nurses and social workers have done case management since the early 1970s. Today the trend in hospitals is toward nurses as case managers:

There is still considerable debate as to whether case managers should come from the nursing field or the social work profession. At this time the trend seems to favor nursing case management. . . . The qualifications of the case manager vary but, according to the American Nurses Association Task Force on Case Management, the baccalaureate degree in nursing with three years of appropriate clinical experience should be the minimum. A master's degree in nursing or a related field is desired. . . . [In the community] a qualified case manager can handle between 30 and 40 active clients at one time.[32 (p. 78)]

Reports indicate that case management contributes to cost containment through its impact on length of stay and decreased costs for care resources. Case management can afford an opportunity for holistic care to be given; it is recommended for illnesses requiring multiple therapies that are also of high cost and required over a period of time.[33]

Nursing diagnoses and medical diagnoses are the critical components of a case management focus. It is the client's diagnoses that the nurse manages in collaboration with the client. Interventions and projected outcomes for conditions that are of therapeutic concern must be clear. As noted earlier, health assessment and planning are important because they are the basis for establishing the networks for care delivery in this coordinated approach.

Patient-focused care

In addition to its more pragmatic goals of cost-saving, restructuring has as its aim "patient-focused care." This focus should provide the appropriate amount of time nurses need to focus on the patient's nursing diagnoses, as opposed to focusing only on disease treatment. This model emphasizes the following (but there are many adaptations): decentralization of support services, expansion of the numbers of support personnel, cross-training, and promotion of teamwork between nursing and allied health care groups.[30 (pp. 26-27)]

One of the areas of concern is cross-training. "Is Everything Everyone's Job?" is the question headlining an editorial by Florence Huey, editor of the *American Journal of Nursing*.[34] This model requires that nurses, radiology technicians, physical therapists, pharmacists, respiratory therapists, and transport personnel take on each others' roles.[34] It specifies that registered nurses are to assume responsibility for the assessment of patients' progress. The Joint Commission on Accreditation, when commenting on this new model, said that "our standards are very prescriptive; only RNs can make nursing diagnoses, prescribe nursing care, and make nursing interventions. . . . Where nursing care is provided there has to be a designated nursing leader."[30 (p. 30)] Some view the patient-focused care model as a return to previous times:

It's hardly unprecedented for RNs to draw blood and administer therapies; 30 years ago, such functions were often part of their job descriptions. With the explosion of technology and specializations, allied professionals took over most of that work. Where patient-focused care prevails, RNs are taking back those tasks and "sharing"

them with other cross-trained workers who in turn help out with bedside care.[30 (p. 27)]

It will be interesting to see how this model facilitates nurses' diagnostic and treatment activities; it may be more cost-saving in the ancillary departments.

Currently there is concern about the ineffective use of nursing personnel, where nurses are doing the work of other departments. The lack of time and its allocation as a resource has always been a problem. Prescott and colleagues have these suggestions:

None of the newer proposals to restructure hospital nursing explicitly emphasizes the need to expand nurse authority over the independent solution of nursing care problems. Lack of attention to this dimension is understandable because physicians have resisted nurses' efforts to decrease physician control of nursing practice along this dimension. . . . Retaining nursing as a clinical profession means that nurses must control the course of restructuring nursing roles. Changes should be evaluated in terms of whether they potentially enhance professional autonomy or the freedom to independently assess and manage nursing care problems.[35 (p. 27)]

NURSING DIAGNOSIS AND HEALTH STATISTICS

Florence Nightingale was the first to devise a system of gathering hospital and death statistics. This work was done in the middle of the nineteenth century. More recently the U.S. National Center for Health Statistics developed the Uniform Minimum Health Data Set. This data set is defined as "a minimum set of items of information with uniform definitions and categories, concerning a specific aspect or dimension of the health care system, which meets the essential needs of multiple data users."[36] Currently health statistics are mainly disease statistics; for example, the number of cases of morbidity and mortality caused by cardiovascular conditions or cancer are counted. Illnesses are classified using the World Health Organization's International Classification of Diseases (ICD). Every U.S. health care agency submits statistics to a national data bank for compilation of national statistics. In medicine, the Uniform Hospital Minimum Data Set consists of the principal diagnosis, other diagnoses, and other relevant data.

A Nursing Minimum Data Set (NMDS) has been proposed for compiling health statistics at a national or international level.[37,38] The data set contains 16 items, 11 of which—such as date of birth and sex—are also included in other sets. The items unique to the nursing minimum data set are listed below:

1. Nursing diagnosis
2. Nursing intervention
3. Nursing outcome
4. Intensity of nursing care
5. Unique identification number of principal registered nurse provider

The proposed NMDS has been submitted to the U.S. Department of Health and Human Services. Before final acceptance the items will have to be field-tested to ensure that they can be retrieved from health care records in all settings. *If the NMDS is accepted nationally, nursing diagnoses must be accurate and must be recorded with the accompanying interventions and outcomes attained. Classification systems would provide measures of intensity of nursing care.* Clearly, computerized nursing information systems would facilitate the collection of statistics at the agency level.

A second needed development in the collection of statistics regarding nursing diagnosis is the request to the World Health Organization to add nursing diagnosis to the ICD. One of the chapters in this system or a separate system might be devoted to nursing diagnoses. This would permit the collection of international statistics on nursing diagnoses. The development of the NMDS and an international classification system are important events in nursing. The reader will want to keep abreast of developments in these two areas.

NURSING DIAGNOSIS AND THE SCOPE OF PRACTICE

What is nursing practice? That question is asked by career-seeking high school students, by legislators who pass laws that regulate practice, and by hardpressed financial vice presidents of agencies delivering nursing care. It is asked by educators designing curricula, by third-party payers, and by research-funding agencies.

Nursing is caring for the whole person. Yet that statement is too vague for those who must decide how many nurses to hire or what courses should be in a curriculum.

In recent years gigantic steps have been taken to define and describe the scope of nursing practice. Many conceptual frameworks have been proposed to clarify the focus, and nurses now lament the proliferation of views. They forget that not long ago nursing was conceptualized only as being a handmaiden to other health care providers, who made all the decisions. The nursing process, requiring actions based on judgment, was "kept in the closet."

Theory and nursing process have led to even clearer articulation of the scope of nursing practice. In 1980 the Congress for Nursing Practice of the ANA defined 11 actual or potential health problem areas that exemplify the focus of nursing practice.[39] Within these areas, theoretical knowledge guides diagnosis and treatment.

The scope of practice will be defined even more clearly as nursing diagnoses are identified, standardized, and classified. Then nurses may point to a taxonomy of actual and potential problems that will clearly state that nurses assume responsibility and accountability for the diagnosis and treatment of these problems. At a very specific, concrete level it can be said that nursing diagnoses are the focus of caring because they represent human health-related responses.

Both the ANA *Social Policy Statement*[39] and the classification of problems in the domain of practice will increase nursing's future scope. If true responsibility is taken for a problem area such as Knowledge Deficit (Health Maintenance), imagine the opportunities for practice that will be open. Clinical research can be done about the quality and quantity of knowledge that correlates with health maintenance behavior. Nurses will be able to lobby for health education and learning centers, the media can be used to reach target populations, and third-party payers can be pressured to reimburse clients for preventive health education. These are only a few examples of what may occur as the domain of independent practice is clearly defined by nursing diagnoses.

NURSING DIAGNOSIS AND NURSING THEORY

The current effort to identify and classify nursing diagnoses has been described as theory development.[40-43] Interestingly, this position can produce various responses. One reaction may be, "If the work on diagnosis is theory development, then it's the *first* useful thing about theory I've seen." People with this point of view usually become involved in diagnostic category identification *even though* it might be theory development! The reaction that rarely leads to involvement is, "Oh, another theory; probably too abstract for practice." Lacking an appreciation of the use of theory in practice, nurses who hold this second view devalue diagnosis because it sounds theoretical.

Probably the most meaningful way for the learner to think about the issue is in the context of practice theory as defined by Dickoff and co-workers.[44] They define four distinct levels of theory, which will structure our discussion of the relationship between nursing diagnosis and theory. We shall see, as these authors propose, that theory begins and ends in practice.

Factor-isolating theory

Identifying and formally labeling phenomena is the first step in the development of a theory in a science. This step is referred to as the *factor-isolating level of theory development.*

Phenomena of concern are isolated and categorized. Then the categories are given names. As previously described, categorization is a method humans use to deal with the otherwise overwhelming complexities of even their simplest environments. Things judged to be similar are given the same name. The names represent concepts or ideas that are the basic building blocks for other levels of theory.

Nursing practice has been commonly represented as a set of tasks related to clients' therapeutic needs. Categorization has been based on terms of needs for nursing, such as "needs suctioning" or "needs emotional support." Grouping clients into a category like "needs emotional support" ignores the diverse health problems that may be present, such as fear, anxiety, and role conflict.

Broad, overinclusive groupings also ignore the different interventions that may be required.

This type of categorization bears a striking resemblance to task-oriented categories in which *things are described by the actions performed in regard to them.*[45] The formal categories of a science are established in quite a different way. Rather than describing phenomena by the response to them, *formal categories specify the intrinsic characteristics of phenomena.* In the case of nursing, intrinsic characteristics would be clusters of client characteristics such as critical defining signs and symptoms. Formal categories such as nursing diagnoses provide a better cognitive focus for determining nursing intervention than do task-oriented categories with their prespecified interventions.

Currently nursing diagnoses describing clients' actual or potential problems are being defined. Thinking of these diagnoses as formal categories or concepts in a clinical science emphasizes the need for a scientific approach to their development. This approach is discussed in Chapter 12, where current identification and classification efforts are also reviewed.

Having seen that the basic building blocks of nursing practice theories are diagnostic concepts, we can now consider other levels of theory. As will be seen, each level of theory presupposes development at lower levels.[44]

Higher levels of theory

Factor-isolating theories are the basis for deriving the familiar concepts taught in courses such as physiology and chemistry. These disciplines isolate phenomena and create concepts such as "chemical," "atom," "organ," and "system." They then proceed to describe these phenomena and predict causal relations. This approach requires three levels of theory development: isolation, description, and prediction. As a practice discipline concerned with intervention, nursing requires higher levels of theory development. Nursing extends beyond description and causal relations to the prescriptive theory level that suggests interventions.[44]

After actual and potential health problems are identified, their natural history can be described. This type of theory is called *descriptive theory.* Descriptive theory allows the depiction of relationships among factors in a client and situation. This description of relationships permits the study and development of third-level theories that are *predictive.* An example is the prediction of the effect A has on B. Situation A may be a nursing intervention and B a health problem (nursing diagnosis). Or A may be some causal factor in the development of B, a health problem.

Predictive theories are indispensable for the fourth level of theory. This is *prescriptive theory,* which assists in producing desired health outcomes:

Prescriptive theories are situation-producing or goal-incorporating theories. They are not satisfied to conceptualize factors, factor relationships, or situation relationships, but go on to attempt conceptualization of desired situations as well as conceptualizing the prescription under which an agent or practitioner must act in order to bring about situations of the kind conceived as desired in the conception of goal.[44] (p. 420)

In summary, identification and naming of health conditions described by nursing diagnoses is the first level of theory development. Building on these diagnostic concepts, higher levels of theory can be developed that will be a basis for treatment. In essence, the identification and classification of nursing diagnoses is the first step in developing a clinical science that can be used by all nursing clinicians. Theory development begins and ends in practice.

SUMMARY

Selected issues of practice have been examined to clarify the relevance of nursing diagnoses. It was argued that because the focus of nursing care is the client's diagnoses, it follows logically that diagnoses can provide a focus for programs designed to assure quality care.

Perhaps an even more basic issue is the availability of and access to professional nursing care in institutions and communities. The suggestion was made that staffing in institutions might be improved if nursing diagnoses were considered in planning nursing staff allocations. In community practice as well as in institutions financial reimbursement for care is an issue. As nursing moves toward third-party payment for services, nursing

diagnoses will be a mechanism upon which to base reimbursement.

For many years it has been difficult to define the scope of nursing practice. Nursing diagnosis may make it possible to arrive at a clearer definition of nursing's domain of responsibility. Once the domain is defined, research and the development of practice theory can be focused on the health problems that are relevant to nursing.

Throughout this and the preceding chapter the reader may have thought that everything is being tied to nursing diagnosis! This observation is true. It suggests that perhaps clients' health problems are the basis for thinking about all nursing issues.

In essence, nursing's main social responsibility is to ensure that nursing services are available, accessible, and of a quality that promotes or maintains health. This is a huge undertaking unless narrowed to those conditions nurses are best able to prevent and treat. The next chapter deals with the way those conditions can be indentified.

NOTES AND REFERENCES

1. Joint Commission on Accreditation of Healthcare Organizations: *Hospital accreditation manual,* Chicago, 1993, The Commission.
2. Agency for Health Care Policy and Research: *Clinical practice guideline, #3: pressure ulcers in adults, prediction and prevention*, Rockville, Md, 1992, U.S. Department of Health and Human Services.
3. Gordon M: Determining study topics, *Nurs Res* 29:83, 1980.
4. McCourt A: Nursing diagnosis: key to quality assurance. In Hurley M, editor: *Classification of nursing diagnoses: proceedings of the sixth conference,* St Louis, 1986, Mosby.
5. Westfall UE: Nursing diagnosis: its use in quality assurance, *Top Clin Nurs* 5:78, 1984.
6. Kessner DM, Kalk CE, Singer J: Assessing health quality: the case for tracers, *N Engl J Med* 288:189, 1973.
7. North American Nursing Diagnosis Association: *NANDA nursing diagnoses: definitions and classifications, 1992,* Philadelphia, 1992, The Association.
8. Gordon M: *Manual of nursing diagnosis,* St Louis, 1993, Mosby.
9. Nurses delivering primary care may have responsibilities for treating some common diseases, but in most settings this treatment is given under physician supervision, orders, or protocols.
10. McCourt A: Personal communication, April 1979.
11. McCloskey J, Bulechek G: *Nursing intervention classification (NIC),* St Louis, 1992, Mosby.
12. Maas M: Personal communication, March 1993.
13. American Nurses Association Steering Committee on Databases to Support Clinical Nursing Practice: Nursing clas-

sification recognized by National Library of Medicine, *Am Nurse,* March 1993, p 9.

14. Lancour J: Nursing diagnosis and the effectiveness initiative, *Nurs Diagn* 2:33, 1991.
15. Readers may be troubled by the name "Uniform *Medical* Language System." Perhaps change will come about, now that nursing is incorporated. Yes, it should be the Uniform Health Care Language System (UHLS).
16. Visiting Nurse Association of Omaha: *Client management information system for community health nursing agencies,* Tech Rep HRP 0907023, Washington, DC, 1986, US Department of Health and Human Services, Division of Nursing.
17. Saba VK: The classification of home health care nursing: diagnoses and interventions, *Caring Magazine* 11:50, 1992.
18. Welch CA: Health care distribution and third-party payment for nurses' services, *Am J Nurs* 75:1844, 1975.
19. Jennings CP: Nursing's case for third party reimbursement, *Am J Nurs* 79:110, 1979.
20. Thompson J, Diers D: DRGs and nursing intensity, *Nursing and Health Care* 6:435, 1985.
21. Social Issues, 1985. Health care costs: the fever breaks, fierce competition—will quality care suffer? *Business Week,* p 86, Oct 21, 1985.
22. Halloran E, Halloran D: Exploring the DRG nursing equation, *Am J Nurs* 85:1093, 1985.
23. Halloran E, Kiley M, Nadzam D: Nursing diagnosis for identification of severity of condition and resource use. In Hurley M, editor: *Classification of nursing diagnoses: proceedings of the sixth conference,* St Louis, 1986, Mosby, p 299
24. McKibbin R et al: Nursing costs and DRG payments, *Am J Nurs* 85:1353, 1985.
25. Halloran E: The challenge for nursing administrators: nursing care, quality and decision support for future delivery systems. In Chaska N, editor: *The nursing profession: turning points,* St Louis, 1990. Mosby.
26. Halloran E: RN staffing: more care—less cost, *Nurs Manage* 14:18, 1983.
27. Halloran E, Kiley M: Nursing dependency, diagnosis-related groups, and length of hospital stay, *Health Care Fin Rev* 8:27, 1987.
28. Simmons DA: *A classification scheme for client problems in community health nursing,* Pub No HRA 80-16, Hyattsville, MD, 1980, US Department of Health and Human Services.
29. Giovanetti P: *Patient classification systems in nursing: a description and analysis,* Pub No HRA 78-22, Washington, DC, 1978, US Department of Health, Education and Welfare.
30. Brider P: The move to patient focused care, *Am J Nurs* 92:26, 1992.
31. Weil M, Karls J: Historical origins and recent developments. In Weil M, editor: *Case management in human service,* San Francisco, 1985, Jossey-Bass.
32. Morrison C: People with AIDS: case management and access to care. In Chinn P, editor: *Health policy: who cares,* Washington, DC, 1991, American Academy of Nursing.
33. Zander K: Nursing case management: strategic management of cost and quality outcomes, *J Nurs Admin* 18:23, 1988.
34. Huey F: Is everything everyone's job? *Am J Nurs* 92:7, 1992.
35. Prescott PA et al: Changing how nurses spend their time, *Image* 23:23, 1991.
36. Health Information Policy Council: *Background paper: uniform minimum health data sets,* Unpublished manuscript, Washington, DC, 1983, US Department of Health and Human Services.
37. Werley H, Lang N: *Nursing minimum data set,* New York, 1987, Springer, p 12.
38. Werley H: Nursing diagnosis and the nursing minimum data set. In McLane A, editor: *Classification of nursing diagnoses: proceedings of the seventh conference,* St Louis, 1987, Mosby.
39. American Nurses Association: *Social policy statement,* Washington, DC, 1980, The Association.
40. Bircher AV: On the development and classification of diagnoses, *Nurs Forum* 14:20, 1975.
41. Henderson B: Nursing diagnosis: theory and practice, *Adv Nurs Sci* 1:75, 1978.
42. Kritek PB: Generation and classification of nursing diagnoses: toward a theory of nursing, *Image* 10:33, 1978.
43. Kritek PB: Commentary: the development of nursing diagnosis and theory, *Adv Nurs Sci* 2:73, 1979.
44. Dickoff J, James P, Wiedenbach E: Theory in a practice discipline. I. Practice oriented theory, *Nurs Res* 17:415, 1968.
45. Bruner JS, Goodnow JJ, Austin GA: *A study of thinking,* New York, 1956, Wiley, pp 5-6.

CHAPTER 12

NURSING DIAGNOSIS: DEVELOPMENT AND CLASSIFICATION

T he focus of this chapter is on the development and classification of nursing diagnoses. Historically the concept has been in the nursing literature for nearly 50 years. Yet just over 20 years have passed since Gebbie and Lavin[1] called the first conference in 1973 to begin identifying and classifying conditions that nurses diagnose and treat.

This conference initiated the development of a language to describe conditions of concern to nurses that were not already classified in health-related taxonomies. Having such a language has had an impact: clinical and educational implementation of nursing diagnosis in the last 20 years has far exceeded its implementation in the first 20 years after its appearance in the literature (1950-1973). Its development and implementation have many facets. They involve a clear definition of nursing diagnosis (what is included in the concept of nursing diagnosis, the generation and labeling of new diagnoses, and the refinement of diagnoses already identified). Indirectly related to development are the implementation of nursing diagnosis in practice, continued development and conceptual analyses of categories,[2] and clinical research. The classification of nursing diagnoses, which follows development, involves the identification of relationships among diagnoses, principles for organizing the categories, and decisions about axes within the system.

A classification system for nursing diagnoses cannot be developed by armchair theorizing. It is the clinicians practicing nursing who identify client conditions and test diagnoses in everyday practice. For these reasons even the beginner should appreciate how classification systems are developed, why they are developed, and what each nurse can contribute. First let us consider nursing diagnosis and diagnostic judgment in professional nursing.

NURSING DIAGNOSIS IN THE PROFESSION

What is the status of nursing diagnosis in the profession, and what work is ahead? It will become evident that nursing diagnosis has been integrated into many areas of professional nursing practice and interest; however, there are controversies that provoke thought. Some argue that nursing diagnosis does not enhance professional practice, and some nurses have difficulty with the term *diagnosis,* although the process of clinical judgment is accepted as being within the scope of nursing practice.

A number of interesting developments have occurred in the last few years. They include the following:

1. The NANDA Taxonomy, which has been incorporated into the nursing Uniform Minimum Data Set (see pp. 269-270). This proposed data set will provide health statistics.
2. Nursing diagnoses have been entered into the National Library of Medicine Metathesaurus of the Unified Medical Language System (UMLS) (see p. 263). This library contains resources for the health professions and is accessible by computer.
3. The identification of clients' nursing diagnoses or other clinical problems is part of the accreditation standards of the Joint Commission on Accreditation of Healthcare Organizations. This commission sets a national standard related to implementation (see p. 255).
4. Most of the leading textbooks include nursing diagnoses, thus allowing the concept to be taught in entry level programs.
5. Each nursing diagnosis is indexed for literature searches in the Cumulative Index to Nursing and Allied Health Literature (CINAL). A clinician, educator, or researcher can look up the literature on a particular nursing diagnosis.
6. Nursing diagnoses are listed in the commonly used *Taber's Cyclopedic Medical Dictionary.*[3]
7. Nursing diagnoses have been the focus for writing national guidelines by the Agency for Health Care Policy and Research (ACHPR) of the U.S. Department of Health and Human Services (Chapter 11). The guidelines are based on a review of relevant research and expert opinion. Nursing experts chaired or co-chaired the Task Forces on Guidelines, which include management of pain, incontinence, and pressure ulcer (see pp. 256-259).
8. The American Nurses Association has submitted the nursing diagnosis taxonomy (Appendix D) to the World Health Organization's Committee on International Classification. Currently the taxonomies

used by member countries are a focus of study by the International Council of Nurses in Geneva.

9. The Association of Francophone European Diagnosis (AFEDI) is an affiliate of NANDA. It held one of the two large conferences on nursing diagnosis in Europe (one in Paris and one in Amsterdam, both in 1992).
10. Translations of nursing diagnoses in textbooks or manuals have been done by nationals in most European and Asian, and in some African, countries. These translations permit nurses to select which diagnoses are applicable to their cultures and to share with English-speaking countries their identification of diagnoses. Outside North America large conferences on nursing diagnosis have been held in Australia, Thailand, Denmark, France, and The Netherlands.
11. The French-speaking committee on Translation has been established and has completed the official French translation of nursing diagnoses from the *NANDA Taxonomy I, Revised, 1992.* This committee comprises nurses from France, Belgium, and Quebec, Canada.
12. The journal *Nursing Diagnosis* began publication in 1990 and contains cutting-edge articles on the development and classification of nursing diagnosis.
13. The NANDA conference in 1994 will mark 21 years of the national effort to develop and classify nursing diagnoses. There have been 11 conferences on the classification of nursing diagnoses.

IMPLEMENTATION IN PRACTICE: VIEWPOINTS

As nursing diagnosis and diagnostic judgment become integrated into professional nursing, questions about issues replace those about implementation. Some suggest that the next focus should be on the quality and accuracy of judgments. Just as the refinement of diagnostic categories must be continuous, the quality and accuracy of judgments must be continuously monitored. This may be the next step beyond implementation.

In this book nursing diagnosis has been viewed as the focus for nurse-initiated treatment intended to resolve a situation or guide clients in resolving those health-related situations they choose to resolve. Nurses assume accountability for outcomes, as the NANDA definition states, until the client can assume that responsibility. Also, diagnoses describe (1) life processes and a desire for a higher level of wellness, (2) potential problems (risk conditions), and (3) actual problems.

This book has focused on issues related to competency in diagnostic and therapeutic judgment. The emphasis has been on judgment rather than on the equally important subject of nurse-client interaction, the context in which nursing judgments are made.

Caring and the philosophical beliefs underlying nursing theories make up an important, but different, area of discourse. They deal with the nurse-client relationship. Some raise the question: Does a theory of caring replace nursing diagnosis? Caring is a critical topic for practice and in the education of nurses. Caring is the energy that motivates diagnosis and treatment. Helping persons to identify their health concerns, solve their health problems, and improve their quality of life are caring behaviors. Theories of caring do not replace diagnosis, because diagnostic judgment is a basic assumption in professional caring. Nursing "connects with the whole *and* serves people."[4] Connection alone is not sufficient. Similarly, merely clinical judgment and technological competency by themselves are not sufficient. Watson expresses it in this way:

The process of human-to-human caring illuminates the mystery of humanity and the possibility of a higher power, order, or energy in the universe that can be activated through the nurse caring process, that can in turn potentiate healing and health and facilitate self-knowledge, self-reverence, self-control, self-care, and possibly even self-healing. Such an orientation requires a certain assumption that fundamental clinical, technological competencies and knowledge underpin nursing practice. The human caring process goes beyond the basic educational competency level toward higher-level, professional care processes that potentiate health and healing in persons and society.[5] (p. 220)

In the process of a nurse's transition from novice to higher levels, the connection between caring and competence becomes a personal reality.

There are other reactions to the use of nursing diagnosis. For example, should goals and objectives for a client's behavior direct nursing care, or should problems (diagnoses) and outcomes? With the emphasis on outcome in today's health care, it is not so much the interventions that are done but the achievement of outcomes relative to an identified problem that are to be demonstrated. Evaluation is outcome oriented rather than process oriented. In comparing goal-oriented treatment (or in the words of Nurcome,[6] "goal-directed treatment") with nursing diagnosis–directed treatment, Seahill states that the use of nursing diagnoses in inpatient child psychiatric nursing should be avoided. A main issue is which language is to be used, nursing or some other. He concludes:

First, child psychiatry is multidisciplinary. Any move by a single discipline to separate itself and use its own lexicon must have compelling reasons to do so. Second, in child psychiatry, there is an emphasis on the whole patient—including the child's response to illness. The claim that nurses evaluate and treat separate problems may be less true in this setting than in general medicine. Third, because child psychiatry is multidisciplinary and because further limitations may be placed on hospital stays, efficient and effective clinical management demands effective information sharing. Hence, the use of nursing diagnoses in inpatient child psychiatric settings could be a retreat from a central role in favor of a more peripheral role.[7] (p. 97).

The concerns about nursing diagnosis can be enumerated:

1. It separates nursing from the medical lexicon and might be a retreat by nursing from a central role to a peripheral role.
2. It does not place emphasis on the whole patient.
3. It has limitations when dealing with short hospital stays.
4. Care delivery is multidisciplinary.

It is difficult to imagine how nursing could "separate itself" from the medical lexicon (if a client has a disease or disorder). This approach has never been recommended; in fact, there are moves to integrate lexicons. The "compelling reason" for developing nursing diagnoses is that the medical classifications do not contain all the conditions that nurses diagnose and treat. It should not be expected that a classification of diseases or a classification of mental disorders would encompass conditions that *nurses* are educated and licensed to treat. The medical and psychiatric lexicons are based on a different perspective; the *Diagnostic and Statistical Manual of Mental Disorders* (DSM III-R)[8] deals with mental disorders and the *International Classifications of Diseases* (ICD) describes anatomical and pathophysiological conditions. The nursing perspective, as reflected in the nursing literature, extends beyond these areas. The DSM III-R listed only one nurse among the 406 members of its advisory committees and consultants for the 1987 revision. The same questions arise in other nursing specialties using the international disease classification: Is the nursing perspective different from that used with diseases and disorders? Do we base interventions on the same conditions? Do we seek the same outcomes? Should we value collaboration to the detriment of our own knowledge development?

Nursing diagnosis is not incompatible with a holistic approach. The "approach" to nurse-client interaction is a philosophical choice. It is how nursing diagnosis is used within the nurse's approach that makes care holistic or not.

Seahill's comments[7] raise some interesting questions and a multitude of issues. Are most nursing diagnoses at a higher level of abstraction than the DSM III-R and in a different domain from the ICD? In other settings where multidisciplinary teams deliver care (e.g., rehabilitation nursing) nursing's diagnostic language is very useful to the team as a supplement to the medical language. What produces the differences in these two specialties? The *NANDA Taxonomy* is not referenced in Seahill's article, causing one to suspect that another classification is being used as a reference for his comments.[9]

Some diagnostic concepts from the nursing diagnosis classification may be useful to teams in child psychiatry. They can be used as the basis for goal-oriented treatment; in fact, outcome-focused treatment is widely emphasized in contemporary health care. In addition, nursing diagnoses have other advantages. Seahill's examples emphasize the need to add to the nursing diagnosis taxonomy; he refers to "pivotal problems" that are formulated by the team "*after a* diagnostic formulation is fashioned."[7] Nurses contribute to the definition of pivotal problems such as "immature ego development," which may "explain poor social judgment, poor impulse control, and risk-taking behavior." Poor social judgment is the base for generating an intervention *goal* of "improve social judgment."

This goal "could foster ego development" and is operationalized by objectives (outcomes). "As a whole, the goals of treatment provide a portrait of the child and family at discharge."[7 (p. 97)] Poor social judgment is not on the listing of nursing diagnoses, but concepts of social judgment might be added. Also, these are not terms in the diagnostic or symptom listing of the DSM III-R.[8] Discharge outcomes are generated from nursing diagnoses, and these outcomes are the bases for designing intervention. Thus the process Seahill describes is really no different. The substantive difference in this author's point of view and others is the language used for "pivotal problems." Should it be uniform so as to be retrieved for knowledge development activities, or should it be individual and specific to the team generating the pivotal problems? Even more basic: "Until this [i.e., that nurses treat different problems in this field] can be shown by rigorous clinical research, it may be premature to use separate nursing diagnoses in the inpatient child psychiatric setting."[7 (p. 97)] Truly, this is the major question raised by Seahill. If a nurse's scope of practice is the same as that of other members of the psychiatric team, then DSM III-R language should suffice and licensure should be similar.

One underlying thread in some literature relates to the quality of professional nursing practice. Critiques that relate nonprofessional and unethical behavior to nursing diagnosis suggest that the problems cited lie at a much deeper level than diagnostic labeling. They may reside in a philosophy or ethic of person, an environment that is not supportive of respect for clients' autonomy and dignity, or both. Is nursing diagnosis the problem, or is it how the concept is used? The latter is emerging as an area of concern as implementation proceeds.

Should collaborative problems (interdependent dimension) be classified as nursing diagnoses? This is a different level of question. It arises from Murphy and Stern's research on nursing diagnosis in critical care.[10] In their study nurses saw *NANDA's Taxonomy* as inadequate because it lacked sufficient collaborative problems. This is similar to the comments of others in this specialty.[11,12] An examination of the "treatment" of subcategories of decreased cardiac output in Kern and Omery's study[13] suggests that nurses should cluster nursing diagnoses under the pathophysiological state. Diagnoses included Pain, Activity Intolerance, Fear, Anxiety, and Knowledge Deficit. Diagnoses in some subcategories are Sensory Overload and High Risk for Hypothermia and Fluid Volume Deficit.

Some nurses do not use nursing diagnoses because diagnoses do not adequately describe their perspective on client's problems or, as has been done traditionally, they are nesting the nursing diagnoses inside the collaborative problem. It may be that disease terms are stressed during learning, which has been the tradition in acute care education, or that the status language in acute care settings and the level of problem conceptualization require the language of disease. Mitchell[14] (p. 100) proposes another reason: the "potential for harm to human beings exposed to the diagnostic encounter." This idea represents an "unclarified ethical dilemma" involving the diagnostic process itself. This might be reduced if "nurses had restricted their practice to the control and management of altered biophysiologic states."[13] (p. 101) (This restriction would not be helpful to psychiatric–mental health nurses, although at one point nursing in mental hospitals was restricted mainly to meeting clients' bodily needs.)

Imaginative extrapolations and premises from Mitchell's[14] theoretical position are used as a basis for conclusions about the "potential" problems in diagnostic judgment and nursing diagnoses. Mitchell projects patients' feelings, such as: "[the] experience of being judged and labeled creates suffering in ways relating to feeling misunderstood, disconnected, and alone."[14] (p. 99) If patients react this way to assessment, it is more than "potentially harmful." Mitchell supposes that this hypothesized reaction occurs because "regardless of the words used in the label, the actual labeling process is reductionistic and objectifying, thus potentially harmful."[14] (p. 100) There are ways around the mind's tendency toward reductionism. Of course, referring to a client as "disconnected" is also labeling; categorization is difficult to avoid.

Mitchell proposes that "harm is made real in the witnessed suffering of downcast eyes, tears, and silent pleas for understanding when individuals are held apart in human encounters."[14] (p. 101) Nonprofessional and unethical behavior and poor nursing care are described and attributed to the fact that the nurse is being forced to use nursing diagnoses, thus causing a "moral dilemma related to the consequences of the diagnostic encounter."[14] (p. 102) Even though the arguments are an appeal to the emotions, the criticism is not to be ignored. There is a justifiable concern if nurses indeed use nursing diagnosis in the manner described. Of even more concern are Mitchell's two examples of disrespect for the client in nurse-client interactions.[14] No comments are made regarding how these unethical incidents of nurse behavior, when and if they occur, are handled.

There have been other similar reports. Hagey and McDonough[15] point out a number of legitimate concerns regarding the social use of nursing diagnoses in labeling clients. Their article should be studied in its entirety, but the ideas of ignoring the client's perspective, imposing erroneous meaning on a situation, and making decisions that implicate clients as the source of the problem, which "absolves staff of their neglect"[15] (p. 153) deserve some reflection when nursing diagnosis is being used. Many comments center around the nurse in a bureaucratic environment where the purpose of using nursing diagnosis is to "save work" or "get the work done." In support of Hagey and McDonough's criticisms, it is not unheard of for some to say they are not interested in nursing diagnosis unless it saves time. The job orientation, or as these authors suggest, the work environment and working conditions "interfere with in-depth problem solving and thoughtful nursing care."[15] (p. 157) It may also be asked why nurses committed to quality professional care tolerate a situation that does not permit time to listen to hidden meanings in clients' conversations and to think about them.

There was a time when nurses were not expected to think and thus were not given time for it because the "orders" for their work were written by others. As nurses change their perception of their role in the health care system, they may have to change the work situation to accommodate their new role perception. Diagnosis requires that time be spent with clients and that the meaning of situations to both client and nurse be thought through. It is not a simple stimulus-response activity.

These last two discussions raise an important question: Is it the concept of nursing diagnosis, or is it the level of professional practice these authors[15] contemplate or have observed that should be implicated? No one would condone the situations these authors relate. It is important that they call this quality of practice to our attention. Again the question: Is it nursing diagnosis that is causing these situations, or is it a philosophy (including ethics) of nurse-client interaction? Probably an equal number of examples can be given in which nurses used diagnoses in the context of holistic, growth-promoting, caring, nurse-client encounters.

The standardized, preprinted care plans that have been adapted to nursing diagnoses are another area of concern. They are seen as "dogma" in nursing practice. Rodgers[16] makes the following comments:

> The growing system of nursing diagnosis presents a similar risk [i.e., similar to standardized care plans]. The taxonomy has not yet achieved the status of dogma, perhaps because of continuing debate and development of the diagnostic statements. However, as nurses increasingly employ nursing diagnoses to guide their thinking, the potential exists for the introduction of another source of dogma as the conceptualization of nursing care situations becomes reduced to a preconceived category system.[16 (p. 180)]

This author makes the point that we can use diagnostic categories in a rigid manner, such as, if a client has had a colostomy, there must be body image disturbance! There is great variation in nursing practice, and nursing diagnoses may be used in the way Rodgers describes. When diagnostic manuals that include nursing diagnosis–medical diagnosis links are used in a preconceived manner, diagnoses for a disease, rather than for a person, may result. Again the question, Is it the nurses' *use* of standardized care plans/guidelines, or is it the concept of nursing diagnoses? Maybe nurses have not been educated to use guidelines in a way that does not standardize their responses to people.

The idea of identifying a client's condition as a basis for planning nursing care is well accepted. That this condition should be conceptualized at a level beyond a set of observations is also accepted. What produces difficulty for some is the name applied to the process. The issue seems to be the word *diagnosis* and its association with medicine. Levine[17] reacted to the term for reasons having to do with its legal implications and suggested *trophicognosis* as a substitute. Her concern was justified, since she conceived of nursing diagnosis as the diagnosis of "disease and its manifestations . . . without using the formal language of medical diagnosis."[17 (p. 58)] Several current diagnoses do fit her definition. These include Fluid Volume Deficit, Impaired Gas Exchange, Alteration in Tissue Perfusion, and Decreased Cardiac Output. If

placed in the position of a consumer, this writer would request a physician rather than a nurse to treat these problems as they are currently defined. The secondary functional problems that occur because of these conditions certainly require nursing treatment.

A second reaction to nursing diagnosis is that it pigeonholes clients. This concept has a negative emotional connotation. Humans are predisposed to categorize experiences in order to choose appropriate behavior in a situation. The need to categorize in order to understand a situation is found in simple societies and even in cultures with a more holistic perception than ours. Nurses categorize clients' behavior; this act did not originate with nursing diagnosis. The categories sometimes used are not very flattering. Admittedly, pigeonholing and stereotyping happens, usually because of inadequate knowledge of the person or family or too-early closure on a diagnosis. Should we blame the nurse or the concept of diagnosis? Perhaps sensitivity to these errors will prevent them.

The negative descriptions of nursing practice serve to raise issues about contemporary nursing care delivery. The argument that any poor nursing practice is due to nursing diagnosis is weak. Yet if diagnoses are being indiscriminately applied without sufficient data and in a standardized manner, the reasons should be investigated. Disrespect for clients and their autonomy should not be sanctioned by colleagues, since such actions are in direct conflict with the professional code of ethics.

IMPLEMENTATION

In this book clinical judgment has been viewed as a predominantly analytical process incorporating intuitive and analogical aspects. Those who take this perspective believe that known components of the diagnostic process can be described in words, learned, and applied in practice to the extent that a person's intelligence allows. Apprenticeship does not need to be the major mode of learning when this is true.

By pulling together what is known about how humans reason, a basis for clinical teaching and learning of diagnosis can be formulated. Helping others to implement nursing diagnosis may be done informally in conversation or formally through conferences. In either case, an awareness of current practice and steps in its implementation are useful. Some comments follow on its implementation in practice education, and programs of research.

Implementation in practice

Professional developments in the health fields do not spread across the nation as fast as some people desire. In medicine the application of new knowledge and techniques is sometimes delayed 5 or more years; the situation is no different in nursing. One indicator of interest in a topic is the frequency of its appearance in journals and textbooks. Since the beginning of nurses' national effort to identify nursing diagnoses in 1973, several hundred articles have appeared in leading journals, and most textbooks include the subject, indicating a reasonably high level of interest.

This interest does not help improve care, at least not until motivation leads to implementation. In some regions the question of implementation has long since been resolved. A 1989 national study of 692 accredited hospitals, each with 400 or more beds, indicated that 53% reported using nursing diagnosis in their documentation system.[18]

Clinicians are using diagnoses in quality assurance programs and clinical research. When a hospital requires that students know and use nursing diagnosis before achieving affiliation for clinical experience, and when another advertises for a clinical specialist knowledgeable in nursing diagnosis, it is clear that diagnosis is established in those places. On the other hand, situations are encountered in which even nursing process is not implemented. Although different levels of competency are currently encountered, those interested in improving their nursing practice are generally enthusiastic about learning nursing diagnosis. It is sometimes said that ideas arise from the academic ivory tower. This was not the case with nursing diagnosis. Clinicians seemed to appreciate its importance more than educators did in the early years.

The literature reflects the impact of organizations on the implementation of diagnosis and responsibility for clinical judgment. The effect of an organization is especially strong when there is an employee or dependency mentality ("They tell me what to do") versus a feeling of professional autonomy in the employee's role. It is an interesting situation when the dependency orientation prevails. Concurrent with the introduction of nursing diagnosis there must be a change in attitude regarding responsibility and accountability as a professional for clinical judgment, justification for particular judgments (the clinical data), and public documentation. It may be necessary to make it clear that nurses have the authority to diagnose and treat (a professional model of practice).[19] In either situation, it may be useful to have nursing diagnosis integrated with quality assurance.[20]

The literature contains a number of tools for implementing nursing diagnosis,[20] methods for implementation,[21] and evaluation to assist in measuring the effect of implementation.[22,23] The literature on the difficulties encountered in the clinical teaching of nursing diagnosis supports the increasing levels of difficulty involved in aspects of clinical judgment.[24,26] For example, observation requires less skill than either making a judgment about the observations or using nursing knowledge to judge that one problem is contributing to another (causal connections).

Implementation in education

Competency in clinical judgment is a continuous learning process during a nurse's career. Thus the subject is of concern to students, in-service educators, and faculty. One important challenge is teaching nursing diagnosis and diagnostic-therapeutic reasoning.

Although interest has increased, diagnostic skills do not always appear "in bold type" in the curricula of professional programs. Looking to the future, educators will have to assure that all students develop beginning competency in diagnosis and in the treatment of common nursing diagnoses. Otherwise new graduates will not be prepared to practice at a level consistent with national standards of care (see the box on p. 218). State board examinations reflect this requirement. Competency in diagnosis is something graduates will use as clinicians the remainder of their professional lives. This "usefulness" criterion alone places nursing diagnosis in the category of essential content in educational programs and in-service education. This is consistent with the American Association of Colleges of Nursing report on the essential content for baccalaureate nursing programs that stresses clinical judgment.[27]

Clinical experiences in disease-related judgments may not be easily transferred to judgments about nursing diagnoses. There are indications that beyond the general diagnostic process, knowledge is a significant factor in success as a diagnostician.[28] Knowledge about nursing diagnoses and reasoning have to be synthesized. Dealing with uncertainties and variability among clients requires repetitive experience in the diagnosis of common problems. Clearly the most economical way to acquire diagnostic skill is under the guidance of faculty. Feedback in the early stages of training and focused clinical experiences offered in the educational setting are critical in developing this competency.

Currently both remedial education and expertise in diagnosis should be built into master's degree and clinical doctoral programs. A nurse's graduation as a clinical specialist or teacher should guarantee to society that the nurse has the ability to diagnose and treat clients with high-incidence nursing diagnoses in his or her specialty. Nurses who hold a master's degree are the ones who will act as consultants in differential diagnosis and complex diagnostic interactions and provide feedback to generalists on the development of their competencies. They are also the more sophisticated clinical experts who have the responsibility for studying new conditions and refining current categories.

In-service educators continually remind us that they must fill in the gaps that result not only from deficiencies in educational programs but also from new developments in practice or nurses' lack of continuing education. Orientation programs, workshops, and even classes in the identification of specific diagnoses and the treatment of clients with these conditions are useful. Many in-service educators find, as Aspinall[29] has remarked, that nursing diagnosis and diagnostic judgment are the "weak link" in nursing process competencies. Clinicians are eager to learn. They find that organizing their care around nursing diagnoses makes practice interesting and challenging and focuses care planning better as well.

The content of learning

The two areas of learning that are basic to beginning competency in diagnostic judgment are critical thinking and the categories used in critical thinking. These areas are similar to the components and definition of critical thinking by the National Council on Education[30]:

Critical thinking is the intellectually disciplined process of actively and skillfully conceptualizing, applying, analyzing, synthesizing, and evaluating information gathered from, or generated by, observation, experience, reflection, reasoning, or communication, as a guide to belief and action.

The question of how to teach and learn critical thinking, or diagnostic-therapeutic reasoning, arises often. The answer is complicated by the multifaceted nature of this ability. A hierarchy of skills is also misleading; complexity depends on the nature of the data and the situation. Nickerson[31] makes an important point about teaching thinking:

We think without being taught to do so; but we do not necessarily become good thinkers without some assistance . . . or by completing traditional content courses. . . . The point is not to get people to do these things at all, but rather to teach them to do them more effectively and more appropriately than they do already.[31 (pp. 25, 29)]

Studying basic processes in the context of nursing knowledge increases students' awareness of critical thinking and helps them to be more aware of intuitive, analytic, and systematic processes in their thinking. For example, diagnostic reasoning entails observation, using relationships, using numbers, measuring, classifying and abstracting, communicating, predicting, and inferring. Methods, programs, difficulties, and results concerning the teaching of diagnostic reasoning are beginning to appear in the literature.[32-36]

Assisting with implementation

Assistance in implementation is a role that may be assumed by both students and clinicians; the usual roles of student and graduate may be reversed where nursing diagnosis is concerned. It is not uncommon to find students helping clinicians learn about nursing diagnosis while clinicians are helping the students perfect other clinical skills. Here we review the implementation process. A knowledge of methods and resources is useful when opportunities to offer help arise. Other people's curiosity should always be used to advantage.

Nurses will encounter care settings in which the

idea of nursing diagnosis is unheard of, controversial, seen as student activity, or considered interesting but unclear. In such settings it is appropriate for a student, if asked, to present a brief description and some examples of nursing diagnosis. This brief description should be followed by suggesting some reading or a conference to discuss the idea. The staff may not be ready to think about diagnosis; a "back-door" approach might include helping the staff plan a conference on any of the following topics:

1. "Are we implementing our institution's philosophy and objectives of nursing on this unit?" (Each person at the meeting should have a copy of the unit's philosophy and objectives to examine.) Usually objectives specify the identification of clients' health problems.
2. "Is our practice on this unit consistent with national standards?" (Each person should have a copy of the generic or specialty ANA Standards of Care to examine and perhaps also an article about legal aspects; see the box on p. 218.)
3. "Is our scope of practice consistent with the scope defined nationally?" (Each person should have a copy of the ANA's *Social Policy Statement* to examine; see p. 5.) Diagnosis lies within the scope of nursing practice.
4. "Is our practice consistent with the law?" (Each person should have copies of the state practice act and the state board of nursing rules and regulations; this approach is useful if diagnosis or judgment is specified in those documents.)

These topics provide a basis for thinking about current practice. The objective is to examine personal role concepts relative to outside criteria. This comparison, combined with a selected reading on the concept of nursing diagnosis, should lead the nurses attending the conference to consider the idea of using diagnoses, which is step one. Conversations with and questions about diagnosis from the nurses at the conference suggest their readiness for step two. The second step in implementation is to provide information. One or more of the following may be helpful:

1. Provide a short bibliography of two or three articles about nursing diagnosis, especially articles that are relevant to the type of cli-

ents the present staff serves. (See Annotated Bibliography at the end of the book.)
2. Secure a speaker who is an expert on nursing diagnosis; the speaker may be either a member of the staff or from another facility in the town or city.
3. Some staff members may be able to attend a continuing education course on nursing diagnosis and then report to the others. Contact the local, state, or regional diagnosis association through NANDA.

If the staff shows an interest in trying nursing diagnosis as a means of organizing nursing care, inform physicians they work with before recording nursing diagnoses on clients' charts. The physicians may not understand the new way of recording. Think about (1) the physicians' level of knowledge and attitudes and (2) how nursing diagnosis might influence client care positively, and be ready with examples relevant to any particular physician's interest. Make sure to gain the support of the nursing staff before informing other professionals.

The group is ready for step three when even a few staff members want to learn more. Step three begins the staff's educational process. The first learning objective is the application of the definition of nursing diagnosis. *Diagnostic reasoning exercises,* such as those found in Appendix Q, should be useful at this point. These exercises require the knowledge and application of the definition of a nursing diagnosis. Recognition of what is and what is not a diagnosis is achieved when discriminations can be made and reasons stated for choosing or not choosing different items.

The group is then ready to move on to *diagnostic selection exercises;* an example is provided in Appendix Q. It is a good idea to prepare exercises of various levels of difficulty. For example, in vignettes the cues might range from obvious, critical defining signs and symptoms to cues that are ambiguous or conflicting. Also, a higher level of difficulty is attained if no diagnoses are provided at the end of the vignette and diagnostic hypotheses must be generated while the vignette is being read. A list of diagnoses and defining characteristics, such as those provided in a manual, are used to assist in problem identification. An example of this second type of diagnostic selection exercise is found in Appendix R. Early diagnostic concept learning is facilitated if (1) a language is provided (diagnostic labels) and (2) vignettes are constructed directly from the defining characteristics of diagnoses. Ambiguities and uncertainties may be introduced after the basic concepts are acquired. First the "textbook picture," or prototype, which consists of the definition and the critical characteristics, must be learned.

The next level of learning, problem formulation, uses total case data rather than vignettes. Learning may be facilitated by *diagnostic formulation exercises.* Examples can be found in Appendixes I and R. This is the most difficult but also the most meaningful exercise. It simulates the process used in actual client care. Answers to the exercises in Appendixes Q and R are provided in Appendix S.

The repetition of diagnostic formulation exercises increases the group's skill in analyzing and integrating clinical data. When the group develops expertise in formulating nursing diagnoses from simulated case data, each participant should be asked to bring in admission data and diagnoses from one of his or her own clients. Deficiencies in assessment, hypothesis generation, testing, and problem formulation can then be discussed; this discussion should benefit both the individual and the group. After one or two experiences, diagnostic process (the hypothesis-testing model discussed in Chapters 8 and 9) should be discussed. This discussion will focus attention on the process being used as well as on the diagnostic labeling of health problems.

Step four involves using the diagnostic process with clients. One of the factors that facilitates the formulation of nursing diagnoses is collecting a *nursing* data base. Difficulties arise if the collected information is more appropriate to medical than to nursing diagnoses. As implementation of the diagnostic process begins, the nurses may become aware of the need to improve their interviewing and assessment skills. In addition, branching, hypothesis testing, and problem formulation usually need to be discussed. Some nurses may not wish to record their first efforts in the client's chart. Provide opportunities for review by the group, a colleague, or whoever is guiding the nurses' learning. Such opportunities help alleviate anxiety about mistakes in labeling and charting.

Step five in implementation may last a year. This is the questioning and doubting phase. Topics usually requiring discussion include physicians' reactions, ways to treat diagnoses, further work on terminology, and the creation of new terms to describe client conditions. The most common cause of discouragement in the novice is the time they take to complete diagnosis and care planning take.

One or more of the following approaches may help the staff get through the phase of feeling that "nursing diagnosis takes too much time":

1. "Can I help? In what area are you having difficulty?"
2. "How many times have you gone through the diagnostic process [systematic health status assessments, problem identification, and care planning]? Oh, just once?"
3. "Do you remember how long it took you to give your first bath and make a bed?"
4. "Have you noticed how long it takes a medical student to do a client history and examination?" [Or] "When you go to a physician for the first time, I imagine the history and examination take at least 30 minutes, and the physician is probably experienced; I guess most of us would not refuse that much attention."
5. "Oh, do you think there are areas in the functional patterns assessment that are not important?" [This approach usually induces conflict.]
6. "Might you be intervening as well as assessing? Oh, that's why it takes so long. Assessment probably takes only half that time."
7. "What nursing diagnoses did your client have? Oh, you wouldn't have wanted to miss these."
8. "Yes, but now you have a base; daily assessments can be done from this base, and look how many problems you can prevent that would take nursing time to treat."
9. "It won't take you that long the next time. This is one of the best ways of establishing a therapeutic relationship with a client or family."
10. "Don't clients deserve the time it takes to do a functional health assessment?" [This is the ethical-moral-legal appeal.]

Learning to assess functional health patterns and identify and label problems, if any, systematically takes time. That is why in other professions the skills have always been developed during the educational program. Nurses who did not have this opportunity to learn diagnostic judgment skills while in school will have to take the time to do so once they start to practice. There is nothing magical that will produce overnight the competency needed in current practice. The consolation is that diagnostic skills have lasting value, in contrast to learning how to use the latest machine, which may be outdated in a year.

The literature contains a number of articles useful for implementing nursing diagnosis in practice settings. Sharing even one of the experiences described in these articles may stimulate the staff's interest. Feild's[36] excellent description of her experience with the change process for implementing diagnosis is a good resource for staff, head nurses, and administrators. Dalton[37] and Weber[38] provide many insights about establishing diagnosis-based care in a community setting and a private practice, respectively. Bruce[39] describes a program of implementation stimulated by nursing administration, and Rantz, Miller, and Jacobs[40] discuss implementation in long-term care. Other sources mentioned previously also provide ideas.[19-21]

As implementation proceeds, resource information from articles listed in the bibliographies of chapters and the annotated bibliography at the end of the book may be helpful. The journal *Nursing Diagnosis* is also very useful.

Clearly the best way to exchange ideas about implementation is to hold local meetings, as is done in some regions. All participants in the monthly meetings comment on what they have learned as a result of discussions with nursing colleagues. The local groups that have been formed in various states can provide leadership through its members' practice and through conferences held in conjunction with state nurses' associations. Most important, a local group offers a forum for nurses to extol or criticize the latest developments in nursing diagnosis. These groups have also contributed greatly to the national effort. What with the international affiliations with NANDA, even more contributions from groups are expected.

In summary, professional education can be designed to enable students to learn beginning diagnostic and therapeutic skills before graduation. When students or staff begin to use nursing diagnoses in obvious areas, such as care plans and charts, other nurses ask questions. To prepare the reader for these questions, a brief overview of the stages of implementation and the available resources has been provided. Introducing the staff to a professional role concept compatible with using nursing diagnosis is a basic step in implementing diagnosis; it leads them to examine the concept. The next steps in implementation center on the use of diagnostic nomenclature and process skills. No one becomes an expert in diagnosis overnight, but once skills are developed they last a lifetime.

Diagnostic judgment is a process that requires a "language" to describe conclusions. In the next section, current developments in naming client conditions encountered in practice are described.

CLASSIFICATION SYSTEM DEVELOPMENT

Diagnostic categories have been discussed throughout this book; at this point the reader needs to know where these categories originated and how they may change or evolve in the future. This brings us to the idea of classification systems in nursing. To understand the development of a diagnostic classification system, or taxonomy, it is necessary to review some terms and their definitions and the purposes of classification. The section on classification ends with diagnostic category development, the contents of the classification system most commonly used in clinical practice. Following this NANDA,[41] the association that assumes responsibility for diagnostic classification, is described. Research on diagnosis ends the chapter.

Nursing classification systems

A diagnostic classification system is only one type used in nursing practice. Classifications of interventions and outcomes are being developed that will interface with a diagnostic system. Clients have been classified to enhance staffing decisions. Except for the system designed by Halloran and colleagues that uses nursing diagnoses (see p. 266 and Appendix O), most systems use therapeutic needs or tasks requiring nursing time. Clients are grouped according to acuteness or intensity of illness. Classifications of nursing care providers have been attempted based on educational levels or roles, and, of course, there are the familiar bureaucratic classifications of nurses along managerial lines, such as head nurse, clinical director, and director of nurses. None of the current classifications of nurses can be integrated with practice-based classifications, because nurses have not been classified according to any diagnostic or therapeutic expertise they have gained other than that inferred by education. Similarly, no work exists on the diagnostic and therapeutic complexity of current diagnostic categories. The emphasis in this section is on diagnostic classification.

Characteristics of a classification system

A classification system is an arrangement of phenomena into groups or sets based on their relationships. For example, in a university, students are classified by educational level: baccalaureate, master's, and doctoral. Students working for a baccalaureate degree are further classified as freshmen, sophomores, juniors, and seniors. In the sciences and professions, classification is used to sort, code, and order the phenomena of interest during first-level theory development, as discussed in Chapter 11. Biology is an example; it names and orders classes of living things. Chemistry classifies elements in a periodic table, and medical science classifies diseases. A *class is a grouping of similar phenomena.* For example, apples are a class of fruit. In using the classification system, a piece of fruit that shares the same, or similar, characteristics with apples would be classified (named) as an apple. In nursing practice a diagnostic class is used to name a cluster of observed signs and symptoms when the observations correspond to the characteristics of the diagnostic class. (The terms *diagnostic category* and *diagnostic class* are used synonomously; they refer to classes at various levels of the taxonomy.)

Taxonomy is another term that is heard in discussions of nursing diagnoses. It is used as a synonym for *classification* but also refers to the science of classification. A provisional diagnostic taxonomy of *human response patterns* is discussed in this section.

Nomenclature is another term that is encountered in discussions of classification. It refers to a *compilation of accepted terms for describing phenomena,* such as the names of nursing diagnoses.

The diagnoses listed in Appendix A represent the currently developed and approved diagnostic nomenclature. Development of a classification system requires that certain conditions be met:

1. The purpose of the system is clear.
2. The conceptual focus and classes of phenomena are identified.
3. Names are given to the phenomena.
4. Classes are systematically ordered according to an organizing principle.

Hangartner,[42] in his discussion of classification systems, uses as an example the common telephone book. The ideas of purpose, focus, and naming, and the ordering principle are illustrated in this example of a simple classification system:

The *NYNEX Yellow Pages* for the Boston area describes a system for classifying large and small businesses that provide a particular product or service. Underlying the structure of this system is the everyday "theory" of classifying businesses according to their services. Purpose, focus, ordering principle, and description are evident if we want to construct a guide to using this classification system:

Purpose: Telephone directories are provided as an aid to good telephone service.

Focus: Exclusively business-related heading: "Product or service."

Ordering principle: Headings are always alphabetical. Think of the heading most likely to carry what you want. Flip to it and you'll find names, addresses and phone numbers of business people ready to serve you. Forgotten the name? Again, turn to the heading best describing the firm's type of business. Glancing down the list (alphabetical) will usually bring the name back to mind.

Listed under "Employment" are, among others, "Employment Agencies," "Employment Contractors—Temporary Help," and "Employment Training Service." Under each is an alphabetical listing of business names. This constitutes a three-level ordering hierarchy.

A classification system of nursing diagnoses has a similar format: broad categories, diagnostic categories, and subcategories. This kind of system provides a hierarchical reference to the health problems within the scope of nursing practice. Nursing diagnoses are arranged at one horizontal level, with similar problems grouped together separately from dissimilar ones.

PURPOSE OF CLASSIFICATION

Why does nursing desire a classification system? What purpose can it serve other than filling the pages of a manual? These are critically important questions that have to be answered before the development of a classification system begins. What is classified—that is, the focus of classification—and how the classes are ordered depend on the purpose of the system.

Classification systems designed for a single purpose are more desirable than multipurpose schemes that have to be accommodated to many types of operations. The initial purpose of developing a classification system in nursing was to facilitate practice. Diagnostic nomenclature did not exist; it was not a situation in which basic-level diagnoses had already been identified and standardized and were just awaiting a system of classification that would be relevant to practice. It was necessary to start "from scratch." The task was to begin to develop a way of naming the client conditions that generated therapeutic concern. In essence, nurses had to sort and code their world of practice.

In their foresight, Gebbie and Lavin,[1] coordinators of the First National Conference for Classification of Nursing Diagnosis, set the focus for classification system development: nursing diagnoses. Several articles had already appeared in the literature, but in the early 1970s most nurses still described their practice in terms of nursing objectives and tasks. The client conditions necessitating care were not articulated. In fact, the first classification system relevant to practice focused on therapeutic objectives, as can be seen in the 21 problems listed in the box on p. 38.

With a diagnostic classification system, or taxonomy, nurses in practice can consult a manual that contains diagnostic nomenclature, enabling them to use words consistently. Each diagnostic term used has a standard definition. This uniformity decreases the probability of communication errors.

A diagnostic classification system may be used to construct other systems with other purposes. There may be systems for computerizing nursing information; one such system of interest to nursing administrators would relate diagnoses to nursing care time. Classifying clients' diagnoses and the time required for intervention would assist in determining staffing patterns and hospital reimbursement. In addition, the development of a clinical science would be facilitated by the classification of those client conditions amenable to nursing therapy.

In summary, current efforts in classification are directed toward establishing a system to facilitate practice. Yet this system may also be used to design others. Let us examine what progress has been made and the methodology used to identify and order diagnostic categories.

CONCEPTUAL FOCUS FOR CLASSIFICATION

A discussion of the conceptual focus of a classification system immediately raises the question, What is being classified? This is a persistent question, and the answer has many consequences. The discussion of the focus and organizing concepts of a classification system is divided into three phases.

The first phase describes the effort to go beyond an alphabetical listing to a conceptual organization of the emerging diagnoses. Since 1973 NANDA's efforts have been directed toward identifying and naming the health-related conditions of clients that nurses reported they actually diagnosed and treated in their practice. Each nurse-participant's personal concept of nursing influenced the identification and development of diagnostic categories; no common conceptual focus was used. The advantage of representing the diversity in nursing is balanced by a disadvantage: diagnoses can be described at various levels of abstraction and are disparate in conceptual focus. In 1977 Sister Callista Roy,[43] a member of the Task Force of the National Group for Classification of Nursing Diagnoses (later NANDA) concerned with diagnostic classification, convened a group of nurse theorists (Appendix E) for the following purpose:

1. To develop a framework for organizing diagnoses in a classification system
2. To make recommendations on the level of abstraction of the diagnostic labels
3. To correlate the group's work with the ongoing development of diagnostic categories
4. To clarify the relevance of the framework for nursing practice

In their first and subsequent reports, the Theorist Group presented a framework with the central concept, health of unitary man (human). Nine patterns of unitary human–environment interaction were identified: exchanging, communicating, relating, valuing, choosing, moving, perceiving, knowing, and feeling. The patterns and early definitions are contained in Appendix F. Currently identified defining characteristics and diagnoses were grouped under these abstract categories that represent unitary patterns of human–environment interaction. It was recognized that each pattern would require an explicit definition. Basic assumptions underlying the framework were prepared by the Theorist Group in 1982[44] and are contained in Appendix T.

The reader may note that the assumptions implicit in the conceptual framework in Appendix T are similar to the work of Rogers, reviewed on pp. 56-58, as well as other associated philosophies of human beings. The nine patterns were identified between 1977 and 1982 by the Theorist Group, not by one theorist, through analysis of the diagnostic list. At this time the dynamically interrelated patterns contained 42 diagnoses. In their 1982 report the Theorists noted that the framework was incomplete and that a gap existed between the framework and the accepted nursing diagnoses.[43] They recommended further refinement and research. Progress reports on the work of the Theorist Group (from 1978 to 1982) may be found in the proceedings of the NANDA conferences.[43,44]

The second phase of the work on focus and classification was directed at linking already identified diagnoses and the conceptual system. Further work on this framework by the NANDA Taxonomy Committee, chaired by Dr. Phyllis Kritek, continued between 1982 and 1986. The committee's proposal to endorse the *NANDA Nursing Diagnosis Taxonomy I* (Appendix C) was accepted by the 1986 General Assembly of NANDA members.[45] The following represent changes and additions to previous work[45]:

1. The nine patterns mentioned above constitute the level 1 concepts, the most abstract level, and are called *human response patterns*. These patterns are the conceptual framework for organizing the taxonomy.
2. Level 2 concepts are less abstract and represent alterations in subcategories of human response patterns. Alterations are defined as "the process or state of becoming or being made different without changing into some-

thing else (see Appendix V)." Levels 2, 3, 4, and 5 contain current diagnoses.
3. Descriptors of actual or potential, acuity, and other qualifiers are defined in Appendix V.

The overall purpose of classifying human response patterns is to describe the structure and order of phenomena. The hierarchical arrangement of concepts identifies previously undiscovered properties of classes. Ordering also assists in the development of research hypotheses about relationships among concepts within the system.[46] Classes are arranged in a hierarchy according to their level of abstraction (see Appendix C). Each higher-level class includes the classes at the lower levels. Consider a familiar example: *fruit* is at a higher level of abstraction than *apples,* but *McIntosh apples* represent a lower level of abstraction than the general class, apples. In diagnosis *alterations in nutrition* is at a higher level of abstraction than *protein deficit.* The reason one class, category, or concept is at a higher or lower level of abstraction than another is the distance from observable characteristics; the greater the distance from its observable characteristics, the more abstract (as opposed to concrete) the idea, *and* the more abstract the category level is, the more it includes. *Fruit* is a highly inclusive category, as is *altered nutrition.* These categories are so inclusive and nonspecific that they are usually useless in determining actions.

The levels within *Taxonomy I* represent a hierarchical ordering from abstract (level 1) to concrete (levels 3, 4, and 5). The example in Table 12-1 of a level 1 concept, "Feeling," illustrates the idea of levels and order within the taxonomy; note that the diagnostic categories from Appendix A that are in boldface are classified at various levels. Thus it is obvious that current diagnoses vary in their level of abstraction. The categories in boldface are used as diagnoses in practice. An examination of this pattern and the eight others in Appendix C makes it clear that further development of the diagnostic nomenclature is necessary. One current difficulty in using some diagnostic categories in practice is that they are too general; further specification is necessary. Revealing problems, of course, is the value of classification as opposed to an alphabetical listing. Classification reveals many problems in the specificity and construction of diagnostic categories. It also reveals missing elements.

Table 12-1 NANDA Taxonomy: Human Response Pattern 9.0: Feeling

Level 1	9.0 FEELING
Level 2	9.1 Altered Comfort
Level 3	**9.1.1 Pain***
	9.1.1.1. Chronic
Level 2	9.2 [Altered emotional integrity]
Level 3	**9.2.1 Grieving**
Level 4	**9.2.1.1. Dysfunctional**
	9.2.1.2. Anticipatory
Level 3	**9.2.2 High Risk for Violence**
	9.2.2.1 High Risk for Self-Mutilation
	9.2.3 Posttrauma Response
Level 4	**9.2.3.1 Rape Trauma Syndrome**
Level 5	**9.2.3.2 Rape Trauma**
	9.2.3.1.1 Compound Reaction
	9.2.3.1.2 Silent Reaction
	9.3 [Altered emotional state]
Level 3	**9.3.1 Anxiety**
	9.2.4 Fear

Excerpted from NANDA: *NANDA nursing diagnoses: definitions and classification*, 1993.
*Diagnoses in bold are those used in clinical documentation.

The third phase of development was guided by Dr. Joyce Fitzpatrick. The Taxonomy Committee has identified the purposes of classification system development as follows:

1. To increase understanding
2. To identify relationships and gaps
3. To facilitate disciplinary communication
4. To systematically organize information[47 (p. 132)]

There have been critiques or comments on most of the above areas in the *Taxonomy*.[48-50] These criticisms are being addressed in the current taxonomy work and involve issues related to internal validity, reliability, and utility.[47]

Diagnostic taxonomy and functional health patterns

Functional health patterns are frequently used as a format for organizing assessment data. The novice diagnostician also finds the functional pattern groupings of diagnostic categories to facilitate the process of going from data (Appendix H) to diagnosis (Appendix B). In addition, in some curricula nursing knowledge is organized within the patterns, and in some cases the patterns have been incorporated into computer software. Let us consider how the functional health patterns are related to the taxonomy.

Level 2 concepts

In this author's opinion *Taxonomy I* is compatible with the functional health patterns. For example, if the term *altered* is removed from level 2 terms in Appendix C, the level 2 concepts are the functional health patterns. Although it is possible to convert the functional patterns to the more specific level 2 concepts (e.g., coping pattern or role pattern), this would increase the memory requirements to nearly 30 areas of assessment.

Note that "Growth and Development" is placed under "Moving" in the *NANDA Taxonomy* in Appendix C. Actually, this "diagnosis" probably should be considered a characteristic of *each* of the nine human response patterns rather than a separate diagnosis. Development is incorporated into the functional patterns. The patterns emerge developmentally based on person-environment interaction (cultural influences are also included in "environment"; they influence development). Separate diagnoses related to growth and development are in the following areas: self-care skills, communication skills, and social skills. Either "Developmental Lag" or "Altered Growth and Development" might be used with these further specifications.

Level 1 concepts

Fig. 12-1 represents this author's idea of how the functional patterns fit with superordinate level 1 patterns. Let us start by examining the relationships proceeding from lower to higher levels. Each of the functional patterns is an integration of lower-level biological, social, and psychological-spiritual functioning. The integration is expressed in each pattern. There is no one-to-one matching or labeling one functional pattern as physiological and another as psychosocial or spiritual. The functional health patterns are interdependent. One pattern cannot be understood by itself; the whole context of client-environment interaction must be considered.

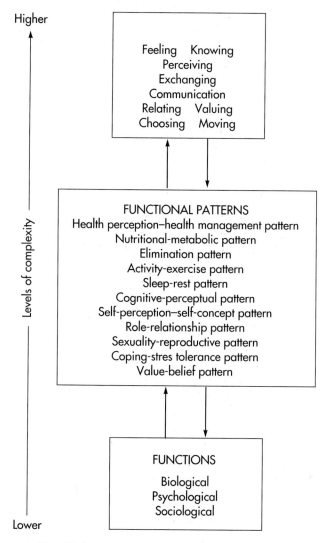

Fig. 12-1 Patterns at various levels of complexity.

Fig. 12-1 illustrates how each functional pattern contributes to and is influenced by a pattern of-knowing, feeling, etc. Think of the nine human response patterns as life processes. Now consider the health perception–health management pattern. Health perception and health management are influenced by a person's pattern of knowing, perceiving, feeling, relating, valuing, choosing, moving, communicating, and exchanging. Each of these is evident in Mrs. B.'s health perception–health management pattern, which was described in a previous chapter:

Mrs. B. has always perceived herself as "healthy"; no colds or infections; was thrown off her bicycle 6 months ago and now rides only on bicycle paths. "I get plenty of exercise and watch my diet. I don't know why the ulcer keeps acting up." In the last 5 months she gained weight from eating ice cream and drinking a lot of milk for an "acidy stomach"; says she looks "terrible" with the extra weight. Severe abdominal pain unrelieved by milk, cream, or antacids in the last week caused her to visit a physician; she was admitted to the hospital on the same day because of a low hemoglobin level and blood in her stool. She delayed seeking

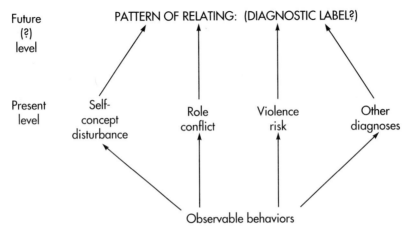

Fig. 12-2   Possible levels of diagnosis.

help because of her busy work schedule; stopped taking pills (name of medication not known) shortly after the last episode of bleeding because she felt better. States she works hard and that "I guess women have to work twice as hard to succeed in some companies." States the doctor is going to try a regimen of "pills and antacids and see how I do for a few days."

What are the consequences of this proposal? Higher-level problems might be found in any one of the human response patterns. A person may have a problem in relating that emerges from the analysis of functional health pattern assessment. Supporting data may be found in several patterns, or a family may have difficulty in a number of functional patterns in the area of choosing. It is the interaction of the parts that makes up the whole; that is, a pattern at a higher, more complex level of human functioning. Is this not the case with the taxonomy-pattern concepts? A higher level of synthesis of human behavior exists within the concepts of choosing, relating, and so forth. It is interesting to consider whether the pattern (e.g., "choosing" or "relating" in the above examples) is treated as the probable cause (etiological or related factors) and thus the focus of intervention.

Taxonomy I: implications for diagnosis

The implications of *Taxonomy I* for diagnosis are both obvious and not so obvious as one looks into the future. As previously suggested, the nine pattern concepts contain health problems at a level higher than that currently identified. Instead of a cluster of signs and symptoms, this level of diagnosis represents a cluster of "diagnoses," or problems with a common causal entity.

A life process may be seen as a thread that ties together and explains current health problems or risk states. Thus envisioned, this level of diagnosis may also explain particular sets of problems. To make this type of diagnosis, it may be necessary to move from assessment data to (1) diagnoses (as currently conceived) and then to (2) a synthesis that results in problem identification (within a category of knowing, choosing, and so forth). Fig. 12-2 illustrates how discernible behavior may be described as self-concept disturbance, role conflicts, violence potential, and other problems. A synthesis of these problems may reveal a larger problem, such as relating, and a diagnosis as yet unnamed in the nomenclature. If intervention focuses on the client's pattern of relating, then all the more concrete diagnoses may be improved.

The identification of more complex patterns has been discussed by others.[51-54] It is unlikely that this level of diagnosis, even if identified, will be resolved in a 2-day hospital stay. It is more likely that this level will need treatment at both the dysfunctional pattern level and the higher level of life pattern/process.

Congruence between Taxonomy I and diagnoses

The reader may be thinking: Will the taxonomy control the acceptance of diagnoses, or will new diagnoses possibly force changes in the taxonomy as needed? As Kritek[55] states:

Generation and classification should occur in tandem. Each process enhances, and challenges, the other. To continue to develop, test, and approve labels in a conceptual vacuum makes little sense.

The NANDA Taxonomy Committee suggests that the answer lies in clinical studies to test both the taxonomy and the diagnostic categories.[47] To identify diagnostic categories at the higher level of human response patterns, research will be needed to identify and label patterns of relating, exchanging, and so forth.

A deeper question plagues taxonomy development. As discussed in earlier chapters, are the human response patterns too abstract to guide identification of client conditions? What exactly is it that we are identifying and classifying—conditions resolved by nursing treatment or all health problems of concern in practice? The concepts of human response patterns, client-environment interactions, unitary human, and so forth still do not provide an answer. Yet there is a distinct feeling that we are getting closer to an answer. Those just entering the profession should be pleased that there still is intellectual work for the next generation of nurses.

The *NANDA Taxonomy* was approved as a "working taxonomy" and will be developed further. Revisions will be presented at NANDA biennial conferences, thus affording opportunities for further comments by the membership and the nursing community between conferences. It is predicted that the taxonomy will keep on evolving through theoretical work and research, as well as through interaction with the diagnostic nomenclature being developed.

Diagnostic category development

As seen in the previous discussion, a taxonomy has various levels. The level that contains diagnostic categories is the one most commonly used. This level contains the classes used in nursing practice to label diagnostic judgments about health-related conditions. Each class, or category, is defined by a cluster of observable characteristics. The characteristics are used in practice as diagnostic criteria to judge whether a particular condition is present or absent.

Since 1973 NANDA has been classifying health-related conditions that nurses say they diagnose and treat in their daily practice. The progress of this work may be seen in Appendix U, which lists the diagnoses by year of acceptance.

The state of development of diagnoses to some degree reflects the overall state of knowledge development in nursing. By no means are all the currently identified diagnostic categories built on a sound conceptual or theoretical base, nor do they include or represent a complete listing of all health-related conditions treated by nurses. Neither are these categories always precise enough to assure agreement among different nurse-diagnosticians viewing the same client. It is encouraging that those just entering the profession can still contribute to and shape the development of diagnostic categories, none of which are carved in stone. A nurse could spend her or his entire career studying one nursing diagnosis and its associated interventions and outcomes in multiple populations and across various cultures!

Current diagnostic categories share the same problems as some of the categories in medicine and psychiatry. Yet with all their deficiencies, clinicians are reporting their usefulness in direct and indirect care activities. This is probably because having language symbols (diagnostic terms) for recognizing and thinking about problems encountered in practice (1) increases sensitivity to cues and awareness of clients' conditions and (2) provides a "resting point" for thinking about how to provide professional help and guidance. The widespread use of diagnostic categories in practice is the reason it is so important for nurses to recognize the need for refinement of categories used in clinical reasoning and to make a concerted effort to improve currently identified categories.

Conceptual and structural aspects of diagnostic categories are examined in the next section. The ideas may prove useful in developing and refining the categories used in clinical practice.

Conceptual basis of a diagnostic category

A diagnostic category represents a conceptual view, or model, for thinking about a set of observations. Previously, the term *conceptual model* was used to refer to a perspective, or way of thinking, about *all of nursing*. The difference in the use of the term here is that now it is applied to *one* phenomenon in nursing; that is, one phenomenon described by one diagnostic concept. Each diagnostic category serves as a model to organize and account for empirical observations.

As the reader has learned, diagnostic concepts are created by nurses, and the "creation" represents the perspective of the "creator." If a diagnostic concept[56] survives in the "marketplace" of clinical practice and is used by others, it may be concluded that that way of thinking about the health problem is useful. That is, it is a useful and meaningful way of thinking about the cluster of observed behaviors. As knowledge increases, models may change and categories will then be changed or modified.

Knowing the conceptual meaning of a diagnostic category permits the use of the category to interpret clinical observations. *Meaning* refers to the conceptual basis of the diagnostic category, that is, the synthesis of theoretical and empirical knowledge about the health problem. There may be a discrepancy between one nurse's idea of the meaning of Separation Anxiety and another nurse's; therefore the meaning needs to be specified to prevent miscommunication and errors in the use of the category.

The conceptual basis of each diagnostic category needs to be specified. Many articles provide guidelines for developing the conceptual basis of each diagnostic category.[57-60] Work in this area leads to clear definitions and permits the development of more precise measurements. One way to approach the refinement of diagnostic categories is described below:

1. What is the current state of knowledge in the area described by a diagnostic category? Review the research literature related to each category; start with high-incidence diagnoses.
2. Write up the conceptual basis, citing references. Point out agreements, disagreements, gaps.
3. Does consistency exist between current concepts and each label, definition, characteristic, and etiological factor? Identify consistencies and inconsistencies.
4. Write up the conceptual analysis of elements in item 3. Identify what further conceptual analysis, research, and development are needed to improve the category. Is there a basis for any immediate improvements? If so, suggest them. Share findings.
5. Begin the analyses and research indicated.

Items 1 to 4, which provide a review of the literature, may in some cases provide sufficient basis for suggesting revisions in current categories to the NANDA Diagnosis Review Committee (Appendix V). Item 5 provides a continual program of theory development and research and can be the basis for further revisions. Revisions and reformulations will continue as long as the condition described by the category is of concern to nurses.

Some current categories might be improved merely by structural analysis and expert opinion. Even improvements in the structure of categories will begin to eliminate one source of diagnostic errors. Yet it is important to be aware that tidiness is only a "minor virtue" compared with the underlying conceptual insights, which are of major concern.

Structure of diagnostic categories

The structure of diagnostic categories refers to the content and format of labels, definitions, major characteristics (diagnostic criteria), minor characteristics (supporting data), and etiological or related factors. These are the elements of a category that are most frequently used in everyday practice. The level of theoretical development of a concept influences what is included in the structural elements. For purposes of discussion let us assume that theoretical development of a concept is sufficient; now let us review some considerations in creating a diagnostic category.

Level of generality

Recall that it was said that patterns, categories, classes, or concepts are found at various levels of

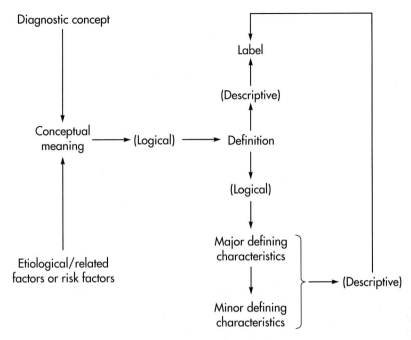

Fig. 12-3   Relationships among components of a diagnostic category.

abstraction. Abstract categories are more general descriptions (e.g., "color") than concrete categories (e.g., "red"). A general term is *inclusive,* that is, it includes many things. Categories at a high level of generality, or inclusiveness, are not useful for planning treatment. For example, a very general category is "dysfunctional elimination pattern." It is so inclusive that it encompasses all the relevant diagnoses and certainly would not be used to plan treatment. "Dysfunctional bowel pattern" includes fewer diagnostic categories and is less abstract but still does not represent a useful level. Moving toward more concrete concepts: Does "intermittent constipation pattern" provide a focus for recognizing a specific condition in clinical situations, clustering observations, and planning treatment? Probably so, because this category is at a useful level of generality.

In previous chapters, groupings such as "Alteration in Parenting or Alterations in Skin Integrity, were used as examples of highly general and inclusive categories. When this type of category is encountered, a logical question to ask is: What kind of alteration? As may be seen in Appendix C, categories at a high level of abstraction (general categories) are at levels 1 and 2, whereas the clinically useful categories are probably at levels 3, 4, and 5. In refining or constructing categories, it is necessary to aim for the level of generality that is "appropriate for using, thinking about, or naming"[60] (p. 24) the condition. This is the level needed for "thinking about" the condition and for "using" the diagnosis in treatment planning.

Naming and defining categories

Consistency should exist between (1) the meaning of the diagnostic concept; (2) its structural elements, which are the category name, the definition, and the major characteristics (the diagnostic criteria for making the diagnosis); and (3) the structural elements themselves. This dictum applies to the categories used to describe an actual or potential problem or to describe an etiological factor, as illustrated in Fig. 12-3.

Consistency is defined as agreement or harmony among (1) parts or features and (2) between parts and the whole. When they are internally consistent, there are no contradictions among the elements in

Fig. 12-3. For example, logical consistency and consistency in description are evident in the following:

1. The conceptual meaning is reflected in the descriptive label (the name).
2. The label concisely summarizes the definition.
3. The major or critical characteristics permit discriminations between the presence or absence of the phenomena described by the definition and name.
4. At least one of the critical characteristics differentiates the category from all others.

Naming a diagnostic category requires a consideration of how the category is to be used in thinking and communicating. As discussed in Chapter 8, categories are used as diagnostic hypotheses. Commonly, several hypotheses will be held in memory while the client is asked questions and observations are made. The limited memory capacity of human beings suggests that names should be concise and descriptive of the diagnostic criteria. The category name should provide a *memory probe* for retrieving knowledge about definition, critical and supporting characteristics, and possible etiological factors. (As the network of knowledge is built up, interventions, outcomes, and other relationships needed for a diagnosis will be retrieved in the same way.)

Consideration should also be given to the overall system of naming categories. Levine[61] has suggested that consultation with language experts is necessary to overcome labeling problems. Communication is a second consideration in naming. The goal is to develop terms that describe the signs and symptoms clearly and concisely. There are advantages and disadvantages to selecting words that have traditional meaning to nurses. One advantage is that the term(s) look familiar and are acceptable. A disadvantage is that old, familiar, personal meanings that are inconsistent with its "scientific" meaning may be attached to the category.

A clear, concise definition must accompany each diagnostic category. The words employed should be consistent with the conceptual meaning of the category and the list of major characteristics. *A definition differentiates a category from all others.*[62] Current definitions may be used as a base for revisions, when indicated. As an example, let

us revise a definition, step by step, according to the following characteristics:

1. Its conceptual meaning
2. The clarity and conciseness of its label and definition
3. Its consistency with diagnostic and supporting criteria

The diagnostic category Activity Intolerance will be used as it serves to demonstrate several points. The definition of Activity Intolerance is given below.

A state in which an individual has **insufficient physiological or psychological energy** to endure or complete **required or desired daily activities.**

The major concepts are in boldface so they stand out from the rest of the sentence. Read the following slowly and think about the ideas:

The definition might be more concise with the deletion of the first seven words. Isn't the following sufficient to express the concept of Activity Intolerance?

Insufficient physiological or psychological energy to endure or complete required or desired activities.

The thought expressed in this definition is highly complex. Complexity results from the two disjunctive concepts, energy and activities. Disjunctions are connected by *or:* (1) "physiological *or* psychological energy" and (2) "endure *or* complete . . . activities." The latter disjunctive concept ("endure or complete activities") may not be intended to be a disjunction. Commas inserted to indicate that *endure* is further explicated by the word *complete* would change the phrase to: "endure, or complete, . . . activities." This is the most likely meaning, since endurance is measured by the ability to complete an activity across time. When the inclination is to write a disjunctive definition, it should be determined whether two distinct entities are being considered under one category.

When the conceptual basis of this diagnostic category is considered, a question arises about the two types of energy: Are the definition and label consistent with the meaning of the concept being described? First we will assume that the label is consistent with the concept it describes, and then we will check the definition for consistency.

The expectation would be to find the meaning of the two words *activity intolerance* and their connection. *Tolerance* is defined as "to endure or complete required or desired daily activities." Toleration of an activity is usually measured by the degree of completion and the deviation from resting levels both during and after activity. A person might very well *endure* an activity until it is completed but exhibit serious signs of Activity Intolerance during and after the activity. Should this be considered in defining the concept of Activity Intolerance? Isn't it interesting to see what is found when one explores the "depths" of these categories and language usage!

The second concept in the diagnostic label is *activity*. Note that the definition is restrictive. It focuses on daily, as opposed to weekly, monthly, or yearly activities. Removing this restriction would result in "insufficient endurance for the completion of required or desired activities."

The definition of *activities* appears sufficiently inclusive; both required and desired activities are specified. The phrase may be made clearer with some minor changes in wording: "insufficient endurance to complete required or desired activities." The problem of using the same word, *activity,* in both the label and the definition still exists. Also, should activities be specified as "energy consuming"? Perhaps not; the usual connotation is that activity *is* energy consuming, and adding modifiers merely increases the complexity of the concept. Thought should also be given to the restriction implied by the word *endurance*. Is endurance the only reason for not completing activities? Strength is another common factor. Whereas endurance is usually associated with cardiac and circulatory factors, strength is associated with muscle mass, tonus, and metabolism. Both strength and endurance interact in "completing activities," and the amounts needed of each vary with the activity. Another consideration is that defining characteristics should specify levels of "insufficient endurance." Such levels might specify degrees of not completing required or desired activities within the time span dictated by the particular activity.

Let us now shift the focus from the label to the definition. Let us assume that the definition captures the essence of the diagnostic concept and examine the label. Consider physiological or psychological energy, which are probably categories that contain reasons for insufficient endurance (or tolerance). A lot of conceptual and format questions arise. Are these categories of etiological or of con-

tributing factors? Are we restricting the use of a diagnostic category if the etiological factors are built into a definition? (This author has been guilty of this in the past.) Yet do the concepts "insufficient physiological energy" or "insufficient psychological energy" provide a clear focus for intervention? Isn't "psychological energy" an umbrella concept for a cluster of signs and symptoms indicating various conditions? Does psychological energy mean *volition,* which is as important in voluntary activity as strength and endurance? It is necessary that both terms be defined operationally before a decision can be made.

In analyzing a diagnostic category, we examined each idea, or concept, in relation to the label and the definition individually and also in relation to each other. What we needed in this examination was the conceptual basis used by the author of the definition. Perhaps proceeding from the conceptual basis to a succinct definition and then to a label is the best way to achieve clarity. The following section further examines the consistency among the defining characteristics, labels, and the definition of *Activity Intolerance.*

Defining characteristics

Structurally a defining characteristic is *a value or an attribute of the client, environment, or both that serves as an indicator of the condition* described by the category.[63] Major characteristics are present in all clients with the condition; thus they would be the *critical characteristics* for making the diagnosis. Major diagnostic criteria require attention because they discriminate between clients who have the condition and those who do not. They also permit the diagnostician to discriminate among conditions. The major characteristics, as previously stated, need to be clear and precise, express the essential nature of the category, and differentiate the category from all others. Each characteristic should be concrete and measurable through observation or client reports. If it is possible to quantify the characteristic, consistency across clients and agreement among diagnosticians will be increased. The following are the major and minor characteristics listed for Activity Intolerance by NANDA[64] (p. 55):

1. Verbal report of fatigue or weakness
2. Abnormal heart rate or blood pressure
3. Exertional discomfort or dyspnea
4. Electrocardiographic changes reflecting arrhythmias or ischemia

In examining the category Activity Intolerance, we began with the definition below:

A state in which an individual has insufficient physiological or psychological energy to endure or complete required or desired activities.

We ended with the definition:

Insufficient endurance to complete required or desired activities.

An examination of the internal consistency of the characteristics and the definition reveals that a critical characteristic is missing: noncompletion of an activity (to some degree). Without this characteristic there is no consistency with the diagnostic label, which includes the word *activity,* or with the definition. A characteristic must be added, such as, "inability to complete an activity (specify activity or activity level)." The "specify" refers to a level of activity or to what activity the person cannot complete. This addition allows designation of the *level* of activity intolerance in the diagnosis. Thus the diagnosis might be documented as Activity Intolerance, Level II. This term has a precise meaning, and improvements could be tracked across time.

Although more might be added to this discussion, there have been sufficient examples of questions to raise in the analysis of a new or current diagnostic category. It should be kept in mind that this writer may have imposed meanings that were not compatible with the intended meaning (unspecified). For example, "to endure" may not have meant endurance in the physiological sense but rather "to bear up under a burden" in the psychological sense. Specifying the conceptual basis and the definition of terms is very important when categories are to be used by thousands of nurses in clinical practice and research.

Etiological or related factors

The discussion above pertaining to concepts also applies to what is commonly called etiological or related factors. These factors are explanatory concepts used to describe a probable cause of a problem. As stated previously, etiological factors and problem statements are related by theoretical knowledge derived from research, logical argument, or personal experience. This knowledge is used to support the judgment that a particular factor(s) is contributing to the problem.

The identification of etiological concepts for each health problem is a major task. It involves discovering the statistical relationship between problems and etiological factors. The first step in dealing with currently specified factors is concept analysis, as discussed above. Once the proposed etiological factors are operationalized, research directed at determining the probability of relationships between a health-related condition and contributing factors can follow.

General criteria for a useful category

Categories must be valid representations of reality and must facilitate clinical reasoning and judgment; otherwise they are not useful. The following criteria may be helpful in developing categories to be used to describe diagnostic judgments:

1. The category is within the conceptual focus of nursing and within the limits set by nurse practice acts. Nursing intervention can usually resolve the problem.
2. The level of generality, or inclusiveness, is appropriate for use in outcome projection (problem statement) and planning intervention (etiological factors).
3. The name given to the category is descriptive, concise, and clear. It conserves memory resources.
4. A specific, concise definition is stated. The definition is consistent with the conceptual or theoretical basis of the concept and the diagnostic criteria that make the definition operational.
5. Valid diagnostic criteria (critical or major characteristics) are designated. These characteristics permit discrimination among categories.
6. Categories designated as etiological factors are valid, conceptually defined, have major characteristics that operationalize their definition, and facilitate therapeutic judgments.

A number of recent articles may be used to guide diagnosis development and classification. (See Annotated Bibliography.)

Standardization of diagnoses

It could be said that the diagnostic labels are standardized. That is, there is an established usage and meaning for each diagnostic label. All those who have been educated in the profession should know the proper usage and employ it. Yet standardization does not imply that labels are written in stone. As with dictionaries, periodic revisions will occur. Also, a great deal of refinement needs to be done, as has been discussed.

Why standardize? Before answering this question directly, let us try something important. Please turn to the back of this pamphlet.

If you are confused, that is not unexpected. The standard usage of the word *pamphlet* was not employed; I described what you are reading as a pamphlet instead of as a book. This resulted in poor communication between us. The situation is similar in nursing practice. Similar phenomena must be called by the same name or communication suffers; different labels generate different meanings.

A related issue in classification is: Are diagnoses human processes or patterns, or are they states? Many of the labels in the current list of diagnoses (Appendix A) describe states; e.g., Constipation, Pain, Fluid Volume Deficit, Knowledge Deficit. Others describe behavioral processes or patterns: Impaired Mobility, Ineffective Coping, Sleep Pattern Disturbance. From a treatment perspective, a clinician changes a state, or at least modifies it. A state closely borders on being an entity or static condition. Medicine also describes states: e.g., cancer or diabetes. Current nursing diagnoses are not as rigid; no client would be called a constipatic or a grievic, in the same way as "diabetic," "schizophrenic," or "asthmatic" is used.

Standard average European English, as our language is called, leads to defining client conditions as if they were concrete, material objects. The idea of change, which we certainly recognize, is not readily expressed in English.[65]

Although diagnoses describe the state of the client at the time of encounter, is that the state of a pattern or process or a state-as-entity? For example, do we treat Pain as an entity? Or do we treat Pain Self-Management Deficit as a subclass of comfort management and a human functional pattern? Do we treat Constipation as an entity or as an intermittent constipation pattern?

Functional patterns or processes are close to the concept of "human responses" found in the ANA statement on the scope of practice.[66] Patterns and processes also approach a more holistic (total person) philosophy, especially when the defining signs and symptoms are biopsychosocial. But can all therapeutic concerns be expressed in one naming format? Will this approach prove useful for treatment decisions? We do not know.

NORTH AMERICAN NURSING DIAGNOSIS ASSOCIATION

NANDA is an organization of nurses (predominantly from the United States and Canada) who have assumed responsibility for the classification of nursing diagnoses. Its history extends back to 1973 and the First National Conference in the United States. This conference was coordinated by two faculty members at St. Louis University, Kristine Gebbie and Mary Ann Lavin. At this conference the Task Force for the Classification of Nursing Diagnosis was formed to continue work on the identification and classification of diagnoses. The Task Force held national conferences in 1975, 1978, 1980, 1982, and every 2 years thereafter.

In 1982 the North American Nursing Diagnosis Association (NANDA) was formed. The name reflected the 9-year history of participation by nurses from Canada and the United States in the development of diagnoses.

Purposes of the association

The purposes of NANDA are to develop, refine, and promote a taxonomy of nursing diagnostic terminology of general use to professional nurses. These purposes are implemented through a set of standing committees chaired by members of the Board of Directors.

Membership

Membership is open to registered nurses; associate memberships are open to professional nursing students and nonnurses. Nurses outside North America may belong individually or as a group.

Liaison activities

Since 1974 NANDA has had a formal liaison with the ANA through its Cabinet for Practice and, more recently, with the Nursing Organizations' Liaison Forum (NOLF). Communication has been instituted with other nursing organizations and groups engaged in classification or related work.

Implementation of purposes

One of NANDA's purposes is classification system development. Diagnoses are submitted to the Diagnostic Review Committee from individuals or groups according to the guidelines and review cycle presented in Appendix V. The final acceptance of a diagnostic category depends on a vote of the membership via mailed ballot. Taxonomy development is an ongoing activity. NANDA sponsored an invitational research conference to identify specific methodologies, which resulted in a very useful monograph.[67] Important issues in diagnosis have been addressed by invited speakers at biennial conferences; however, basic educational programs are viewed as a responsibility of regions or localities. The address of NANDA is

North American Nursing Diagnosis Association
1211 Locust Avenue
Philadelphia, PA 19107

Groups have formed in many parts of the United States—regional, state, and local—in some regions and provinces in Canada, and one in Europe. These groups provide a mechanism for discussion of issues related to development, implementation, and research at the local level. Some groups have begun their own newsletters to promote communication.

The nurses working on identification, development, and classification are an enthusiastic group who see the potential for nursing diagnosis in clinical practice, theory development, and the organization of nursing knowledge. This group of nurses is committed to the improvement of nursing care delivery through clarification of that area of nursing practice that involves diagnosis and treatment.

RESEARCH ON NURSING DIAGNOSIS

Clinical opportunities are plentiful for collecting data that might be used in clinical studies of nursing diagnoses. Students in professional education programs may have opportunities to do a clinical study as part of a research or senior elective course, or within a faculty's research project. After graduation opportunities will arise for collaboration or independent research; in some settings research is required for promotion to senior staff levels.

The work associated with development and classification of diagnoses has gone through a period of identifying the common conditions nurses said they diagnosed and treated in their practice. It was important to describe nurses' perceptions of these conditions and publish a listing that could be used to focus research on each diagnostic category. The problem of credibility arises if the acceptance and revision of categories is based on opinion. As Fuller[68] has suggested, basing acceptance of diagnoses on nurses' recall and opinions

runs the risk of defining nursing practice by consensus rather than by inquiry . . . . If unity and order are to be identified in the practice of nursing, the identification will surely come from the quiet pursuit of knowledge using the scientific method.[68] (p. 701)

Most agree that research and field testing are the necessary criteria for substantiating proposals of new diagnoses and revisions. Expert opinion may be used to evaluate the research base.

Research focused on diagnostic categories has increased considerably but still falls below what is needed. There is nearly an equal distribution of nurse consensus studies and clinical data-based studies of categories. Epidemiological research has been reported; studies in the medical-surgical setting are most common. There also have been some studies in the area of nurse staffing, quality assurance, and other areas of application.

The next section provides a brief introductory overview of the types of studies needed in nursing diagnosis and related areas. No attempt is made to review particular studies. The identification of new diagnoses, and testing and refinement of current diagnoses are considered. Epidemiological surveys and studies in related areas conclude the section.

Identification studies

Most agree that the current listing of diagnostic categories is incomplete. When a clinician repeatedly observes a condition that cannot be labeled with a current diagnosis, attention should be paid to the manifestations observed in the client-environment pattern. Both a conceptual analysis of the set of manifestations and studies to further describe the phenomenon are indicated at this point. Either qualitative, quantitative, or both types of methodologies may be employed to study the condition. It is advisable to report the condition in a journal such as *Nursing Diagnosis*. This will alert others to the condition and simultaneous research can begin.

Some have suggested that diagnoses seem to cluster in a pattern, somewhat like a syndrome. Chronic Pain, Activity Intolerance, and Impaired Physical Mobility each seem to be associated with a particular set of dysfunctional patterns (other diagnoses). Studies are needed to identify clusters of problems that are associated with a common etiological factor. Whether or not the cluster is more useful for care planning than each single problem is another question for study that would determine if these syndromes should be given a diagnostic label. The currently listed categories Rape Trauma Syndrome, Disuse Syndrome and Relocation Stress Syndrome, are examples of this type of category.

Each category should be examined for reliability and validity. These dimensions of a category specify its dependability and applicability. In one sense reliability and validity are a test of the conceptual clarity of the diagnostic concept; problems in attaining an acceptable level usually are solved by further concept development. Reliability and validity are described in the next section, when refinement studies are considered.

Qualitative (descriptive) research methods are useful within the factor-isolating phase of category development, as discussed in Chapter 11. Logan and Jenny[69,70] identified Dysfunctional Ventilatory Weaning Response using this method.

Refinement studies

There is a critical need for the refinement of categories that are widely used in practice. Many of the categories need the conceptual work outlined in the previous section.[59,62] After a category has been developed, the next step toward refinement is to establish validity and reliability. Quantitative research methods have been used in validating defining characteristics.[71-73]

Reliability

Whereas the credibility of a category is determined by its validity, its dependability is determined by its reliability; that is, during the diagnostic process, a category must have defining characteristics that can be used by one or more nurses to arrive at the same judgment; this is referred to as *interdiagnostician reliability*. Also, it is important that an individual nurse be able to use a particular diagnosis consistently to describe the same condition in various clients; this is called *intradiagnostician reliability*. These terms are the equivalent of *interrater* and *intrarater reliability*. Reliability is important in preventing diagnostic errors.

A group of experts skilled in the diagnostic process measures the degree to which the defining characteristics of a category can be used to arrive consistently at the same diagnosis.[74] The degree of reliability may be established by presenting such a group with a list of defining characteristics and requesting a diagnostic judgment. Interdiagnostician agreement is a measure of the reliability of the characteristics. Another method is to use written or videotaped cases to determine the agreement among the diagnoses formulated. The problem with using clinical situations is that all the raters will have to be present during assessment if there is a possibility that the client's condition will change before all assessments are done. Also, the concern about exposing a client to repeated assessments makes the simulated situation more attractive as a method. Reliability is a necessary but not sufficient condition for validity.

Validity

Studies are needed that will focus on the validity of, or the accuracy with which, a new or current diagnosis describes a condition occurring in practice. It should be noted that the label and definition are not the subject for research. These components are created by the category developer. *Validity* is the degree to which a cluster of defining characteristics describes a reality that can be observed in a client-environment interaction. Researchers should be concerned with the extent to which observations (which are later formulated as the characteristics of a category) are authentic representations of what exists in clinical practice; this measure refers to the *internal validity* of a category. The degree to which the characteristics may be used legitimately to diagnose the condition across various groups of clients is the *external validity* of a diagnostic category. These two measures establish *construct validity*.

Clinton[75] suggests that the construct, predictive, and discriminant validity of a diagnostic category should be established. *Predictive validity* refers to the degree to which the cluster of defining characteristics (derived from descriptive studies and concept analysis) is associated with other theoretically related phenomena. The degree to which the cluster of characteristics can detect differences between groups of clients is a test of *discriminant validity*. The known-groups technique provides a measure to detect differences between a group of clients expected to have a particular condition and a group expected not to have the condition.

Fehring[76] provides a model for establishing the content validity index (CVI) of diagnostic categories. He suggests each diagnostic category should have standardized validity measures, including diagnostic content validity (DCV), clinical diagnostic validity (CDV), and etiological correlation rating (ECR). The DCV is a CVI using experts' ratings of characteristics relative to the conceptual definition.

Experts' observations of the characteristics in a clinical situation are the basis for a category's CDV index. Using the DCV and CDV indices, the major characteristics (diagnostic criteria) of a category can be designated. Correlations describing the strength of association between problems and their etiological factors are represented by the ECR. The validity of categories must be determined before correlations between or among categories are noted; thus it is important to know the DCV and CDV before giving attention to the problem–etiological factor relationship.

Asking nurses or using the data of nursing assessments to establish validity requires some thought. Expert raters and astute clinical observers should be consulted. It may also be important to establish the reliability of the clinical data collectors' interviewing and examination skills and their sensitivity to cues. Other principles of validity testing also apply. Examples of studies using different methodologies may be found in the literature.[77]

Validity provides a measure of the confidence that should be placed in the accuracy of a category in depicting reality. Of course, conceptual reality is relative to the perceiver. It may be found that the characteristics are (1) present as a pattern in the client-environment interactions that are being measured and (2) related to the conceptual definition of the diagnosis, yet nurses may not agree that

the diagnosis is within the conceptual or legal focus of nursing practice. As Fehring[76] suggests, a study of the consensual validity of the category using a random sampling of the population of nurses may be necessary. On the other hand, if the investigator has confidence in the category's conceptual and legal dimensions, survival in the "marketplace" of clinical practice will provide an indication of nurses' consensus about the category.

Epidemiological studies

Epidemiological studies are designed to document the base-rate occurrence of diagnoses in the population. A review of research from 1953 to 1983 reveals several studies and many methodological problems,[78] which in recent years have been addressed. Unless an acceptable level of reliability and validity is established for diagnostic categories, the dependability of both the categories and the judgments employing the categories may be open to question.

Various populations may be studied to determine the epidemiology of nursing diagnoses. Populations may be selected by medical groupings such as disease or diagnosis-related groups or by gender, ethnicity, culture, setting, phase of illness, and other variables. Table 12-2 shows a comparison of high-frequency, high-treatment priority nursing diagnoses in three specialties.[79] If diagnoses 2, 4, 6, and 7 in the critical care listing were categorized separately, the following diagnoses would be raised in rank: Anxiety, Sleep-Pattern Disturbance, High Risk for Fluid Volume Deficit, and Ineffective Breathing Pattern.

It would also be interesting to select a nursing diagnostic population, such as clients with immobility, and determine the co-occurring nursing diagnoses that cluster with this condition in various age groups. Epidemiological studies add to the nursing knowledge base. In practice the knowledge is used in the following areas:

1. The diagnostic process, to predict likely possibilities and increase sensitivity to cues
2. To predict the nursing care requirements of specific populations
3. To guide the selection of the essential content of in-service and formal education programs

The concurrence of medical and nursing diag-

Table 12-2 Comparison of the Eight High-Frequency–High-Treatment Priority Nursing Diagnoses in Rehabilitation Nursing, Critical Care Nursing, and Neonatal Intensive Care Nursing*

Rank	Rehabilitation nursing	Critical care nursing	Neonatal intensive care nursing
1.	Impaired Physical Mobility	Pain (specify location)	Impaired Gas Exchange
2.	Knowledge Deficit	Impaired Gas Exchange	High Risk for Altered Body Temperature
3.	Self-Care Deficit: Bathing/Hygiene	High Risk for Infection	Ineffective Airway Clearance
4.	Self-Care Deficit: Dressing/Grooming	Decreased Cardiac Output	Ineffective Breathing Pattern
5.	Self-Care Deficit: Toileting	High Risk for Impaired Skin Integrity	High Risk for Infection
6.	Transfer Deficit (Specify Level)	Fluid Volume Excess	Nutritional Deficit
7.	High Risk for Injury	Altered Cardiopulmonary Tissue Perfusion	Impaired Skin Integrity
8.	High Risk for Impaired Skin Integrity	Ineffective Airway Clearance	High Risk for Impaired Skin Integrity

*High-frequency nursing diagnoses are those rated as nearly always or frequently present in the practice of 75% or more of a national sample of rehabilitation nurses (N = 720), critical care nurses (N = 678), and neonatal intensive care nurses (N = 408). All diagnoses were rated as nearly always or frequently a treatment priority in the specialty.

noses is of particular interest because of the current practice of prospective payment based on diagnostic-related groupings. Concurrence studies would help establish the approximate cost of medical and nursing resources used by a population of clients (see Chapter 11). With the emphasis on cost containment and early discharge, it would be helpful to study nursing diagnoses at discharge and correlate them with the community nursing services available. Cross-cultural epidemiological studies are also needed; they would contribute to further development of categories.

Diagnostic process studies

The process of how nurses collect, interpret, cluster, and give names to their diagnostic judgments requires a great deal more investigation. Studies are needed of the aspects of the process,[80] diagnostic errors,[81] the effect of initial impressions and other potential biases, and the influence of various

educational strategies on competency. Task, personality, and setting variables should also be foci of research.

This area of research will continue to grow. It will be influenced by the emphasis placed on clinical judgment skills by the Association of Colleges of Nursing and the National League for Nursing's accreditation criteria related to critical thinking.

Diagnostic outcome and process studies

The determination of realistic diagnostic outcomes for specified time periods (e.g., discharge) would be a fruitful area of study. Research of this type could guide individual practitioners as well as quality assurance reviews. Experimental research on treatments for nursing diagnoses is critically needed to determine which interventions lead to desired outcomes in the most cost-efficient and

Table 12-3   High Risk for Infection: Diagnosis-Intervention-Outcome Links*

Diagnosis	Outcome	Intervention
High Risk for Infection 1. Tissue destruction 2. Immunosuppression 3. Increased environmental exposure to pathogens	Absence of signs of infection (specify; e.g., lungs clear, afebrile, negative cultures)	Ensure use of aseptic technique (catheters, tubes, lines, etc.) Provide adequate nutrients. Teach methods of preventing infection to visitors (precautions, etc.) Explain methods of preventing infection to patient (precautions, etc.) Immunosuppressive precautions (specify)

*Based on a national survey of critical care nurses, outcomes were rated as nearly always or usually achieved by more than 68% of 145 nurses. Interventions were rated as critically important or important for achieving these outcomes by more than 70% of the 163 nurses.

humanistic manner. Retrospective studies of treatments provided and outcomes attained would provide data on outcome-process linkages for each diagnosis. Also, the many variables that influence outcomes and treatments need to be identified. Some current diagnoses may be sufficiently reliable and valid for investigators to proceed with outcome and treatment studies. The increased use of computers in health care institutions should facilitate large-scale studies on each diagnosis, on outcomes, and on treatment. These studies should provide a research base for diagnosis-based outcome and process standards and provide data for cost-benefit analyses.

In a study of diagnosis-intervention outcome links,[82] it was assumed there is a core set of achievable outcomes in a particular setting and a core set of interventions that are critically important for achieving those outcomes. After identifying high-frequency diagnoses and their critical defining characteristics, a national sample of critical care nurses rated the achievability of outcomes and the criticality of interventions to achieve those outcomes. Table 12-3 provides an example of these linkages: they are the critical outcomes and inter-

ventions for this particular diagnosis. It is also probable that the diagnosis should be more precise. Support for this supposition was found in the clusters of defining characteristics that suggested three specific diagnoses: High Risk for Respiratory Infection, Skin Infection, and Urinary Tract Infection. A fourth diagnosis, High Risk for Maternal or Infant Infection, is suggested by one NANDA defining characteristic, rupture of amniotic membranes.[79]

Studies of the ethics of diagnosis and treatment

Most studies in nursing ethics focus on the collaborative area of practice with physicians or with nurses' ethical responsibilities in personal-professional-bureaucratic conflicts. Research is needed on ethical issues in nursing diagnosis and treatment but may have to await an increased consciousness of moral responsibilities in this area of practice. For example, many nurses state they do not have time for assessment beyond that required in their collaborative role. "No time for nursing assessment and diagnosis" is stated as a fact and does not seem to be viewed as a dilemma in the allocation of resources. Respect for the autonomy of clients, informed consent, and other issues are also relevant in the domain of practice described by nursing diagnoses.

Nursing diagnosis can help focus clinical research and provide a way of organizing knowledge gleaned from clinical studies of "problems," interventions, results of interventions, and the variables that influence any of these. Perhaps investigators will become sufficiently interested in one or more diagnoses to begin a program of research that will extend beyond the initial studies of a category to its use in nursing process.

SUMMARY

In this final chapter, four issues critical to the future development of nursing diagnosis are discussed: acceptance of diagnosis, current status of implementation, problems and prospects in classification, and research. For various reasons not everyone accepts the idea of nursing judgment beyond those described by the traditional medical concepts. At this point the reader should have sufficient background in the subject to take a position on what the direction of the profession should be.

The implementation of nursing diagnosis and the diagnostic process is not seen in every clinical setting in North America. Yet if outside accreditors cite the organized approach to care resulting from diagnosis, nurses may consider the concept. Nurses who become bored with a routine approach to every "gallbladder patient" may consider using the diagnostic process, which can reveal the individuality of persons and families. Diagnosis-based care planning may become so habitual during educational programs that new graduates will be unable to consider any other way of determining nursing interventions.

The classification of nursing diagnoses and related research have been reviewed. The problems and prospects are evident. The development of nomenclature and a classification system for nursing practice will not be done by an elitist group. Clinicians, clinical specialists, theorists, educators, and researchers all have much to offer. It is hoped that this review will stimulate more nurses to become enthusiastic about contributing to the future direction of nursing diagnosis.

FUTURE DIRECTIONS

Many forces within and external to nursing will influence the future direction of nursing diagnosis both in North America and in other areas of the world. Nurses using diagnosis and those with whom they communicate in practice settings will encourage a clearer definition of the concept. It may be expected that potential problems, requiring preventive nursing intervention, will continue to be defined as nursing diagnoses. As primary care specialists become more involved in identifying these high-risk health patterns, additional nomenclature will be devised, followed by research to identify methods of helping clients decrease health risks. When risk reduction and health promotion can be demonstrated and related to cost and quality of life, the public may be persuaded to finance preventive care.

Financing nursing care will be a major factor influencing the development of a diagnostic classification system. As it is now, hidden within the costs of room and board or medical care, nursing is not clearly perceived by the public. What nurses do and why they do it will become obvious when direct reimbursement is a reality. At that point it will become necessary to articulate which actual or potential problems are to be treated, what outcomes will result, and how these health outcomes will contribute to goals that society values.

In acute and long-term care settings, nursing's concern with the quality of life will encourage assessment of functional patterns. The resident minimum data set in current use is very similar to functional health patterns. The recognition of actual or potentially dysfunctional patterns should stimulate experimental studies of nursing intervention. Diagnosis-intervention-outcome links will be established to enhance decision making in care planning.

The aged will comprise a high percentage of clients in health care settings. Ways will have to be found to sustain their optimal function and quality of life. Otherwise, the dire predictions for the year 2000 made by some analysts of health care—financial collapse of the health care system and euthanasia—may come true. Nurses focus on optimal patterns of functioning; this focus is especially useful in the health care of the elderly. If nursing's domain of practice is established as the detection of potential problems and the restoration of integrated function after dysfunctional patterns occur, nurses may be the health care providers who assume the major responsibility for meeting the health care needs of the elderly population. The beliefs and values traditionally held by nurses may influence society to recognize the aged for their wisdom, rather than for their disabilities.

One of the areas of immediate concern is the validity and reliability of diagnostic categories. What would reliability studies accomplish? If a sign or symptom can be demonstrated to occur in 95 out of 100 persons, it is a reliable predictor of a condition. Nurses caring for clients need clusters of highly reliable cues to diagnose actual or potential problems with confidence and accuracy. Without these predictors, diagnostic errors occur. Diagnostic errors lead to inadequate care plans and interventions. In turn, inadequate interventions rarely permit health outcomes to be attained and may result in harm and suffering.

Establishing the level of reliability of current lists of defining characteristics would greatly facilitate education. Students could then learn the few critical cues that reliably predict the presence of a diagnosis. Other currently listed cues may be useful in supporting a judgment but are not critical. Noncritical cues may be learned later, as clinical experience in diagnosing a condition accumulates.

Another major effort in conjunction with the ANA is the development of a uniform nursing language. The distinct similarities among the classification systems widely used or recently developed are striking. The *NANDA Taxonomy,*[47] the SABA Classification of Home Health Nursing Diagnoses, and the Omaha Community Health Classification System overlap a great deal. This may be seen by comparing Appendixes A and W. An in-depth analysis of the similarities among the terms and their definitions is the first step in determining overlap. In addition, dieticians are now in the process of coding the conditions they encounter in their practice. Appendix W contains a sample of their coding system.

Future graduates of professional nursing programs should demonstrate competence in using diagnostic categories to organize client data and plan care. This will occur only if both diagnostic process and diagnostic categories are integrated into educational programs, if increased skills in critical thinking are developed, and if a respect for this dimension of practice is acquired. Clinical studies of the diagnostic process used by health care providers will increase. The search for knowledge to increase diagnostic efficiency and validity of diagnosis will be influenced by a continued emphasis on cost and quality control, with attention to outcomes. Expanding knowledge of the diagnostic process will facilitate its teaching. Studies will test the application of knowledge of cognitive processes to specific diagnostic situations in nursing. As faculty appreciate the need for training in uncertainty-based judgment, methods of controlling uncertainties in this dimension of practice will be learned.

Several issues that will influence the future direction of nursing diagnosis have been briefly reviewed in this book. To those in this and other countries who see beyond the mere obvious, wonder why, and reason how, is left the future of nursing and nursing diagnosis.

NOTES AND REFERENCES

1. Gebbie KA, Lavin MA: Classifying nursing diagnoses, *Am J Nurs* 44:250, 1974.
2. The term *category* refers to a diagnosis in the classification system. Each category has a conceptual base that represents the knowledge about the phenomena; thus each diagnosis may also be referred to as a concept.
3. Thomas CL: *Taber's cyclopedic medical dictionary*, ed 17, rev, Philadelphia, 1992, Davis.
4. Barnum BJ: On nursing, *Nurs Health Care* 11:227, 1990 (editorial).
5. Watson J: Watson's philosophy and theory of human caring in nursing. In Riehl-Sisca J, editor: *Conceptual models for nursing practice,* Norwalk, CT, 1989, Appleton & Lange.
6. Nurcombe R: Goal directed treatment planning and the principles of brief hospitalization, *J Am Acad Child Adolesc Psychiatry* 28:26, 1989.
7. Seahill L: Nursing diagnosis versus goal-oriented treatment planning in inpatient child psychiatry, *Image* 23:95, 1991.
8. American Psychiatric Association: *Diagnostic and statistical manual of mental disorders,* ed 3, rev, Washington, DC, 1987, The Association.
9. Loomis ME et al: Development of a classification system for psychiatric–mental health nursing: individual response class, *Arch Psychiatr Nurs* 4:16, 1987. Proposal by the ANA Council of Psychiatric–Mental Health Nurses on psychiatric nursing diagnoses. Presentation of a classification system.
10. Murphy G, Stern P: Applying nursing diagnosis in critical care, *Can Nurse* 89:28, 1993. Grounded theory approach was used to determine the processes critical care nurses use

to describe their practice and to define and use nursing diagnoses. Includes a list of difficulties encountered in using diagnoses and recommendations, a useful listing for implementors.

11. Steel D, Whalen J: A proposal for two new nursing diagnoses: potential for organ failure and potential for tissue destruction, *Heart Lung* 4:426, 1987.

12. Miller E, Williams S: Alteration in cerebral perfusion: clinical concept or nursing diagnosis? *J Neurosci Nurs* 19:183, 1987.

13. Kern L, Omery A: Decreased cardiac output in the critical care setting, *Nurs Diagn* 3:94, 1992.

14. Mitchell G: Nursing diagnosis: an ethical analysis, *Image* 23:99, 1991.

15. Hagey RS, McDonough P: The problem of professional labeling, *Nurs Outlook* 32:151, 1984.

16. Rodgers BL: Deconstructing the dogma in nursing knowledge and practice, *Image* 23:177, 1991.

17. Levine M: Trophicognosis: an alternative to nursing diagnosis. In American Nurses Association, editor: *Exploring progress in medical-surgical nursing,* Kansas City, MO, 1966, The Association.

18. Brunckhorst L et al: Who's using nursing diagnoses? *Am J Nurs* 389:267, 1989.

19. Maas M: Organizational characteristics that facilitate the use of nursing diagnoses, *Nurs Clin North Am* 22:881, 1987.

20. McCourt A: Implementation of nursing diagnoses through integration with quality assurance, *Nurs Clin North Am* 22:899, 1987.

21. Greenlee K: Effects of implementation of an operational definition of nursing diagnoses in a critical care setting. In Carroll-Johnson R, editor: *Classification of nursing diagnoses: proceedings of the ninth conference,* Philadelphia, 1992, Lippincott.

22. Bulechek G et al: An evaluation guide to assist with implementation of nursing diagnosis, *Nurs Diagn* 1:18, 1990.

23. Minton J, Creason N: Evaluation of admission nursing diagnoses, *Nurs Diagn* 2:119, 1991.

24. Thomas N, Newsome G: Factors affecting the use of nursing diagnosis, *Nurs Outlook* 40:182, 1992.

25. Hanson M et al: Education in nursing diagnosis: evaluating clinical outcomes, *J Contin Educ Nursing* 21:79, 1990.

26. Woolley N: Nursing diagnosis: exploring the factors which may influence the reasoning process, *J Adv Nurs* 15:110, 1990.

27. American Association of Colleges of Nursing: *Essentials of college and university education for nursing,* Washington, DC, 1986, The Association.

28. Elstein M, Schulman LS, Sprafka SA: *Medical problem solving: an analysis of clinical reasoning,* Cambridge, MA, 1978, Harvard University Press.

29. Aspinall MJ: Nursing diagnosis: the weak link, *Nurs Outlook* 24:433, 1976.

30. National Council on Education: Critical thinking, *Chronicle of Higher Education* 2:345, 1992.

31. Hedley C, Houtz J, Baratta A, editors: *Cognition, curriculum, and literacy,* Norwood, NJ, 1990, Ablex.

32. Corcoran S, Narayan S, Moreland H: "Thinking aloud" as a strategy to improve clinical decision making, *J Crit Care* 17:463, 1988.

33. Dunn J, Crosby F: Teaching nursing diagnoses to school nurses: a curriculum plan, *J Contin Educ Nurs* 19:205, 1988.

34. Tanner C: Teaching clinical judgment, *Ann Rev Nurs Res* 153,

35. Lunney M: Educating nurse diagnosticians, *Nurse Educ* 13:24, 1988.

36. Feild LM: Implementation of nursing diagnosis in clinical practice, *Nurs Clin North Am* 14:525, 1979.

37. Dalton JM: Nursing diagnosis in a community health setting, *Nurs Clin North Am* 14:525, 1979.

38. Weber S: Nursing diagnosis in private practice, *Nurs Clin North Am* 14:533, 1979.

39. Bruce J: Implementation of nursing diagnosis: an administrator's perspective, *Nurs Clin North Am* 14:509, 1979.

40. Rantz M, Miller T, Jacobs C: Nursing diagnoses in long term care, *Am J Nurs* 85:916, 1986.

41. NANDA, The North American Nursing Diagnosis Association, was formerly the National Conference Group for Classification of Nursing Diagnoses (1973-1982).

42. Hangartner C: Principles of classification. In Gebbie K, Lavin M, editors: *Classification of nursing diagnoses: proceedings of the first national conference on classification of nursing diagnoses,* St Louis, 1975, Mosby.

43. Roy C: Framework for classification systems development: progress and issues. In Kim MJ, McFarland G, McLane A, editors: *Classification of nursing diagnoses: proceedings of the fifth national conference,* St Louis, 1984, Mosby.

44. Roy C: Theoretical framework for classification of nursing diagnoses. In Kim MJ, Moritz DA, editors: *Classification of nursing diagnoses: proceedings of the third and fourth national conferences,* New York, 1982, McGraw-Hill.

45. McLean A: Minutes and summary of the General Assembly. In McLean A, editor: *Classification of nursing diagnoses: proceedings of the seventh conference,* St Louis, 1987, Mosby.

46. Sokal RR: Classification: purposes, principles, progress, prospects, *Science* 185:1115, 1974.

47. Kerr M et al: Committee report: from Taxonomy I to Taxonomy II, *Nurs Diagn* 2:131, 1991; Hoskins L et al: Axes: focus of Taxonomy II, *Nurs Diagn* 3:117, 1992.

48. Porter E: Critical analysis of NANDA Nursing Diagnosis, Taxonomy I, *Image* 18:136, 1986.

49. Rasch R: The nature of taxonomy, *Image* 19:147, 1987.

50. England M: Nursing diagnosis: a conceptual framework. In Fitzpatrick J, Whall A, editors: *Conceptual models of nursing,* Norwalk, CT, 1989, Appleton & Lange.

51. Rossi L, Krekeler K: Small group reactions to the theoretical framework of unitary man. In Kim MM, Moritz DA, editors: *Classification of nursing diagnoses: proceedings of the third and fourth national conferences,* St Louis, 1982, Mosby, p 274.

52. Feild LM: Comments of clinical specialists on the unitary man framework. In Kim MJ, Moritz DA, editors: *Classification of nursing diagnoses: proceedings of the third and fourth national conferences,* St Louis, 1982, Mosby, p 265.

53. Weber S: Comments of clinical specialists on the unitary man framework. In Kim MJ, Moritz DA, editors: *Classification of nursing diagnoses: proceedings of the third and fourth national conferences,* St Louis, 1982, Mosby, p 270.

54. Kirk LW: The design for relevance revisited: an elaboration of the conceptual framework for nursing diagnosis. In Hurley M, editor: *Classification of nursing diagnoses: proceedings of the sixth conference,* St Louis, 1986, Mosby.

55. Kritek A: NANDA Taxonomy I. In McLean A, editor: *Classification of nursing diagnoses: proceedings of the seventh conference,* St Louis, 1987, Mosby.

56. It is more appropriate to use the term *diagnostic concept* in this discussion; recall that the terms *category* and *concept* refer to the same thing but are used in different contexts.

57. Norris CA: *Concept clarification in nursing,* Rockville, MD, 1982, Aspen Systems.

58. Nicoll LH: *Perspectives on nursing theory,* Boston, 1986, Little, Brown.

59. Gordon M: Toward theory-based diagnostic categories, *Nurs Diagn* 1:5, 1990.

60. Rosch E: Basic level categories. In Tosch E, Llloyd B, editors: *Cognition and categorization,* Hillsdale, NJ, 1978, Erlbaum.

61. Levine ME: Taxonomy development. In McLane A, editor: *Classification of nursing diagnoses: proceedings of the seventh conference,* St Louis, 1987, Mosby.

62. Avant KC: The art and science in nursing diagnosis development, *Nurs Diagn* 1:51, 1990; Avant K: Paths to concept development in nursing diagnosis, *Nurs Diagn* 2:105, 1991.

63. Previously, when the clinical practice context was considered, defining characteristics were called *signs* and *symptoms.* Two types of defining characteristics are identified by NANDA: (1) major characteristics, which are present in *all* clients with the condition and (2) minor characteristics, which are present in *most* clients with the condition. Under the diagnosis Activity Intolerance, "verbal report of fatigue or weakness" now carries an asterisk because it is designated as the major critical defining characteristic or diagnostic criterion.

64. North American Nursing Diagnosis Association: *NANDA nursing diagnoses: definitions and classification,* Philadelphia, 1992, The Association, p 55.

65. Warner R: Relationship between language and disease concepts, *Int J Psychiatry Med* 7:57, 1976.

66. American Nurses Association: Nursing: a social policy statement, Washington, DC, 1980, The Association.

67. North American Nursing Diagnosis Association: *Invitational conference monograph. Research methods for validating nursing diagnoses,* Philadelphia, 1989, The Association.

68. Fuller SS: Holistic man and the science and practice of nursing, *Nurs Outlook* 26:701, 1978.

69. Logan J, Jenny J: Deriving a new diagnosis through qualitative research: dysfunctional ventilatory weaning response, *Nurs Diagn* 1:37, 1990.

70. Jenny J, Logan J: Analyzing expert nursing practice to develop a new nursing diagnosis: dysfunctional ventilatory weaning response. In Carroll-Johnson R, editor: *Classification of nursing diagnoses: proceedings of the ninth conference,* Philadelphia, 1991, Lippincott, pp 133-140.|

71. Summers S et al: Validation of the nursing diagnosis hypothermia. In Carroll-Johnson R, editor: *Classification of nursing diagnoses: proceedings of the ninth conference,* Philadelphia, 1991, Lippincott, pp 97-104.

72. Kelly D: The identification and clinical validation of the defining characteristics of alteration in cardiac tissue perfusion. In Carroll-Johnson R, editor: *Classification of nursing diagnoses: proceedings of the ninth conference,* Philadelphia, 1991, Lippincott, pp 105-111.

73. Anderson J, Thomson A: Impaired Skin Integrity: clinical validation of the defining characteristics. In Carroll-Johnson R, editor: *Classification of nursing diagnoses: proceedings of the ninth conference,* Philadelphia, 1991, Lippincott, pp 126-132.

74. Gordon M, Sweeney MA: Methodological issues in nursing diagnosis research, *Adv Nurs Sci* 20:1, 1979.

75. Clinton J: Nursing diagnoses research methodologies. In Hurley M, editor: *Classification of nursing diagnoses: proceedings of the sixth conference,* St Louis, 1986, Mosby, pp 159-167.

76. Fehring RJ: Validating diagnostic labels: standardized methodology. In Hurley M, editor: *Classification of nursing diagnoses: proceedings of the sixth conference,* St Louis, 1986, Mosby, pp 183-190.

77. Lackey NR: Use of Q methodology in validation of defining characteristics of specified nursing diagnoses. In Hurley M, editor: *Classification of nursing diagnoses: proceedings of the sixth national conference,* St Louis, 1986, Mosby, pp 191-206; Lo CK, Kim MJ: Construct validity of sleep pattern disturbance: a methodological approach. In Hurley M, editor: *Classification of nursing diagnoses: proceedings of the sixth national conference,* St Louis, 1986, Mosby, pp 207-215; Vincent KG: Validation of a nursing diagnosis: a nurse consensus survey. In Hurley M, editor: *Classification of nursing diagnoses: proceedings of the sixth national conference,* St Louis, 1986, Mosby, pp 207-214; Mehmert P, Delaney C: Validating impaired physical mobility, *Nurs Diagn* 2:143, 1991; Thomas MD, Sanger E, Whitney, J: Nursing diagnosis of depression, *J Psychosocial Nurs* 24:6, 1986.

78. Gordon M: Nursing diagnosis. In Werley HH, Fitzpatrick JJ, editors: *Annual review of nursing research,* vol 3, New York, 1985, Springer.

79. Gordon M: *Comparison of high frequency nursing diagnoses in three nursing specialties,* Boston College School of Nursing, Chestnut Hill, Mass 02167 (in press).

80. Gordon M: High risk nursing diagnoses in critical care. In Carroll-Johnson R, editor: *Classification of nursing diagnoses: proceedings of the tenth conference,* Philadelphia, 1993, Lippincott.

81. Tanner C: Thinking about critical thinking, *J Nurs Ed* 32:99, 1993 (editorial).

82. Lunney M: Accuracy of nursing diagnoses: concept development, *Nurs Diagn* 1:12, 1990.

APPENDIX A

ALPHABETICAL LISTING OF NANDA's ACCEPTED NURSING DIAGNOSES, 1992

Definitions, defining characteristics, and related factors are included in *NANDA Taxonomy I,* revised June 1992.

Activity Intolerance (Specify Level)
Activity Intolerance, High Risk for
Adjustment, Impaired
Airway Clearance, Ineffective
Anxiety
Aspiration, High Risk for
Body Image Disturbance
Bowel Incontinence
Breastfeeding, Effective
Breastfeeding, Ineffective
Breastfeeding, Interrupted
Breathing Pattern, Ineffective
Cardiac Output, Decreased
Communication, Impaired Verbal
Conflict, Decisional (Specify)
Conflict, Parental Role
Constipation
Constipation, Colonic
Constipation, Perceived
Coping, Defensive
Coping, Ineffective (Individual)
Coping, Ineffective Family: Compromised
Coping, Ineffective Family: Disabling
Coping, Family: Potential for Growth
Denial, Ineffective
Diarrhea
Disuse Syndrome, High Risk for
Diversional Activity Deficit
Dysreflexia
Family Processes, Altered
Fatigue
Fear (Specify)
Feeding Pattern, Ineffective Infant
Fluid Volume Deficit
Fluid Volume Deficit, High Risk for

Fluid Volume Excess
Gas Exchange, Impaired
Grieving, Anticipatory
Grieving, Dysfunctional
Growth and Development, Altered
Health Maintenance, Altered
Health-Seeking Behaviors (Specify)
Home Maintenance Management, Impaired
Hopelessness
Hyperthermia
Hypothermia
Identity Disturbance, Personal
Incontinence, Functional
Incontinence, Reflex
Incontinence, Stress
Incontinence, Total
Incontinence, Urge
Infection, High Risk for
Injury, High Risk for
Knowledge Deficit (Specify)
Mobility, Impaired Physical
Neglect, Unilateral
Neurovascular Dysfunction, High Risk for Peripheral
Noncompliance (Specify)
Nutrition, Altered: Less than Body Requirements
Nutrition, Altered: More than Body Requirements
Nutrition, Altered: High Risk for More than Body Requirements
Oral Mucous Membrane, Altered
Pain
Pain, Chronic
Parenting, Altered
Parenting, High Risk for Altered
Poisoning, High Risk for
Post-Trauma Response
Powerlessness
Protection, Altered
Rape Trauma Syndrome

Rape Trauma Syndrome: Compound Reaction
Rape Trauma Syndrome: Silent Reaction
Relocation Stress Syndrome
Role Conflict, Parental
Role Performance, Altered
Role Strain, Caregiver
Role Strain, Caregiver, High Risk for
Self-Care Deficit: Bathing/Hygiene (Specify Level)
Self-Care Deficit: Dressing/Grooming (Specify Level)
Self-Care Deficit: Feeding (Specify Level)
Self-Care Deficit: Toileting (Specify Level)
Self-Care Deficit, Total
Self-Esteem Disturbance
Self-Esteem, Chronic Low
Self-Esteem, Situational Low
Self-Mutilation, High Risk for
Sensory-Perceptual Alteration
Sexual Dysfunction
Sexuality Patterns, Altered
Skin Integrity, Impaired

Skin Integrity, Impaired, High Risk for
Sleep Pattern Disturbance
Social Interaction, Impaired
Social Isolation
Spiritual Distress (Distress of the Human Spirit)
Suffocation, High Risk for
Swallowing, Impaired
Temperature, Altered Body, High Risk for
Therapeutic Regimen, Ineffective Management of
Thermoregulation, Ineffective
Thought Processes, Impaired
Tissue Integrity, Impaired
Tissue Perfusion, Altered (see types)
Trauma, High Risk for
Urinary Elimination, Altered
Urinary Retention
Ventilation, Inability to Sustain Spontaneous
Violence, High Risk for (Self-Directed or Directed at Others)
Ventilatory Weaning Response, Dysfunctional (DVWR)

APPENDIX B

DIAGNOSTIC CATEGORIES GROUPED BY FUNCTIONAL HEALTH PATTERNS, 1993-1994

HEALTH PERCEPTION–HEALTH MANAGEMENT PATTERN (N = 12)

Altered Health Maintenance*
Ineffective Management of Therapeutic Regimen
Total Health Management Deficit
Health Management Deficit (Specify)
Noncompliance (Specify)
High Risk for Noncompliance (Specify)
Health-Seeking Behaviors (Specify)
High Risk for Infection
High Risk for Injury (Trauma)
High Risk for Poisoning
High Risk for Suffocation
Altered Protection

NUTRITIONAL-METABOLIC PATTERN (N = 21)

Altered Nutrition: Potential for More than Body Requirements *or* High Risk for Obesity
Altered Nutrition: More than Body Requirements *or* Obesity (Exogenous)
Altered Nutrition: Less than Body Requirements *or* Nutritional Deficit (Specify)
Ineffective Breastfeeding
Effective Breastfeeding
Interrupted Breastfeeding
Ineffective Infant Feeding Pattern
High Risk for Aspiration
Impaired Swallowing
Altered Oral Mucous Membrane
High Risk for Fluid Volume Deficit
Fluid Volume Deficit

Diagnoses in boldface are from *NANDA Taxonomy I, Revised, June 1992*, North American Nursing Diagnosis Association. Others are from Gordon M: *Manual of nursing diagnoses*, St Louis, 1993, Mosby.

Fluid Volume Excess
High Risk for Impaired Skin Integrity
Impaired Skin Integrity
Pressure Ulcer (Specify Stage)
Impaired Tissue Integrity
High Risk for Altered Body Temperature
Ineffective Thermoregulation
Hyperthermia
Hypothermia

ELIMINATION PATTERN (N = 12)

Constipation *or* Intermittent Constipation Pattern
Colonic Constipation
Perceived Constipation
Diarrhea
Bowel Incontinence
Altered Urinary Elimination Patterns
Functional Incontinence
Reflex Incontinence
Stress Incontinence
Urge Incontinence
Total Incontinence
Urinary Retention

ACTIVITY-EXERCISE PATTERN (N = 24)

High Risk for Activity Intolerance
Activity Intolerance (Specify Level)
Fatigue
Impaired Physical Mobility (Specify Level)
High Risk for Disuse Syndrome
High Risk for Joint Contractures
Total Self-Care Deficit (Specify Level)
Self-Bathing Hygiene Deficit (Specify Level)
Self-Dressing Grooming Deficit (Specify Level)
Self-Feeding Deficit (Specify Level)
Self-Toileting Deficit (Specify Level)

Altered Growth and Development: Self-Care Skills (Specify)
Diversional Activity Deficit
Impaired Home Maintenance Management (Mild, Moderate, Severe, High Risk, Chronic)
Dysfunctional Ventilatory Weaning Response (DVWR)
Inability to Sustain Spontaneous Ventilation
Ineffective Airway Clearance
Ineffective Breathing Pattern
Impaired Gas Exchange
Decreased Cardiac Output
Altered Tissue Perfusion (Specify)
Dysreflexia
High Risk for Peripheral Neurovascular Dysfunction
Altered Growth and Development

SLEEP-REST PATTERN (N = 1)

Sleep Pattern Disturbance

COGNITIVE-PERCEPTUAL PATTERN (N = 12)

Pain
Chronic Pain
Pain Self-Management Deficit (Acute, Chronic)
Uncompensated Sensory Deficit (Specify)
Sensory-Perceptual Alterations: Input Deficit *or* Sensory Deprivation
Sensory-Perceptual Alterations: Input Excess *or* Sensory Overload
Unilateral Neglect
Knowledge Deficit (Specify)
Impaired Thought Processes
Uncompensated Short-Term Memory Deficit
High Risk for Cognitive Impairment
Decisional Conflict (Specify)

SELF-PERCEPTION–SELF-CONCEPT PATTERN (N = 15)

Fear (Specify Focus)
Anxiety
Mild Anxiety
Moderate Anxiety
Severe Anxiety (Panic)
Anticipatory Anxiety (Mild, Moderate, Severe)
Reactive Depression (Situational)
Hopelessness
Powerlessness (Severe, Low, Moderate)
Self-Esteem Disturbance
Chronic Low Self-Esteem
Situational Low Self-Esteem
Body Image Disturbance

High Risk for Self-Mutilation
Personal Identity Disturbance

ROLE-RELATIONSHIP PATTERN (N = 20)

Anticipatory Grieving
Dysfunctional Grieving
Disturbance in Role Performance
Unresolved Independence-Dependence Conflict
Social Isolation *or* Social Rejection
Social Isolation
Impaired Social Interaction
Altered Growth and Development: Social Skills (Specify)
Relocation Stress Syndrome
Altered Family Processes
High Risk for Altered Parenting
Altered Parenting
Parental Role Conflict
Parent-Infant Separation
Weak Mother-Infant Attachment *or* Parent-Infant Attachment
Caregiver Role Strain
High Risk for Caregiver Role Strain
Impaired Verbal Communication
Altered Growth and Development: Communication Skills (Specify)
High Risk for Violence

SEXUALITY-REPRODUCTIVE PATTERN (N = 5)

Sexual Dysfunction (Specify Type)
Altered Sexuality Patterns
Rape-Trauma Syndrome
Rape-Trauma Syndrome: Compound Reaction
Rape-Trauma Syndrome: Silent Reaction

COPING–STRESS-TOLERANCE PATTERN (N = 9)

Ineffective Coping (Individual)
Avoidance Coping
Defensive Coping
Ineffective Denial *or* Denial
Impaired Adjustment
Post-Trauma Response
Family Coping: Potential for Growth
Ineffective Family Coping: Compromised
Ineffective Family Coping: Disabling

VALUE-BELIEF PATTERN (N = 1)

Spiritual Distress (Distress of the Human Spirit)

APPENDIX C

NANDA TAXONOMY I REVISED (1992)

Taxonomy I Revised (1992) includes the nursing diagnoses accepted for clinical use and testing at the tenth conference. The bracketed items and blank spaces found within the Taxonomy represent areas that are yet to be named, described, or voted on.

Approved nursing diagnoses are placed by the Taxonomy Committee based on the following considerations:

1. Level of abstraction
2. Consistency with current theoretical views in nursing
3. Consistency with basic definitions within each pattern area

The order of numbers within a level is not determined by priority or importance. Brackets clarify the placement of diagnoses within the patterns.

I. EXCHANGING

1.1. Altered Nutrition
  1.1.1.
  1.1.2. [Systemic]
    1.1.2.1. More than Body Requirements
    1.1.2.2. Less than Body Requirements
    1.1.2.3. High Risk for More than Body Requirements
1.2 [Altered Physical Regulation]
  1.2.1. [Immunologic]
    1.2.1.1. High Risk for Infection
  1.2.2. [Temperature]
    1.2.2.1. High Risk for Altered Body Temperature
    1.2.2.2. Hypothermia
    1.2.2.3. Hyperthermia
    1.2.2.4. Ineffective Thermoregulation
  1.2.3. [Neurologic]
    1.2.3.1. Dysreflexia
1.3 Altered Elimination
  1.3.1. Bowel

Adapted from North American Nursing Diagnosis Association: *NANDA nursing diagnoses: definitions and classifications,* Philadelphia, 1992, The Association.

    1.3.1.1. Constipation
      1.3.1.1.1. Perceived
      1.3.1.1.2. Colonic
    1.3.1.2. Diarrhea
    1.3.1.3. Bowel Incontinence
  1.3.2. Altered Urinary Elimination
    1.3.2.1. Incontinence
      1.3.2.1.1. Stress
      1.3.2.1.2. Reflex
      1.3.2.1.3. Urge
      1.3.2.1.4. Functional
      1.3.2.1.5. Total
    1.3.2.2. Retention
1.4 [Altered Circulation]
  1.4.1. [Vascular]
    1.4.1.1. Tissue Perfusion
      1.4.1.1.1. Renal
      1.4.1.1.2. Cerebral
      1.4.1.1.3. Cardiopulmonary
      1.4.1.1.4. Gastrointestinal
      1.4.1.1.5. Peripheral
    1.4.1.2. Fluid Volume
      1.4.1.2.1. Excess
      1.4.1.2.2. Deficit
        1.4.1.2.2.1. Actual
        1.4.1.2.2.2. High Risk for
  1.4.2. [Cardiac]
    1.4.2.1. Decreased Cardiac Output
1.5 [Altered Oxygenation]
  1.5.1. [Respiration]
    1.5.1.1. Impaired Gas Exchange
    1.5.1.2. Ineffective Airway Clearance
    1.5.1.3. Ineffective Breathing Pattern
      1.5.1.3.1. Inability to Sustain Spontaneous Ventilation
      1.5.1.3.2. Dysfunctional Ventilatory Weaning Response (DVWR)
1.6 [Altered Physical Integrity]
  1.6.1. High Risk for Injury
    1.6.1.1. High Risk for Suffocation
    1.6.1.2. High Risk for Poisoning
    1.6.1.3. High Risk for Trauma
    1.6.1.4. High Risk for Aspiration

1.6.1.5. High Risk for Disuse Syndrome
1.6.2. Altered Protection
  1.6.2.1. Impaired Tissue Integrity
    1.6.2.1.1. Oral Mucous Membranes
    1.6.2.1.2. Skin Integrity
      1.6.2.1.2.1. Impaired
      1.6.2.1.2.2. High Risk for

2. COMMUNICATING

2.1. Altered Communication
  2.1.1. Verbal
    2.1.1.1. Impaired

3. RELATING

3.1. [Altered Socialization]
  3.1.1. Impaired Social Interaction
  3.1.2. Social Isolation
3.2. [Altered Role]
  3.2.1. Altered Role Performance
    3.2.1.1. Parenting
      3.2.1.1.1. Altered
      3.2.1.1.2. High Risk for
    3.2.1.2. Sexual
      3.2.1.2.1. Dysfunction
  3.2.2. Altered Family Processes
    3.2.2.1. Caregiver Role Strain
    3.2.2.2. High Risk for Caregiver Role Strain
  3.2.3. [Altered Role Conflict]
    3.2.3.1. Parental Role Conflict
3.3. Altered Sexuality Patterns

4. VALUING

4.1. [Altered Spiritual State]
  4.1.1. Spiritual distress

5. CHOOSING

5.1. Altered Coping
  5.1.1. Individual Coping
    5.1.1.1. Ineffective
      5.1.1.1.1. Impaired Adjustment
      5.1.1.1.2. Defensive Coping
      5.1.1.1.3. Ineffective Denial
  5.1.2. Family Coping
    5.1.2.1. Ineffective
      5.1.2.1.1. Disabled
      5.1.2.1.2. Compromised
    5.1.2.2. Potential for Growth
5.2. [Altered Participation]
  5.2.1. Ineffective Management of Therapeutic Regimen
    5.2.1.1. Noncompliance (Specify)
5.3. [Altered Judgment]

5.3.1. [Individual]
  5.3.1.1. Decisional Conflict
5.4. Health-Seeking Behaviors (Specify)

6. MOVING

6.1. [Altered Activity]
  6.1.1. Physical Mobility
    6.1.1.1. Impaired
      6.1.1.1.1. High Risk for Peripheral Neurovascular Dysfunction
    6.1.1.2. Activity Intolerance
      6.1.1.2.1. Fatigue
    6.1.1.3. High Risk for Activity Intolerance
6.2. [Altered Rest]
  6.2.1. Sleep Pattern Disturbance
6.3. [Altered Recreation]
  6.3.1. Diversional Activity
    6.3.1.1. Deficit
6.4. [Altered ADL]
  6.4.1. Home Maintenance Management
    6.4.1.1. Impaired
  6.4.2. Altered Health Maintenance
6.5. Self-Care Deficit
  6.5.1. Feeding
    6.5.1.1. Impaired Swallowing
    6.5.1.2. Ineffective Breastfeeding
    6.5.1.2.1. Interrupted Breastfeeding
    6.5.1.3. Effective Breastfeeding
    6.5.1.4. Ineffective Infant Feeding Pattern
  6.5.2. Bathing/Hygiene
  6.5.3. Dressing/Grooming
  6.5.4. Toileting
6.6. Altered Growth and Development
6.7. Relocation Stress Syndrome

7. PERCEIVING

7.1. Altered Self-Concept
  7.1.1. Body Image Disturbance
  7.1.2. Self-Esteem Disturbance
    7.1.2.1. Chronic Low Self-Esteem
    7.1.2.2. Situational Low Self-Esteem
  7.1.3. Personal Identity Disturbance
7.2. Altered Sensory Perception (Specify)
  7.2.1. Visual
    7.2.1.1. Unilateral Neglect
  7.2.2. Auditory
  7.2.3. Kinesthetic
  7.2.4. Gustatory
  7.2.5. Tactile
  7.2.6. Olfactory
7.3. [Altered Meaningfulness]
  7.3.1. Hopelessness
  7.3.2. Powerlessness

8. KNOWING

8.1. [Altered Knowing]
   8.1.1. Knowledge Deficit (Specify)
8.2. Altered Thought Processes

9. FEELING

9.1. Altered Comfort
   9.1.1. Pain
      9.1.1.1. Chronic
9.2. [Altered Emotional Integrity]
   9.2.1. Grieving

9.2.1.1. Dysfunctional
   9.2.2.2. Anticipatory
9.2.2. High Risk for Violence
   9.2.3.1. High Risk for Self-Mutilation
9.2.3. Posttrauma Response
   9.2.3.1. Rape Trauma Syndrome
      9.2.3.1.1. Compound Reaction
      9.2.3.1.2. Silent Reaction
9.3. [Altered Emotional State]
   9.3.1. Anxiety
   9.3.2. Fear

APPENDIX D

PROPOSED ICD-10 VERSION OF NANDA'S TAXONOMY I REVISED (1992): CONDITIONS THAT NECESSITATE NURSING CARE

HUMAN RESPONSE PATTERN: CHOOSING

*Y00 Family Coping, Impaired
    Y00.0   Compromised
    Y00.1   Disabled
Y01 [Health-Seeking Behavior]
    Y01.09   Health-Seeking Behaviors (Specify)
*Y02 Individual Coping, Impaired
    Y02.0   Adjustment, Impaired
    Y02.1   Conflict, Decisional
    Y02.2   Coping, Defensive
    *Y02.3   Denial, Impaired
    Y02.4   Noncompliance
    Y02.5   Ineffective Management of Therapeutic Regime

COMMUNICATING

Y10 [Communication, Impaired]
    Y10.0   Verbal

EXCHANGING

Y20 [Bowel Elimination, Altered]
    Y20.0   Bowel Incontinence
    Y20.1   Constipation, Colonic
    Y20.2   Constipation, Perceived
    Y20.3   Diarrhea
*Y21 Cardiac Output, Altered
Y22 [Fluid Volume, Altered]
    Y22.0   Deficit
    Y22.1   Deficit, Risk
    Y22.2   Excess
*Y23 Injury, Risk
    *Y23.0   Aspiration
    *Y23.1   Disuse Syndrome
    *Y23.2   Poisoning
    *Y23.3   Suffocation
    *Y23.4   Trauma
    Y23.5   Altered Protection
Y24 [Nutrition, Altered]
    Y24.0   Less than Body Requirement
    Y24.1   More than Body Requirement
    Y24.2   More than Body Requirement: Risk
Y25 [Physical Regulation, Altered]
    Y25.0   Dysreflexia
    Y25.1   Hyperthermia
    Y25.2   Hypothermia
    *Y25.3   Infection: Risk
    *Y25.4   Thermoregulation, Impaired
Y26 [Respiration, Altered]
    *Y26.0   Airway Clearance, Impaired
    *Y26.1   Breathing Pattern, Impaired
    Y26.2   Gas Exchange, Impaired
    Y26.3   Dysfunction Ventilatory Weaning Response (DVWR)
    Y26.4   Inability to Sustain Spontaneous Ventilation
Y27 Tissue Integrity, Altered
    *Y27.0   Oral Mucous Membrane, Impaired
    Y27.1   Skin Integrity, Impaired
    Y27.2   Skin Integrity, Impaired: Risk
Y28 [Tissue Perfusion, Altered]
    Y28.0   Cardiopulmonary

Prepared by the NANDA Board of Directors, Taxonomy Committee, and ANA Liaison, January 28, 1989. Diagnoses accepted in 1992 have been added by the author to the classifications. The "Y" coding is a chapter in the international classification. (From North American Nursing Diagnosis Association: *NANDA nursing diagnoses: definitions and classification,* Philadelphia, 1992, The Association.) Items in brackets are not NANDA-accepted diagnoses. Items with an asterisk (*) are changes in terminology from NANDA diagnostic labels made by the NANDA-ANA Liaison in order to meet the requirements of the ICD system. NANDA diagnoses not specifically identified are embedded in the coding system.

Y28.1   Cerebral
Y28.2   Gastrointestinal
Y28.3   Peripheral
Y28.4   Renal
Y29   Urinary Elimination, Altered
Y29.0   Incontinence, Functional
Y29.1   Incontinence, Reflex
Y29.2   Incontinence, Stress
Y29.3   Incontinence, Urge
Y29.4   Incontinence, Total
Y29.5   Retention

FEELING
Y30   Anxiety
Y31   [Comfort, Altered]
Y31.0   Pain [Acute]
Y31.1   Pain, Chronic
Y32   Fear
Y33   [Grieving]
Y33.0   Anticipatory
Y33.1   Dysfunctional
Y34   Posttrauma Response
Y34.0   Rape Trauma Syndrome
Y34.1   Rape Trauma Syndrome: Compound Reaction
Y34.2   Rape Trauma Syndrome: Silent Reaction
*Y35   Violence: Risk
Y35.1   Self-Mutilation: Risk

KNOWING
Y40   [Knowledge Deficit]
Y40.0   Knowledge Deficit (Specify)
Y41   Thought Processes, Altered

MOVING
Y50   [Activity, Altered]
Y50.0   Activity Intolerance
Y50.1   Activity Intolerance: Risk
Y50.2   Diversional Activity Deficit
Y50.3   Fatigue
Y50.4   Mobility, Impaired Physical
Y50.5   Sleep Pattern Disturbance
Y50.6   Peripheral Neurovascular Dysfunction: Risk
*Y51   Bathing/Hygiene Deficit
*Y52   Dressing/Grooming Deficit

*Y53   Feeding Deficit/Nondeficit
*Y53.0   Breastfeeding, Impaired
Y53.01   Breastfeeding, Effective
Y53.02   Breastfeeding, Interrupted
Y53.1   Swallowing, Impaired
Y53.2   Feeding Pattern, Ineffective Infant
Y54   Growth and Development, Altered
Y55   Health Maintenance, Altered
Y56   Home Maintenance Management, Impaired
*Y57   Toileting Deficit
Y58   Relocation Stress Syndrome

PERCEIVING
Y60   [Meaningfulness, Altered]
Y60.0   Hopelessness
Y60.1   Powerlessness
Y61   [Self-Concept, Altered]
Y61.0   Body Image Disturbance
Y61.1   Personal Identity Disturbance
Y61.2   Self-Esteem Disturbance, Chronic Low
Y61.3   Self-Esteem Disturbance, Situational
*Y62   [Sensory Perception, Altered]
Y62.0   Auditory
Y62.1   Gustatory
Y62.2   Kinesthetic
Y62.3   Olfactory
Y62.4   Tactile
Y62.5   Visual
Y62.6   Unilateral Neglect

RELATING
Y70   Family Processes, Altered
Y71   Role Performance, Altered
Y71.0   Parental Role Conflict
Y71.1   Parenting, Altered
Y71.2   Parenting, Altered: Risk
Y71.3   Sexual Dysfunction
Y72   Sexuality Patterns, Altered
Y73   [Socialization, Altered]
Y73.0   Social Interaction, Impaired
Y73.1   Social Isolation

VALUING
Y80   [Spiritual State, Altered]
Y80.0   Spiritual Distress

APPENDIX E

MEMBERS OF THE THEORIST GROUP, 1977-1982

Andrea Bircher, R.N., Ph.D.
University of Oklahoma
College of Nursing

Rosemary Ellis, R.N., Ph.D.
Case Western Reserve University
School of Nursing

Joyce Fitzpatrick, R.N., Ph.D.
Wayne State University
School of Nursing

Marjory Gordon, R.N., Ph.D.
Boston College
Graduate Medical-Surgical Nursing

Margaret Hardy, R.N., Ph.D.
Boston University
School of Nursing

Imogene King, R.N., Ph.D.
University of South Florida

Rose McKay, R.N., Ph.D.
University of Colorado
School of Nursing

Margaret A. Newman, R.N., Ph.D.
The Pennsylvania State University
College of Human Development

Dorothea Orem, R.N., Ph.D.
Consultant

Rose Marie Parse, R.N., Ph.D.
Duquesne University
School of Nursing

Martha Rogers, R.N., Sc.D.
New York University
Department of Nursing

Sr. Callista Roy, R.N., Ph.D.
Mount St. Mary's College
Department of Nursing

M. J. Smith, R.N., Ph.D.
Duquesne University
School of Nursing

Gertrude Torres, R.N., Ed.D.
Consultant

316

APPENDIX F

DEFINITIONS OF HUMAN RESPONSE PATTERNS (OCTOBER 1989)

Choosing To select between alternatives; the action of selecting or exercising preference in regard to a matter in which one is a free agent; to determine in favor of a course; to decide in accordance with inclinations.

Communicating To converse; to impart, confer, or transmit thoughts, feelings, or information, internally or externally, verbally or nonverbally.

Exchanging To give, replenish, or lose something while receiving something in return; the substitution of one element for another; the reciprocal act of giving and receiving.

Feeling To experience consciousness, sensation, apprehension, or sense; to be consciously or emotionally affected by a fact, event, or state.

Knowing To recognize or acknowledge a thing or a person; to be familiar with by experience or through information or report; to be cognizant of something through observation, inquiry, or information; to be conversant with a body of facts, principles, or methods of action; to understand.

Moving To change the place or position of a body or any member of the body; to put and/or keep in motion; to provoke an excretion or discharge; the urge to action or to do something; to take action.

Perceiving To apprehend with the mind; to become aware of by the senses; to apprehend what is not open or present to observation; to take in fully or adequately.

Relating To connect; to establish a link between; to stand in some association to another thing, person, or place; to be born or thrust in between things.

Valuing To be concerned about; to care; the worth or worthiness; the relative status of a thing, or the esteem in which it is held, according to its real or supposed worth, usefulness, or importance; one's opinion of linking for a real person or thing; to equate in importance.

From Carroll-Johnson RM, editor: *Classification of nursing diagnoses: proceedings of the ninth conference,* Philadelphia, 1991, Lippincott, p 464.

APPENDIX G

FUNCTIONAL HEALTH PATTERNS TYPOLOGY: DEFINITIONS

TYPOLOGY

Functional health patterns of clients, whether individuals, families, or communities, evolve from client-environment interaction. Each pattern is an expression of biopsychosocial integration. No one pattern can be understood without knowledge of the other patterns. Functional patterns are influenced by biological, developmental, cultural, social, and spiritual factors. Dysfunctional health patterns (described by nursing diagnoses) may occur with disease; dysfunctional health patterns also may lead to disease.

The judgment of whether a pattern is functional or dysfunctional is made by comparing assessment data to one or more of the following: (1) individual baselines, (2) established norms for age groups, (3) cultural, social, or other norms. A particular pattern must be evaluated in the context of other patterns and its contribution to optimal function of the client assessed.

HEALTH PERCEPTION–HEALTH MANAGEMENT PATTERN

Describes the client's perceived pattern of health and well-being and how health is managed. Includes the individual's perception of health status and its relevance to current activities and future planning. Also included is the individual's health risk management and general health care behavior, such as adherence to mental and physical health promotion activities, medical or nursing prescriptions, and follow-up care.

NUTRITIONAL-METABOLIC PATTERN

Describes pattern of food and fluid consumption relative to metabolic need and pattern indicators of local nutrient supply. Includes the individual's patterns of food and fluid consumption: daily eating times, the types and quantity of food and fluids consumed, particular food preferences, and the use of nutrient or vitamin supplements. Describes breastfeeding and infant feeding patterns. Includes reports of any skin lesions and general ability to heal. The condition of skin, hair, nails, mucous membranes, and teeth and measures of body temperature, height, and weight are included.

ELIMINATION PATTERN

Describes patterns of excretory function (bowel, bladder, and skin). Includes the individual's perceived regularity of excretory function, use of routines or laxatives for bowel elimination, and any changes or disturbances in time pattern, mode of excretion, quality, or quantity. Also included are any devices employed to control excretion.

ACTIVITY-EXERCISE PATTERN

Describes pattern of exercise, activity, leisure, and recreation. Includes activities of daily living requiring energy expenditure, such as hygiene, cooking, shopping, eating, working, and home maintenance. Also included are the type, quantity, and quality of exercise, including sports, which describe the typical pattern for the individual. Factors that interfere with the desired or expected pattern for the individual (such as neuromuscular deficits and compensations, dyspnea, angina, or muscle cramping on exertion, and cardiac/pulmonary classification, if appropriate) are included. Leisure patterns are also included and describe the activities the individual undertakes as recreation either with a group or as an individual. Emphasis is on the activities of high importance or significance to the individual.

SLEEP-REST PATTERN

Describes patterns of sleep, rest, and relaxation. Includes patterns of sleep and rest-relaxation periods during the 24-hour day. Includes the individual's perception of the quality and quantity of sleep and rest and perception of energy level. Included also are aids to sleep such as medications or nighttime routines that the individual employs.

COGNITIVE-PERCEPTUAL PATTERN

Describes sensory-perceptual and cognitive pattern. Includes the adequacy of sensory modes, such as vision, hearing, taste, touch, or smell, and the compensation or prothetics utilized for disturbances. Reports of pain perception and how pain is managed are also included when appropriate. Also included are the cognitive functional abilities, such as language, memory, and decision making.

SELF-PERCEPTION–SELF-CONCEPT PATTERN

Describes self-concept pattern and perceptions of self. Includes the individual's attitudes about himself or herself, perception of abilities (cognitive, affective, or physical), body image, identity, general sense of worth, and general emotional pattern. Pattern of body posture and movement, eye contact, voice, and speech pattern are included.

ROLE-RELATIONSHIP PATTERN

Describes pattern of role engagements and relationships. Includes the individual's perception of the major roles and responsibilities in current life situation. Satisfaction or disturbances in family, work, or social relationships and responsibilities related to these roles are included.

SEXUALITY-REPRODUCTIVE PATTERN

Describes patterns of satisfaction or dissatisfaction with sexuality; describes reproductive pattern. Includes the individual's perceived satisfaction with or disturbances in his or her sexuality. Included also is the female's reproductive stage, pre- or postmenopause, and any perceived problems.

COPING–STRESS-TOLERANCE PATTERN

Describes general coping pattern and effectiveness of the pattern in terms of stress tolerance. Includes the individual's reserve or capacity to resist challenge to self-integrity, modes of handling stress, family or other support systems, and perceived ability to control and manage situations.

VALUE-BELIEF PATTERN

Describes patterns of values, goals, or beliefs (including spiritual) that guide choices or decisions. Includes what is perceived as important in life, quality of life, and any perceived conflicts in values, beliefs, or expectations that are health related.

APPENDIX H

FUNCTIONAL HEALTH PATTERNS: ASSESSMENT GUIDELINES FOR ADULT, INFANT, AND EARLY CHILDHOOD, FAMILY, COMMUNITY, CRITICALLY ILL

ADULT ASSESSMENT
Nursing history

1. *Health perception–health management pattern*
   a. How has general health been?
   b. Any colds in past year? If appropriate, absences from work/school?
   c. Most important things you do to keep healthy? Think these things make a difference to health? (Include family folk remedies, if appropriate.) Breast self-examination? Use cigarettes? Drugs? Ever had a drinking problem? When was your last drink?
   d. Accidents (home, work, driving)?
   e. In past, been easy to find ways to follow things doctors or nurses suggest?
   f. If appropriate: What do you think caused this illness? Action taken when symptoms perceived? Results of action?
   g. If appropriate: Things important to you while you're here? How can we be most helpful?
2. *Nutritional-metabolic pattern*
   a. Typical daily food intake? (Describe.) Supplements?
   b. Typical daily fluid intake? (Describe.)
   c. Weight loss/gain? (Amount.) Height loss/gain? (Amount.)
   d. Appetite?
   e. Food or eating: Discomfort? Swallowing? Diet restrictions? If appropriate: Breastfeeding? Problems?
   f. Heal well or poorly?
   g. Skin problems: Lesions, dryness?
   h. Dental problems?
3. *Elimination pattern*
   a. Bowel elimination pattern. (Describe.) Frequency? Character? Discomfort? Problem in control? Laxatives?
   b. Urinary elimination pattern. (Describe.) Frequency? Problem in control?
   c. Excess perspiration? Odor problems?
4. *Activity-exercise pattern*
   a. Sufficient energy for desired/required activities?
   b. Exercise pattern? Type? Regularity?
   c. Spare-time (leisure) activities? Child: Play activities?
   d. Perceived ability for: (code for level)
      Feeding _____   Grooming _____
      Bathing _____   General mobility _____
      Toileting _____   Cooking _____
      Bed mobility _____ Home maintenance _____
      Dressing _____   Shopping _____
      Functional Levels Code
      Level 0:   Full self-care
      Level I: Requires use of equipment or device
      Level II: Requires assistance or supervision from another person
      Level III: Requires assistance or supervision from another person and equipment or device
      Level IV: Is dependent and does not participate
5. *Sleep-rest pattern*
   a. Generally rested and ready for daily activities after sleep?
   b. Sleep-onset problems? Aids? Dreams (nightmares)? Early awakening?
   c. Rest/relaxation periods?
6. *Cognitive-perceptual pattern*
   a. Hearing difficulty? Aid?
   b. Vision? Wear glasses? When last checked?
   c. Any change in memory lately?

d. Easy/difficult to make decisions?

e. Easiest way for you to learn things? Any difficulty learning?

f. Any discomfort? Pain? How do you manage it?

7. *Self-perception–self-concept pattern*

a. How would you describe yourself? Most of the time, feel good (not so good) about yourself?

b. Changes in your body or the things you can do? Problem to you?

c. Changes in way you feel about yourself or your body (since illness started)?

d. Find things frequently make you angry? Annoyed? Fearful? Anxious? Depressed? What helps?

e. Ever feel you lose hope? Not able to control things in life? What helps?

8. *Role-relationship pattern*

a. Live alone? Family? Family structure (diagram)?

b. Any family problems you have difficulty handling (nuclear/extended)?

c. How does family usually handle problems?

d. Family depend on you for things? How managing?

e. If appropriate: How do family/others feel about your illness/hospitalization?

f. If appropriate: Problems with children? Difficulty handling?

g. Belong to social groups? Close friends? Feel lonely (frequency)?

h. Things generally go well for you at work? (School?) If appropriate: Income sufficient for needs?

i. Feel part of (or isolated in) neighborhood where living?

9. *Sexuality-reproductive pattern*

a. If appropriate to age/situation: Sexual relationships satisfying? Changes? Problems?

b. If appropriate: Use of contraceptives? Problems?

c. Female: When menstruation started? Last menstrual period? Menstrual problems? Para? Gravida?

10. *Coping–stress-tolerance pattern*

a. Any big changes in your life in the last year or two? Crisis?

b. Who is most helpful in talking things over? Available to you now?

c. Tense a lot of the time? What helps? Use any medicines, drugs, alcohol?

d. When (if) have big problems (any problems) in your life, how do you handle them?

e. Most of the time, is this (are these) way(s) successful?

11. *Value-belief pattern*

a. Generally get things you want out of life? Important plans for the future?

b. Religion important in your life? If appropriate: Does this help when difficulties arise?

c. If appropriate: Will being here interfere with any religious practices?

12. *Other*

a. Any other things that we haven't talked about that you'd like to mention?

b. Questions?

Screening examination format

(May add other pattern indicators to expand the examination)

General appearance, grooming, hygiene _____

Oral mucous membranes (color, moistness, lesions) __

Teeth: Dentures __ Cavities __ Missing _____

Hears whisper? _____

Reads newsprint? __ Glasses? __

Pulse (rate) __ (rhythm) __ (strength) _____

Respiration _ (depth) _ (rhythm) _ Breath sounds _

Blood pressure ____

Hand grip __ Can pick up pencil? __

Range of motion (joints) __ Muscle firmness __

Skin: Bony prominences _ Lesions _ Color changes __

Gait __ Posture __ Absent body part _____

Demonstrated ability for: (Code for level)

Feeding __   Grooming __

Bathing __   General mobility __

Toileting __   Cooking __

Bed mobility __   Home maintenance __

Dressing __   Shopping __

Intravenous, drainage, suction, etc. (specify) _____

Actual weight __ Reported weight __

Height __ Temperature __

During history and examination:

Orientation __ Grasps ideas and questions (abstract, concrete)? __

Language spoken __ Voice and speech pattern _____

Vocabulary level ____

Eye contact __ Attention span (distraction) _____

Nervous or relaxed (rate from 1 to 5) __

Assertive or passive (rate from 1 to 5) __

Interaction with family member, guardian, other (if present) _____

INFANT AND YOUNG CHILD ASSESSMENT

When a new infant or child is added to a nurse's caseload, a comprehensive assessment is done to establish a data base for developmental assessment and for nursing diagnosis and treatment. Information is needed on (1) the development of each functional pattern/anatomical growth, (2) current health patterns, and (3) family health/home environment in which the infant/child is developing. Minimally, the admission nursing history/examination should screen for high-incidence problems. The questions/items listed below may be used as a guide for a comprehensive parent-child health history or used selectively for problem screening.

Nursing history

1. *Health perception–health management pattern*
   Parents' report of:
   a. Mother's pregnancy/labor/delivery history (of this infant, of others)?
   b. Infant's health status since birth?
   c. Adherence to routine health checks for the infant/child? Immunizations?
   d. Infections in the infant/child? Child's absences from school?
   e. If applicable: Infant's/child's medical problem, treatment, and prognosis?
   f. If applicable: Actions taken by parents when signs/symptoms perceived?
   g. If appropriate: Has it been easy to follow doctors' or nurses' suggestions?
   h. Preventive health practices (e.g., diaper change, utensils, and clothes)?
   i. Do parents smoke? Around children?
   j. Accidents? Frequency?
   k. Infant's crib toys (safety)? Carrying safety? Car safety?
   l. Parents' safety practices (e.g., household products, medicines)
   Parents (self):
   a. Parents'/family's general health status?
2. *Nutritional-metabolic pattern*
   Parents' report of the infant's/child's:
   a. Breast/bottle feeding? Intake (estimated)? Sucking strength?
   b. Appetite? Feeding discomfort?
   c. Twenty-four-hour intake of nutrients? Supplements?
   d. Eating behavior? Food preferences? Conflicts over food?
   e. Birth weight? Current weight?
   f. Skin problems: Rashes, lesions, etc.?
   Parents (self):
   a. Parents'/family's nutritional status? Problems?
3. *Elimination pattern*
   Parents' report of the infant's/child's:
   a. Bowel elimination pattern? (Describe.) Frequency? Character discomfort?
   b. Diaper changes? (Describe routine.)
   c. Urinary elimination pattern? (Describe.) Number of wet diapers per day? (Estimate amount.) Stream (strong, dribble)?
   d. Excess perspiration? Odor?
   Parents (self):
   a. Elimination pattern? Problems?
4. *Activity-exercise pattern*
   Parents' report of:
   a. Bathing routine? (When, how, where, and what type of soap?)
   b. Dressing routine? (Clothing worn, changes inside/outside home)
   c. Typical day's activity for the infant/child (hours spent in crib, being carried, playing, etc.; type of toys used)?
   d. Infant's/child's general activity level? Tolerance?
   e. Perception of infant's/child's strength (strong or fragile)?
   f. Child's self-care ability (bathing, feeding, toileting, dressing, grooming)?
   Parents (self):
   a. Activity/exercise/leisure pattern? Child care? Home maintenance?
5. *Sleep-rest pattern*
   Parents' report of:
   a. Sleep pattern of the infant/child: Estimated hours?
   b. Infant's/child's restlessness? Nightmares? Nocturia?
   c. Infant's sleep position? Body movements?
   Parents (self):
   a. Sleep pattern?
6. *Cognitive-perceptual pattern*
   Parents' report of:
   a. General responsiveness of the infant/child?
   b. Infant's response to talking? Noise? Objects? Touch?
   c. Infant's following of objects with eyes? Response to crib toys?
   d. Learning (changes noted)? What is being taught to the infant/child?
   e. Noises/vocalizations? Speech pattern? Words? Sentences?
   f. Use of stimulation: Talking, games, etc.?
   g. Vision, hearing, touch, kinesthesia of the infant/child?
   h. Child's ability to tell name, time, address, telephone number?
   i. Infant's/child's ability to identify needs (hunger, thirst, pain, discomfort)?
   Parents (self):
   a. Problems with vision, hearing, touch, etc.?
   b. Difficulties making decisions? Judgments?

7. *Self-perception–self-concept pattern*
Parent's report of:
  a. Infant's/child's mood state (irritability)?
  b. Child's sense of worth, identity, competency?
Child's report of:
  a. Mood state?
  b. Many/few friends? Liked by others?
  c. Self-perception ("good" most of time? Hard to be "good"?)
  d. Ever lonely?
  e. Fears (transient/frequent)?
Parents (self):
  a. General sense of worth, identity, competency?
  b. Self-perception as parents?

8. *Role-relationship pattern*
Parent's report of:
  a. Family/household structure?
  b. Family problems/stressors?
  c. Interactions between family members and infant (or child)?
  d. Infant's/child's response to separation?
  e. Child: Dependency?
  f. Child: Play pattern?
  g. Child: Temper tantrums? Discipline problems? School adjustment?
Parents (self):
  a. Role engagements? Satisfaction?
  b. Work/social/marital relationships?

9. *Sexuality–reproductive pattern*
Parents' report of child's:
  a. Feeling of maleness/femaleness?
  b. Questions regarding sexuality? How parent responds?
Parents (self):
  a. If applicable: Reproductive history?
  b. Sexual satisfaction/problems?

10. *Coping–stress-tolerance pattern*
Parents' report of:
  a. What produces stress in child? Level of stress tolerance?
  b. Child's pattern of handling problems, frustrations, anger, etc.?
Parents (self):
  a. Life stressors? Family stress?
  b. Strategies for handling problems? Support systems?

11. *Value-belief pattern*
Parents' report of:
  a. Child's moral development, choice behavior, commitments?
Parents (self):
  a. Things important in life (values, spirituality)? Desires for the future?
  b. If appropriate: Perceived impact of disease on goals?

12. *Other*
  a. Any other things that we haven't talked about that you'd like to mention? Any questions?

Screening examination format

  a. General appearance of infant/child _____
  b. General appearance of parent(s) _____
  c. Child's height/weight _____ Structural growth and development _____
  d. Skin color, hydration, rashes, lesions _____
  e. If warranted: Child's/infant's urine and stool ___
  f. Reflexes (appropriate to age) _____
     Blood pressure _____
  g. Breathing pattern; rate, rhythm _____
  h. Heart sounds; rate, rhythm _____
  i. Infant/child: Responsiveness, cognitive-perceptual development _____
  j. Child: Eye contact, speech pattern, posturing ___
  k. Smiling response (infant) _____
  l. Social interaction (child): Aggressive/withdrawn? _____
  m. Response to vocalizations? Requests? _____

FAMILY ASSESSMENT

The 11 functional health pattern areas are applicable to the assessment of families. Families are the primary client in community health nursing. In some cases a family assessment may be indicated (1) in the care of an infant or child whose development is influenced by family health patterns or (2) when an adult has certain health problems that can be influenced by family patterns. The following guidelines provide information on family functioning:

1. *Health perception–health management pattern*
History:
  a. How has family's general health been (in last few years)?
  b. Colds in past year? Absence from work/school?
  c. Most important things you do to keep healthy? Think these make a difference to health? (Include family folk remedies, if appropriate.)
  d. Members' use of cigarettes, alcohol, drugs?
  e. Immunizations? Health care provider? Frequency of check-ups? Accidents (home, work, school, driving)? (If appropriate: Storage of drugs, cleaning products, scatter rugs, etc.)
  f. In past, been easy to find ways to follow things doctors, nurses, social workers (if appropriate) suggest?
  g. Things important in family's health that I could help with?
Examination:
  a. General appearance of family members and home.

b. If appropriate: Storage of medicines, cribs, playpens, stove, scatter rugs, hazards, etc.

2. *Nutritional-metabolic pattern*
   History:
   a. Typical family meal pattern/food intake? (Describe.) Supplements (vitamins, types of snacks, etc.)?
   b. Typical family fluid intake? (Describe.) Supplements: type available (fruit juices, soft drinks, coffee, etc.)?
   c. Appetites?
   d. Dental problems? Dental care (frequency)?
   e. Anyone have skin problems? Healing problems?
   Examination:
   a. If opportunity available: Refrigerator contents, meal preparation, contents of meal, etc.

3. *Elimination pattern*
   History:
   a. Family use of laxatives, other aids?
   b. Problems in waste/garbage disposal?
   c. Pet animals waste disposal (indoor/outdoor)?
   d. If indicated: Problems with flies, roaches, rodents?
   Examination:
   a. If opportunity available: Examine toilet facilities, garbage disposal, pet waste disposal; indicators of risk for flies, roaches, rodents.

4. *Activity-exercise pattern*
   History:
   a. In general, does family get a lot of/little exercise? Type? Regularity?
   b. Family leisure activities? Active/passive?
   c. Problems in shopping (transportation), cooking, keeping up the house, budgeting for food, clothes, housekeeping, house costs?
   Examination:
   a. Pattern of general home maintenance, personal maintenance.

5. *Sleep-rest pattern*
   History:
   a. Generally, family members seem to be well rested and ready for school/work?
   b. Sufficient sleeping space and quiet?
   c. Family find time to relax?
   Examination:
   a. If opportunity available: Observe sleeping space and arrangements.

6. *Cognitive-perceptual pattern*
   History:
   a. Visual or hearing problems? How managed?
   b. Any big decisions family has had to make? How made?
   Examination:
   a. If indicated: Language spoken at home.

b. Grasp of ideas and questions (abstract/concrete).
c. Vocabulary level.

7. *Self-perception–self-concept pattern*
   History:
   a. Most of time family feels good (not so good) about themselves as a family?
   b. General mood of family? Happy? Anxious? Depressed? What helps family mood?
   Examination:
   a. General mood state: nervous (5) or relaxed (1); rate from 1 to 5.
   b. Members generally assertive (5) or passive (1); rate from 1 to 5.

8. *Role-relationship pattern*
   History:
   a. Family (or household) members? Member age and family structure (diagram).
   b. Any family problems that are difficult to handle (nuclear/extended)? Child rearing? If appropriate: Spouse ever get rough with you? With the children?
   c. Relationships good (not so good) among family members? Siblings? Support each other?
   d. If appropriate: Income sufficient for needs?
   e. Feel part of (or isolated from) community? Neighbors?
   Examination:
   a. Interaction among family members (if present).
   b. Observed family leadership roles.

9. *Sexuality-reproductive pattern*
   History:
   a. If appropriate (sexual partner within household or situation): Sexual relations satisfying? Changes? Problems?
   b. Use of family planning? Contraceptives? Problems?
   c. If appropriate (to age of children): Feel comfortable in explaining/discussing sexual subjects?
   Examination: None

10. *Coping–stress-tolerance pattern*
    History:
    a. Any big changes within family in last few years?
    b. Family tense or relaxed most of time? When tense what helps? Anyone use medicines, drugs, alcohol to decrease tension?
    c. When (if) family problems, how handled? Most of the time is this way (or ways) successful?
    Examination: None

11. *Value-belief pattern*
    History:
    a. Generally, family get things they want out of life?
    b. Important things for the future?

c. Any "rules" in the family that everyone believes are important?

d. Religion important in family? Does this help when difficulties arise?

Examination: None

COMMUNITY ASSESSMENT*

Communities develop health patterns. In some practice settings the community is the primary client. In other cases an individual client or a family may have, or be predisposed to, certain problems that require an assessment of certain community patterns. The following are guidelines for a comprehensive community assessment, but selected patterns can also be assessed, depending on the focus of care delivery:

1. *Health perception–health management pattern*

   History (community representatives):

   a. In general, what is the health/wellness level of the population on a scale of 1 to 5, with 5 being high? Any major health problems?

   b. Any strong cultural patterns influencing health practices?

   c. Do people feel they have access to health services?

   d. Is there a demand for any particular health services or prevention programs?

   e. Do people feel fire, police, safety programs are sufficient?

   Examination (community records):

   a. Morbidity, mortality, disability rates (by age group, if appropriate)?

   b. Accident rates (by district, if appropriate)?

   c. Currently operating health facilities (types)?

   d. Ongoing health-promotion–prevention programs; utilization rates?

   e. Ratios of health professionals to population?

   f. Laws regarding drinking age?

   g. Arrest statistics for drug use/drunk driving by age group?

2. *Nutritional-metabolic pattern*

   History (community representatives):

   a. In general, do most people seem well nourished? Children? Elderly?

   b. Food supplement programs? Food stamps: Rate of use?

   c. Is cost of foods reasonable in this area relative to income?

   d. Are stores accessible for most? "Meals on Wheels" available?

   e. Water supply and quality? Testing services (if most have own wells)? (If appropriate: Water usage cost? Any drought restrictions?)

   f. Any concern that community growth will exceed good water supply?

   g. Are heating/cooling costs manageable for most? Programs?

   Examination:

   a. General appearance (nutrition, teeth, clothing appropriate for climate)? Children? Adults? Elderly?

   b. Food purchases (observations at food store checkout counters)?

   c. "Junk" food (machines in schools, etc.)?

3. *Elimination pattern*

   History (community representatives):

   a. Major kinds of wastes (industrial, sewage, etc.)? Disposal systems? Recycling programs? Any problems perceived by community?

   b. Pest control? Food service inspection (restaurants, street vendors, etc.)?

   Examination:

   a. Communicable disease statistics?

   b. Air pollution statistics?

4. *Activity-exercise pattern*

   History (community representatives):

   a. How do people find the transportation here? To work? For recreation? To health care?

   b. Do people (senior, others) have/use community centers? Recreation facilities for children? Adults? Seniors?

   c. Is housing adequate (availability, cost)? Public housing?

   Examination:

   a. Recreation/cultural programs?

   b. Aids for the disabled?

   c. Residential centers, nursing homes, rehabilitation facilities relative to population needs?

   d. External maintenance of homes, yards, apartment houses?

   e. General activity level (e.g., bustling, quiet)?

5. *Sleep-rest pattern*

   History (community representatives):

   a. Generally quiet at night in most neighborhoods?

   b. Usual business hours? Are industries round-the-clock?

   Examination:

   a. Activity/noise levels in business district? In residential areas?

---

*Community assessment items are adapted from Gikow F, Kucharski P: *Functional health pattern assessment of a community.* Paper presented at the 112th annual meeting of the American Public Health Association, Anaheim, CA, November 13, 1984. Gikow and Kucharski used the assessment to evaluate health-related needs of a community served by their agency.

6. *Cognitive-perceptual pattern*
   History (community representatives):
   a. Do most groups speak English? Bilingual?
   b. Educational level of population?
   c. Schools seen as good/needing improvement? Adult education desired/available?
   d. Types of problems that require community decisions? Decision-making process? What is best way to get things done/changed here?
   Examination:
   a. School facilities? Dropout rate?
   b. Community government structure; decision-making lines?

7. *Self-perception–self-concept pattern*
   History (community representatives):
   a. Good community to live in? Going up in status, down, or about the same?
   b. Old community? Fairly new?
   c. Does any age group predominate?
   d. People's mood, in general: Enjoying life, stressed, feeling "down"?
   e. People generally have the kinds of abilities needed in this community?
   f. Community/neighborhood functions? Parades?
   Examination:
   a. Racial, ethnic mix (if appropriate)?
   b. Socioeconomic level?
   c. General observations of mood?

8. *Role-relationship pattern*
   History (community representatives):
   a. Do people seem to get along well together here? Places where people tend to go to socialize?
   b. Do people feel they are heard by the government? High/low participation in meetings?
   c. Enough work/jobs for everybody? Are wages good/fair? Do people seem to like the kind of work available (happy in their jobs/job stress)?
   d. Any problems with riots, violence in the neighborhoods? Family violence? Problems with child/spouse/elder abuse?
   e. Does community get along with adjacent communities? Do people collaborate on any community projects?
   f. Do neighbors seem to support each other?
   g. Community get-togethers?
   Examination:
   a. Observation of interactions (generally or at specific meetings)?
   b. Statistics on interpersonal violence?
   c. Statistics on employment, income/poverty?
   d. Divorce rate?

9. *Sexuality-reproductive pattern*
   History (community representatives):
   a. Average family size?
   b. Do people feel there are any problems with pornography, prostitution, or other?
   c. Do people want/support sex education in schools/community?
   Examination:
   a. Family sizes and types of households?
   b. Male/female ratio?
   c. Average maternal age? Maternal mortality rate? Infant mortality rate?
   d. Teen pregnancy rate?
   e. Abortion rate?
   f. Sexual violence statistics?
   g. Laws/regulations regarding information on birth control?

10. *Coping–stress-tolerance pattern*
    History (community representatives):
    a. Any groups that seem to be under stress?
    b. Need/availability of phone help lines? Support groups (health related, other)?
    Examination:
    a. Statistics on delinquency, drug abuse, alcoholism, suicide, psychiatric illness?
    b. Unemployment rate by race/ethnic group/sex?

11. *Value-belief pattern*
    History (community representatives):
    a. Community values: What seem to be the top four things that people living here see as important in their lives? (Note health-related values, priorities.)
    b. Do people tend to get involved in causes/local fund-raising campaigns? (Note if any are health related.)
    c. Are there religious groups in the community? Churches available?
    d. Do people tend to tolerate/not tolerate differences or socially deviant behavior?
    Examination:
    a. Zoning/conservation laws?
    b. Scan of community government health committee reports (goals, priorities)?
    c. Health budget relative to total budget?

If a community health nurse or agency does not wish an in-depth study of a community, screening of functional patterns is possible by selecting items from the examination sections.

ASSESSMENT OF THE CRITICALLY ILL

Clients who are critically ill, such as those with *severe* respiratory, cardiac, neurological, or psychological instability, are unable to respond to a full functional health pattern assessment. At times, examination and observation are the major data collection methods used during the critical phase of an illness if the client does not have the energy, capacity, or attention span to provide a health history. Nurses caring for critically ill individuals need to use screening techniques and be sensitive to cues of high-incidence diagnoses. The following may occur in homes or hospital settings:

Health perception–health management pattern

High Risk for Infection
High Risk for Injury
High Risk for Suffocation

Nutritional-metabolic pattern

High Risk for Nutritional Deficit
High Risk for Pressure Ulcer
Hypothermia
Ineffective Thermoregulation
High Risk for Fluid Volume Deficit
High Risk for Aspiration
Hyperthermia

Elimination pattern

High Risk for Constipation/Impaction
Constipation
Diarrhea

Activity-exercise pattern

High Risk for Activity Intolerance
Activity Intolerance
Ineffective Airway Clearance
High Risk for Joint Contractures
Ineffective Breathing Pattern
Dysfunctional Ventilatory Weaning Response (DVWR)
Total Self-Care Deficit (Level III or IV)
Impaired Bed Mobility
High Risk for Disuse Syndrome
Dysreflexia
Inability to Sustain Spontaneous Ventilation
High Risk for Peripheral Neurovascular Dysfunction

Sleep-rest pattern

Sleep-Pattern Disturbance

Cognitive-perceptual pattern

Uncompensated Sensory Deficit (specify)
Decisional Conflict
High Risk for Cognitive Impairment
Sensory Deprivation/Overload
Impaired Thought Processes
Pain

Self-perception–self-concept pattern

Fear
Powerlessness
Self-Esteem Disturbance
Anxiety
Hopelessness

Role-relationship pattern

Alteration in Family Processes
Unresolved Independence-Dependence Conflict
Anticipatory Grieving
Dysfunctional Grieving
Altered Role Performance
Impaired Communication
Weak Parent-Infant Attachment
Parental Role Conflict

Coping–stress tolerance pattern

Ineffective Coping
Compromised Family Coping
Avoidance Coping
Post-Trauma Response

Value-belief pattern

Spiritual Distress

Nursing History and Examination Documentation: An Example

NURSING HISTORY AND EXAMINATION

First hospital admission of a 55-year-old married, obese white male, administrator of a Spanish center. Sitting upright in bed, tense posture and expression. Five-year history of slightly elevated blood pressure. One year before admission had 12-hour episode of dizziness and was started on medication; two other episodes relieved by rest. Presented at emergency room with dizziness and numbness of left arm.

Health Perception—Health Management Pattern. Viewed health as good until 1 year ago when was diagnosed as "having high blood pressure." States job "stressful," but "the people need me." Has had headaches for last 6 months and two episodes of dizziness, one at work and one at home lasting about 2 hours. Rested and symptoms went away. Delayed seeking care because was "too busy." Thought it was "overwork," not blood pressure. Discontinued blood pressure medication and physician visits about 6 months ago, "when blood pressure came down and I felt better"; states medicine caused impotence. To emergency room today because of left arm numbness and fear of stroke. Mother died of "stroke" 15 months ago. Concerned that he hasn't been taking care of himself and "I need to learn about what to do." Wants to know "everything."

Asked if would be O.K. to do some job-related paper work if someone brought it in. Takes no medicine currently, except Alka-Seltzer and a laxative; doesn't smoke; social drinking.

Nutritional-Metabolic Pattern. Sample diet related: MDR intake of protein, excess carbohydrate and fat; minimal high-roughage foods (fruits and vegetables), approximately 3 cups of coffee/day, fluid intake low, no history of lesions at mouth corners or mucous membranes; has gained weight gradually last 15 years. Some indigestion and heartburn after lunch attributed to days with multiple problems; takes Alka-Seltzer; dieting unsuccessful; problem is "probably stress of job; I get home and eat big supper and snacks in evening";

no food dislikes. Takes lunch (sandwich and cake) to work and eats at desk; restaurants in area not good.

Elimination Pattern. Daily bowel movement pattern with two to three episodes of constipation/month, each lasting 2 days; hard stools; straining; laxatives used. Attributes this pattern to his diet; knows he should eat better. Reports no problems voiding or in control of elimination.

Activity-Exercise Pattern. Spectator sports, uses car, minimal walking due to time schedule, sedentary job, considers self too old for exercise. Increasing fatigue last few weeks, noted less energy 2 months before admission; no self-care deficit. Recreation consists of reading novels, watching TV, dinner with other couples. Lives in first-floor apartment in city and drives ¾ mile to work.

Sleep-Rest Pattern. Average 4-6 hours sleep/night, quiet atmosphere, own room with wife, double bed, uses bed board. Presleep activities include watching TV or completing paper work from job; difficulty with sleep onset for 1 month; awakens in morning many times thinking about job-related problems.

Cognitive-Perceptual Pattern. Sight corrected with glasses, changed 1 year ago; no change in hearing, taste, smell. No perceived change in memory: "I couldn't take it if I started losing my mind, like with a stroke." Learning ability: sees self as slower than when in college, alert manner, grasps questions easily. Takes no sedatives, tranquilizers, other drugs. No headache at present.

Self-Perception–Self-Concept Pattern. Sees self as needing to do things well (job, father, husband); "sometimes I don't think I'm doing well with my family, having them live in this area, but in my job you have to be near when people need help. . . . It will be just great if I get sick and they have to take care of me, instead of me taking care of them."

Role-Relationship Pattern. Describes family as happy and understanding of his job commitments; wife former social worker; "kids good," "but I know we'll have trouble as Joe (10 years old) gets older." "Maybe I should move out of [lower socioeco area in city cited]." 10-year-old assaulted 4 months ago; 14-year-old boy interested in sports and "keeps out of trouble, so far." Family usually "sits down together" to handle problems. Social relationships confined to "a few other couples," finds this sufficient. Job demanding 9-10 hours/day "always trying to get money to keep the center solvent" (assistant taking over while client is in hospital); enjoys job and helping people; co-workers are "good to work with." Wife states they are close; worried about husband's health; states he is more concerned with other people than himself; she admires him for this. Wife able to handle home responsibilities during hospitalization. States she and children had physical exams recently; no health problems; no elevation in their blood pressure.

Sexuality-Reproductive Pattern. Two children; states impotent when on BP medication. When "BP went down" stopped meds; potency returned. No problems perceived in sexual relationship.

Coping–Stress-Tolerance Pattern. Feels tense at work; has tried relaxation exercises with some alleviation; doesn't always have time. States the best way to deal with problems is to "attack them." Afraid of having a stroke and being dependent: "This thing today has really scared me." ". . . I have too many things to think about at work and at home and now this blood pressure thing." Life changes: Father died 3 years ago; mother died of stroke 15 months ago. Took job at Spanish center 2 years ago to be near mother who "was getting old." Pleased he did this and feels good about it.

Value-Belief Pattern. "Life has been good to me"; feels deeply about "injustices in society" and wants to do something about them. States family is important to him. Religion (Catholic) important to him; would like to be active in church affairs.

Examination

Blood pressure __205/118__   Temperature   __99.8°F__
Pulse rate __Regular and strong__
Respirations __18__
Nutritional-Metabolic Pattern
Skin No area of redness over bony prominences; no lesions; dryness, callouses on feet, and discomfort
Oral mucous membranes Moist, no lesions
Actual wt 230 lb Reported wt 220 lb Ht 5'11"

Activity-Exercise Pattern

Gait Steady   Posture Well balanced
Muscle tone, strength-coordination Hand grip firm, left and right; lifts legs; can pick up pencil; tenseness in neck and shoulder muscles

Range of motion (joints) Some tightness in bending forward
Prostheses-assistive devices __None__
Absence of body part __No__
Demonstrated ability for:
Feeding __0__   Grooming __0__
Bathing __0__   General mobility __0__
Toileting __0__   Dressing __0__
(0 = full self-care)

Cognitive-Perceptual Pattern

Perceptual: Hears whisper __Yes__
Reads newsprint with glasses
Language: __English; grasps ideas, abstract and concrete; speech clear; attention span good__

Self-Perception–Self-Concept Pattern

General appearance Well groomed, good hygiene
Nervous/relaxed 2 (scale of 1-5) Tense; some relaxation during history taking
Eye contact __Yes__ Attention span __Good__
Assertive/Passive 3 (scale of 1-5)

Role-Relationship Pattern

Interactions: Communications with wife supportive; both somewhat tense, children not present.

DATA RECORDING SHEET

The admission assessment data recording sheet is placed in the client's chart. It becomes part of the permanent health care record. The following format with additional lines for recording can be imprinted on a permanent record sheet.

Nursing History and Examination

General description of client (age, general appearance, chief concerns, etc.) ⎯⎯⎯⎯⎯

Health perception–health management pattern ⎯⎯

Nutritional-metabolic pattern ⎯⎯⎯⎯

Elimination pattern ⎯⎯⎯⎯

Activity-exercise pattern ⎯⎯⎯⎯

Sleep-rest pattern ⎯⎯⎯⎯

Cognitive-perceptual pattern ⎯⎯⎯⎯

Self-perception–self-concept pattern ⎯⎯⎯⎯

Role-relationship pattern ⎯⎯⎯⎯

Sexuality-reproductive pattern _____

Coping–stress-tolerance pattern _____

Value-belief pattern _____

Nursing diagnoses (Use problem-oriented recording: see Chapter 10)*

_____

_____

_____

*See answers in Chapter 10 text.

APPENDIX J

VALIDITY, RELIABILITY, AND RELEVANCE: THE "GOOD" CUES

Two of the most important characteristics of data used in diagnosis are validity and reliability. Accurate diagnoses depend on these characteristics. As previously discussed in uncertainty-geared situations, the best and most reliable indicators facilitate accurate judgments.

VALID CUES

A cue is valid if it represents the properties of what is being judged. For example, the description of food and fluid intake represents one property of a nutritional-metabolic pattern; thus it is one piece of information that is valid for making a judgment about this pattern. Is the client's description of what her husband cooks for each meal valid information about her dietary pattern? No; information on the type of meals prepared does not provide direct information about intake and leads to risky judgments based on assumptions.

There are degrees of validity. *Highly valid data represent critical properties of a functional health pattern. Information of lower validity requires assumptions that may or may not be true.* The clearer the definition of functional health patterns, the easier it is to seek valid data with which to make judgments about patterns. Thus definitions of the critical properties of a pattern are continually improved as new knowledge accumulates. In addition, during assessment keep in mind the definition and components of each health pattern so that the data collected is relevant. This leads to a valid, functional assessment.

Let us now apply this information on validity to diagnostic categories and their defining characteristics (cues). A cue to a health problem is highly valid if it contains information on the critical properties of a diagnostic category. It is a highly sensitive indicator if when the condition is present it is nearly always present. In the example above, the actual food ingested would be a more valid indicator of nutritional deficit than the husband's cooking practices. (The cooking practices may be further explored when the search for etiological factors begins.) Refinement of diagnostic categories

needs to center on identifying the most valid characteristics and their reliability. For example, one study focused on the 15 currently identified characteristics (cues) of the diagnosis High Risk for Aspiration.[1] More than 75% of a national sample of 188 critical care nurses rated 3 of the 15 cues as nearly always or frequently present when High Risk for Aspiration was present. These 3 cues can be thought of as the highly valid risk factors in this setting:[2]

1. Depressed cough and gag reflex
2. Reduced level of consciousness
3. Impaired swallowing

Impaired swallowing results from depressed cough and gag reflexes. Thus this cue does not add information if the other two cues are present. This critical care study suggests that in preventative care, cues 1 and 2 above are highly valid for this condition; the other 12 cues may or may not be present as co-occurring risk factors.[3]

RELIABLE CUES

Reliable information is also valued as "good." *Information is reliable if it is (1) a dependable indicator of a functional pattern or of a diagnosis and (2) obtained through accurate measurement.* For example, in the list below, which measure of food and fluid intake is most dependable and therefore most reliable as data for assessing the nutritional-metabolic pattern?

1. A client's description of food and fluid intake
2. A nurse's daily observation of fluid and fluid intake
3. The husband's description of the meals served to the client

To make a judgment about food and fluid intake, most would prefer to use the second option, the nurse's observations. This preference is based on the idea that an outside observer (who is also a professional) is free of

331

bias and more accurate. It may be that the client is just as accurate as the nurse, but we do not know this. The husband's description of meals served to the client has the lowest reliability; we do not know if the client eats all of her meals. If the diagnosis being investigated was Health Management Deficit (salt-free diet), the client's report of her food and fluid intake would be important information in assessing her knowledge and practices.

The example above has further implications. The cost of obtaining information through observation is high. If there is no reason to suspect the client is unreliable, her verbal report may be accepted. In some situations observation is impossible; client reports are then accepted as the most reliable information obtainable. In other situations judgments are so important that, irrespective of time and costs, direct measurements are performed. Situations must be judged individually.

Reliable cues are dependable. A cue is a highly specific indicator if it is present when the condition is present and does not occur with any other conditions. Reliability, in addition to validity, is a dimension of critical defining characteristics (diagnostic criteria). As work on nursing diagnoses progresses, the critical cues will be specified in manuals and will be the most dependable information for accurate diagnosis.

The second feature of reliability, accuracy of measurement, contributes to "good" information. This is why the following points should always be considered during information collection:

1. Observational and interviewing skills
2. Accurate measuring devices (e.g., equipment)
3. Good lighting for observation
4. Well-formulated questions
5. Careful listening to verbal cues
6. Communication of acceptance, interest, and caring

In summary, valid and reliable cues obtained by accurate measures provide a data base for judgments about functional health patterns and diagnoses.

In the next section, relevant and irrelevant cues are discussed; highly valid and reliable cues are the relevant data for assessment and diagnosis. Sometimes in practice this comment is heard: "There isn't much relevant information in that note (on the client's chart)." Consider now what that comment might mean.

RELEVANT CUES

The key to efficiency (saving time) and effectiveness (accuracy) in functional health pattern assessment and diagnosis is to focus on relevant information. The terms *relevant* and *irrelevant* are used frequently to pertain to validity. Relevance of a cue depends on the purpose of information collection, such as health status evaluation. Specific information about the essential properties of

each pattern is considered relevant data. This information is what makes the data base informative.

For example, if the health perception–health management pattern is being assessed, relevant cues will be found in the following:

1. The client's perception of his/her/family's general health
2. General level of resistance (e.g., to colds, infections)
3. Health practices (things done to keep healthy, including taking any prescribed drugs; treatments, tests, and immunizations)
4. Health beliefs (perception of whether health practices make a difference)
5. Use of tobacco, alcohol, drugs
6. Compliance, adherence, management of therapeutic regimen
7. If illness is present: perceived cause, actions taken, results of action; if no illness is present: management of everyday health problems[4]

In contrast, irrelevant information for the health perception–health management pattern includes repeating the physician's history of the illness from the care provider's perspective; in most settings this information may be found on the client's record. The nurse is interested in how the client perceives the illness (if present) and manages both health and illness. The second purpose of assessment is to identify dysfunctional patterns (nursing diagnoses) if they are present. Early data may suggest a tentative diagnosis. The cue search then becomes focused on the highly valid, relevant, critical characteristics (signs and symptoms) that define the diagnoses under consideration.

Irrelevant information may produce interference. A great deal of irrelevant information causes cognitive processes to become overloaded with noncontributory or redundant information: the "chaff" as opposed to the "wheat." For example, before the assessment of a client's nutritional pattern is completed, there should be sufficient data to determine whether any type of nutritional deficit or excess is present and how the client manages this health pattern. This necessary information is the "wheat." It may be interesting to know also that the client's father was a good cook, but this information in isolation is probably irrelevant.

Studies have shown that adding a lot of irrelevant information increases errors, takes more time, and increases difficulty.[5,6] These findings may be explained by the difficulty human beings have in holding large amounts of information in working memory. When searching for cues to support or reject a possible diagnosis, zero in on the critical defining characteristics and, one by one, assess for their presence or absence. As frequently stated: "Go where the money is." (Sutton's law: the notorious Willie Sutton, when asked why he robbed banks, replied, "That's where the money is.")

The advantage of focusing on relevant data is that less time is needed for the assessment. For example, the client might be asked five separate questions about his or her sleep pattern. Suppose instead the client is asked, "Most mornings when you get up, do you feel rested and ready for the day?" If the response to this question is yes, is it relevant in a screening assessment to know the hours of sleep and other particulars? These details would be relevant only if a problem were present. Each new piece of clinical data should provide additional information relevant to judgment about functional health patterns or diagnoses.

On occasion a client may provide a great deal of unsolicited irrelevant information, with discussion of each pattern, such as stories about the life successes of each of his or her children. Be aware this may signal: (1) a need for attention, (2) a need to impress (be alert for self-perception–self-concept data), (3) unclear orientation of the client at the beginning of an admission assessment, or (4) the nurse's hesitancy in conducting the admission interview. In handling this type of situation consider that increased amounts of irrelevant data can interfere with information processing and cause errors in judgment. To interrupt tactfully, a nurse might say: "Your children's success must give you a lot of pleasure (supportive, interested comment); tell me, when you . . . [go on to a related question in the history]."

CUE VALUES: QUANTITY AND QUALITY

Cues may take on different values. For example, the characteristic "marital status" has six values: married, divorced, separated, widowed, single, and never married. Some cues—for example, blood pressure or heart rate—have numerical values. Quantification (numerical values) allows more precise measurement. Yet many cues to a client's health status are subjective impressions of quality or quantity, such as estimates of respiratory depth, moistness of the skin, or severity of discomfort.

As Norris[7] has pointed out, many of the common conditions encountered in practice have not been adequately described or have had precise measures developed; fatigue, restlessness, and nausea are examples. As much as possible, data should be scaled (and the scales carefully defined) or quantified numerically. Quantification increases the reliability of measures and, subsequently, the reliability of judgments and communications.

CUE TYPES: INFLUENCE ON JUDGMENT

Different types of clinical information are used in different phases of the diagnostic process and in establishing a level of confidence in the diagnostic judgment. Diagnostic and supporting cues, subjective and objective cues, and historical and current cues as well as examples of their use, are discussed in the following sections.

Diagnostic and supporting cues

As previously mentioned, diagnostic cues, or criteria, are the critical characteristics of a diagnostic category. They are the cues that must be present if the diagnostic label is used, because they coincide with the formal definition of the category. When diagnostic cues (critical characteristics) are fully identified by NANDA, it is expected they will be highly valid and reliable, limited in number, and relevant to only one diagnostic category. For example, when a client repeatedly verbalizes negative feelings about an actual or perceived change in the structure or function of his or her body or a body part, this is a *diagnostic cue* to Body Image Disturbance. Other cues may be present in the situation, such as anxiety, fear, or hiding/overexposing/ignoring a body part. These are *supporting cues* that increase the diagnostician's confidence and serve to validate a client's verbal expression of feelings. Supporting cues may be useful, but not highly reliable, indicators of a diagnosis. There are two reasons for the low reliability of supporting cues:

1. Supporting cues usually describe behaviors that are not always present with the condition.
2. Supporting cues may be indicators of other conditions and therefore do not permit discrimination among conditions.

The situation in diagnosis is similar to everyday tasks of discrimination, such as telling "this from that"; we learn which cues to rely on and which are variable in different situations.

In general, there are three types of cues or clusters of cues that require attention and are important in diagnosis:

1. Cues to a change in a client's functional patterns
2. Deviation from pattern norms (population, cultural-ethnic, baseline)
3. Cues to delays or to dysfunctional pattern development (developmental assessment)

The first type is the cue that signifies a change in a client's usual patterns that is unexplained by expected norms for growth and development. A change may be positive and health supporting or negative and potentially dysfunctional. An example of the latter is a change in the role-relationship pattern so that the client becomes socially isolated.

The second type of cue that requires attention is deviation from an appropriate population norm. For example, a person may have no change in frequency of elimination but may depend on laxatives and enemas to maintain regularity. This represents a deviation from "normality." In another situation, a client may act within the norms of his or her ethnic group but be deviant in terms of the general or dominant social norms. This situation may produce problems for the person in one or many functional pattern areas, a possibility that requires validation with the client. A person may have no change in nutritional pattern, but this does not mean the pattern is productive for the person. It may be causing an elimination problem, or a nutritional deficit may be present if the person's requirements have increased. These problems are detected only by evaluating information relative to the whole.

The third type of cue or cue cluster important for nursing diagnosis is that which indicates pattern development. Each of the functional health patterns is continually evolving as the person grows older. For example, it is expected that a young child's activity-exercise pattern will evolve as his or her neurological development permits more coordinated movement. Similarly, value-belief patterns change with life experiences, including experiences with death. Cues to the development of functional health patterns are important. They may signify developmental lags or evolving patterns that are dysfunctional for the client.

Describing signs and symptoms only from the viewpoint of the nurse may lead to errors of omission. The way a client "defines the situation" must be taken into account. For example, it may be "apparent" that a particular mother and father are very concerned, caring, and capable. But if their child says, "Mommy doesn't love me," this statement should be recognized as a cue; it should not be brushed aside with some superficial reassurance. If that is how the child defines the situation, that is how it is for him or her. Similarly, a person who says there is no other recourse but suicide may truly perceive there is no other way. When a person newly diagnosed as diabetic says, "I can't manage," the response, "Of course you can," may cut off critically important diagnostic cues.

Dismissing cues with superficial reassurance may decrease the nurse's anxiety and the time spent in assessment. Yet the underlying problem will not go away. It will probably come back to haunt the staff in a different guise because the original communication was not attended to. A client's "uncooperative" behavior (from the nurse's or doctor's perspective), frequent calls, and repeated visits to an emergency room are common ways clients express unresolved problems.

Any discussion of important cues must take into consideration the cues that define currently accepted nursing diagnoses. These are health problems within the scope of nursing practice, and cues to their presence must not be missed. For example, if a client's dietary pattern, body weight, and other characteristics are not assessed, a nutritional deficit may be missed. A dilemma exists: Many diagnoses are not well defined. Therefore, what are the "important" cues? At this stage of development, the list of accepted diagnoses (Appendix A) and their defining criteria (with their deficiencies) are the best available in the nursing literature.[7,8] A discussion about what needs to be done to ensure that critical criteria for using diagnostic labels are available is contained in Chapter 12.

Subjective and objective cues

Frequently in practice a subjective-objective classification of cues is used. This is probably a false distinction. All observations have some subjectivity because the stimulus has been processed through the observer's mind. Common usage defines *objective data* as care provider observations and laboratory and other tests, whereas *subjective data* refers to perceptions, feelings, and other reports of the client, including subjective perceptions and feelings, such as self-concept or pain. In contrast are the so-called objective data the nurse observes, such as skin color, heart rate, or parent-child interaction. In many health care agencies, clinical data are commonly categorized as subjective or objective within the format of the problem-oriented recording system.[9]

The objective-subjective designation is relevant to the processing of information. The trained observer credits himself or herself with more objectivity than the client. Thus objective data are considered to be free from personal biases, emotions, and the like, which can influence information processing. This supposition, of course, is not always true; many times people, nurses included, see what they are ready to see. Yet the clinician *tries* to put aside biases or predispositions and be objective when analyzing clinical data. Some are more successful than others.

It is well to recognize there are two primary value systems that relate to subjective and objective data. In the diagnosis of disease or disease complications, objective data are valued for their diagnostic significance. Thus, when a nurse records or reports data to a physician to help in medical diagnosis, the emphasis is usually on objective data, for example, blood pressure or skin color. Objective and subjective data are of equal diagnostic significance to nurses. Some examples will clarify these two sets of values.

In the process of diagnosing disease, the physician considers subjective reports to be tentative until verification can be obtained by objective measures. In the extreme case, physical symptoms may be categorized as hypochondria if objective measurement does not support subjective reports. A somewhat paradoxical situation exists: If a lesion is observed on an x-ray film, the situation is reversed; support for the presence of the lesion is sought in subjective data from the client. For example, if a pathological lung condition is found by objective x-ray examination, the patient is asked whether pain, dyspnea, or other subjective symptoms have been experienced. A conflict between the two types of data is resolved either by greater reliance on objective measurements or, in some cases, a "wait-and-see" attitude. In psychiatric diagnosis, subjective data are essential but are complemented by objective examination to rule out a pathological condition in an organ. For example, signs of a behavioral disorder are not given a psychiatric label without ruling out organic problems, such as a brain tumor.

Nurses are equally concerned with objective and subjective data. They shuttle back and forth between their own observations (the so-called objective data) and the subjective reports of the client. Many manage to arrive at a synthesis. For example, a nurse may objectively measure the size of a pressure sore. Yet there is equal diagnostic concern about the individual's coping response to this condition and the personal and environmental factors that brought it about. Subjective client reports have diagnostic value because they help the nurse understand the client's perspective. These subjective data are valued because nurses' primary emphasis is on people and their total situation, including, but not limited to, the client's disease. Medical care providers, of course, do not totally ignore the person's ideas, actions, feelings, values, or beliefs, but these entities are not diagnostic of disease.

When a nurse acts within a nursing framework, the concerns, the data, and the diagnoses are different from those of physicians. When a nurse operates within a biomedical framework and transmits data to a physician, objective data are valued more than subjective reports. Both frameworks are used in nursing practice.

A related typology of clinical cues is the sign-and-symptom classification. The term *symptom* designates an experience related by a client. Information about symptoms is subjective. It includes the client's perceptions of body temperature, skin sensations, palpitations, feelings of competency or esteem, beliefs, attitudes, and values. In contrast, a *sign* is an objective indicator of a health problem. A symptom may also be a sign, and a client may perceive a sign but may not be able to interpret it. From this discussion, which may confuse some, the reader will appreciate why the terms *sign* and *symptom* are frequently used interchangeably. For the reader who wishes to pursue the distinction further, King's treatment of the subject[10] will be of interest.

Historical and current cues

Another useful way of thinking about the clinical data collected for purposes of nursing diagnosis is from a time perspective. An understanding of a client's functional patterns is constructed from historical and current cues. This way of classifying clinical data permits the

cues used in nursing diagnoses to be examined. Are they based on historical information, current information, or both? Second, are diagnoses based only on cues to the client's state or also on cues about the situational or environmental context?

To appreciate the distinction between historical and current information, keep in mind that current data come from "the here and now." Historical data may pertain to last night, 2 days ago, or 10 years ago. Their importance lies in the person(s)-environment interaction that is characteristic of the nursing focus in health care. In addition, the distinction between historical and current cues influences diagnostic thinking.

Historical state cues

Historical cues about the state of the person, family or community provide an individualized baseline for interpreting the current state. These baselines are within the context of the client's own functional patterns. One common example is blood pressure. What does a current value of 95/78 mean? If the value for the past 2 years has been 150/90, the interpretation is different than if blood pressure has been consistently in the 96/70 to 100/80 range. In another example, knowing how many hours of sleep a night a client has gotten in the past helps the nurse interpret and evaluate the present value of this characteristic. A nursing diagnosis should never be made exclusively from historical cues. Why is this so, and how might it occur?

Inferences about a particular client's behavior may be derived deductively by combining information (in this case, historical data) and generalizations from memory. For example, a nurse may infer that because a patient was "angry and complaining about the staff" on the day of admission (historical information), that is also the client's current emotional state ("complaining") 2 weeks later. In a sense the client is never allowed to escape the history. Using only historical cues predisposes to diagnostic error; for example, a person who has had a colostomy immediately brings to the nurse's mind the diagnosis of Body Image Disturbance. Clearly the current state of the client must be assessed and, in this case, subjective reports must be obtained. Also, the inference or assumption created in the mind of the clinician may or may not stand up to the test of reality. This discussion contains ideas so important in avoiding diagnostic errors that it warrants rereading.

Current state cues

To identify emerging patterns and detect changes, cues to a client's current state in combination with his or her historical state baselines are used. Current state cues should always be sought before making diagnoses. The reason for a self-care deficit, or any other problem, is determined by current or historical cues to causal factors. To determine whether a change in pattern has been abrupt or gradual, historical data are used.

In addition to collecting information about the state of the person, the nurse measures characteristics of the client's situation. These characteristics describe the context within which functional patterns evolve. Attention is focused on both historical and current situational cues.

Historical contextual cues

Events that have already occurred are part of a person's life history. Not only are they history, they are also the *context* (not the *state*) out of which the person's current functional patterns have evolved. It is worthwhile to consider a few examples, since this type of cue is very useful in diagnosis. First consider an obvious relationship. During assessment, the nurse elicits the information that the client avoids high-roughage foods. For example, no bran, leafy vegetables, nuts, or other foods with bulk are reported in the diet. This has been the pattern for a decade or more. (Note the historical and current state information.) The nurse believes the client is missing a good source of vitamins and is susceptible to constipation because of the lack of bulk in the diet.

The nurse has two options: one is to plunge ahead and try to correct this behavior; the other is to wonder why the client avoids roughage. Choosing the latter option, the nurse can ask questions to determine whether there is any explanation in the client's past history. The nurse learns that about 15 years earlier the client was diagnosed as having diverticulosis[11] and was told to avoid high-roughage foods. This contextual event (being diagnosed and instructed) happened in the past but is the reported reason for the current dietary pattern.

Historical contextual cues (situational context) not only are helpful in understanding functional patterns but also play an important role in prediction. There is an indication from research[6] that nurses use situational cues to predict the most likely health problems. In an admission assessment, prediction is necessary because the universe of possibilities is open. To fully investigate every conceivable diagnosis is impossible. Therefore predictions (inferences, or hypotheses) are made about the likelihood of various problems. Problems estimated to be highly probable are investigated first. Predictions are made on the basis of historical contextual cues and the knowledge of relationships stored in the nurse's memory. For example, a recent historical event in the life of a person, such as a first heart attack, is information that can be used to predict the likelihood of certain dysfunctional problems the nurse knows are often associated with heart attack.

Historical information about the environmental context also helps in the understanding of the background from which functional health patterns arise and develop.

This information includes the client's prior living environments, economic conditions, health and welfare resource systems, and interpersonal and sociocultural environments. In addition to contributing to the nurse's understanding of clients' health patterns, this information may be useful in predicting problems.

The reader may wonder, Why bother to think about possibilities? Why not just collect the assessment data? The perceptually sensitive observer anticipates. An inference is made from relationships stored in the observer's memory. This inference then forms the basis for a set of probing questions and the search for further cues. *Predictive inference* is anticipation, and it largely depends on contextual cues. Assumptions or inferences drawn on the basis of the person's history are helpful but must be used with caution if incorporated without validation into diagnosis. Although a historical event (one that occurred 2 days earlier) of having an amputation or breast removal may be associated with an alteration in body image, leg amputation is an insufficient rationale for making the diagnosis of Body Image Disturbance. Rather, a tentative diagnostic hypothesis (Body Image Disturbance) should be generated to guide the search for cues. Diagnoses based only on historical cues about the situation may result in errors of historical stereotyping.

Current contextual cues

Current contextual cues have two main uses in diagnosis. When examined in a situational context, the meaning of a cue to the state of a client may become clear. This type of cue is mainly used in interpretation and in combination with the historical context to assess the evolution of the client's situational or environmental pattern.

In this discussion, the types of client and environmental cues have been separated out in order to define, analyze, and bring attention to them. In actual practice these cues are not collected in separate packages but are obtained as part of the assessment sequence. What usually happens is that a piece of information is collected and attended to; then the question arises: What kind of information is necessary to derive meaning from this cue? One may branch to historical information about the client and the client's past environment. This information is usually obtained by questions posed to the client or others possessing the historical data. Branching may also point toward the need for more current data. Current data are obtained by questions aimed at eliciting subjective reports about the client's state. The nurse may also need to examine the current situational context, such as the client's home environment. Obviously, if the type of information needed (historical or current) is known, assessment proceeds more rapidly.

NOTES AND REFERENCES

1. North American Nursing Diagnosis Association: *NANDA taxonomy I, revised 1992,* Philadelphia, 1993, Nursecom.

2. Gordon M: *High frequency, high treatment priority nursing diagnoses in critical care,* Manuscript submitted for publication, 1993.

3. It might be argued that if a reduced level of consciousness were present, cough and gag reflexes would probably be depressed. Yet it is not clear how much reduction "reduced" means. If cough and gag reflexes were tested and found to be depressed, that would be an important risk factor, irrespective of the level of consciousness. Testing the cough and gag reflexes would be more invasive than assessing the level of consciousness, but if the level of consciousness were unstable, depressed cough and gag reflexes would be the better cue.

4. This list comprises components of a screening assessment; components of other patterns may be found in Chapter 5 and Appendix H.

5. Ciafrani KL: The influence of amounts and relevance of data on identifying health problems. In Kim MJ, McFar-land G, McLane A, editors: *Classification of nursing diagnoses: proceedings of the fifth national conference,* St Louis, 1984, Mosby.

6. Gordon M: Predictive strategies in diagnostic tasks, *Nurs Res* 29:39, 1980.

7. Norris CM: *Concept clarification in nursing,* Rockville, MD, 1982, Aspen Systems.

8. Gordon M: *Manual of nursing diagnosis 1993-1994,* St Louis, 1993, Mosby.

9. The problem-oriented recording system is a charting format that requires the separation of objective observations and subjective reports. Its use with nursing diagnoses is discussed in Chapter 10.

10. King LS: Signs and symptoms, *JAMA* 206:1063, 1968.

11. Diverticulosis is a condition in which there are small outpouches and weak points in the wall of the colon. Older methods of treatment included the avoidance of high-roughage foods.

APPENDIX K

HYPOTHESIS TESTING STRATEGIES

SIMULTANEOUS HYPOTHESIS SCANNING

The multiple hypothesis testing procedure is useful if (1) a number of hypotheses (possibilities) have been generated, as occurs early in assessment of a pattern area or (2) diagnoses represented in the hypotheses share the same cue but different values. A clinically significant change in blood pressure, for example, is a critical cue in hypertension and hemorrhagic shock. The value for blood pressure is elevated in hypertension but considerably reduced in shock.

Cognitive requirements are high when multiple hypotheses are tested simultaneously, because the number of hypotheses to which information must be related increases. Inductive and deductive inferences are required to relate the cues obtained to each hypothesis being tested and to increase or decrease hypothesis probabilities as a result of the information obtained. Yet unlikely diagnoses are eliminated, and the memory and inferential strain is reduced quickly.

Cognitive strain may occur if memory and inferential requirements exceed the diagnostician's capacity. Strain on cognitive capacities is manifested as forgetting information and as inferential errors. One reason for cognitive strain is prolonged holding of a large initial pool of hypotheses because of poor selection of predictive cues. To identify highly probable diagnostic hypotheses quickly requires a clinical knowledge of predictors and optimal decisions about the sequence of information collection.

A second, but related, reason for cognitive strain is prolonged multiple testing of hypotheses. Highly valid predictors may have been collected, but the diagnostician attempts to reduce uncertainty even further. Usually the continued search for predictive cues is due to a lack of understanding of the probabilistic nature of clinical information. It should be recognized that uncertainty in prediction cannot be totally eliminated. The diagnostician should rely on good predictive cues and begin to test likely diagnostic hypotheses; it is always possible to return to the unlikely hypotheses if necessary.

The need to scan multiple hypotheses simultaneously can be expected to lessen or disappear after (1) the most probable diagnoses to explain a dysfunctional pattern have been identified, and (2) the values of the defining characteristics shared by two or more diagnoses have been obtained. After the likely possibilities are identified, a decided shift in procedure occurs.[1] Thereafter the data sought are specific to the remaining hypotheses and each is tested, one by one.

Collecting information that differentiates among the remaining hypotheses requires a search for diagnostic cues. These are the critical cues that define and differentiate among diagnoses. Single-hypothesis testing is useful at this point.

SUCCESSIVE HYPOTHESIS SCANNING

The successive scanning of hypotheses involves assessing a client or situation to test one hypothesis at a time. This is a reasonable approach when critical, differentiating cues apply to only one diagnosis. Moreover, if only one or two hypotheses remain, they can be tested individually. The main advantage of testing hypotheses one at a time is that memory strain and inferential strain do not increase over the base level. Easing these strains is particularly welcome if the processes of generating hypotheses, predictive testing, and testing overlapping cues were prolonged early in the assessment of the pattern area. Another advantage is that the potential for forgetting or for inferential errors is low when only a few hypotheses need be considered. The use of cues to test hypotheses individually ensures accuracy. No risk is taken, because *all* hypotheses in the pool are tested. For this reason, confidence in the results of assessment should be high.

To use single-hypothesis testing exclusively throughout the entire admission assessment is an inefficient diagnostic strategy. Maximum information is not obtained from answers to each question in this procedure. If only one hypothesis is generated and tested at a time, information relevant to other possibilities is lost. On the other hand, the information could be held in memory; but this approach removes one of the major advantages of this procedure, which is low memory strain.

Single-hypothesis testing is a costly procedure if used exclusively. It increases the total time needed for assessment and requires repetitious questioning and observations, which creates the impression of disorganization. Yet when memory strain and inferential strain are high and when time and resources for testing are unlimited, this procedure is useful. If the assessment situation is problem focused (Chapter 7), as is the case after diagnoses are established, the procedure is certainly ideal. The successive investigation of single hypotheses is a "safe but slow" way of proceeding.[1] The major shift to successive scanning within a strategy appears to occur when the diagnostician is confident (for the moment) that the most probable diagnoses have been identified. Consider an example: The sleep-rest pattern of a 40-year-old client is being assessed. A question has been posed and the client has responded that she has not been sleeping too well. This cue indicates a diagnosis of Sleep-Pattern Disturbance; a diagnostic strategy for investigating the cue is needed. The data on the client reveals the change to a dysfunctional pattern occurred about 2 weeks before hospital admission. Background information and the pattern areas already assessed suggest one etiological cue: This client has realistic health concerns; about 2 weeks earlier she was told she might have cancer.

The diagnostic hypotheses generated were as follows:

1. Sleep Onset Disturbance
2. Sleep Pattern Disturbance (Early Awakening)
3. Sleep Pattern Interruption
4. Sleep Pattern Reversal

The interventions for each of these four hypotheses are different; thus it is important to identify which one is truly the problem. The only causal hypothesis at the moment is broad and vague: health concerns—cancer.

A cue was sought to predict the probabilities of each of the hypotheses generated. The client was asked for a specific description of her sleep pattern. Simultaneous testing of the four diagnostic hypotheses revealed that Sleep Onset Disturbance and Early Awakening Disturbance were most likely. Data about the number of hours the client was sleeping did not support either hypothesis 3 or hypothesis 4; the client sleeps 3 to 4 hours per night. The etiological hypothesis (the client's concern about having cancer) and two of the four hypotheses about the problem remain at this point.

A focused single-hypothesis testing strategy is appropriate. Sleep Onset Disturbance and Early Awakening Disturbance are the diagnoses still under consideration. Now the critical differentiating cues must be obtained. The probability of Early Awakening Disturbance decreases when the nurse obtains the answer to a clarifying question: The client says the reason she awakens early is that at home the whole household always retires at 10 PM and arises at 5 AM. The next question is designed to elicit data to support or reject the remaining diagnostic possibility, Sleep Onset Disturbance.

What type of data should be collected to test this single hypothesis? The diagnostic cues of Sleep Onset Disturbance are listed below:

1. Report of difficulty falling asleep
2. A 15-minute or longer sleep delay after attempts to go to sleep
3. Consecutive episodes of delayed sleep onset[2]

Knowing these diagnostic cues, the nurse can formulate questions to elicit the pertinent data. As previously discussed, measures of client characteristics must be reliable and valid. Which of the following questions would elicit the most reliable and valid data?

1. "When you have difficulty getting to sleep, how many minutes would you estimate it takes to fall asleep? Does this occur frequently?"
2. "When you have difficulty getting to sleep, how long do you lie awake? Does it happen every night?"

The first option focuses on the data needed, whereas the second is less specific. The client might respond, "A long time." A time-consuming second question would then have to be asked. Moreover, the question about consecutive episodes is leading the client to a particular response in the second option. As experience is gained in formulating good questions, the time required for assessment decreases. In this case, the client responded that most nights it takes 3 or 4 hours for her to fall deeply asleep. The diagnostic hypothesis of Sleep Onset Disturbance is supported. Now the probable cause of this sleep problem must be determined.

In summary, hypothesis testing procedures differ from hypothesis-generation procedures. This appears to be the case both in actual and potential problem identification and in the identification of etiological factors. After likely diagnoses have been identified, procedures within an analytic strategy shift. The most probable diagnostic hypotheses become the bases for a focused cue search. Unless diagnostic cues overlap (i.e., they have differing values that distinguish one diagnosis from another), the procedure of choice is to investigate the remaining hypotheses one by one.

The type of data sought is specific to each diagnostic hypothesis. These data are the diagnostic cues that constitute the critical defining signs and symptoms of each nursing diagnosis. Without the presence of these specific cues, the diagnostic category name should not be used. (As previously stated, work is in progress to identify critical signs and symptoms.) There are usually few critical diagnostic cues, but they differentiate one diagnosis from another. Supporting data may also be sought. Supporting data influence confidence in a diagnosis when cues are uncertainty based or when available measures are only partially reliable.

REFERENCES

1. Gordon M: Predictive strategies in diagnostic tasks, *Nurs Res* 29:39, 1980.
2. Schwartz AK, Aaron NS: *Somniquest,* New York, 1979, Berkeley Books.

APPENDIX L

NANDA Descriptors for Constructing Diagnostic Categories

Diagnostic labels may include but *are not limited to* the following qualifiers:

Altered A change from baseline.

Impaired Made worse, weakened; damaged, reduced; deteriorated.

Depleted Emptied wholly or partially; exhausted of.

Deficient Inadequate in amount, quality, or degree; defective; not sufficient; incomplete.

From North American Nursing Diagnosis Association: *NANDA nursing diagnoses, definitions, and classification,* Philadelphia, 1992, the Association, pp 85-86.

Excessive Characterized by an amount or quantity that is greater than is necessary, desirable, or useful.

Dysfunctional Abnormal; incomplete functioning.

Disturbed Agitated; interrupted, interfered with.

Ineffective Does not produce the desired effect.

Decreased Lessened, lesser in size, amount, or degree.

Increased Greater in size, amount, or degree.

Acute Severe but of short duration.

Chronic Lasting a long time; recurring; habitual; constant.

Intermittent Stopping and starting again at intervals; periodic; cyclic.

Potential for Enhanced (wellness diagnosis) Enhanced is defined as made greater; to increase in quality or more desired.

APPENDIX M

EXAMPLE OF A NATIONAL TREATMENT GUIDELINE: PRESSURE ULCER TREATMENT

RISK ASSESSMENT TOOLS AND RISK FACTORS

Goals: Identify at-risk individuals and the specific factors placing them at risk.

1. Bed- and chair-bound individuals or those with impaired ability to reposition should be assessed for additional factors that increase the risk for developing pressure ulcers. These factors include immobility, incontinence, nutritional factors such as inadequate dietary intake and impaired nutritional status, and altered level of consciousness. Individuals should be assessed on admission to acute care and rehabilitation hospitals, nursing homes, home care programs, and other health care facilities. A systematic risk assessment can be done by using a validated risk assessment tool such as the Braden Scale or Norton Scale. Pressure ulcer risk should be reassessed at periodic intervals. (Strength of evidence = A.) All assessments of risk should be documented. (Strength of evidence = C.)

SKIN CARE AND EARLY TREATMENT

Goal: Maintain and improve tissue tolerance to pressure in order to prevent injury.

1. All individuals at risk should have a systematic

Excerpted from the U.S. Department of Health and Human Services, Agency for Health Care Policy and Research: *Clinical practice guidelines: pressure ulcer in adults,* Rockville, Md, 1992.
Strength of Evidence refers to the strength of the research evidence that supports the recommendation. *A* and *B* refer to research, and *C* refers to expert opinion.

skin inspection at least once a day, with particular attention to the bony prominences. Results of skin inspection should be documented. (Strength of evidence = C.)

2. Skin should be cleansed at the time of soiling and at routine intervals. The frequency of skin cleansing should be individualized according to need and/or patient preference. Avoid hot water and use a mild cleansing agent that minimizes irritation and dryness of the skin. During the cleansing process, care should be taken to minimize the force and friction applied to the skin. (Strength of evidence = C.)

3. Minimize environmental factors leading to skin drying, such as low humidity (less than 40%) and exposure to cold. Dry skin should be treated with moisturizers. (Strength of evidence = C.)

4. Avoid massage over bony prominences. (Strength of evidence = B.)

5. Minimize skin exposure to moisture due to incontinence, perspiration, or wound drainage. When these sources of moisture cannot be controlled, use underpads or briefs made of materials that absorb moisture and present a quick-drying surface to the skin. For information about assessing and managing urinary incontinence, refer to *Urinary Incontinence in Adults: Clinical Practice Guideline* (available from USDHHS). Topical agents that act as barriers to moisture may also be used. (Strength of evidence = C.)

6. Skin injury due to friction and shear forces should be minimized through proper positioning, transferring, and turning techniques. In addition, friction injuries may be reduced by the use of lubricants (such as corn starch and creams), protective films (such as transparent film dressings and skin sealants), protective dressings (such as hydrocolloids),

and protective padding. (Strength of evidence = C.)

7. When apparently well-nourished individuals develop an inadequate dietary intake of protein or calories, caregivers should first attempt to discover the factors that are compromising intake and offer support with eating. Other nutritional supplements or support may be needed. If dietary intake remains inadequate and if consistent with the overall goals of therapy, more aggressive nutritional intervention, such as enteral or parenteral feedings, should be considered. (Strength of evidence = C.)

   For nutritionally compromised individuals, a plan of nutritional support and/or supplementation should be implemented that meets the individual's needs and is consistent with the overall goals of therapy. (Strength of evidence = C.)

8. If there is a potential for improving an individual's mobility and activity status, rehabilitation efforts should be instituted if consistent with the overall goals of therapy. Maintaining current activity level, mobility, and range of motion is an appropriate goal for most individuals. (Strength of evidence = C.)

9. Interventions and outcomes should be monitored and documented. (Strength of evidence = C.)

MECHANICAL LOADING AND SUPPORT SURFACES

Goal: Protect against the adverse effects of external mechanical forces: pressure, friction, and shear.

1. Any individual in bed who is assessed to be at risk for developing pressure ulcers should be repositioned at least every 2 hours if consistent with overall patient goals. A written schedule for systematically turning and repositioning the individual should be used. (Strength of evidence = B.)

2. For individuals in bed, positioning devices such as pillows or foam wedges should be used to keep bony prominences (e.g., knees or ankles) from direct contact with one another, according to a written plan. (Strength of evidence = C.)

3. Individuals in bed who are completely immobile should have a care plan that includes the use of devices that totally relieve pressure on the heels, most commonly by raising the heels off the bed. Do not use donut-type devices. (Strength of evidence = C.)

4. When the side-lying position is used in bed, avoid positioning the individual directly on the trochanter. (Strength of evidence = C.)

5. Maintain the head of the bed at the lowest degree of elevation consistent with medical conditions and other restrictions. Limit the amount of time the head of the bed is elevated. (Strength of evidence = C.)

6. Use lifting devices such as a trapeze or bed linen to move (rather than drag) individuals in bed who cannot assist during transfers and position changes. (Strength of evidence = C.)

7. When lying in bed, any individual assessed to be at risk for developing pressure ulcers should be placed on a pressure-reducing device, such as a foam, static air, alternating air, gel, or water mattress. (Strength of evidence = B.)

8. For any person at risk for developing a pressure ulcer uninterrupted sitting in a chair or wheelchair, should be avoided. The individual should be repositioned so that the points under pressure are shifted at least every hour, or should be put back to bed if consistent with overall patient management goals. Individuals who are able to do so should be taught to shift their weight every 15 minutes. (Strength of evidence = C.)

9. For chair-bound individuals, the use of a pressure-reducing device such as those made of foam, gel, air, or a combination is indicated. Do not use donut-type devices. (Strength of evidence = C.)

10. The positioning of chair-bound individuals in chairs or wheelchairs should include consideration of postural alignment, distribution of weight, balance and stability, and pressure relief. (Strength of evidence = C.)

11. A written plan for the use of positioning devices and schedules may be helpful for chair-bound individuals. (Strength of evidence = C.)

EDUCATION

Goal: Reduce the incidence of pressure ulcers through educational programs.

1. Educational programs for the prevention of pressure ulcers should be structured, organized, and comprehensive and directed at all levels of health care providers, patients, and family or caregivers. (Strength of evidence = A.)

2. The educational program for the prevention of pressure ulcers should include information on the following items (Strength of evidence = B):
   - Etiology and risk factors for pressure ulcers
   - Risk assessment tools and their application
   - Skin assessment
   - Selection and/or use of support surfaces
   - Development and implementation of an individualized program of skin care

- Demonstration of positioning to decrease the risk of tissue breakdown
- Instruction on accurate documentation of pertinent data

3. The educational program should identify those responsible for pressure ulcer prevention, describe each person's role, and be appropriate to the audience in terms of level of information presented and expected participation. The educational program should be updated regularly to incorporate new and existing techniques or technologies. (Strength of evidence = C.)

4. Educational programs should be developed, implemented, and evaluated using principles of adult learning. (Strength of evidence = C.)

APPENDIX N

NURSING INTERVENTION CLASSIFICATION

DEFINITIONS AND EXAMPLES

Taxonomy of nursing interventions A systematic organization of the intervention labels into what can be considered a conceptual framework with rules and principles for ordering the labels clearly articulated.

Nurse-initiated treatments Interventions initiated by the nurse in response to a nursing diagnosis: "an autonomous action based on scientific rationale that is executed to benefit the client in a predicted way related to the nursing diagnosis and the stated goals." Examples might include patient contracting, counseling, reminiscence therapy, preparatory sensory information, and oral health promotion.

Physician-initiated treatments Interventions that are initiated by a physician in response to a medical diagnosis but are carried out by a nurse in response to a "doctor's order." Examples might include Medication Administration, Electrolyte Monitoring, and IV Therapy.

INTERVENTION LABELS

Abuse protection management
Acidosis management
Acid-base management: metabolic alkalosis
Acid-base management: respiratory acidosis
Acid-base management: respiratory alkalosis
Acid-base monitoring
Active listening
Activity therapy
Admission care
Airway insertion and stabilization
Airway management: acid-base
Airway suctioning
Allergy management
Amputation care
Analgesic administration
Anesthesia administration
Anger control assistance
Animal assisted therapy
Anticipatory guidance
Anxiety reduction

Area restriction
Art therapy,
Artificial airway management
Aspiration precautions
Assertiveness training
Attachment promotion
Autogenic training
Bathing
Bed rest care
Behavior management
Behavior modification
Bibliotherapy
Biofeedback
Birthing
Bleeding precautions
Bleeding reduction
Bleeding reduction: nasal
Bleeding reduction: wound
Blood products administration
Body image enhancement
Body mechanics promotion
Bottle feeding
Bowel incontinence care
Bowel irrigation
Bowel management
Bowel training
Calming technique
Cardiac care
Cardiac care: acute

Cardiac care: rehabilitative
Cardiac precautions
Caregiver support
Cast care: maintenance
Cast care: wet
Cerebral edema management
Cesarean section care
Chemotherapy management
Chest physiotherapy,
Childbirth preparation
Circulatory care
Circulatory precautions
Code management
Cognitive restructuring
Cognitive stimulation
Communication enhancement
Communication enhancement: hearing deficit
Communication enhancement: visual deficit
Confusion management
Constipation/impaction management
Contact lens care
Cough enhancement
Counseling
Crisis intervention
Culture brokerage
Cutaneous stimulation

Excerpted from McCloskey JC, Bulechek GM: *Nursing interventions classification (NIC)*, St Louis, 1992, Mosby, pp xvii, xx-xxiv.

Decision-making support
Delirium management
Diarrhea management
Diet staging
Discharge planning
Dying care
Dysreflexia management
Dysrhythmia management
Ear care
Eating disorders management
Electrolyte management
Electrolyte management:
  hypercalcemia
Electrolyte management:
  hyperkalemia
Electrolyte management:
  hypermagnesemia
Electrolyte management:
  hypernatremia
Electrolyte management:
  hyperphosphatemia
Electrolyte management:
  hypocalcemia
Electrolyte management:
  hypokalemia
Electrolyte management:
  hypomagnesemia,
Electrolyte management:
  hyponatremia
Electrolyte management:
  hypophosphatemia
Electrolyte monitoring
Embolus care: peripheral
Embolus care: pulmonary
Embolus precautions
Emergency care
Emotional support
Energy management
Enteral tube feeding
Environmental management
Environmental management:
  attachment process
Environmental management:
  comfort
Environmental management:
  safety
Environmental management:
  violence prevention
Epidural analgesia administra-
  tion
Exercise promotion
Exercise therapy: ambulation
Exercise therapy: balance
Exercise therapy: joint mobility

Exercise therapy: muscle con-
  trol
Eye care
Fall prevention
Family integrity promotion
Family integrity promotion:
  childbearing family
Family involvement
Family mobilization
Family planning; contraception
Family planning: infertility,
  unplanned pregnancy
Family process maintenance
Family support
Family therapy
Feeding
Fetal monitoring
First aid
Flatulence reduction
Fluid/electrolyte management
Fluid management
Fluid monitoring
Fluid resuscitation
Foot care
Gastrointestinal intubation
Genetic counseling
Grief work facilitation
Hair care
Hallucination management
Health screening
Health system guidance
Heat exposure treatment
Heat/cold application
Hemodialysis therapy
Hemodynamic regulation
Hemorrhage control
Home maintenance assist-
  ance
Hope instillation
Humor
Hyperglycemia management
Hypervolemia management
Hypnosis
Hypoglycemia management
Hypothermia treatment
Hypovolemia management
Immunization/vaccination ad-
  ministration
Incision site care
Infant care
Infection control
Infection protection
Intracranial pressure (ICP)
  monitoring
Intrapartal care

Intravenous (IV) insertion
Intravenous (IV) therapy
Invasive hemodynamic monitor-
  ing
Lactation management
Lactation suppression
Learning readiness enhancement
Limit setting
Mechanical ventilation
Mechanical ventilatory weaning
Medication administration: en-
  teral
Medication administration: fever
  treatment
Medication administration: in-
  terpleural
Medication administration: oral
Medication administration: par-
  enteral
Medication administration: topi-
  cal
Medication management
Memory training
Milieu therapy
Music therapy
Mutual goal setting
Nail care
Neurological monitoring
Newborn care
Newborn monitoring
Nonnutritive sucking manage-
  ment
Nutrition management
Nutrition therapy
Nutritional counseling
Nutritional monitoring
Oral health maintenance
Oral health promotion
Oral health restoration
Ostomy care
Oxygen therapy
Pain management
Parent education: adolescent
Parent education: childbearing
  family
Parent education: child-rearing
  family
Patient contracting
Patient controlled analgesia
  (PCA) assistance
Patient rights protection
Perineal care
Peripheral sensation manage-
  ment
Peripherally inserted central
  (PIC) catheter care

Peritoneal dialysis therapy
Physical restraint
Play therapy
Positioning
Positioning: neurological
Positioning: wheelchair
Postmortem care
Postpartal care
Pregnancy termination care
Prenatal care
Preparatory sensory information
Presence
Pressure management
Pressure ulcer care
Pressure ulcer prevention
Progressive muscle relaxation
Prosthesis care
Radiation therapy management
Rape-trauma treatment
Reality orientation
Recreation therapy
Referral
Reminiscence therapy
Respiratory monitoring
Respite care
Resuscitation
Risk identification
Risk identification: childbearing
  family
Role enhancement
Seclusion
Security enhancement
Seizure management
Seizure precautions
Self-awareness enhancement
Self-care assistance: bathing/
  hygiene
Self-care assistance: dressing/
  grooming
Self-care assistance: feeding
Self-care assistance: toileting
Self-esteem enhancement
Self-modification assistance
Self-responsibility facilitation

Sexual counseling
Shock management
Shock management: cardiac
Shock management: vasogenic
Shock management: volume
Shock prevention
Sibling support
Simple guided imagery
Simple massage
Simple relaxation therapy
Skin care: topical treatments
Skin surveillance
Sleep enhancement
Smoking cessation assistance
Socialization enhancement
Specimen management
Spiritual support
Splinting
Subarachnoid hemorrhage pre-
  cautions
Substance use prevention
Substance use treatment
Substance use treatment: Alco-
  hol withdrawal
Substance use treatment: drug
  withdrawal
Substance use treatment: over-
  dose
Suicide prevention
Support group
Support system enhancement
Surgical assistance: circulating
Surgical assistance: scrubbing
Surgical preparation
Surveillance
Surveillance: safety
Sustenance support
Suturing
Swallowing therapy
Teaching: disease process
Teaching: group
Teaching: individual
Teaching: infant care
Teaching: preoperative

Teaching: prescribed activity/
  exercise
Teaching: prescribed diet
Teaching: prescribed medication
Teaching: procedure/treatment
Teaching: psychomotor skill
Teaching: safe sex
Technology management
Temperature regulation
Therapeutic touch
Therapy group
Total parenteral nutrition (TPN)
  administration
Touch
Traction care
Transcutaneous electrical nerve
  stimulation (TENS)
Transport
Triage
Truth telling
Tube care
Tube care: chest
Tube care: gastrointestinal
Tube care: urinary
Tube care: ventriculostomy/
  lumbar drain
Urinary catheterization
Urinary catheterization: inter-
  mittent
Urinary elimination manage-
  ment
Urinary incontinence care
Urinary retention care
Values clarification
Ventilation assistance
Visitation facilitation
Vital signs monitoring
Weight gain assistance
Weight management
Weight reduction assistance
Wound care
Wound care: closed drainage
Wound irrigation

APPENDIX O

PATIENT CLASSIFICATION: DEVELOPED AT UNIVERSITY HOSPITALS OF CLEVELAND

Courtesy University Hospitals of Cleveland. (Form no longer used by University Hospitals of Cleveland.)

UNIVERSITY HOSPITALS OF CLEVELAND
NURSE/PATIENT SUMMARY

	RN Code Number	Other Code Number	Consultant Code Number
TODAY			
LAST NIGHT			
LAST EVENING			

Primary Nurse Code Number _____

Date Today
DIRECTIONS: Check the items below if Actually or Potentially Present.

HEALTH PERCEPTION-MANAGEMENT
Potential for Injury . . . . _____001
Noncompliance . . . . _____002
Infection/Contagion . . . . _____003
Prolonged Disease/Disability . . . . _____004
Instability . . . . _____005
Impaired Life Support Systems . . . . _____006
Sanitation Deficit . . . . _____007
Socio-cultural-economic Considerations . . . . _____008

NUTRITIONAL-METABOLIC
Fluid
   Excess Volume . . . . _____009
   Volume Deficit . . . . _____010
   Potential Volume Deficit . . . . _____011
   Bleeding . . . . _____012
Nutrition
   Less Nutrition than Required . . . . _____013
   More Nutrition than Required . . . . _____014
   Potential for Excess . . . . _____015
Skin Integrity
   Actual Skin Impairment . . . . _____016
   Potential Skin Impairment . . . . _____017
   Alterations in Oral Mucous Membrane . . . . _____018
Altered Body Temperature . . . . _____019

ELIMINATION
Urinary
   Incontinence . . . . _____020
   Other Altered Urinary Elim. Pattern . . . . _____021
Bowel
   Constipation . . . . _____022
   Diarrhea . . . . _____023
   Incontinence . . . . _____024

ACTIVITY-EXCERCISE
Activity Intolerance . . . . _____025
Ineffective Airway Clearance . . . . _____026
Altered Breathing Pattern . . . . _____027
Impaired Gas Exchange . . . . _____028
Altered Tissue Perfusion . . . . _____029
Decreased Cardiac Output . . . . _____030
Diversion Activity Deficit . . . . _____031

Altered Health Maintenance . . . . _____032
Impaired Mobility . . . . _____033
Self-Care Deficit . . . . _____034
Impaired Home Maintenance Mgmt . . . . _____035

COGNITION-PERCEPTION
Altered Comfort
   Discomfort . . . . _____036
   Pain . . . . _____037
Altered Level of Consciousness . . . . _____038
Altered Thought Process . . . . _____039
Impulsivity/Hyperactivity . . . . _____040
Altered Sensory Perception . . . . _____041
Knowledge Deficit . . . . _____042
Growth and Development Deficit . . . . _____043

SLEEP-REST
Sleep Disturbance . . . . _____044

SELF-PERCEPTION/SELF-CONCEPT
Anxiety . . . . _____045
Disturbed Self-Concept . . . . _____046
Depression . . . . _____047
Fear . . . . _____048
Powerlessness . . . . _____049

ROLE RELATIONSHIPS
Grieving . . . . _____050
Altered Family Process . . . . _____051
Altered Parenting . . . . _____052
Social Isolation . . . . _____053
Impaired Verbal Communication . . . . _____054
Potential for Violence . . . . _____055

SEXUALITY-REPRODUCTION
Sexual Dysfunction . . . . _____056
Rape-Trauma Syndrome . . . . _____057

COPING-STRESS TOLERANCE
Ineffective Individual Coping . . . . _____058
Ineffective Family Coping . . . . _____059
Potential for Growth in Family Coping . . . . _____060

VALUE-BELIEF
Spiritual Distress . . . . _____061

APPENDIX P

PRACTICE-BASED COMPONENTS FOR A COMPUTERIZED NURSING INFORMATION SYSTEM

DATA SET ITEMS AND DEFINITIONS

The data set items that follow can be logically derived (1) from current models and standards of nursing practice and (2) from reflection on the information needed to support cognitive processes involved in patient care. Identification, demographic, medical, setting, and care provider items are required but are not unique to a nursing practice data set.

Identification variables

1. Patient identification
   Item-categories: Name and assigned number.
   Definition: The legal name and assigned agency number of the patient.
   Rationale: Required for discrimination among patients during care.

Demographic variables

2. Age
   Item-categories: Newborn to 120 (month/years); date of birth (month, day, year).
   Definition: Chronological age of the patient at admission and date of birth.
   Rationale: Required for application of developmental norms, health statistics, and individualization of treatment.
3. Sex
   Item-categories: Male or female.
   Definition: Predominant sexual classification based on physical characteristics.
   Rationale: Required for application of norms, health statistics, and individualization of treatment.
4. Race/ethnicity
   Item-categories: DHHS or concise categories in current use.

Definition: Subdivision of human population based on genetic and/or geocultural characteristics.
Rationale: Required for application of norms, health statistics, and individualization of treatment.
5. Marital status
   Item-categories: Never married, married, separated, widowed, divorced, not determined.
   Definition: Current marital status on admission.
   Rationale: Required as contextual data relative to diagnosis; treatment; and, in some cases, discharge planning.
6. Principal residence
   Item-categories: Dwelling number, street address, city/town, state or foreign country, zip code.
   Definition: Primary, current mailing address of the patient. If no address, specify categories: city, state. If institution, specify name in addition to address.
   Rationale: Required for discharge planning and identification of environmental variables in diagnosis and treatment.

Setting and care provider identification variables

7. Agency subdivision
   Item-categories: Name of agency subdivision (determined locally).
   Definition: Name of recognized geographic agency subdivision (e.g., unit, clinic, or district name).
   Rationale: Required for further patient identification.
8. Admission and discharge date
   Item-categories: Month, day, year of admission and discharge.
   Definition: Actual month, day, year in which patient began to receive health services at the agency and month, day, year in which patient was discharged or transferred to another facility or agency.
   Rationale: Required variable in some instances of diagnosis and treatment. Specifies the onset and termination of nursing services.

Excerpted from Gordon M: Practice-based data set for a nursing information system, *J Med Syst* 9:45, 1985.

9. Primary nurse identification
Item-categories: Name or other identification of nursing care provider.
Definition: Name of professional nursing care provider who is primarily responsible for care of patient from admission to discharge.
Rationale: Required for designation of responsibility for diagnosis, treatment, and evaluation.

Care provision variables

10. Next of kin/guardian
Item-categories: Name, street address, city/town, state, zip code, telephone area code, number.
Definition: Name, mailing address, and telephone number of kin, close friend, or guardian.

Rationale: Designation required for emergency notification. Guardian participation in treatment planning (parents) or discharge planning.
11. Functional health status
Item-categories: See Table P-1.
Definition: Eleven categories and assessment parameters for admission-baseline data on functional health patterns.
Rationale: Required as baseline and for evaluating any change that may occur during the period of hospital/clinic/community care. Documented information for legal and accreditation purposes.
12. Nursing diagnoses (See Appendix B)
Item-categories: Problem, etiological or related factors, and supporting data.

Table P-1   Item-Categories and Parameters: Functional Health Status Nursing History/Examination

I. Health perception–health management pattern
  a. Perception of general health status
  b. Colds in past year; work/school absences
  c. Health practices and effect
  d. Ease of adherence to medical/nursing suggestions
  e. Perceived cause of present illness
  f. Actions taken when illness perceived; results
  g. Personal requests regarding health management
II. Nutritional-metabolic pattern
  a. Typical daily food intake; supplements
  b. Typical daily fluid intake
  c. Weight change
  d. Appetite
  e. Perceived diet restrictions
  f. Associated discomfort: foods, eating
  g. Perceived healing ability
  h. Perceived problems
  i. Perceived dental problems; dentures
  j. Skin color, turgor, lesions
III. a. Description of bowel elimination pattern: frequency, character, discomfort, control
  b. Description of urinary elimination pattern: frequency, character, discomfort, control
  c. Perspiration/odor
IV. Activity-exercise pattern
  a. Perceived energy level
  b. Type and regularity of exercise pattern
  c. Spare time/play activities
  d. Self-care level (see code); feeding, bathing, toileting, bed mobility, dressing, grooming, general mobility, cooking, home maintenance, shopping
  e. Gait, posture, ROJM, coordination
V. Sleep-rest pattern
  a. Perceived readiness for day's activities
  b. Sleep problems: onset, early awakening, interrupted, reversal

Continued.

Table P-1 Item-Categories and Parameters: Functional Health Status Nursing History/Examination—cont'd

VI. Cognitive-perceptual pattern
- a. Hearing; aids
- b. Vision; glasses, last check
- c. Memory; attention
- d. Learning style; difficulties
- e. Perceived discomfort or pain
- f. Insight, judgment, decision making
- g. Level of consciousness, orientation
- h. Language spoken

VII. Self-perception–self-concept pattern
- a. Self-description and evaluation
- b. Body/physical ability changes and self-competency evaluation
- c. Frequency of anger, fear, anxiety, depression; what helps
- d. Nervousness/relaxed (rating)

VIII. Roles-relationship pattern
- a. Live alone/family, family structure
- b. Family problems (nuclear/extended)
- c. Family problem-solving pattern
- d. Family dependency needs, management
- e. Family reaction to illness
- f. Child-rearing/relationship patterns (problems)
- g. Social group membership; frequency of loneliness
- h. Perceived work/school relationship
- i. Perception of neighborhood (isolated/integrated feelings)
- j. Assertive/passive (rating)

IX. Sexuality-reproductive pattern
- a. Perceived changes/problems in sexuality, sexual relations
- b. Use of contraceptives; problems
- c. Menstruation onset and pattern (female)
- d. Para, gravida (female)

X. Coping–stress-tolerance pattern
- a. Tension/stress management; use of drugs, alcohol, etc.
- b. Significant other during stress; availability
- c. Changes in life last 1-2 years
- d. Problem-solving strategies; effect

XI. Value-belief pattern
- a. Goal achievement; goals in life
- b. Perceived importance of religion
- c. Desired religious practices (during hospital stay)

Definition: Actual or potential health problems for which the professional nurse is primarily accountable for the diagnosis, plan of treatment, and treatment outcomes between admission and discharge/transfer. Includes the problem, etiological or related factors, supporting data. Includes active diagnoses, conditions that develop subsequent to admission, and discharge diagnoses. Etiological categories describe the factors contributing to the problem that can be influenced by nursing intervention (e.g., probable cause). Supporting data are the assessment findings that validate the presence of the problem and etiological factors.

Rationale: Required as a basis for treatment planning (etiological factors) and projecting outcomes (problems). Required for accreditation purposes, professional standards, and, in some states, legal purposes. Supporting data (subjective and objective) are required until diagnoses are standardized to assure common understanding of the diagnoses. (Supporting data may always be required in teaching institutions with nursing and medical student affiliations.)

13. Projected and discharge outcomes
    Item-categories: Projected treatment outcomes and means of indicating presence or absence of projected outcomes at discharge.
    Definition: Projected outcomes are indicators of problem resolution. They are *predicted* to be attained (prognostic indicators) by discharge or other designated periods. Discharge (or periodic) outcomes are the *actual* outcomes attained by the patient. Both projected and discharge outcomes are indicators of resolution relative to the diagnoses; they are coded by diagnosis.
    Rationale: Desired goals or outcomes are required information for treatment planning and accreditation purposes. Projected and discharge outcome information is required for treatment evaluation and quality care review.

14. Nursing treatment orders
    Item-categories: Nursing treatment orders and means of designating treatments received.
    Definition: Definitive treatment orders coded for nursing diagnostic categories. Includes active orders, discontinued orders, and discharge orders between admission and discharge/transfer. Treatment orders are coded for the nursing diagnoses and medical diagnoses in Item 14 if the medical diagnosis or therapeutic regimen requires secondary nursing orders (e.g., observations, or individualizing of treatment or diagnostic procedures). Symbols are used to designate time (or visit) in which treatment was received by patient and for care provider identification.
    Rationale: Required for legal and accrediting purposes and for care and continuity of care. Required for judging responses to treatment.

15. Medical diagnosis
    Item-categories: From ICDA, APA, or other nomenclature system used by agency.
    Definition: All physician-identified diagnoses including the primary medical diagnosis or problem, coexisting diagnoses, conditions that develop subsequent to admission, and discharge diagnoses.
    Rationale: Required for predicting dysfunctional health patterns, for understanding the basis for medical treatment orders, and for discharge planning.

16. Medical treatment orders
    Item-categories: Medical treatment, taxonomy in use, and means of designating treatments received (time and care provider identification).
    Definition: Primary treatment orders, discontinued orders, and discharge orders formulated by a physician between admission and discharge/transfer. Symbols are used to designate time (or visit) in which treatment was received by patient and care provider designation.
    Rationale: Required for legal and accrediting purposes and for care and continuity of care. Required for judging responses.

17. Diagnostic and surgical procedures
    Item-categories: Diagnostic procedure taxonomy, including x-rays and lab tests; surgical procedure taxonomy (ICDA); dates of procedures and means of designating completion of procedures (time and care provider identification).
    Definition: Primary diagnostic and surgical procedure orders, discharge orders, and discontinued orders between admission and discharge. Symbols are used to designate time (or clinic visit) of order, time of completion (especially with delayed reports), and care provider identification designation.
    Rationale: Required for legal, accrediting, and accounting purposes and for care and continuity of care. Required for judging health status and responses.

APPENDIX Q

DIAGNOSTIC REASONING EXERCISES: LEVEL 1

A. DIAGNOSTIC RECOGNITION EXERCISE

Which of the following are useful descriptions of client problems/etiological factors on which to base nursing care?

1. Needs occupational therapy/boredom
2. Impaired verbal communication/uncompensated aphasia
3. Altered tissue perfusion: (cerebral)/arteriosclerosis
4. Altered nutrition: less than body protein requirements/low financial resources
5. High risk for fluid volume deficit
6. Chest pain/myocardial infarction
7. Stress

B. DIAGNOSTIC SELECTION EXERCISE, TYPE I

Select the best nursing diagnosis on which to base care for this client:

Mr. G., aged 58, complains of increased, frequent urination and general malaise. He appears flushed and is having difficulty remembering events of the past 24 hr. He is exhibiting Kussmaul respirations. Blood sugar level is 800 mg/dL. Mr. G.'s wife died 1½ years ago. His son reports that "since then he's been low and drinking more heavily." There have been frequent crying episodes, eating and sleeping patterns are poor, and he has been neglecting personal hygiene. Mr. G. says he's "so lonely" without his wife.

1. Depression/loss of wife
2. Self-neglect syndrome/loss
3. Loneliness/loss of wife
4. Health management deficit/delayed grief resolution
5. Grief/loss of wife
6. Diabetes mellitus

C. DIAGNOSTIC SELECTION EXERCISE, TYPE II

Generate and evaluate diagnostic hypotheses after each set of data using the list of diagnoses in Appendix A:

Mrs. A. is a 39-year-old woman. It is 9 AM on her second day after a hysterectomy. When you walk in the room she is wearing her own nightgown and lying supine in the bed. The bed is in disarray. Her face is flushed, she's crying, and she turns away as you approach.

Diagnostic hypotheses to be investigated?

You touch her arm in a gentle way, find the skin slightly warm to the touch. She says she is having pain at the operative site.

Diagnostic hypotheses to be investigated?

She begins to tell you about her husband's visit last night. She says she felt so angry but "there was no reason"; refused to kiss her husband and even "told him to go and find another woman." You recall from admission nursing history and assessment that she described her family and sexual relationships as good but that she had anticipatory anxiety, etiology undiagnosed.

Diagnostic hypotheses to be investigated?

You say very gently, "When you think about it now, why do you think you were so angry?" She says, crying, "He reminds me how incomplete I am now; I'm finished as a female." You say, "Oh, no wonder you feel upset. I think we should talk about this. But first let me take your temperature and then let's sit and talk."

Diagnostic hypotheses to be investigated?

T = 101° F

Diagnostic hypotheses to be investigated?

See Appendix S for answers.

D. DIAGNOSIS EXERCISE: USING VALID AND RELIABLE CUES

Does this person have an intermittent constipation pattern? If so, what cues are absolutely necessary for making this diagnosis? For the moment, disregard the etiological or related factors. The task is to select information that is absolutely necessary for the accurate diagnosis of an intermittent constipation pattern. These are the cues:

1. Decreased activity level
2. Hard, formed stool today
3. Palpable mass in abdomen
4. Reports feeling of pressure or fullness in rectum
5. Reports history of frequent straining at stool
6. Appetite impairment
7. Headache
8. Reports two or three episodes per month (history) of hard, formed stool following period of no bowel movement

After finishing your analysis of the cues above, read on.

What needs to be determined are the necessary and sufficient criteria for diagnosing an intermittent constipation pattern that will reduce uncertainty and attain a confidence level sufficient for making the judgment. The inference in item 1, "decreased activity level," is obviously insufficient for making the diagnosis; it may be either a factor contributing to the severity or an etiological (causative) factor in this diagnosis. "Hard, formed stool today," item 2, indicates the possibility of the presence of constipation. It does not provide data about an intermittent pattern. A cue such as this should be investigated in terms of its frequency and precipitating factors.

The third cue, "palpable mass in the abdomen," is not definitive. It does not differentiate between stool and a tumor. The fourth cue is similar; a rectal tumor could cause the same sensation but would usually also be associated with other symptoms. Item 5 is "history of frequent straining at stool"; this indeed does provide a valid cue. Is it sufficient information? No, but it is a key piece of information that will be held aside for the moment.

The sixth cue, "appetite impairment," is interesting; it may be secondary to constipation but deserves investigation to ensure that it is not a cue to another condition. It could be a predisposing or causative factor of constipation if sufficient fluids and bulky foods are not being ingested. "Headache," item 7, is not unusual with constipation but is not diagnostic. However, it does deserve explanation even in isolation. Thus far we have one cue; the rest of the information might be signs or symptoms of other conditions. Therefore the cues represent unreliable and nondifferentiating evidence for the diagnosis under consideration. They might be supporting cues for a current state of constipation but not for an intermittent pattern.

Item 8, a "history of hard, formed stool two or three times per month following a period of no bowel movement," is a highly valid predictor of the diagnosis being entertained. It is a verbal report; unless the reliability of the client is questionable, it does provide sufficient confidence for the diagnosis. Is this one cue sufficient to identify the health problem? Is it a necessary or critical cue, without which the validity of the diagnosis would be questionable? Is it a conclusive sign? The answer to each of these questions is yes. Item 5, frequent straining, is redundant; it really does not provide any further information but only supports the probability that the stool, as described in item 8, is hard to evacuate. Redundant cues do, however, serve a function. They provide a check or support for a diagnostic judgment and can increase the confidence level when information is uncertain. Up to a point, redundant cues are probably psychologically necessary. In excess, they provide quantity, not quality, in a data base.

The etiology of this health problem is still to be identified. A number of options are open. If the eight pieces of data were actually collected in a real situation, certain questions would arise. Should etiological factors be investigated immediately? Or should the problem be referred to a physician for differential medical diagnosis?

The cues "appetite impairment" and "palpable mass," in conjunction with the problem of intermittent constipation, suggest the need for a differential medical diagnosis. Might a tumor be present? It is highly advisable to refer the problem to a physician if the nurse is not competent to discriminate among the etiological factors of intermittent constipation, especially a tumor. A second option is to discuss with a physician the findings and the possibility of administering an enema. The palpable mass may be stool accumulated in the colon; if so, it would disappear when the enema was expelled. In the absence of abdominal tumor, the client's constipation problem may be amenable to nursing intervention. Etiological factors to be investigated by the nurse include dietary patterns, abdominal muscle tone, bowel habits, anxiety, and decreased activity.

This example illustrates the need to examine the data collected, predict alternative explanations, and test possibilities. It also demonstrates the uncertain nature of clinical data. Essentially, two main factors should influence the nurse's judgment: the validity and reliability of information available *and* the theoretical knowledge the nurse brings to bear in interpretation.

DIAGNOSTIC REASONING EXERCISES: LEVEL 2

DIAGNOSTIC FORMULATION EXERCISES

The following three cases illustrate a basic data base collected at admission when the clients were added to a nurse's caseload. To simulate the way data were collected and hypotheses generated, stop at the end of each pattern area assessment (e.g., health-perception–health-management, nutritional-metabolic) to formulate any tentative nursing diagnoses that may be indicated by cues. Discard, revise, or reformulate diagnoses as you continue reading. At the end of each case, state the nursing diagnoses and data that support your admission diagnoses. Diagnostic terms appear in Appendix B; diagnostic terms should be generated if the list is inadequate. Defining signs and symptoms are found in the *Manual** or in NANDA publications. Answers (suggested diagnoses) to the following cases appear in Appendix S.

Case 1

Nursing history and examination

First prenatal clinic visits of a 24-year-old, married former secretary with no history of chronic disease. Last menstrual period, February; expected date of confinement November 15; 5 weeks pregnant. Husband is 25-year-old machine operator who receives health care at company clinic and is in "good health."

Health Perception–Health Management Pattern. Sees self as healthy and pleased about pregnancy. Usual childhood diseases, including chicken pox, measles, mumps. No recent colds or other illnesses. Keeps healthy by "eating right" and "supporting each other." Sees this making a difference compared with other families she knows. No use of cigarettes or drugs; one glass wine per week, socially. No pattern of breast self-examination; doesn't know how. No delay in coming to clinic when missed first period; came to clinic because parents use this hospital clinic for care.

---

*Gordon M: *Manual of nursing diagnosis, 1993-1994,* St Louis, 1993, Mosby.

Nutritional-Metabolic Pattern. Typical diet: *Breakfast:* orange juice, cereal with fruit, coffee, toast and butter; *Lunch:* alternate lunch-meat or cheese sandwich and salads, soft drink (no-cal) or coffee; *Dinner:* two vegetables, meat, rolls and butter, coffee, dessert or fruit; *Snacks:* 1 cookie or fruit, coffee, or soft drink. No vitamin supplements. Fluids: 1-2 glasses water, three to four cups coffee. Appetite good; tries to restrict calories; states has gained about 1 lb. No nausea, dental problems, or skin dryness. Some tingling and fullness of breasts; lotions helpful.

Elimination Pattern. Regular bowel movements every day. No changes or discomfort. Knows she must maintain roughage and fluid intake. Slight increase in urinary frequency; realizes this is due to enlarging uterus; no problems in control. No excess perspiration or odor.

Activity-Exercise Pattern. Resigned secretarial job because of pregnancy and time pressures in job. Worked for busy executive who wanted her to stay another 4 to 6 months. Does housework; has restricted other exercise; drives car instead of walking; stopped playing tennis; wants to be "careful and sure nothing happens to baby." States too much activity could cause miscarriage, but doesn't know exactly how. Leisure activities: TV, movies with husband, and visiting friends. Has felt more fatigue since she stopped working; attributes this to pregnancy.

*Reported functional level**

Feeding __0__ Dressing __0__ Home maintenance __0__

Bathing __0__ Grooming __0__ Shopping __0__

Functional level code

Level 0: Full self-care

Level I: Requires use of equipment or device

Level II: Requires assistance of supervision from another person

Level III: Requires assistance or supervision from another person *and* equipment or device

Level IV: Is dependent and does not participate

Toileting __0__ General mobility __0__
Bed mobility __0__ Cooking __0__

Sleep-Rest Pattern. Feels rested in AM. Tires by afternoon and takes 2-hr nap. Sleep onset delayed since stopped work; states due to excitement of being pregnant and starts thinking about plans; can't get to sleep. No history of sleep disturbances.

Cognitive-Perceptual Pattern. No perceived hearing or vision problems, discomfort, memory changes. Learns "easily"; likes to read and then discuss questions.

Self-Perception–Self-Concept Pattern. Feels she is "easy to get along with," "bright," and "reasonably good-looking." Thinks she will be a "good, careful" mother. "Excited about changes" in her body and has been looking at maternity clothes; doesn't want to wait until dresses or slacks get tight and press on baby. No feelings of anger, depression. States that "every new mother is a little fearful and anxious in case something happens to baby." Has stopped work; will devote time to "getting things ready," but friends and neighbors all work and she has few to talk to; day "seems long."

Role-Relationship Pattern. Lives with husband; 25-year-old machine operator; married 3 years; he "is excited about baby." Both hope it is a boy. Perceives no family problems. Handles problems by "attacking them"; discusses things. Social activities at tennis club; have close friends, couples same age. Moved into neighborhood 3 years ago, people friendly and help each other. No perceived financial problems. Parents and in-laws live in same town. She and husband are only children, so this will be first grandchild. Client's mother had two miscarriages and client does not want this to happen to her. Parents available to help after baby born. Gets on well with parents and in-laws.

Sexuality-Reproductive Pattern. Sexual relations decreased so "nothing happens to baby." Told husband this was important and he agrees. Previous sexual pattern: no perceived problems. Stopped contraceptives 6 months ago; wants three children. Menses started age 13, regular cycle 30 days; length 4 days. Last menstrual period 5 weeks ago. Para 0, Gravida 0. Plans to breastfeed.

Coping–Stress-Tolerance Pattern. Feels "a little tense about a miscarriage." Hasn't talked to anyone about this. Usually talks over problems with husband; very supportive; but doesn't want to worry him. States they "deal with problems, don't shove them under the table." Perceives this as successful but has had no big problems. No other life changes in last few years.

Value-Belief Pattern. Thinks "do what you can in this life; we've no aspirations to be rich." Comes from close family and learned "family important." Methodist; practices religion and finds it supportive.

Examination

General appearance, grooming, hygiene __Good__

Oral mucous membranes (color, moistness, lesions) __Normal__

Teeth: dentures __0__ Cavities __0__ Missing __0__

Hears whisper? __Yes__

Reads newsprint? __Yes__ Glasses __No__

Pulse (rate) __84__ (rhythm) __Reg__

Respirations __18__ (depth) __Normal__ (rhythm) __Reg__

Breath sounds __Normal__

Blood pressure __118/70__ Hand grip __Strong__ Can pick up pencil? __Yes__

Range of motion (joints) __Full__ Muscle firmness) __Firm__

Skin: bony prominence: __0__ Lesions __0__ Color changes __0__

Breasts __Firm, developed, areolas darkened, no tenderness__

Pelvis: __gynecoid (see medical examination)__

Gait __Reg__ Posture __Good__ Absent body part __0__

Intravenous, drainage, suction, etc. (specify) __0__

Actual weight __120 lb__ Reported weight Pregravida 119

Height __5'6"__

Temperature __98.6° F__

During history and examination:

Orientation __Yes__ Grasp ideas and questions? (Abstract, concrete) __Both__

Language spoken __Eng__ Voice and speech pattern __Normal__

Vocabulary __Good__

Eye contact __Yes__ Attention span (distraction) __Good span__

Nervous or relaxed __3__
1 _____ 5

Assertive or passive __3__
1 _____ 5

Interaction with family member, guardian, other (if present)   Husband not present; at work

Nursing diagnoses

(See Appendix S for answers.)

Case 2

Nursing history and examination

First admission of unconscious 6-year-old boy, with facial lacerations and linear skull fracture. To Emergency Room by ambulance after car accident; accompanied by anxious, distraught father who was not injured and provided history. Mother out of town visiting sister. (Screening assessment because of father's anxiety.)

Health Perception–Health Management Pattern. Previously alert, healthy child. Has had usual childhood diseases and immunizations, including tetanus; no colds this winter. Father states hasn't insisted son use seat belt when riding in front seat.

Nutritional-Metabolic Pattern. Appetite has been good; no vitamin supplements, no weight loss; seen by pediatrician 2 weeks ago; told developing normally.

Elimination Pattern. Bowel movements regular; no nighttime incontinence.

Activity-Exercise Pattern. Energetic 6-year-old boy; plays actively with children in neighborhood; baseball favorite sport.

*Reported functional level**
Pretrauma:
Feeding   0   Dressing   0   Home maintenance   —
Bathing   2   Grooming   2   Shopping   —
Toileting   0   General mobility   0
              Bed mobility   —   Cooking   —

Sleep-Rest Pattern. No sleep problems; stopped naps at 4 years old.

Cognitive-Perceptual Pattern. Comatose since accident; no convulsions. No previous hearing, vision, or

---

*Functional level code
Level 0: Full self-care
Level I: Requires use of equipment or device
Level II: Requires assistance or supervision from another person
Level III: Requires assistance or supervision from another person *and* equipment or device
Level IV: Is dependent and does not participate

learning problems. Until accident, speech had been clear.

Self-Perception–Self-Concept Pattern. Described as generally outgoing and friendly with strangers. Recently began calling self "bad boy" when things go wrong. Made "big fuss" last week over skinned knee and whether it "would get better."

Role-Relationship Pattern. Looking forward to school in fall. Has three good friends in neighborhood. At times takes older brother's clothes to try on, but relationship perceived as good. Family structure: two brothers 14 and 16 years old, mother, father; paternal grandmother lives next door; other grandparents deceased. Family relationships good; no perceived problems. Father states he feels "guilty," about accident; "although not my fault"; hit from rear by another car; "Why couldn't I be the one to die?" (relates unconsciousness to approaching death of child). Father pacing in room.

Sexuality-Reproductive Pattern. Deferred.

Coping–Stress-Tolerance Pattern. Seeks parents for security when situations stressful. Father states he and wife are supportive of each other. He'll "feel better when she gets here."

Value-Belief Pattern. Religion: Episcopal. Assessment deferred.

Examination

General appearance, grooming, hygiene   —

Oral mucous membranes (color, moistness, lesions)   Normal color; no lesions

Teeth: dentures   0   Cavities   0   Missing   2 upper front

Hears whisper?   No

Reads newsprint?   Comatose   Glasses   No

Pulse (rate)   100   (rhythm)   Reg

Respirations   20   (depth)   Deep   (rhythm)   Reg

Breath sounds   clear   Blood pressure   98/58
   Po$_2$ 78 mm Hg

Hand grip   Absent   Can pick up pencil?   No

Voluntary movement   Absent LL, LA, RL, RA
   Functional Level   4

Range of motion (joints)   Full involuntary   Muscle firmness   Tone decreased

Skin: bony prominence   Intact   Lesions   Facial lacerations

Color changes __0__ Gait __—__ Posture __—__ Absent body part __0__

Intravenous, drainage, suction, etc. (specify) __IV__

Actual weight __—__ Reported weight __49__

Height __36″__

Temperature __99° F__

During history and examination:

Orientation __No response to stimuli__ Pupils __Equal; react to light__

Convulsions __None__ Grasp ideas and questions (abstract, concrete)? __0__

Language spoken __Eng__ Voice-speech pattern __—__ Vocabulary __—__

Eye contact __—__ Attention span (distraction) __—__

Nervous or relaxed __(Comatose)__

1 _____ 5

Assertive or passive __(Comatose)__

1 _____ 5

Interaction with family member, guardian, other (if present)

Nursing diagnoses

(See Appendix S for answers).

Case 3

Nursing history and examination 10/27/81

Sixth admission for diabetic ketoacidosis of a 19-year-old white female with juvenile onset diabetes mellitus since age 5. Admitted with nausea and vomiting, abdominal pain, and blood glucose level of 505 mg/dL. Medical evaluation states there is no obvious predisposing physical cause of ketoacidosis; admissions attributed to "noncompliance." Did not take insulin for 2 days prior to this admission.

Health-Perception–Health-Management Pattern. States that diet, exercise, and insulin are "all important" to her health, yet doesn't follow prescribed diet, does no exercise, and takes insulin only sporadically. Feels she understands the aspects of her disease well; has been able to understand instructions given to her by doctors and nurses. Does not follow recommendations; sometimes "forgets" to take insulin or because it is "too much of a pain." She states that she probably would be healthier if she were "a good little diabetic" but that she knows she isn't. Believes she is susceptible to diabetic ketoacidosis since she has had five previous admissions; says this admission was due to a "virus"; doesn't believe that not taking insulin for last 2 days could cause current problem; states she over-

slept (11 AM) and it was too late to take insulin. Takes "night dose" at 5 PM. States once went for a week without taking insulin. Doesn't consider herself to be very healthy, would give herself a "2 on a scale of 1 to 10."

Nutritional-Metabolic Pattern. Does not follow prescribed diet or count calories. *Breakfast:* Eats cereal with tea or toast, butter, and tea. *Lunch:* Eats peanut butter and butter sandwich with iced tea; usually has cereal or peanut butter again for dinner. States eats about 10 pieces of bread per day, since this is what she eats whenever she gets hungry. She drinks six glasses sugar-free iced tea per day. Dislikes meat of any kind; doesn't care for poultry or fish. States that her family does not eat meals together; she gets her own meals. If her mother prepares a meat meal, she usually goes to her bedroom and feeds the meat to her cats. Usually eats alone; if does eat with parents, it's only when she makes the dessert, the only thing she knows how to cook. Has bought a vegetarian cookbook but says that she's too "lazy" to learn how to cook. Asked to see a dietician so that she can lose weight. Reports 5′3″, 135 lbs.

Elimination Patterns. No difficulty with bowels or urination, takes no laxatives. Does not complain of polyuria despite large fluid intake (approximately 2000 mL per day reported).

Activity-Exercise Pattern. Reports no daily exercise pattern. Does not walk; feels she is weak and isn't able to do any activities. No activities outside her home. Has no physical disabilities but does not perform any activities other than watching TV or reading. Attended college for one semester but left and has no plans to return; unemployed.

Sleep-Rest Pattern. Usually retires at 1 or 2 AM, gets up at 7 AM to take insulin and eat. Usually naps in the afternoon for 2 hours when has nothing to do. Feels she is adequately rested. Takes no sleeping meds; no problems getting to sleep.

Cognitive-Perceptual Pattern. Reports no hearing difficulties. Wears glasses all the time for nearsightedness. No difficulty with recall. Considers herself to be "rather intelligent with IQ of 126," yet not "smart enough to be super like 140, the gifted." States has no difficulty learning and learns well with reading materials, since things that she's told sometimes "slip right through" and must be interesting and challenging in order for her to give any attention to them. Points out that English and literature are her favorite subjects; reports pleasure in getting a 750 score on her SAT.

Reported functional level*

Feeding	0
Bathing	0 in bed
Toileting	0 in bed
Dressing	0
Grooming	0
General mobility	(Bed rest)
Bed mobility	0
Home maintenance	0
Shopping	0
Cooking	0

Self-Perception–Self-Concept Pattern. Considers herself to be physically weak and this prohibits her from doing things, such as joining the Army; doesn't think she could make it through basic training. She becomes annoyed at herself; considers herself to be "lazy." Believes parents are supportive enough when she needs them but states she usually doesn't tell them when things bother her and therefore remains "independent."

Role-Relationship Pattern. Lives with her parents; has a brother who is in the Air Force. Related that once she told her guidance instructor that she was living as a hermit after school and then the instructor picked "up the cue and had my whole family see the school psychologist." States that psychologist helped her mother to "change a lot and stop nagging" but that it did nothing for her. Reports no family problems but states that her family is "a bunch of strangers living under the same roof." Describes family as one that doesn't outwardly show emotions, but feels that they give her what she wants (such as money). Feels her family gives her enough attention but "probably I could get used to receiving more from them." States her diabetes is "no big thing" to her family, since she's had it since age 5; "it is considered just the way it is." Family usually doesn't visit her in the hospital unless she asks them to, says she likes it this way. Has no friends, doesn't belong to any social groups, because she "has nothing in common with people her age." Likes to talk about herself; says enjoys talking

---

*Functional level code
Level 0: Full self-care
Level I: Requires use of equipment or device
Level II: Requires assistance or supervision from another person
Level III: Requires assistance or supervision from another person *and* equipment or device
Level IV: Is dependent and does not participate

about the "concepts" she is reading (Greek mythology), whereas girls her age like to talk "about boys or what clothes are 'in' this fall." She sees her life as being "boring."

Sexuality-Reproductive Pattern. Reports normal menstrual cycle 28 days for 5 days duration. Presently on 2nd day of menstrual cycle. Has had no sexual relations. Dated in high school but no dating since graduation.

Coping–Stress-Tolerance Pattern. States she has learned that "you can't do too much about things"; "you just wait and see what happens." Voice low during this discussion and sad facial expression. Regained composure quickly and changed subject.

Value-Belief Pattern. States that she has not yet "gotten anything out of life that I have wanted"; says she would like "to do something useful and challenging with my life" but hasn't been able to identify these things. Might consider teaching. Won't be satisfied until able to "physically do something both useful and challenging." Doesn't want to waste time doing things aimlessly.

Examination

General appearance, grooming, hygiene __Obese teenager in no acute distress; disheveled; hair dull and oily (unclean), uncombed__

Oral mucous membranes (color, moistness, lesions): __Pink, moist, no lesions__

Teeth: dentures __none__ Cavities __multiple cavities__ Missing __none__

Hears whisper? __Yes__

Reads newsprint? __Yes__ Glasses __for reading and distance__

Pulse (rate) __100__ (rhythm) __Regular__

Respirations __20__ (depth) __Normal__ (rhythm) __Regular__

Breath sounds __No wheezes, rales__

Blood pressure __130/86__ Hand grip __Strong__ Can pick up pencil? __Yes__

Range of motion (joints) __Within normal limits__ Muscle firmness __Firm__

Skin: bony prominence; __Intact__ Lesions __Knotty cutaneous deposits on arms and thighs from injections__

Gait __not observed__ Posture __Relaxed upright posture in bed__

Absent body part __0__

Intravenous, drainage, suction, etc. (specify) __0__

Actual weight ___135___ Reported
weight ___135___ Height ___5'3"___

Temperature ___99° F___

During history and examination:

Orientation: ___Yes___

Grasp ideas and questions (abstract, concrete)? ___Both;
good abstract ability___

Language spoken ___English___ Voice and speech pattern ___Normal___

Vocabulary ___Extensive___

Eye contact ___Yes___ Attention span (distraction): ___Good attention span; very interested in sharing information about self___

Nervous or relaxed ___4___

1 _____ 5

Assertive or passive ___3___

1 _____ 5

Interaction with family member, guardian, other (if present) ___None present___

Nursing diagnoses

(See Appendix S for answers.)

APPENDIX S

Answers to Diagnostic Reasoning Exercises

DIAGNOSTIC REASONING EXERCISE (APPENDIX Q)

Item 1. *Needs occupational therapy/boredom* is not a nursing diagnosis. Need for care is described before describing the problem. If signs of boredom are present, further investigation is required.

Item 2. *Impaired Verbal Communication/Uncompensated Aphasia* represents a useful description on which to base care; it is a nursing diagnosis. The client would be helped to compensate for aphasia.

Item 3. *Altered tissue perfusion (cerebral)/arteriosclerosis* is a serious condition but usually not within the diagnostic competencies of a nurse. If this diagnostic judgment is made, the client should be referred for medical evaluation. Probably the client has nursing diagnoses but they are not described by this label. Altered Tissue Perfusion is accepted for clinical testing (see Appendix A), but it is difficult to justify that nursing care can resolve this problem.

Item 4. *Altered Nutrition: Less than Body Protein Requirements/Low Financial Resources* is a nursing diagnosis that employs accepted diagnostic labels. A more concise description would be "protein deficit/low financial resources."

Item 5. *High Risk for Fluid Volume Deficit* is a well-formulated potential problem that provides a basis for care when risk factors are delineated.

Item 6. *Chest pain/myocardial infarction* is a concise expression of the accepted diagnostic category, Pain. A modifier "chest" is employed to specify anatomical location. The stated etiology does not provide a basis for nursing intervention because nurses do not treat a myocardial infarction. If chest pain is a new symptom, or if current orders for pain medication or other drugs are inadequate to control pain, these observations should be referred to the physician. The pain may also signify increased Activity Intolerance or Pain Self-Management Deficit, requiring health education. Further data are needed to determine if this is chronic pain (angina) or a sign of a complication. "Chest pain/myocardial infarction" represents inadequate for-

mulation of a nursing diagnosis and inadequate assessment.

Item 7. *Stress* is not a useful description of a problem. The term represents an inference that requires further exploration to identify the problem and etiology before a plan of care can be designed.

DIAGNOSTIC SELECTION EXERCISE, TYPE I (APPENDIX Q)

Item 1. *Depression/loss of wife* represents inadequate problem formulation. Data suggest depression is a sign of another problem.

Item 2. *Self-neglect syndrome/loss* represents superficial problem formulation. Data suggest this is a sign of another problem.

Item 3. *Loneliness/loss of wife* represents superficial problem formulation. Does not provide a basis for clustering all the related data.

Item 4. *Health Management Deficit/Delayed Grief Resolution* is the best nursing diagnosis within the set on which to base care. Permits clustering all data in one concise expression and focusing nursing care on grief resolution.

Item 5. *Grief/loss of wife* does not adequately represent the data available; grief is an expected reaction to loss of a wife; therefore no problem is communicated on which to base care.

Item 6. *Diabetes mellitus* is a medical diagnosis, not a nursing diagnosis. Disease-related nursing care can be organized on the basis of this description.

DIAGNOSTIC SELECTION EXERCISE, TYPE II (APPENDIX Q)

Diagnostic hypotheses generated from the first set of data include: (1) *wound infection* (Is flush due to fever and a possible wound infection?); (2) *atelectasis* (Is flush due to fever and possible pulmonary complications? This complication is of low probability in lower abdominal surgery.); (3) *Urinary Retention* (Are the cues—"bed in disarray," "lower abdominal surgery," "crying," and "face flushed"—signs of discomfort due to retention? This is a low probability on the second day unless there has been a postoperative history of retention.); (4) *incisional pain* (Are the signs of discomfort caused by pain? A likely pain site is the operative wound.); or (5) *Fluid Volume Deficit* (are flush and signs of discomfort on the second postoperative day caused by a history of low fluid intake?). The cues "bed in disarray," "face flushed," and "crying at 9 AM" suggest the possibility of Sleep-Pattern Disturbance related to any of the above hypotheses. Adding the cues "turns away as you approach" and "hysterectomy" suggests unexpressed anger and situational depression over loss. A hypothesis to direct cue search could be formulated broadly as *Ineffective Coping Related to Loss* or, more specifically, as *perceived sexuality impairment.*

The test for skin warmth evident in the second set of data further supports the hypotheses of wound infection, pulmonary complications and Fluid Volume Deficit. Pain at the operative site is a cue that also points to wound infection or to incisional pain without the presence of infection.

The third set of cues supports the hypothesis of *perceived sexuality impairment.* Information in the fourth data set suggests the nurse is testing the hypothesis of perceived sexuality (or reproductive) impairment. A likely etiological hypothesis is *loss (hysterectomy).* Note the priority for hypothesis investigation; the plan is to investigate previously generated hypotheses related to conditions manifesting fever—wound infection, atelectasis, and Fluid Volume Deficit.

In the fifth data set, information is obtained to support the hypotheses of *wound infection, Fluid Volume Deficit,* and the low-probability hypothesis of *pulmonary complications.* Knowing the amount and sufficiency of last voiding would decrease the risk of missing the problem of Urinary Retention. The nurse would then quickly collect further data on these possibilities and call a physician.

Pain perception may be heightened by the psychological problem. A judgment must be made whether to: (1) collect further data related to pain management, (2) offer the client the postoperative narcotic ordered, (3) offer the opportunity to discuss the client's perceptions and feelings about sexuality or reproductive loss, or (4) a combination of these actions.

The data support the tentative nursing diagnoses formulated either as *perceived sexuality or reproductive impairment/loss (hysterectomy)* or as *ineffective coping/perceived loss of sexuality.* Further data would help formulate the diagnosis more specifically or may support the possibility of a normal process of grieving. Pain management and any surgical-related care would be determined after medical evaluation of the client.

DIAGNOSTIC FORMULATION EXERCISES (SEE APPENDIX R)
Case 1: Nursing diagnoses

1. Problem: Anticipatory Anxiety (Miscarriage)
   Etiological factors: Identification with mother's miscarriage; Knowledge Deficit (Activity Tolerance and Health Management during Pregnancy)
   - States too much activity could cause miscarriage; activity (tennis, walking, sexual) self-restricted "so nothing happens to baby."
   - Client's mother had two miscarriages and client doesn't want this to happen.
   - Wants to be "careful and sure nothing happens to baby."
   - Resigned secretarial job because of pregnancy, time pressures in job; expected date of confinement—35 weeks.
   - Sleep onset delayed "since stopped work."
   - Increase of fatigue attributed to pregnancy.
   - Thinks she will be "good, careful mother."
   - Using maternity clothes to avoid ordinary clothes getting tight and pressing on baby.
   - "Every new mother is a little fearful and anxious in case something happens to baby."
   - Medical examination: no health problems; pregnancy progressing normally.
   - Will devote time to "getting things ready"; friends and neighbors work; few people to talk to; days "seem long"; afternoon naps, 2 hr.
2. Problem: *Health Management Deficit/Lack of Knowledge* (Breast Self-Examination)
   - No pattern of breast self-examination.
   - States she doesn't know how to examine.

Case 2: Nursing diagnoses

1. Problem: High Risk for Airway Obstruction
   - Comatose
   - Drooling at intervals
   - Unresponsive to stimuli
   - Po_2 78 mm Hg
2. Problem: *Total Self-Care Deficit (Level IV)*
   Etiological factors: *Comatose state*
   - Unresponsive to stimuli
   - No voluntary movement of extremities
3. Problem: *Parental guilt*
   Etiological factors: *Perceived responsibility (accident); fear of child's death*
   - Hadn't insisted son use seat belts.
   - States feels "guilty about accident, although not my fault."
   - "Why couldn't I be the one to die"; relates son's coma to approaching death.
   - Father pacing in room states will "feel better" when mother returns from out-of-town trip to visit sister.

Case 3: Nursing diagnoses

These data describe a complex client situation. Although a great deal of information was collected, more is needed for diagnosis. The case demonstrates that in complex situations, all the data needed cannot be collected in a busy hospital unit at admission. Also, it takes time to think about alternative interpretations and what diagnostic hypotheses would direct further cue search.

Further data on family dynamics, support systems, and client's insight and inclination to deal with problems are needed. Historically, focusing on the diagnosis Noncompliance/Knowledge Deficit has not been effective (sixth admission for ketoacidosis). Underlying problems exist.

Ethically it is important to remember that this 19-year-old client's rights should not be violated in data collection. Calling the family to verify data or to gather further information without this client's knowledge could be viewed as a violation of rights. It may also jeopardize the nurse-client relationship. When encountering a client who volunteers the type and amount of information presented in this case the question *why* should be raised. Does the behavior signify a plea for help, a testing of the nurse's reaction, or both? Mutual understanding is needed regarding the client's choice to deal with her life situation. If the client is requesting help, the problems interfering with her disease management, as well as her general health management, can be further explored and identified. At some point the client and nurse may decide that one or both parents should be included.

Noncompliance (Disease Management) is a presenting problem but is probably only a sign of more serious problems. Nurses perceiving themselves to have inadequate diagnostic or treatment skills in the possible developmental problems this client and family exhibit may seek consultation. A mental health–clinical nursing specialist may be consulted.

Two possible hypotheses that can serve as a basis for (1) clustering current data and (2) guiding further cue search are listed below.

Chronic situational depression

19-year-old female
Disheveled; hair dull and oily (unclean)
Sixth admission for diabetic ketoacidosis (blood glucose level: 505 mg/dL)
Doesn't consider self healthy; would give herself "2 on a scale of 1 to 10"
Usually eats alone
States she has learned that "you can't do too much about things, you just wait and see what happens."

Voice low and sad facial expression during this discussion
Feels she is physically weak and not able to do any activities
Not yet "gotten anything out of life that I have wanted"
Would like to do something "useful and challenging with my life," but hasn't been able to identify these things
No friends; doesn't belong to any social groups because "has nothing in common with people her age"
Perceives her life as "boring"
No insulin taken for 2 days prior to admission; doesn't believe this could cause her current problem
Overslept (11 AM), so too late to take insulin; night dose at 5 PM
States once went a week without taking insulin
States diet, exercise, insulin important to health
States doesn't follow diet; forgets to take insulin; too much of a "pain"
No exercise; takes insulin sporadically
States understands her disease
Believes herself susceptible to ketoacidosis (five previous admissions)
Knotting, cutaneous deposits on arms and thighs from injections
No daily exercise
Asked to see dietician so that she can lose weight
Weight (reported 135 lbs.); Height 5′ 3″
Attended college for one semester; no plans to return
Unemployed 19-year-old
Considers self "rather intelligent; IQ of 126; not smart enough to be super like 140, the gifted"
Pleased with 750 score on SAT
States things must be interesting and challenging in order to hold her attention
English and literature are her favorite subjects
Might consider teaching
Not satisfied until able to "physically do something both useful and challenging"
Doesn't want to waste time doing things aimlessly
Likes to talk about self and "concepts" she is reading about (e.g. Greek mythology); girls her age talk "about boys, clothes"
Dated in high school; not dating since graduation

Dysfunctional family dynamics

Perceives family as "a bunch of strangers living under the same roof"; don't show emotions but give her material things she wants (such as money)
States family gives enough attention but "probably I could get used to receiving more from them"
Usually eats alone
No activities outside home
Psychologist helped mother to "change a lot and stop nagging"

Lives with parents; brother in Air Force

Believes parents are supportive when she needs them

Usually doesn't tell parents when things bother her and therefore remains "independent"

States family does not eat meals together; gets own meals

Bought vegetarian cookbook (doesn't eat meat); says too "lazy" to learn to cook

Diabetes "no big thing" to family, as she has had it since age 5

Family doesn't visit hospital unless asked; she likes it that way

EARLY DEVELOPMENT OF DIAGNOSTIC CLASSIFICATION SYSTEM

PATTERNS OF UNITARY MAN-ENVIRONMENT

Exchanging Mutual giving and receiving.
Communicating Sending messages.
Relating Establishing bonds.
Valuing Assigning relative worth.
Choosing Selecting alternatives.
Moving Activity.
Perceiving Reception of information.
Knowing Meaning associated with information.
Feeling Subjective awareness of information.

BASIC ASSUMPTIONS UNDERLYING THE FRAMEWORK, FROM A NARRATIVE PREPARED BY THE THEORIST GROUP IN 1982

The first basic assumption about unitary man/human is the belief that unitary man/human is an open system, that is, a system of mutual interaction with the environment. Negentropy, a characteristic of open systems, is a process of continuous development toward increasing com-

From Roy, C Sr: Framework for classification system development: progress and issues. In Kim MJ, McFarlane A, McLane A, editors: *Classification of nursing diagnoses: proceedings of the fifth national conference,* St Louis, 1984, Mosby, p 29.

plexity and diversity. This process can be seen in observations of individuals throughout the life process and observations from generation to generation.

The second basic assumption is that unitary man/human is a four-dimensional energy field characterized by pattern and organization. Each human field has a unique pattern. The uniqueness of the pattern and organization of each field is manifest in nine man/human-environment interactional patterns. The basic assumptions about health are that (1) it is a value, (2) it is a pattern of energy exchange, (3) this pattern enhances the field integrity of unitary man/human (field integrity is denoted by completeness, efficiency, clarity, accuracy, and authenticity), and (4) it is manifested through nine man human/environment interactional patterns.

Nursing diagnosis

Nursing is concerned with the health of unitary man/human. Nursing diagnosis is an integral component of the science and practice of nursing. It is a judgment about health based on data relevant to the conceptual framework of nine patterns. Diagnosis requires refinement of the patterns through identification of the characteristics.

APPENDIX U

Nomenclature Development, 1973-1992

NOMENCLATURE DEVELOPMENT, 1973-1992

1973	1975	1978	1980
Adjustment to Illness, Impairment of Significant Others'	Adjustment to Illness, Impairment of Significant Others'	Adjustment to Illness, Impairment of Significant Others'	
Adjustment to Illness, Impairment of All Significant Others'			
Adjustment to Illness, Impairment of Spouse's			
Adjustment to Illness, Impairment of Child's			
Adjustment to Illness, Impairment of Nonfamily's			
Anxiety, Mild	Anxiety, Mild	Anxiety, Mild	
Anxiety, Moderate	Anxiety, Moderate	Anxiety, Moderate	
Anxiety, Severe	Anxiety, Severe	Anxiety, Severe	
Panic	Panic	Panic	
Body Fluids, Depletion of	Body Fluids, Depletion of	Fluid Volume Deficit	Fluid Volume Deficit
	Body Fluids, Excess	Fluid Volume Deficit, Potential	Fluid Volume Deficit, Potential
	Body Fluid, Excess	Body Fluids, Excess	
Bowel Function, Irregular: Constipation	Bowel Elimination, Alteration in: Constipation	Bowel Elimination, Alteration in: Constipation	Bowel Elimination, Alteration in: Constipation
Bowel Function, Irregular: Diarrhea	Bowel Elimination, Alteration in: Diarrhea	Body Elimination, Alteration in: Diarrhea	Bowel Elimination, Alteration in: Diarrhea
	Bowel Elimination, Alteration in: Impaction	Bowel Elimination, Alteration in: Impaction	
	Bowel Elimination, Alteration in: Incontinence	Bowel Elimination, Alteration in: Incontinence	Bowel Elimination, Alteration in: Incontinence

1982 and 1984	1986	1988	1990	1992
Activity Intolerance Activity Intolerance, Potential	Activity Intolerance Activity Intolerance, Potential	Activity Intolerance Activity Intolerance, Potential Fatigue	Activity Intolerance Activity Intolerance, Potential Fatigue	Activity Intolerance Activity Intolerance, High Risk for Fatigue
	Post-trauma Response Adjustment, Impaired	Post-trauma Response, Adjustment, Impaired	Post-trauma Response, Adjustment, Impaired	Post-trauma Response, Adjustment, Impaired
Anxiety	Anxiety	Anxiety	Anxiety	Anxiety
		Aspiration, Potential for	Aspiration, Potential for	Aspiration, High Risk for
Fluid Volume Deficit, Actual Fluid Volume Deficit, Potential Fluid Volume, Alteration in: Excess	Fluid Volume Deficit, Actual Fluid Volume Deficit, Potential Fluid Volume, Alteration in: Excess	Fluid Volume Deficit Fluid Volume Deficit, Potential Fluid Volume, Alteration in: Excess	Fluid Volume Deficit Fluid Volume Deficit, Potential Fluid Volume, Excess	Fluid Volume Deficits Fluid Volume Deficit, High Risk for Fluid Volume, Excess
Bowel Elimination, Alteration in: Constipation Bowel Elimination, Alteration in: Diarrhea	Bowel Elimination, Alteration in: Constipation Bowel Elimination, Alteration in: Diarrhea	Bowel Elimination, Alteration in: Constipation Bowel Elimination, Alteration in: Diarrhea	Colonic Constipation, Perceived Constipation, Colonic Diarrhea	Constipation, Colonic Constipation, Perceived Diarrhea
Bowel Elimination, Alteration in: Incontinence	Bowel Elimination, Alteration in: Incontinence	Bowel Elimination, Alteration in: Incontinence	Bowel Incontinence	Bowel Incontinence

Continued.

NOMENCLATURE DEVELOPMENT, 1973-1992—cont'd

1973	1975	1978	1980
	Cardiac Output, Alteration in: Decreased	Cardiac Output, Alteration in: Decreased	Cardiac Output, Alteration in: Decreased
	Circulation, Interruption of	Circulation, Interruption of Tissue Perfusion, Chronic, Abnormal	Tissue Perfusion, Alteration (Subcategories: see Appendix A)
Cognitive Functioning, Alteration in Level of Distractibility Hypovigilance Hypervigilance Cognitive Dissonance Inappropriate and Unrealistic-Based Thinking			
		Consciousness, Altered Levels of	
Decreased Capacity for Abstract Conceptualization Inaccurate Interpretation of Environment Increased Egocentricity Thought Processes Impaired	Thought Processes Impaired	Thought Processes Impaired	Thought Processes, Alteration in
Impaired Perception Impaired Retention Impaired Reflection Impaired Decision Making Impaired Judgment Confusion	Confusion		
Comfort Level, Alterations in Physiological Comfort Level, Alterations in Psychological Comfort Level, Alterations in Environmental Comfort Level, Alterations in Spiritual Comfort Level, Alterations in	Alterations in Comfort: Discomfort	Comfort, Alterations in: Pain	Comfort, Alterations in: Pain
Communication, Impairment of Verbal Nonverbal Communication, Impairment of		Communication, Impaired Verbal	Communication, Impaired Verbal

1982, 1984	1986	1988	1990	1992
		Breastfeeding, Ineffective	Breastfeeding, Ineffective Breastfeeding, Effective	Breastfeeding, Ineffective Breastfeeding, Effective Breastfeeding, Interrupted
Cardiac Output, Alteration in: Decreased	Cardiac Output, Alteration in: Decreased	Cardiac Output, Alteration in, Decreased	Decreased Cardiac Output	Decreased Cardiac Output
Tissue Perfusion, Alteration (Subcategories: see Appendix A)	Tissue Perfusion, Alteration (Subcategories: see Appendix A)	Tissue Perfusion, Alteration (Subcategories: see Appendix A)	Tissue Perfusion, Altered (see Subcategories: Appendix A)	Tissue Perfusion, Altered Neurovascular Dysfunction, High Risk for Peripheral
Thought Processes, Alteration in	Thought Processes, Alteration in	Thought Processes, Alteration in	Thought Processes, Altered	Thought Processes, Altered
Comfort, Alterations in: Pain	Comfort, Alterations in: Pain Comfort, Alterations in: Chronic Pain	Comfort, Alterations in: Pain Chronic Pain Comfort, Alterations in:	Pain Chronic Pain	Pain Chronic Pain
Communication, Impaired Verbal	Communication, Impaired Verbal	Communication, Impaired Verbal	Communication, Impaired Verbal	Communication, Impaired Verbal

Continued.

NOMENCLATURE DEVELOPMENT, 1973-1992—cont'd

1973	1975	1978	1980
		Coping Patterns, Mal-adaptive (Individual) Coping Patterns, Ineffec-tive, Family	Coping, Ineffective (Individual) Coping, Ineffective Family: Disabling Coping, Ineffective Family: Compro-mised Coping, Family: Po-tential for Growth
Digestion, Impairment of (Impaired Digestion)			
			Diversional Activity Deficit
Faith, Alterations in Faith in Self, Alterations in Faith in Others, Alterations in		Spirituality: Spiritual Concern Spirituality: Spiritual Dis-tress Spirituality: Spiritual De-spair	Spiritual Distress (Dis-tress of the Hu-man Spirit)
Fear Functional Fear, Mild Functional Fear, Moderate Functional Fear, Severe Functional Fear, Panic Nonfunctional Fear, Mild Nonfunctional Fear, Moder-ate Nonfunctional Fear, Severe Nonfunctional Fear, Panic			Fear (Specify)
		Functional Performance, Variations in *or* Self-Care Activities, Al-terations in Ability to Perform	

1982, 1984	1986	1988	1990	1992
		Decisional Conflict (Specify)	Decisional Conflict (Specify)	Decisional Conflict (Specify)
Coping, Ineffective (Individual)	Coping, Ineffective (Individual)	Coping, Ineffective (Individual)	Coping, Ineffective (Individual)	Coping, Ineffective (Individual)
Coping, Ineffective Family: Disabling	Coping, Ineffective Family: Disabling	Coping, Ineffective Family: Disabling	Coping, Ineffective Family: Disabling	Coping, Ineffective Family: Disabling
Coping, Ineffective Family: Compromised	Coping, Ineffective Family: Compromised	Coping, Ineffective Family: Compromised	Coping, Ineffective Family: Compromised	Coping, Ineffective Family: Compromised
Coping, Family: Potential for Growth	Coping, Family: Potential for Growth	Coping, Family: Potential for Growth	Coping, Family: Potential for Growth	Coping, Family: Potential for Growth
		Denial, Ineffective	Denial, Ineffective	Denial, Ineffective
		Coping, Defensive	Coping, Defensive	Coping, Defensive
Diversional Activity Deficit	Diversional Activity Deficit	Diversional Activity Deficit	Diversional Activity Deficit	Diversional Activity Deficit
		Dysreflexia	Dysreflexia	Dysreflexia
	Hopelessness	Hopelessness	Hopelessness	Hopelessness
Spiritual Distress (Distress of the Human Spirit)	Spiritual Distress (Distress of the Human Spirit)	Spiritual Distress (Distress of the Human Spirit)	Spiritual Distress (Distress of the Human Spirit)	Spiritual Distress (Distress of the Human Spirit)
Fear (Specify)	Fear (Specify)	Fear (Specify)	Fear (Specify)	Fear (Specify)
				Feeding Pattern, Ineffective Infant

Continued.

NOMENCLATURE DEVELOPMENT, 1973-1992—cont'd

1973	1975	1978	1980
		Home Maintenance Management, Impaired	Home Maintenance Management, Impaired
Self-Care Activities, Altered Ability to Perform	Self-Care Activities, Alteration in Ability to Perform	Total Self-Care Deficit	
Self-Care in All Spheres, Altered Ability to Perform			Total Self-Care Deficit (Specify Level)
Impairment in Performance of Established Hygiene Activities	Self-Care Activities, Alteration in Ability to Perform: Hygiene		Self-Bathing/ Hygiene Deficit (Specify Level)
			Self-Dressing/ Grooming Deficit (Specify Level)
		Self-Feeding Deficit	Self-Feeding Deficit (Specify Level)
		Self-Toileting Deficit (Specify Levels)	Self-Toileting Deficit (Specify Level)
Grieving	Acute Grieving	Grieving	
Normal Grieving			
Normal Grieving, Potential			
	Grieving, Anticipatory		Grieving, Anticipatory
Arrested Grieving	Delayed Grieving		Grieving, Dysfunctional
Arrested Grieving, Potential			
Delayed Onset of Grieving			
Delayed Onset of Grieving, Potential			
Injury, Potential for		Injury, Potential for	Injury, Potential for
Susceptibility to Hazards		Accidental Falling, Potential for	(see Subcategories, Appendix A)
		Knowledge, Lack of (Specify Area)	Knowledge Deficit (Specify)

1982, 1984	1986	1988	1990	1992
Home Maintenance Management Impaired	Home Maintenance Management Impaired	Home Maintenance Management Impaired	Home Maintenance Management Impaired	Home Maintenance Management Impaired
Total Self-Care Deficit (Specify Level) Self-Bathing/ Hygiene Deficit (Specify Level) Self-Dressing/ Grooming Deficit (Specify Level) Self-Feeding Deficit (Specify Level) Self-Toileting Deficit (Specify Level)	Total Self-Care Deficit (Specify Level) Self-Bathing/ Hygiene Deficit (Specify Level) Self-Dressing Grooming Deficit (Specify Level) Self-Feeding Deficit (Specify Level) Self-Toileting Deficit (Specify Level)	Total Self-Care Deficit (Specify Level) Self-Bathing/ Hygiene Deficit (Specify Level) Self-Dressing/ Grooming Deficit (Specify Level) Self-Feeding Deficit (Specify Level) Self-Toileting Deficit (Specify Level)	Total Self-Care Deficit (Specify Level) Self-Bathing/ Hygiene Deficit (Specify Level) Self-Dressing/ Grooming Deficit (Specify Level) Self-Feeding Deficit (Specify Level) Self-Toileting Deficit (Specify Level)	Self-Care Deficit (Specify Level) Self Bathing/Hygiene Deficit (Specify Level) Self-Dressing/Grooming Deficit (Specify Level) Self-Feeding Deficit (Specify Level) Self-Toileting Deficit (Specify Level)
Grieving, Anticipatory Grieving, Dysfunctional	Grieving, Anticipatory Grieving, Dysfunctional	Grieving, Anticipatory Grieving, Dysfunctional	Grieving, Anticipatory Grieving, Dysfunctional	Grieving, Anticipatory Grieving, Dysfunctional
	Growth and Development, Altered	Growth and Development, Altered	Growth and Development, Altered	Growth and Development, Altered
	Health Maintenance Alteration	Health Maintenance Alteration	Health Maintenance Alteration	Health Maintenance Alteration
		Health-Seeking Behaviors (Specify)	Health-Seeking Behaviors (Specify)	Health-Seeking Behaviors (Specify)
Injury, Potential for (see Subcategories, Appendix A)	Injury, Potential for (see Subcategories, Appendix A)	Injury, Potential for (see Subcategories, Appendix A)	Injury, Potential for (see Subcategories, Appendix A)	Injury, High Risk for (see Subcategories, Appendix A)
	Infection, Potential for	Infection, Potential for	Infection, Potential for	Infection, High Risk for
Knowledge Deficit (Specify)	Knowledge Deficit (Specify)	Knowledge Deficit (Specify)	Knowledge Deficit (Specify)	Knowledge Deficit (Specify)

Continued.

NOMENCLATURE DEVELOPMENT 1973-1992—cont'd

1973	1975	1978	1980
Understanding of State of Health, Lack of Understanding of Etiology of State of Health, Lack of Understanding of Preventive Health Measures, Lack of Understanding of Therapy, Lack of			
Manipulation, Verbal Manipulation, Nonverbal	Manipulation		
Mobility, Impaired Mobility, Impaired Physical	Mobility, Impairment of	Mobility, Impairment of	
			Mobility, Impaired Physical
Mobility, Impaired Social Mobility, Impaired Emotional Mobility, Impaired Intellectual Mobility, Impaired Developmental Motor Incoordination Motor Incoordination, Gross Motor Incoordination, Fine			
Noncompliance	Noncompliance	Noncompliance	Noncompliance (Specify)
Noncompliance with Diet Noncompliance with Drug Therapy Noncompliance with Environmental Therapy Noncompliance with Activity Regimen			
Nutrition, Alterations in: Undernutrition	Nutritional Alteration: Less than Required (MDR)	Nutritional Alteration: Less than Body Requirements	Nutrition, Alteration in: Less than Body Requirements
Nutrition, Alterations in: Obesity	Nutritional Alteration: More than Required	Nutritional Alteration: More than Body Requirements	Nutrition, Alteration in: More than Body Requirements
	Nutritional Alteration: Potential	Nutritional Alteration: Related to Changes in Body Requirements	Nutrition, Alteration in: Potential for More than Body Requirements

1982, 1984	1986	1988	1990	1992
Mobility, Impaired Physical	Mobility, Impaired Physical	Mobility, Impaired Physical	Mobility, Impaired Physical	Mobility, Impaired Physical
		Disuse Syndrome, Potential for	Disuse Syndrome, Potential for	Disuse Syndrome, High Risk for
Noncompliance (Specify)	Noncompliance (Specify)	Noncompliance (Specify)	Noncompliance (Specify)	Noncompliance (Specify)
				Ineffective Management of Therapeutic Regimen
Nutrition, Alteration in: Less than Body Requirements Nutrition: Alteration in: More than Body Requirements Nutrition, Alteration in: Potential for More than Body Requirements	Nutrition, Alteration in: Less than Body Requirements Nutrition, Alteration in: More than Body Requirements Nutrition, Alteration in: Potential for More than Body Requirements	Nutrition, Alteration in: Less than Body Requirements Nutrition, Alteration in: More than Body Requirements Nutrition, Alteration in: Potential for More than Body Requirements	Nutrition, Altered: Less than Body Requirements Nutrition, Altered: More than Body Requirements Nutrition, Altered: Potential for More than Body Requirements	Nutrition, Altered: Less than Body Requirements Nutrition, Altered: More than Body Requirements Nutrition, Altered: Risk for More than Body Requirements

Continued.

NOMENCLATURE DEVELOPMENT, 1973-1992—cont'd

1973	1975	1978	1980
		Parenting, Alterations in: Actual	Parenting, Alterations in: Actual
		Parenting, Alterations in: Potential	Parenting, Alterations in: Potential
Respiration, Impairment of	Respiratory Dysfunction	Respiratory Dysfunction	Airway Clearance, Ineffective
			Breathing Pattern, Ineffective
Respiratory Distress			Gas Exchange, Impaired
			Rape Trauma Syndrome
			Rape Trauma, Compound Reaction
			Rape Trauma, Silent Reaction
Role Disturbance			
Altered Relationships with Self and Others			
Family Process, Inadequate			
Group Relations, Noneffective			
Regulatory Functions, Altered External			
Social Isolation			

1982, 1984	1986	1988	1990	1992
Parenting Alterations in: Actual Parenting, Alterations in: Potential	Parenting, Alterations in: Actual Parenting, Alterations in: Potential	Parenting, Alterations in: Actual Parenting, Alterations in: Potential	Parenting, Altered Parenting, Potential for Altered	Parenting, Altered Parenting, High Risk for Altered
Oral Mucous Membranes, Alteration in	Oral Mucous Membranes, Alteration in	Oral Mucous Membranes, Alteration in	Oral Mucous Membrane, Altered	Oral Mucous Membrane, Altered
			Protection, Altered	Protection, Altered
				Relocation Stress Syndrome
Airway Clearance, Ineffective Breathing Pattern, Ineffective Gas Exchange, Impaired	Airway Clearance, Ineffective Breathing Pattern, Ineffective Gas Exchange, Impaired	Airway Clearance, Ineffective Breathing Pattern, Ineffective Gas Exchange, Impaired	Airway Clearance, Ineffective Breathing Pattern, Ineffective Gas Exchange, Impaired	Airway Clearance, Ineffective Breathing Pattern, Ineffective Gas Exchange, Impaired Weaning Response, Dysfunctional Ventilatory Ventilation, Inability to Sustain Spontaneous
Rape Trauma Syndrome Rape Trauma, Compound Reaction Rape Trauma, Silent Reaction	Rape Trauma Syndrome Rape Trauma, Compound Reaction Rape Trauma, Silent Reaction	Rape Trauma Syndrome Rape Trauma, Compound Reaction Rape Trauma, Silent Reaction	Rape Trauma Syndrome Rape Trauma, Compound Reaction Rape Trauma, Silent Reaction	Rape Trauma Syndrome Rape Trauma, Compound Reaction Rape Trauma, Silent Reaction
	Role Performance, Disturbance in	Role Performance, Disturbance in Role Conflict, Parental	Role Performance, Disturbance in Role Conflict, Parental	Role Performance, Disturbance in Role Conflict, Parental Role Strain, Caregiver Role Strain, High Risk for Caregiver
Powerlessness	Powerlessness	Powerlessness	Powerlessness	Powerlessness
Family Process, Alteration in	Family Process, Alteration in	Family Process, Alteration in	Family Processes, Altered	Family Processes, Altered
Social Isolation	Social Interaction, Impaired Social Isolation	Social Interaction, Impaired Social Isolation	Social Interaction, Impaired Social Isolation	Social Interaction, Impaired Social Isolation

Continued.

NOMENCLATURE DEVELOPMENT, 1973-1992—cont'd

1973	1975	1978	1980
Self-Esteem or Self-Actualization, Impairment of Self-Concept, Altered		Self-Concept, Alterations in: (Self-Esteem, Role Performance, Personal Identity, Body Image)	Self-Concept, Disturbance in (see Subcategories, Appendix A)
Altered Body Image	Self-Concept: Alterations in: Body Image		
Depersonalization Identity Conflict			
Sensory Disturbance Sensory Deprivation Sensory Overload Sensory Impairment	Sensory-Perceptual Alterations	Sensory-Perceptual Alterations	Sensory-Perceptual Alterations (see Subcategories, Appendix A)
Disturbances in Visual Perception Disturbances in Auditory Perception Disturbances in Gustatory Perceptions Disturbances in Tactile Perception			
		Sexuality, Alterations in Patterns of	Sexual Dysfunction
Skin Integrity, Impairment of	Skin Integrity, Impairment of: Actual Skin Integrity, Impairment of: Potential	Skin Integrity, Impairment of: Actual Skin Integrity, Impairment of: Potential	Skin Integrity, Impairment of: Actual Skin Integrity, Impairment of: Potential
Skin, Impairment of Regulatory Function of Altered Internal Regulatory Function			
Sleep-Rest Patterns, Ineffective	Sleep-Rest Activity, Rhythm of	Sleep-Rest Activity, Dysrhythm of	Sleep Pattern Disturbance

1982, 1984	1986	1988	1990	1992
		Self-Esteem Disturbance	Self-Esteem Disturbance	Self-Esteem Disturbance
Self-Concept, Disturbance in (see Subcategories, Appendix A)	Self-Concept Disturbance in (see Subcategories, Appendix A)	Chronic Low Self-Esteem	Chronic Low Self-Esteem	Chronic Low Self-Esteem
		Situational Low Self-Esteem	Situational Low Self-Esteem	Situational Low Self-Esteem
		Body Image Disturbance	Body Image Disturbance	Body Image Disturbance
Personal Identity Disturbance	Personal Identity Disturbance	Personal Identity Disturbance	Personal Identity Disturbance	Personal Identity Disturbance
	Hopelessness	Hopelessness	Hopelessness	Hopelessness
Sensory Perceptual Alterations (see Subcategories, Appendix A)	Sensory Perceptual Alterations (see Subcategories, Appendix A)	Sensory Perceptual Alterations (see Subcategories, Appendix A)	Sensory Perceptual Alterations (see Subcategories, Appendix A)	Sensory Perceptual Alterations (see Subcategories, Appendix A)
	Unilateral Neglect	Unilateral Neglect	Unilateral Neglect	Unilateral Neglect
Sexual Dysfunction	Sexual Dysfunction	Sexual Dysfunction	Sexual Dysfunction	Sexual Dysfunction
	Sexuality Patterns, Altered	Sexuality Patterns, Altered	Sexuality Patterns, Altered	Sexuality Patterns, Altered
Skin Integrity, Impairment of: Actual	Skin Integrity, Impairment of: Actual	Skin Integrity, Impairment of: Actual	Skin Integrity, Impaired	Skin Integrity, Impaired
Skin Integrity, Impairment of: Potential	Skin Integrity, Impairment of: Potential	Skin Integrity, Impairment of: Potential	Skin Integrity, Impairment of: Potential	Skin Integrity, High Risk for
	Tissue Integrity, Impaired	Tissue Integrity, Impaired	Tissue Integrity, Impaired	Tissue Integrity, Impaired
Sleep Pattern Disturbance	Sleep Pattern Disturbance	Sleep Pattern Disturbance	Sleep Pattern Disturbance	Sleep Pattern Disturbance

Continued.

NOMENCLATURE DEVELOPMENT, 1973-1992—cont'd

1973	1975	1978	1980
Urinary Elimination, Impairment of	Urinary Elimination, Impairment of: Alterations in Patterns	Urinary Elimination, Impairment of: Alterations in Patterns	Urinary Elimination, Alteration in Patterns
Inability to Control Initiation of Urine Flow	Urinary Elimination, Impairment of: Incontinence	Urinary Elimination, Impairment of: Incontinence	
Inability to Control Cessation of Urine Flow			
Inability to Generate Urine flow	Urinary Elimination, Impairment of: Retention	Urinary Elimination, Impairment of: Retention	
			Violence, Potential for

The books containing the lists from which this table was prepared are:

Gebbie KM, Lavin MA, editors: *Proceedings of the first national conference on classification of nursing diagnoses,* St Louis, 1975, Mosby.

Gebbie KM, editor: *Summary of the second national conference on classification of nursing diagnoses,* St Louis, 1976, Clearing House for the National Group for Classification of Nursing Diagnoses.

Kim MJ, Moritz DA, editors: *Classification of nursing diagnoses: proceedings of the third and fourth conferences,* New York, 1982, McGraw-Hill.

Kim MJ, McFarlane G, McLane A, editors: *Classification of nursing diagnoses: proceedings of the fifth national conference,* St Louis, 1984, Mosby.

Harley M, editor: *Classification of nursing diagnoses: proceedings of the sixth conference,* St Louis, 1986, Mosby.

McLane A, editor: *Classification of nursing diagnoses: proceedings of the seventh conference,* St Louis, 1987, Mosby.

Carroll-Johnson R, editor: *Classification of nursing diagnoses: proceedings of the eighth conference,* St Louis, 1989, Mosby.

Carroll-Johnson R, editor: *Classification of nursing diagnoses: proceedings of the ninth conference,* Philadelphia, 1991, Lippincott.

Carroll-Johnson R, editor: *Classification of nursing diagnoses: proceedings of the tenth conference,* Philadelphia, 1994, Lippincott.

1982, 1984	1986	1988	1990	1992
	Swallowing, Impaired	Swallowing, Impaired	Swallowing, Impaired	Swallowing, Impaired
	Body Temperature, Potential Alteration in	Body Temperature, Potential Alteration in	Body Temperature, Potential Alteration in	Body Temperature, High Risk for Altered
	Hyperthermia	Hyperthermia	Hyperthermia	Hyperthermia
	Hypothermia	Hypothermia	Hypothermia	Hypothermia
	Thermoregulation, Ineffective	Thermoregulation, Ineffective	Thermoregulation, Ineffective	Thermoregulation, Ineffective
Urinary Elimination, Alteration in Patterns	Urinary Elimination, Alteration in Patterns	Urinary Elimination, Alteration in Patterns	Urinary Elimination, Altered	Urinary Elimination, Altered
	Incontinence, Functional	Incontinence, Functional	Incontinence, Functional	Incontinence, Functional
	Incontinence, Reflex	Incontinence, Reflex	Incontinence, Reflex	Incontinence, Reflex
	Incontinence, Stress	Incontinence, Stress	Incontinence, Stress	Incontinence, Stress
	Incontinence, Total	Incontinence, Total	Incontinence, Total	Incontinence, Total
	Incontinence, Urge	Incontinence, Urge	Incontinence, Urge	Incontinence, Urge
	Urinary Retention	Urinary Retention	Urinary Retention	Urinary Retention
Violence, Potential for	Violence, Potential for	Violence, Potential for	Violence, Potential for	Violence, High Risk for Self-Mutilation

APPENDIX V

NANDA DIAGNOSTIC CATEGORY REVIEW GUIDELINES, 1993

NEWLY PROPOSED DIAGNOSES

The North American Nursing Diagnosis Association (NANDA) solicits newly proposed nursing diagnoses for review by the Association. Such proposed diagnoses undergo a systematic review process for inclusion in NANDA's approved list of diagnoses. Approval indicates that NANDA endorses the diagnosis for clinical testing and continuing development by the discipline.

To assist with the submission of proposed diagnoses, the NANDA Diagnosis Review Committee (DRC) has prepared a set of guidelines. These guidelines are designed to promote the consistency, clarity, and quality of submissions. Diagnoses that are submitted but do not meet the guidelines will be returned to the submitter for appropriate revision. Questions regarding the submission process may be forwarded to NANDA Office, 1211 Locust Street, Philadelphia, PA 19107.

NURSING DIAGNOSIS: DEFINITION

(Approved at 9th Conference, 1990)

A nursing diagnosis is a clinical judgment about individual, family, or community responses to actual or potential health problems/life processes. Nursing diagnoses provide the basis for the selection of nursing interventions to achieve outcomes for which the nurse is accountable.

ACTUAL NURSING DIAGNOSIS

1. **Label:** The label provides a name for the diagnosis, a concise phrase or term that represents a pattern of related cues. Diagnostic labels may include *but are not limited* to the following qualifiers:

Check with NANDA Office for current guidelines. Used with permission of North American Nursing Diagnosis Association, 1993.

Altered A change from baseline.

Impaired Made worse; weakened; damaged; reduced; deteriorated.

Depleted Emptied wholly or partially; exhausted of.

Deficient Inadequate in amount, quality, or degree; defective; not sufficient; incomplete.

Excessive Characterized by an amount or quantity greater than is necessary, desirable, or useful.

Dysfunctional Abnormal; incomplete functioning.

Disturbed Agitated; interrupted, interfered with.

Ineffective Not producing the desired effect.

Decreased Lessened; lesser in size, amount, or degree.

Increased Greater in size, amount, or degree.

Acute Severe but of short duration.

Chronic Lasting a long time; recurring; habitual; constant.

Intermittent Stopping and starting again at intervals; periodic; cyclic.

2. **Definition:** The definition of the diagnosis provides a clear, precise description. The definition delineates its meaning and helps differentiate this diagnosis from similar diagnoses.

3. **Defining characteristics:** Defining characteristics are clinical cues that cluster as manifestations of a nursing diagnosis. Diagnostic cues are clinical evidence that describe a cluster of behaviors or signs and symptoms that represent a diagnostic label. Diagnostic cues are concrete and measurable through observation or client/group reports. Diagnostic cues may be either major or minor.

Major diagnostic cues are critical indicators of the diagnosis. Minor diagnostic cues are supporting indicators that are not always present but that complete the clinical picture and increase the diagnostician's confidence in making the diagnosis.[1] The differentiation of major from minor characteristics should be logically depended. If appropriate, the submitter may designate a diagnostic cue as major if it occurs 80% to 100% of the time and minor if it occurs 50% to 79% of the time.

4. **Related factors:** Related factors are conditions or circumstances that may cause or contribute to the development of a diagnosis. Factors that are related to the proposed diagnosis must be listed and supported by an accompanying literature review.

5. **Literature/clinical validation:** A narrative review of the relevant literature is required to support the rationale for the diagnosis, the defining characteristics, and the related factors. If the diagnosis is similar to an approved NANDA diagnosis, the reason for its usefulness must be addressed. Literature citations for defining characteristics are required and should be cited for each cue. If defining characteristics are not supported by the literature, an explanation for their inclusion is required. In addition, the designation of major versus minor defining characteristics must be supported by clinical data. These data may be derived from case studies, nurse consensus, retrospective chart reviews, and/or other appropriate validation methods. A sample three-part (label, related factors, and signs and symptoms) nursing diagnostic statement with the associated outcome criteria and nurse-prescribed interventions must accompany the submission.

Sample

Activity intolerance **related to** deconditioned status as evidenced by inability to wash body or body parts without tachycardia, dyspnea, and fatigue. *(Author's note: deconditioned status is, in part, activity intolerance. Thus it is difficult to view this as also a related factor.)*

Outcome criteria

Bathes independently without tachycardia or dyspnea

Interventions

Position to minimize energy requirements; assist to recondition; teach energy conservation techniques-pacing techniques; provide assistance as indicated

HIGH-RISK NURSING DIAGNOSIS

(NANDA-approved diagnoses previously designated as "Potential for" were labeled "High Risk for" in 1992.)

A high-risk nursing diagnosis is a clinical judgment that an individual, family, or community is more vulnerable to develop the problem than others in the same or similar situation. High-risk nursing diagnoses are supported by risk factors that guide nursing interventions to reduce or prevent the occurrence of the problem.

1. **Label:** The label provides a name for the diagnosis, a concise phrase or term that represents a pattern of related cues. Diagnostic labels may include *but are not limited* to the following qualifiers:

Altered A change from baseline.
Impaired Made worse; weakened; damaged, reduced; deteriorated.
Depleted Emptied wholly or partially; exhausted of.
Deficient Inadequate in amount, quality, or degree; defective; not sufficient; incomplete.
Excessive Characterized by an amount or quantity greater than is necessary, desirable, or useful.
Dysfunctional Abnormal; incomplete functioning.
Disturbed Agitated; interrupted, interfered with.
Ineffective Not producing the desired effect.
Decreased Lessened: lesser in size, amount, or degree.
Increased Greater in size, amount, or degree.
Acute Severe but of short duration.
Chronic Lasting a long time; recurring; habitual; constant.
Intermittent Stopping and starting again at intervals; periodic; cyclic.

2. **Definition:** The definition of the label provides a clear, precise description. The definition delineates its meaning and helps differentiate this diagnosis from all others.

3. **Risk factors:** Risk factors identify behaviors, conditions, or circumstances that render an individual, family, or community more vulnerable to a particular problem than others in the same or similar situation. There are no signs and symptoms for high-risk diagnoses.

4. **Literature/clinical validation:** A narrative review of the literature is required to support the rationale for the diagnosis and the risk factors. Literature citations for each risk factor are required. If the diagnosis is similar to an approved NANDA diagnosis, the reason for its usefulness must be addressed. The submission must include a sample two-part high-risk nursing diagnostic statement (including label and risk factors) with related outcome criteria and nursing-prescribed interventions.

Sample

High Risk for Injury: Fall related to fatigue and altered gait *(Author's note: Not clear if these are risk factors, e.g., a history of falls. "Related to" factors in specifying high-risk diagnoses were dropped in 1986.)*

Outcome criteria

Describes or demonstrates necessary safety measures

Interventions

Teach measures to prevent falls; instruct to request assistance when needed

WELLNESS NURSING DIAGNOSIS

A wellness nursing diagnosis is a clinical judgment about an individual, family, or community in transition from a specific level of wellness to a higher level of wellness.

1. **Label:** The term *Potential for Enhanced* will be the designated qualifier. *Enhanced* is defined as "made greater, to increase in quality, or more desired." Wellness diagnoses will be one-part statements.
2. **Definition:** The definition of the label provides a clear, precise description. The definition delineates its meaning and helps differentiate this diagnosis from all others.
3. **Literature/clinical validation:** A narrative review of the literature is required to support the rationale for the diagnosis. A sample one-part wellness nursing diagnostic statement with related outcome criteria and nursing-prescribed interventions must accompany the submission.

Sample

Potential for Enhanced Parenting.

Outcome criteria

Will practice listening without advice-giving with children

Interventions

Describe active listening; differentiate between listening and advice-giving

REVISION OF NANDA-APPROVED NURSING DIAGNOSES

Changes may be proposed for the label, the definition, and/or the defining characteristics of a NANDA-approved nursing diagnosis. In order for any NANDA-approved nursing diagnosis to be refined or revised, the proposal must contain the following:

1. A narrative describing the rationale for the proposed change.
2. Research findings to support the proposed changes. These findings may be the results of research by the submitter or from research reported in the literature.

DELETION OF NANDA-APPROVED NURSING DIAGNOSES

Proposals may be submitted to delete a NANDA-approved nursing diagnosis. The proposal must contain a narrative describing the rationale for the proposed deletion. The rationale must be supported by the following:

1. Logical justification.
2. Research findings and/or relevant literature review.

DIAGNOSIS REVIEW COMMITTEE REVIEW CYCLE

1. Submission deadline: March 1 (of the year prior to a conference, e.g., 1995; check with NANDA Office).
2. Initial review by the DRC chairperson to ascertain whether required components are present.
3. Incomplete submissions returned with a resubmission deadline date of July 1.
4. Submissions with all the required components reviewed by the DRC. One of the following decisions will be made for each submission:
   a. *Not accepted:* The proposed diagnosis has not been accepted for review by the Expert Advisory Panel. Reasons for "Not Accepted" are listed below:
      - Represents a medical diagnosis
      - Represents a treatment or procedure
      - Does not represent a human response
      - Defining characteristics for actual nursing diagnosis are not cues or signs/symptoms
      - Defining characteristics for high-risk nursing diagnosis are not risk factors
   b. *Hold for Revisions:* The proposed diagnosis will be returned to the submitter for revisions. Listed below are examples of needed revisions:
      - Research population was not representative for conclusions drawn
      - Inadequate literature support for proposed diagnosis
   c. *Accepted for Expert Advisory Panel Review*
5. After the Expert Advisory Panel and the DRC reviews, each proposed diagnosis or proposal (revisions or deletions) will receive one of the following designations:
   a. *Returned to Be Developed (TBD):* This decision delineates submitted work as promising but requiring substantive development. This work will require resubmission in its entirety to the DRC. This category acknowledges promising work in need of substantive revisions.
   b. *Conditional Accept:* This category indicates a provisional acceptance of the submitted work pending receipt of revisions agreed on by the committee and the submitter.
   c. *Accepted:* This category indicates that the submitted work is accepted.
6. Accepted diagnoses or proposals for revisions/deletions will be forwarded to the Board of Directors for approval.
7. Board-approved proposed diagnoses or proposals for revisions/deletions will be presented at the NANDA Conference and will be subject to membership mail vote.

APPENDIX W

SABA AND OMAHA DIAGNOSTIC CLASSIFICATION SYSTEMS

SABA CLASSIFICATION SYSTEM*[1]

A. Activity component

01. Activity Alteration
    01.1. Activity Intolerance
    01.2. Activity Intolerance Risk
    01.3. Diversional Activity Deficit
    01.4. Fatigue
    01.5. Physical Mobility Impairment
    01.6. Sleep-Pattern Disturbance
02. Musculoskeletal Alteration

B. Bowel elimination component

03. Bowel Elimination Alteration
    03.1. Bowel Incontinence
    03.2. Colonic Constipation
    03.3. Diarrhea
    03.4. Fecal Impaction
    03.5. Perceived Constipation
    03.6. Unspecified Constipation
04. Gastrointestinal Alteration

C. Cardiac component

05. Cardiac Output Alteration
06. Cardiovascular Alteration
    01.1 Blood Pressure Alteration

D. Cognitive component

07. Cerebral Alteration
08. Knowledge Deficit (of:)
    08.1. Diagnostic (Laboratory Test)
    08.2. Dietary Regimen
    08.3. Disease Process
    08.4. Fluid Volume
    08.5. Medication Regimen
    08.6. Safety Precaution
    08.7. Therapeutic Regimen

09. Thought Processes Alteration

E. Coping component

10. Dying Process
11. Family Coping Impairment
    11.1. Compromised Family Coping
    11.2. Disabled Family Coping
12. Individual Coping Impairment
    12.1. Adjustment Impairment
    12.2. Decisional Conflict
    12.3. Defensive Coping
    12.4. Denial
13. Posttrauma Response
    13.1. Rape-Trauma Syndrome
14. Spiritual State Alteration
    14.1. Spiritual Distress

F. Fluid volume component

15. Fluid Volume Alteration
    15.1. Deficit of Fluid Volume
    15.2. Deficit Risk of Fluid Volume
    15.3. Excess of Fluid Volume
    15.4. Excess Risk of Fluid Volume

G. Health behavior component

16. Growth and Development Alteration
17. Health Maintenance Alteration
18. Health-Seeking Behaviors
19. Home Maintenance Management Impairment
20. Noncompliance (of:)
    20.1. Diagnostic (Laboratory Test)
    20.2. Dietary Regimen
    20.3. Fluid Volume
    20.4. Medication Regimen
    20.5. Safety Precaution
    20.6. Therapeutic Regimen

H. Medication component

21. Medication Risk
    21.1. Polypharmacy

*From Saba VK: *Classification of home health care nursing diagnoses and interventions,* Washington, DC, 1990, Author.

I. Metabolic component
22. Endocrine Alteration
23. Immunologic Alteration
    23.1. Protection Alteration

J. Nutritional component
24. Nutrition Alteration
    24.1. Less than Body Requirement
    24.2. Less than Body Requirement Risk
    24.3. More than Body Requirement
    24.4. More than Body Requirement Risk

K. Physical regulation component
25. Physical Regulation Alteration
    25.1. Dysreflexia
    25.2. Hyperthermia
    25.3. Hypothermia
    25.4. Thermoregulation Impairment
    25.5. Infection Risk
    25.6. Infection Unspecified

L. Respiratory component
26. Respiration Alteration
    26.1. Airway Clearance Impairment
    26.2. Breathing Pattern Impairment
    26.3. Gas Exchange Impairment

M. Role relationship component
27. Role Performance Alteration
    27.1. Parental Role Conflict
    27.2. Parenting Alteration
    27.3. Sexual Dysfunction
28. Communication Impairment
    28.1. Verbal Impairment
29. Family Processes Alteration
30. Grieving
    30.1. Anticipatory Grieving
    30.2. Dysfunctional Grieving
31. Sexuality Patterns Alteration
32. Socialization Alteration
    32.1. Social Interaction Impairment
    32.2. Social Isolation

N. Safety component
33. Injury Risk
    33.1. Aspiration
    33.2. Disuse Syndrome
    33.3. Poisoning
    33.4. Suffocation
    33.5. Trauma
34. Violence Risk

O. Self-care component
35. Bathing/Hygiene Deficit
36. Dressing/Grooming Deficit
37. Feeding Deficit
    37.1. Breastfeeding Impairment
    37.2. Swallowing Impairment
38. Self-Care Deficit
    38.1. Activities of Daily Living (ADLs) Alteration
    38.2. Instrumental Activities of Daily Living (IADLs) Alteration
39. Toileting Deficit

P. Self-concept component
40. Anxiety
41. Fear
42. Meaningfulness Alteration
    42.1. Hopelessness
    42.4. Powerlessness
43. Self-Concept Alteration
    43.1. Body Image Disturbance
    43.2. Personal Identity Disturbance
    43.3. Chronic Low Self-Esteem Disturbance
    43.4. Situational Self-Esteem Disturbance

Q. Sensory component
44. Sensory/Perceptual Alteration
    44.1. Auditory
    44.2. Gustatory[2]
    44.3. Kinesthetic
    44.4. Olfactory
    44.5. Tactile
    44.6. Unilateral Neglect
    44.7. Visual
45. Comfort Alteration
    45.1. Acute Pain
    45.2. Chronic Pain
    45.3. Unspecified Pain

R. Tissue integrity component
46. Tissue Integrity Alteration
    46.1. Oral Mucous Membranes Impairment
    46.2. Skin Integrity Impairment
    46.3. Skin Integrity Impairment Risk
    46.4. Skin Incision
47. Peripheral Alteration

S. Tissue perfusion component
48. Tissue Perfusion Alteration

T. Urinary elimination component
49. Urinary Elimination Alteration
    49.1. Functional Incontinence
    49.2. Reflex Incontinence
    49.3. Stress Incontinence

49.4. Total Incontinence
49.5. Urge Incontinence
49.6. Retention
50. Renal Alteration

OMAHA CLASSIFICATION SYSTEM*
Domain I. Environmental

01.   Income: Deficit
02.   Sanitation: Deficit
03A. Safety Hazards: Residence
03B. Safety Hazards: Neighborhood
04.   Other:

Domain II. Psychosocial

05.   Communication with Community Resources: Impairment
06.   Isolation: Social
07.   Behavior Pattern: Impairment
08.   Role Change: Impairment
09.   Interpersonal Conflict
10.   Grief
11.   Confusion
12.   Depression
13.   Anxiety
14.   Human Sexuality: Impairment
15.   Parenting: Impairment
16.   Neglect: Child-Adult
17.   Abuse: Child-Adult
18.   Growth and Developmental Lag
19.   Other:

Domain III. Physiologic

20.   Hearing: Impairment
21.   Vision: Impairment
22.   Speech and Language: Impairment

*From Martin KS, Scheet N: *Omaha system: application for community health nursing,* Philadelphia, 1992, Saunders.

23.   Dentition: Impairment
24.   Respiration: Impairment
25.   Circulation: Impairment
26.   Neuromusculoskeletal Function: Impairment
27.   Digestive Function: Impairment
28A. Reproductive Function: Family Planning
28B. Reproductive Function: Pregnancy
28C. Reproductive Function: Impairment
29.   Bowel Function: Impairment
30.   Urinary Function: Impairment
31.   Integument: Impairment
32.   Pain
33.   Consciousness: Impairment
34.   Other:

Domain IV. Health Behaviors

35.   Nutrition: Impairment
36.   Sleep and Rest Patterns: Impairment
37.   Physical Activity: Impairment
38.   Personal Hygiene: Deficit
39.   Substance: Misuse
40A. Therapeutic Regime Noncompliance: Medical-Dental Supervision
40B. Therapeutic Regime Noncompliance: Prescribed Treatment Plan
40C. Therapeutic Regime Noncompliance: Prescribed Medications
40D. Therapeutic Regime Noncompliance: Prescribed Diet
41.   Technical Procedure: Deficit
42.   Other:

NOTES

1. SABA Classification: Terminology modifications made in collaboration with Sheila M. Sparks, D.N.Sc., R.N., C.S., Assistant Professor, School of Nursing, Georgetown University, Washington, DC.—V.K. Saba

Annotated Bibliography

The following references to nursing diagnosis and related areas supplement the chapter references. Citations are organized within three broad areas: diagnosis, process, and application.

DIAGNOSIS
Concept of nursing diagnosis

Baer CL: Nursing diagnosis: a futuristic process for nursing practice, *Top Clin Nurs* 5:89, 1984. Discussion of nursing diagnosis and the criteria for a profession. Views nursing diagnosis as having the potential to influence nursing autonomy. Includes a summary of advantages and disadvantages of using nursing diagnosis.

Bircher A: On the development and classification of diagnoses, *Nurs Forum* 14:10, 1975. Proposes a mastery-competency classification system based on the organizing principle of Maslow's hierarchy of human needs. Defines nursing diagnosis, discusses the potential problems and dangers inherent in making a diagnosis, and outlines the values of nursing diagnosis.

Bonney V, Rothberg J: *Nursing diagnosis and therapy: an instrument for evaluation and assessment,* New York, 1963, National League for Nursing. Contains an early definition of nursing diagnosis and a tool for assessment of functional problems. The assessment form was developed to facilitate planning for nurse staffing for chronically ill and disabled clients.

Carnevali DL: Nursing diagnosis: an evolutionary view, *Top Clin Nurs* 5:10, 1984. Discussion of the evolution of nursing diagnosis, the nursing domain for diagnosis, the evolution of the diagnostic reasoning process, and the relation of nursing values to nursing diagnosis. Offers predictions regarding the future of nursing diagnosis.

Carpenito LJ: Altered thoughts or altered perceptions? *Am J Nurs* 85:1283, 1985. An examination of two nursing diagnoses and suggestions for their use in clinical settings.

Chambers W: Nursing diagnosis, *Am J Nurs* 62:102, 1962. Early article on diagnosis that emphasizes the elements of observation, interpretation, and identifying nursing problems.

Clark J: Should nurses diagnose and prescribe? *J Adv Nurs* 4:485, 1978. Discusses the value of nursing diagnoses and concludes that nurses should diagnose and prescribe if competent.

Craig JL: Ten reasons why we need nursing diagnosis, *RNABC News* (Canada), p 9, September, 1983. Good summary of the reasons nursing diagnosis is needed for professional activities.

Donnelly E: Health promotion, families, and the diagnostic process, *Fam Comm Health* 12:12, 1990. Analyzes diagnostic categories and diagnostic process in the context of family care and makes recommendations for diagnostic category development.

Gebbie KM: Nursing diagnosis: what is it and why does it exist? *Top Clin Nurs* 5:1, 1984. Discussion of the concept of nursing diagnosis; the reasons for its emergence; the contribution it has made to nursing care; and the consequences, both positive and negative, of its use.

Gebbie KA, Lavin MA: Classifying nursing diagnoses, *Am J Nurs* 44:250, 1974. Report of the first national conference on nursing diagnosis and the diagnoses identified.

Gleit CJ, Tatro S: Nursing diagnoses for healthy individuals, *Nurs Health Care* 2:456, 1981. Suggests more liberal use of nursing diagnosis with well clients, which will promote high-level wellness and a more cost-effective health care system.

Gordon M: Conceptual issues in nursing diagnosis. In N, editor: Chaska *The nursing profession: a time to speak,* New York, 1982, McGraw-Hill. Identifies issues in the identification, standardization, and classification of nursing diagnoses. States the first step in implementing nursing diagnosis is for nurses to recognize their autonomy and accountability in practice.

Gordon M: The concept of nursing diagnosis, *Nurs Clin North Am* 14:487, 1979. Discussion of the concept of nursing diagnosis and related issues. Progress up to 1979 in identification and classification is summarized; resources for implementation are cited.

Gordon M: Classification of nursing diagnosis, *J NY State Nurses Assoc* 9:5, 1978. Identifies four major areas of nursing practice that require clinical diagnosis and eight issues in practice that would be clarified by the use of standardized nomenclature.

Gordon M: Nursing diagnosis and the diagnostic process, *Am J Nurs* 76:1276, 1976. Defines nursing diagnosis in terms of concept and structure (PES) and discusses the diagnostic process.

Gordon M, Sweeney MA, McKeehan K: Development of nursing diagnoses, *Am J Nurs* 80:699, 1980. Discusses historical development of nursing diagnosis from 1960 to 1980. Traces changes in form and focus.

Hardy E: The diagnostic wheel: identifying care that is unique to nursing, *Can Nurse* 79:38, 1983. Describes the implementation of an experimental nursing assessment form and diagnostic wheel composed of 15 alterations in living patterns divided into 4 major areas of concern. Examples of its use are given.

Jacoby M: The dilemma of physiological problems: eliminating the double standard, *Am J Nurs* 85:281, 1985. Explores the conceptual focus of nursing diagnosis, particularly the issue of physiological problems. Stresses the need for clinical research to validate the situations and populations in which nurses diagnose and independently treat physiological malfunctions and potential malfunctions.

Kim MJ: The dilemma of physiological problems: without collaboration, what's left? *Am J Nurs* 85:281, 1985. Discusses the need for the identification and classification of physiological problems nurses use in practice. Stresses the need to represent the diversity in nursing practice by including the collaborative, or interdependent, domain of practice.

King LS: What is a diagnosis? *JAMA* 202:714, 1967.Examines the concept of diagnosis and presents the view that diagnosis is not confined just to medicine.

Lash AA: Reexamination of nursing diagnosis, *Nurs Forum* 17:332, 1978. Reviews differences between medical diagnosis and nursing diagnosis in the literature from 1953 to 1976. Views nursing diagnosis as offering autonomy and independent decision making and as necessary to a profession and professional nursing practice.

Levine M: Trophicognosis: an alternative to nursing diagnosis. In American Nurses Association: *Exploring progress in medical-surgical nursing. ANA regional clinical conference* 2:55, 1965. Early paper on nursing diagnosis advocating the use of a different term.

Mills W: Why a classification system? In Carroll-Johnson R, editor: *Classification of nursing diagnoses: proceedings of the ninth conference,* Philadelphia, 1991, Lippincott, (pp. 3-5). Explores the reasons for generating a taxonomy. Six objectives for classification in science are related to nursing as an evolving discipline.

Mundinger M, Jauron G: Developing a nursing diagnosis, *Nurs Outlook* 23:94, 1975. Proposes a two-part structure for nursing diagnosis and the use of "related to" instead of "due to." Discusses problems encountered in defining and instituting nursing diagnosis and gives examples of mistakes made by beginning diagnosticians.

Myers N: Nursing diagnosis, *Nurs Times* 69:1299, 1973. Emphasizes the importance of diagnosis; defines nursing diagnosis.

Popkess-Vawter S: Wellness nursing diagnoses: to be or not to be? *Nurs Diagn* 2:19, 1991. Discusses how the new nursing diagnosis definition provides the opportunity to incorporate a wellness perspective into the nursing diagnosis movement.

Price MR: Nursing diagnosis: making a concept come alive, *Am J Nurs* 80:668, 1980. Discussion of structural components of nursing diagnoses, common errors in diagnosis, steps in the diagnostic process, and how to use a diagnosis.

Proder B: What you should know about nursing diagnosis, *Med Rec News,* p 87, August 1975. Supports the need for a classification system and presents an approach to manual collection of data on patients with nursing diagnoses.

Randell B: Nursing theory: the 21st century, *Nurs Sci Q* 5:176, 1992. UCLA Neuropsychiatric Institute panel discussion by leading nursing theorists who responded to questions. One question directed to the theorists was on nursing diagnoses and their theories; typically, few theorists support nursing diagnosis "nonsense." No substitutes are provided.

Reimer M, Mills W, Letourneau S, editors: *Clinical judgment and decision making: the future with nursing diagnosis,* New York, 1987, Wiley. Papers from many countries about the development, research, implementation, and application of nursing diagnoses. Includes proceedings of a conference.

Rothberg JS: Why nursing diagnosis? *Am J Nurs* 67:1040, 1967. Argues that diagnosis is essential to professional practice and that nursing diagnosis ensures focus on the individual. Presents an early definition of the concept.

Soares CA: Nursing and medical diagnoses: a comparison of essential and variant features. In Chaska N, editor: *The nursing profession: views through the mist,* New York, 1978, McGraw-Hill. Outlines the diagnostic process in nursing and compares it with the diagnostic process in medicine. States that a nursing diagnosis must include the statement of the problem (a conflict in needs) and the indirect or direct causes associated with the problem.

Whitbeck C: What is a diagnosis? Some critical reflections, *Metamedicine* 2:319, 1981. Contrasts philosophical views of diagnosis and argues that it should be viewed within the context of clinical reasoning, intervention, and outcome.

See References, Chapters, 1, 2, and 3.

Legal and professional accountability in nursing diagnosis

Bruce JA, Snyder M: The legal side: the right and responsibility to diagnose, *Am J Nurs* 82:645, 1979. Discusses the legal applicability of nursing diagnosis and the professional right to use nursing diagnosis.

Connecticut Nurses Association: Do nurses diagnose? *Conn Nurs News* 48:7, 1975. Discusses the confusion that has resulted in various court cases due to the absence of a uniform definition for *diagnosis.*

Cushing M: Expanding the meaning of accountability, *Am J Nurs* 83:1202, 1983. Description of three court cases showing the increase in court decisions in favor of holding nurses accountable for exercising their judgment as health care professionals.

Cushing M: Matter of judgment, *Am J Nurs* 82:990, 1982. Discussion and examples of the legal aspects of clinical judgment.

Hershey N: The influence of charting upon liability determinations, *J Nurs Admin* 6:35, 1976. Discusses the importance of charting when a legal issue arises.

Hull RT: Responsibility and accountability analyzed, *Nurs Outlook* 29:707, 1981. An examination of the structure and function of responsibility that leads to a scheme to help clarify some current questions and issues.

Newton LH: To whom is the nurse accountable? A philosophical perspective, *Conn Med Suppl* 43:7, 1979. Discusses the dilemmas of accountability with which nurses are faced because of six types of accountability applicable in four different conceptions of health care.

Shoemaker J: How nursing diagnosis helps focus your care, *RN* 42:56, 1979. Describes nursing diagnosis as a simple, practical way of improving care. Steps in the diagnostic process and required diagnostic skills are discussed.

Warren JJ: Accountability and nursing diagnosis, *J Nurs Admin* 83:34, 1983. Addresses the fact that a taxonomy of nursing diagnoses improves communication within the domain of nursing practice and when implemented could improve nursing care and document nursing accountability.

See References, Chapter 10.

Diagnostic categories: research and development

Alexander CS, Becker HJ: The use of vignettes in survey research, *Pub Opin Q* 42:93, 1978. Methodology applicable to the study of nursing diagnosis is discussed.

Anderson J, Thomson A: Impaired skin integrity: clinical validation of the defining characteristics. In Carroll-Johnson R, editor: *Classification of nursing diagnoses: proceedings of the ninth conference,* Philadelphia, 1991, Lippincott, pp 126-132. Study involved assessing patients with impairments of the skin to develop a list of defining characteristics that would contribute to these validation efforts. A model of clinical inference is presented. Implications for developing diagnostic and taxonomic tools to guide holistic judgments are explored.

Avant K: Paths to concept development in nursing diagnosis, *Nurs Diagn* 2:105, 1991. Three pathways to diagnostic concept development are proposed. The principles and methods that operate on each path are presented.

Avant K: The art and science in nursing diagnosis development, *Nurs Diagn* 1(2):51, 1990. Examines issues confronting nurse clinicians, educators, and scientists interested in continued efforts to generate and validate diagnoses. Suggests tasks necessary for sound diagnosis development.

Berry K: Let's create diagnoses psych nurses can use, *Am J Nurs* 87:707, 1987. Points out the diagnoses that are not useful clinically because of their abstract nature and the lack of differential cues for certain diagnoses. Also points to the need for specific etiologies in order to guide intervention. Content provides ideas for conceptual work and clinical studies.

Brown M: The epidemiological approach to the study of clinical nursing diagnosis, *Nurs Forum* 13:346, 1974. Discusses the epidemiological method for establishing the prevalence, distribution, and causality of a nursing diagnosis. Outlines five criteria for the development of a taxonomy of nursing diagnoses.

Carpenito L: The NANDA definition of nursing diagnosis. In Carroll-Johnson R, editor: *Classification of nursing diagnoses: proceedings of the ninth conference,* Philadelphia, 1991, Lippincott, pp 65-71. Explores the elements of the NANDA definition of nursing diagnosis, drawing from both lay and nursing literature.

Fehring RJ: Validating diagnostic labels: standardized methodology. In Hurley M, editor: *Classification of nursing diagnoses: proceedings of the sixth conference,* St Louis, 1986, Mosby, pp 183-190. Discusses methods to establish reliability and validity estimates for diagnostic categories. Presents methods of handling data that result in reliability and validity scores for diagnostic categories.

Gordon M: Nursing diagnosis. In Werley HH, Fitzpatrick JJ, editors: *Annual review of nursing research,* vol 3, New York, 1985, Springer-Verlag. Reviews major studies in nursing diagnosis (large-sample studies). Concludes that diversity in aspects of methodology, analysis, and reporting does not facilitate combining results on the clinical validity and epidemiology of nursing diagnoses.

Gordon M: Predictive strategies in diagnostic tasks, *Nurs Res* 29:39, 1980. Report of a study of diagnostic strategies used to identify postsurgical complications. Methods are applicable to the study of nursing diagnostic reasoning.

Gordon M, Sweeney M, McKeehan K: Methodological problems and issues in identifying and standardizing nursing diagnosis, *Adv Nurs Sci* 2:1, 1980. Identifies conceptual issues in research on nursing diagnosis and presents three models for identifying and validating diagnostic categories. Interrater reliability of diagnosticians is discussed.

Gould MT: Nursing diagnoses concurrent with multiple sclerosis, *J Neurosurg Nurs* 15:339, 1983. A descriptive study identifying nursing diagnoses that are concurrent with the medical diagnosis of multiple sclerosis.

Goyette-Vincent K: Defining characteristics: general or population specific. In Carroll-Johnson R, editor: *Classification of nursing diagnoses: proceedings of the ninth conference,* Philadelphia, 1991, Lippincott, pp 76-78. Describes the debate surrounding defining characteristics: should those within a diagnosis remain general or should they identify population-specific differences?

Grant J, Kinney M: Using the Delphi technique to examine the content validity of nursing diagnoses, *Nurs Diagn* 3:12, 1992. Describes characteristics, background, advantages, and disadvantages of the Delphi technique. Contains suggested strategies for validating nursing diagnoses using this method.

Grant J, Kinney M, Guzzetta C: Using magnitude estimation scaling to examine the validity of nursing diagnoses, *Nurs Diagn* 1:64, 1990. Describes the use of magnitude estimation scaling as a methodologic strategy for validating the critical defining characteristics of nursing diagnoses.

Halloran EJ: Analysis of variation in nursing workload by patient medical and nursing condition, doctoral dissertation, Chicago, University of Illinois, College of Nursing, *Dissertation Abstracts International* 41:3385B, 1980. Presents data that contribute to information about epidemiology of nursing diagnoses; major purpose was to study nurse workload.

Hoskins LM, McFarlane EA, Rubenfeld MG et al: Nursing diagnosis in the chronically ill: methodology for clinical validation, *Adv Nurs Sci* 8:80, 1986. Describes a study that identified fifty nursing diagnoses in a chronically ill population, validated the diagnoses, and identified the defining characteristics of these diagnoses. Focuses on the methods used to derive and validate the nursing diagnoses.

Jones PE, Jakob DF: *Definition of nursing diagnosis, phase 3 and final report,* Toronto, 1983, Faculty of Nursing, University of Toronto. Presents a detailed report of a study of clinicians' diagnoses.

Kim MJ: Integrated methods for nursing diagnosis research. In Carroll-Johnson R, editor: *Classification of nursing diagnoses: proceedings of the ninth conference,* Philadelphia, 1991, Lippincott, pp 201-206. Suggests an integrated approach, using both qualitative and quantitative methods, as an ideal way to conduct nursing diagnosis validation research. A brief description of the theoretical distinctions between qualitative and quantitative approaches addresses potential variations in integrated approaches.

Logan J, Jenny J: Deriving a new nursing diagnosis through qualitative research: dysfunctional ventilatory weaning response, *Nurs Diagn* 1:37, 1990. Discusses the rationale for the diagnostic label of dysfunctional ventilatory weaning response and describes salient characteristics and interventions related to the diagnosis.

Loomis M, Conco D: Patients' perceptions of health, chronic illness, and nursing diagnoses, *Nurs Diagn* 2:162, 1991. Descriptive exploratory study that sought to determine how persons with chronic health problems define their experiences of health and illness and to determine their ability to identify their health problems using the list of NANDA-approved nursing diagnoses.

Maas M, Hardy M, Craft M: Some methodological considerations in nursing diagnosis research, *Nurs Diagn* 1:24, 1990. Methodological problems and issues are discussed and illustrated in the context of a descriptive study of the nursing diagnoses of patients at a large long-term care facility.

McCourt A: Syndromes in nursing: a continuing concern. In Carroll-Johnson R, editor: *Classification of nursing diagnoses: proceedings of the ninth conference,* Philadelphia, 1991, Lippincott, pp 79-82. Discusses concerns surrounding the application of the term *syndrome* to nursing; specifically, the concern regarding the definition of *syndrome* is addressed.

McFarlane E: Qualitative methods for nursing diagnosis research. In Carroll-Johnson R, editor: *Classification of nursing diagnoses: proceedings of the ninth conference,* Philadelphia, 1991, Lippincott, pp 185-191. Summarizes three papers presented at the conference that addressed specific qualitative methods, the responses that presented ways in which a specific method could be applied to nursing diagnosis research, and a synthesis of the conference's qualitative session.

Miers L: NANDA's definition of nursing diagnosis: a plea for conceptual clarity, *Nurs Diagn* 2:9, 1991. Concerns and questions regarding the conceptual, logical, and grammatical clarity of essential elements in the NANDA definition of nursing diagnosis are posed. Suggestions for clarification are offered.

Mills W: Nursing diagnosis: the importance of a definition, *Nurs Diagn* 2:3, 1991. Terminology that lacks clarity leads to difficulty in operationalizing definitions for taxonomic efforts and research. Suggestions are made to alleviate these difficulties.

Minton J, Creason N: Evaluation of admission nursing diagnoses, *Nurs Diagn* 2:119, 1991. Charts of 33 adult orthopedic patients were evaluated for the type, frequency, and quality of admission nursing diagnoses. Factors that affect the quality of nursing diagnoses and the need for tool refinement are discussed, and research recommendations are made.

Nurs Clin North Am 20: 609, 1985. Entire issue on studies of diagnostic categories.

Pierson M: Identification of a cluster of nursing diagnoses for a caregiver support group, *Nurs Diagn* 3:36, 1992. Identifies a cluster of nursing diagnoses thought to represent the problems and needs encountered by the community of caregivers. The process and content of the NANDA Taxonomy Committee's translation of nursing diagnoses into ICD code is presented.

Pinkley C: Exploring NANDA's definition of nursing diagnosis: linking diagnostic judgments with the selection of outcomes and interventions, *Nurs Diagn* 2:26, 1991. Explores the definition of nursing diagnosis from various perspectives.

Randell R: Signs and symptoms, etiologies, diagnostic labels: what do we mean and where do we want to go? In Carroll-Johnson R, editor: *Classification of nursing diagnoses: proceedings of the ninth conference,* Philadelphia, 1991, Lippincott, pp 72-75. Suggests that the Diagnosis Review Committee intends to clarify issues around signs/symptoms and etiologies so that submitters can address these dilemmas prior to submission, thereby facilitating the review process.

Rodgers BL: Deconstructing the dogma in nursing knowledge and practice, *Image* 23:177, 1991. Cites various areas of dogma in nursing and the risk that the taxonomy will achieve the status of dogma. States this has not yet occurred because of the continuing debate about and development of diagnostic statements.

Rottkamp B, Hurley M: Placement of diagnoses within Taxonomy II: development and process. In Carroll-Johnson R, editor: *Classification of nursing diagnoses: proceedings of the ninth conference,* Philadelphia, 1991, Lippincott, pp 30-34. The major focus of this paper is the conjunction and disjunction between and among diagnoses and their categorization in Taxonomy II.

Sawin K, Heard L: Nursing diagnoses used most frequently in rehabilitation nursing practice, *Rehabil Nurs* 17:256, 1992. Describes a study identifying nursing diagnoses used most frequently in rehabilitation nursing practice. Etiologies of the diagnoses are identified, and patterns of the use of diagnoses in community and inpatient settings are discussed.

Schroeder M: Quantitative methods for nursing diagnosis research. In Carroll-Johnson R, editor: *Classification of nursing diagnoses: proceedings of the ninth conference,* Philadelphia, 1991, Lippincott, pp 192-200. Presents a synthesis of quantitative methods presented at the Conference on Research Methods for Validating Nursing Diagnoses. Major topics addressed reliability and validity issues related to nursing diagnoses, the potential for the use of epidemiological research designs to validate nursing diagnoses, and the need for more sophisticated statistics for validation research.

Smith BA: When is "confusion" translocation syndrome? *Am J Nurs,* 86:1280, 1986. Raises questions about the differential diagnosis between the two conditions.

Tanner CA, Geddis-Hughes AM: Nursing diagnosis: issues in clinical practice research, *Top Clin Nurs* 5:30, 1984. Stresses that if nursing diagnosis is to influence practice positively, the existing nomenclature must be critically evaluated and systematically tested. Stresses that the measurements used to identify diagnoses must be relevant to everyday practice, reliable, valid, and sensitive.

Titler et al: Classification of nursing interventions for care of the integument, *Nurs Diagn* 2:45, 1991. Twelve nursing interventions and their associated activities for care of the integument were extracted from a large data base and validated through a two-round Delphi survey. Definitions, critical activities, and supporting activities were developed for each of these interventions.

Warren J: Implications of introducing axes into a classification system. In Carroll-Johnson R, editor: *Classification of nursing diagnoses: proceedings of the ninth conference,* Philadelphia, 1991, Lippincott, pp 38-44. Highlights some possible implications for the diagnoses and for the users of Taxonomy II. Proposes four axes: unit of analysis, age group, wellness, and illness.

Woodtli A: Validation of defining characteristics: clinical design, *J Neurosc Nurs* 20:324, 1988. Presents the need to determine the clinical validity of defining characteristics and discusses practical and design considerations.

See References, Chapter 11.

Specific diagnoses: research and development

Anderson J, Thomson A: *Impaired skin integrity:* clinical validation of the defining characteristics. In Carroll-Johnson R, editor: *Classification of nursing diagnoses: proceedings of the ninth conference,* Philadelphia, 1991, Lippincott, pp 126-132. Study involved assessing patients with impairments of the skin to develop a list of defining characteristics that would contribute to these validation efforts.

Capuano T, Hitchings K, Johnson S: Respiratory nursing diagnoses: practicing nurses' selection of defining characteristics, *Nurs Diagn* 1:169, 1990. Identifies which defining characteristics professional nurses working in acute care settings associate with each of the three respiratory nursing diagnoses identified by NANDA.

Evans SL: Descriptive criteria for the concept of depleted health potential, *Adv Nurs Science* 1:67, 1979. Presents the concept of depleted health potential, its criteria, and suggestions for its use as a diagnosis.

Gift A, Nield M: Dyspnea: a case for nursing diagnosis status, *Nurs Diagn* 2:66, 1991. Reviews the research concerning dyspnea and proposes this symptom for consideration as a nursing diagnosis.

Hardy M: A pilot study of the diagnosis and treatment of impaired skin integrity: dry skin in older persons, *Nurs Diagn* 1:57, 1990. Discusses a pilot study conducted to isolate the clinical indicators of dry skin in the elderly, test an instrument used to measure the dryness of skin, analyze the importance of factors thought to contribute to dry skin, test the effectiveness of an intervention for treating dry skin, and determine the feasibility of clinical implementation of the protocol.

Janken J, Cullinan C: A nursing diagnosis validation study: defining characteristics of spiritual distress. In Carroll-Johnson R, editor: *Classification of nursing diagnoses: proceedings of the ninth conference,* Philadelphia, 1991, Lippincott, pp 120-125. Descriptive study in which major defining characteristics for *Sensory Perceptual Alteration* are operationalized.

Janken J, Cullinan C: Auditory sensory/perceptual alteration: suggested revision of defining characteristics, *Nurs Diagn* 1:147, 1990. This correlational study of acutely ill geriatric patients suggests that a more accurate diagnosis of Sensory/ Perceptual Alteration can be made by knowing the patient's age and self-rating of hearing, and by checking ear canals for impacted cerumen, rather than by identifying currently accepted defining characteristics.

Jenny J, Logan J: Analyzing expert nursing practice to develop a new nursing diagnosis, dysfunctional ventilatory weaning response. In Carroll-Johnson R, editor: *Classification of nursing diagnoses: proceedings of the ninth conference,* Philadelphia, 1991, Lippincott, pp 133-140. Addresses the development of a new nursing diagnosis, dysfunctional ventilatory weaning response; the methodology, conceptual underpinnings, and rationale for the label; its definition; and its diagnostic attributes.

Kern L, Omery A: Decreased cardiac output in the critical care setting, *Nurs Diagn* 3:94, 1992. Suggests that the diagnosis Decreased Cardiac Output contains at least seven separate and specific components. Results of this exploratory descriptive study support six of these labels.

LeMone P: Analysis of a human phenomenon: self-concept, *Nurs Diagn* 2:126, 1991. Supports the use of the label *self-concept* as a broad category that encompasses the self-esteem, identity, and body-image nursing diagnoses within *Taxonomy I.*

Logan J, Jenny J: Interventions for the nursing diagnosis *dysfunctional ventilatory weaning response: a qualitative study.*

In Carroll-Johnson R, editor: *Classification of nursing diagnoses: proceedings of the ninth conference,* Philadelphia, 1991, pp141-147. Explores the knowledge, judgments, and actions used by expert critical care nurses to wean adult patients from mechanical ventilation. A new nursing diagnosis—*Dysfunctional Ventilatory Weaning Response*—is proposed. Describes actions used by nurses to treat dysfunctional responses seen during the weaning process.

McHolm F: A nursing diagnosis validation study: defining characteristics of spiritual distress. In Carroll-Johnson R, editor: *Classification of nursing diagnoses: proceedings of the ninth conference,* Philadelphia, 1991, Lippincott, pp 112-119. Identifies the defining characteristics of *Spiritual Distress* and compares them with the list presently approved by NANDA.

McKeighen R, Mehmert P: Bathing/Hygiene Self-Care Deficit: defining characteristics and related factors across age groups and diagnosis-related groups in an acute care setting, *Nurs Diagn* 1:155, 1990. Purpose was to validate the nursing diagnosis Bathing/Hygiene Self-Care Deficit. Strong support was found for two defining characteristics. The diagnosis was found among 80 diagnosis-related groups and across all age groups.

Mehmert P, Delaney C: Validating impaired physical mobility, *Nurs Diagn* 2:143, 1991. A study of the clinical presence of *Impaired Physical Mobility* documented in acute-care patients. Defining characteristics documented as empirical referents for the diagnosis were examined.

Ouellet L, Rush K: A synthesis of selected literature on mobility: a basis for studying impaired mobility, *Nurs Diagn* 3:72, 1992. Presents a consolidated multidisciplinary review of the literature related to the concept of mobility. Nursing's perspective is examined, including measurement of the concept.

Rakel B, Bulechek G: Development of alterations in learning: examination of nursing diagnoses for adults hospitalized with acquired immunodeficiency syndrome, *Nurs Diagn* 2:111, 1990. Literature on nursing care of the hospitalized adult with acquired immunodeficiency syndrome indicates that five of the nine highest-frequency problems in this population are physiological.

Rantz M: Reducing death from translocation syndrome, *Am J Nurs* 87:1351, 1987. Describes relationship between mortality statistics and moving long-term residents.

Summers S: Inadvertent hypothermia: clinical validation in postanesthesia patients, *Nurs Diagn* 3:54, 1992. Examines inadvertent hypothermia in postanesthesia patients. Findings indicate that its characteristics are distinctly different from the global nursing diagnosis of hypothermia. A review of the literature on hypothermia showed three distinct types of hypothermia: inadvertent, accidental, and intentional. Each type is distinguished by etiologies and defining characteristics and presented using the hypothetic model case approach.

Summers S et al: Validation of the nursing diagnosis *Hypothermia.* In Carroll-Johnson R, editor: *Classification of nursing diagnoses: proceedings of the ninth conference,* Philadelphia, 1991, Lippincott, pp 97-104. A validation of the nursing diagnosis *Hypothermia* is attempted. The researchers strongly urge consideration for the replacement of the nursing diagnosis of *Hypothermia* with *Alteration in Thermal Comfort.*

Thomas MD, Sanger E, Whitney JD: Nursing diagnosis of depression: clinical identification on an inpatient unit, *J Psy-*

chosoc Nurs Ment Health Serv 34:6, 1986. Identification of depression.

Thomas MD, et al: Nursing diagnosis of patients with manic and thought disorders, *Arch Psychiatr Nurs* 2:339, 1988. Presents diagnoses co-occuring with these disorders.

Wake M, Fehring R, Fadden T: Multinational validation of anxiety, hopelessness, and ineffective airway clearance, *Nurs Diagn* 2:57, 1991. Three diagnoses were tested—Anxiety, Hopelessness, and Ineffective Airway Clearance—through multinational validation. Defining characteristics rated as critical are presented.

Whitley G: Concept analysis of anxiety, *Nurs Diagn* 3:107, 1992. The nursing diagnosis of Anxiety is clarified through concept analysis. Antecedents and consequences are discussed. Empirical referents demonstrating the occurrence of Anxiety are determined, classified, and related to critical attributes.

Woods NF: Toward a holistic perspective of human sexuality: alterations in sexual health and nursing diagnoses, *Holistic Nurs Pract* 1:1, 1987. Discusses sexual development, response, and aging and sexuality. Maps out sexual function, self-concept, and role-relationships across the life span and comments on their integration. Five alterations in sexual health (possible nursing diagnoses) are discussed and interventions suggested.

DIAGNOSTIC CLASSIFICATION SYSTEM DEVELOPMENT
Process of development

Adelotte MK: Nursing taxonomies: state of the art. In McLane A, editor: *Classification of nursing diagnoses: proceedings of the seventh conference,* St Louis, 1987, Mosby, pp 1-16. Comprehensive review of taxonomy development and the difficulties in developing the discipline of nursing. Places taxonomy development in the context of the development of nursing knowledge, its domains, its classifications, and its language.

Beyea S: Concept analysis of feeling: a human response pattern, *Nurs Diagn* 3:97, 1990. Explores the concept of feeling, its historical foundations, and the use of this construct by other disciplines. An operational definition for feeling is proposed to facilitate the classification of nursing diagnoses in regard to the holistic nature of persons.

Burns C: Development and content validity testing of a comprehensive classification of diagnoses for pediatric nurse practitioners, *Nurs Diagn* 2:93, 1991. A conceptual framework was derived that identified, listed, and defined three domains of diagnoses: developmental problems, diseases, and daily living problems. A new method was used to sort diagnoses in a way that decreased overlaps among the domains.

Chang B et al: Self-care deficit with etiologies: reliability of measurement, *Nurs Diagn* 1:31, 1990. Examines the reliability of items in an assessment guide for the diagnostic label Self-Care Deficit and its etiologies/contributing factors.

Dickoff J, James P: Theoretical pluralism for nursing diagnosis. In Carroll-Johnson R, editor: *Classification of nursing diagnoses: proceedings of the eighth conference,* Philadelphia, 1987, Lippincott, pp 98-125. Proposes that the framework for nursing diagnosis should remain open. Pluralism

with an openness to all ideas about the focus of diagnosis is suggested.

Feinstein AR: Clinical biostatistics: what are the criteria for criteria? *Clin Biostat* 25:108, 1979. Presents an outline of the criteria for developing diagnostic criteria used in clinical decision making, many of which are adaptable to nursing diagnosis.

Fitzpatrick J: Taxonomy II: definitions and development. In Carroll-Johnson R, editor: *Classification of nursing diagnoses: proceedings of the ninth conference,* Philadelphia, 1991, Lippincott, pp 23-29. Provides background information about the nature and purposes of taxonomies or classification systems, representing scholarly opinions that guided the deliberations of the Taxonomy Committee. Describes the principles and processes that were part of the development of *Taxonomy II, Draft I,* including the new and expanded human response pattern definitions and the first draft of *Taxonomy II.*

Fitzpatrick J: The translation of NANDA Taxonomy I into ICD code. In Carroll-Johnson R, editor: *Classification of nursing diagnoses: proceedings of the ninth conference,* Philadelphia, 1991, Lippincott, pp 19-22. Presents the taxonomy submitted to WHO and the process of coding the diagnoses in the international format. Also presents the process and content of the NANDA Taxonomy Committee's translation of nursing diagnoses into ICD code. Introduction of the concept Conditions that Necessitate Nursing Care.

Fitzpatrick J: Conceptual basis for the organization and advancement of nursing knowledge: nursing diagnosis/taxonomy, *Nurs Diagn* 1:102, 1990. Analyzes the conceptualization embedded within the development of nursing diagnoses, including the historical perspective on this process.

Gebbie KA: Development of a taxonomy of nursing diagnoses. In Walter J, Pardee G, Molmo D, editors: *Dynamics of problem-oriented approaches: Patient care and documentation,* Philadelphia, 1976, Lippincott. Advocates development of nomenclature by utilizing inductive and deductive reasoning and a classification system for taxonomy preparation.

Gebbie K, Lavin MA: Classifying nursing diagnosis, *Mo Nurse* 42:10, 1973. The first contemporary article suggesting classification of nursing diagnoses. Defines nursing diagnosis, reviews status, and makes recommendations for future development.

Gordon M: Toward theory-based diagnostic categories, *Nurs Diagn* 1:5, 1990. Focuses on the need for four phases for developing the theoretical basis of each diagnostic category: diagnostic concept identification, concept analysis-model development, clinical validation, and construction/reconstruction of diagnostic categories.

Gordon M: Structure of diagnostic categories. In Hurley M, editor: *Classification of nursing diagnoses: proceedings of the sixth conference,* St Louis, 1986, Mosby, pp 39-49. Suggests considerations for developing and refining diagnostic categories. Examines current listing of diagnostic categories from the perspective of the diagnostic process in which they are used.

Goyette-Vincent K: Defining characteristics: general or population specific. In Carroll-Johnson R, editor: *Classification of nursing diagnoses: proceedings of the ninth conference,* Philadelphia, 1991, Lippincott, pp 76-78. Describes the debate surrounding defining characteristics: Should those within a diagnosis remain general or should they identify population-specific differences?

Grant J, Kinney M: The need for operational definitions for defining characteristics, *Nurs Diagn* 2:171, 1991. Argues for the need to develop operational definitions for defining characteristics to provide a reference for recognizing whether they are present in clinical practice.

Hoskins L: What is the focus of taxonomy II? Nursing diagnosis axes. In Carroll-Johnson R, editor: *Classification of nursing diagnoses: proceedings of the ninth conference,* Philadelphia, 1991, Lippincott, pp 35-37. Theoretical definitions are provided for the unit of analysis axis (individual, family, and community), the age-group axis, and for wellness and illness.

Hoskins L et al: Axes: focus of taxonomy II, *Nurs Diagn* 3:117, 1992. Describes the process and development of the proposed axes within the NANDA Taxonomy Committee.

Jones PE: A terminology for nursing diagnosis, *Adv Nurs Sci* 2:1, 1979. Reviews methods of describing nursing practice and taxonomy development. Describes a study to identify and validate diagnostic categories.

Jones PE, Jakob DF: *Definition of nursing diagnosis, phase 3 and final report,* 1983, Faculty of Nursing, University of Toronto. Defines nursing diagnosis and presents a detailed report of a study of clinicians' diagnoses. Presents a listing of nursing diagnoses, many of which are currently classified by the NANDA.

Kerr M: Validation of taxonomy. In Carroll-Johnson R, editor: *Classification of nursing diagnoses: proceedings of the ninth conference,* Philadelphia, 1991, Lippincott, pp 6-13. Several types and methods of developing and validating a taxonomic or classification structure are discussed. Highlights those used most frequently by a variety of disciplines, including nursing.

Kerr M et al: Development of definitions for *Taxonomy II, Nurs Diagn* 3:65, 1992. Outlines the process and decisions by which *Taxonomy II* of NANDA is evolving. Identifies specific problems encountered in the development of previous taxonomies and describes the steps in establishing the validity of the nine human response patterns.

Kritek PB: The generation and classification of nursing diagnoses: toward a theory of nursing, *Image* 10:33, 1978. Describes the current effort to classify diagnoses as first-level theory building.

Loomis M, Conco D: Patients' perceptions of health, chronic illness, and nursing diagnoses, *Nurs Diagn* 2:162, 1991. Descriptive exploratory study to determine how persons with chronic health problems define their experiences of health and illness and to determine their ability to identify their health problems on the list of NANDA-approved nursing diagnoses.

McCourt A: Syndromes in nursing: a continuing concern. In Carroll-Johnson R, editor: *Classification of nursing diagnoses: proceedings of the ninth conference,* Philadelphia, 1991, Lippincott, pp 79-82. Discusses concerns surrounding the application of the term *syndrome* to nursing. Reviews interdisciplinary literature and presents a definition of *syndrome.*

McKay RP: Research Q & A: what is the relationship between the development and utilization of a taxonomy and nursing theory? *Nurs Res* 26:222, 1977. Defines *taxonomy* and *clas-*

sification system. Discusses the major tasks in the development of a taxonomy of nursing diagnoses and its relevance to theory development.

Neumann PG: An attribute frequency model for the abstraction of prototypes, *Memory and Cognition* 2:241, 1974. Discussion and results of research to abstract prototype categories.

Porter E: Critical analysis of NANDA's Nursing Diagnosis Taxonomy I. *Image* 18:136, 1986. *NANDA Taxonomy I* is analyzed in relation to standards of taxonomy, its application to practice, and nursing theory. Presents an alternative scheme and the possibility of focusing on "ranges of appropriate nursing processes."

Randall R: Signs and symptoms, etiologies, diagnostic labels: what do we mean and where do we want to go? In Carroll-Johnson R, editor: *Classification of nursing diagnoses: proceedings of the ninth conference,* Philadelphia, 1991, Lippincott, pp 72-75. Suggests that the Diagnosis Review Committee intends to clarify issues around signs/symptoms and etiologies so that submitters can address these dilemmas prior to submission, thereby facilitating the review process.

Rasch R: The nature of taxonomy, *Image* 19:147, 1987. Proposes that Porter's identification of problems with the NANDA taxonomy reflects some general misunderstandings in nursing about taxonomy. Discusses the nature of and approaches to taxonomic development. (See also McCloskey J: *Image* 19:216, 1987 (letter). Corrects some "misconceptions" in the Porter and Rasch articles.)

Roy C: A diagnostic classification system for nursing, *Nurs Outlook* 23:90, 1975. Explores the rationale for a classification system in nursing. Lists principles of ordering a taxonomy and the deductive approach to its development. Discusses the implications of a diagnostic classification system in nursing practice, education, and research.

Vincent K, Coler M: A unified nursing diagnostic model, *Image* 22:93, 1990. A proposal to connect the taxonomic systems of NANDA and the ANA Council of Psychiatric-Mental Health Nursing.

Warren J: Implications of introducing axes into a classification system. In Carroll-Johnson R, editor: *Classification of nursing diagnoses: proceedings of the ninth conference,* Philadelphia, 1991, Lippincott, pp 38-44. Highlights some possible implications for the diagnoses and for the users of *Taxonomy II.* Proposes four axes: unit of analysis, age group, wellness, and illness.

Warren J, Hoskins L: The development of NANDA's nursing diagnosis taxonomy, *Nurs Diagn* 1:162, 1990. Details of the development of *Taxonomy I* are abstracted from the proceedings of the nine conferences and minutes of the Taxonomy Committee. Rules for the classification are presented, along with suggestions for taxonomic development and collaboration with other health care professions.

See References, Chapter 12.

Considerations in development

Briody M et al: Toward further understanding of nursing diagnosis: an interpretation, *Nurs Diagn* 3:124, 1992. Commentary on the direction of diagnostic category development. In defining phenomena of concern, the authors observe two types of conditions: nursing diagnoses and other responses requiring physician-prescribed interventions. They suggest that the NANDA list might be entitled "Conditions that Necessitate Nursing Care, with "Nursing Diagnoses" and "Collaborative Diagnoses" as subtitles.

Douglas D, Murphy EK: Nursing process, nursing diagnosis, and emerging taxonomies. In McCloskey J, Grace H, editors: *Current issues in nursing practice,* ed 2, Boston, 1985, Blackwell Scientific. Identifies issues in taxonomy development. Views current taxonomy development as expanding, clarifying, and defining the concepts underlying nursing process and nursing diagnosis.

Dracup K: Nursing diagnosis: a rose by any other name, *Heart and Lung* 12:211, 1983 (editorial). Comments on the use of terminology in a profession. Includes questions raised at a critical care conference regarding "physiological diagnoses."

Edel MK: Noncompliance: an appropriate nursing diagnosis? *Nurs Outlook* 33:183, 1985. Discusses compliance and its interpretations to evaluate Noncompliance as a nursing diagnosis. Concludes that elimination of Noncompliance as a nursing diagnosis would encourage greater therapeutic alliances with patients, giving patients greater choices in alternative treatments.

Fawcett J: The metaparadigm of nursing: present status and future refinements, *Image* 16:84, 1984. The central concepts and themes of the discipline of nursing are identified and formalized as nursing's metaparadigm. Examples are given, and refinements are proposed.

Field L, Winslow EH: Moving to a nursing model, *Am J Nurs* 85:1100, 1985. Presents excerpts and a summary of a position paper on medical-surgical nursing that describes the current transition from a medical to a nursing model of practice. Views the nursing model as the focus for nursing diagnosis. Notes that the medical model is useful in working with physicians in the diagnosis and treatment of disease but that it is the nursing model that will help nurses achieve autonomy and control of their practice.

Geissler E: Nursing diagnoses: a study of cultural relevance, *J Prof Nurs* 8:301, 1992. Reports a study of three diagnoses that points to the work needed on defining characteristics and etiological factors and the need to select research problems carefully. Uses one diagnosis, Impaired Verbal Communication related to Cultural Differences, which leads to problems in formulation. The implication is that "cultural differences" is the focus for intervention.

Gleit CJ, Tatro S: Nursing diagnoses for healthy individuals, *Nurs Health Care* 2:456, 1981. Suggests a classification of wellness diagnoses and that an emphasis on wellness can lead to a more cost-effective health care system.

Good M: Noncompliance may be an appropriate diagnosis, *Nurs Outlook* 33:267, 1985 (letter). Response to the paper by Edel cited above. Suggests that nurses let go of their negative view of the word *compliance* and view it from the perspective of self-care. Also see the letter by R (Toth) Haddon in the same issue.

Gordon M: Diagnostic category development. In McCloskey J, Grace H, editors: *Current issues in nursing practice,* ed 2, Boston, 1985, Blackwell Scientific. Discusses category development in the context of clinical reasoning and the factors that require attention in development and refinement.

Hagey RS, McDonough P: The problem of professional labeling, *Nurs Outlook* 32:151, 1984. Discusses the problems that can occur in diagnostic labeling when it is used to save time or meet institutional obligations. Provides many ideas for thought and discussion.

Hinshaw AS: Nursing diagnosis: forging the link between theory and practice. In Carroll-Johnson R, editor: *Classification of nursing diagnoses: proceedings of the eighth conference,* Philadelphia, 1989, Lippincott, pp 3-10. Points to the need for research on each diagnosis and encourages this line of development.

Jacoby M: The dilemma of physiological problems: eliminating the double standard, *Am J Nurs* 85:281, 1985. Explores the conceptual focus of nursing diagnosis, particularly the issue of physiological problems. Stresses the need for clinical research to validate the situations and populations in which nurses diagnose and independently treat physiological malfunctions and potential malfunctions.

Jones PE, Jakob DF: *Definition of nursing diagnosis, phase 3 and final report,* 1983, Faculty of Nursing, University of Toronto. Defines nursing diagnosis and presents a detailed report of a study of clinicians' diagnoses. Presents a listing of nursing diagnoses, many of which are currently classified by NANDA.

Jones PE, Jakob D: Nursing diagnosis: differentiating fear and anxiety, *Nurs Papers (McGill Univ)* 14:20, 1981. Results of a study that suggests nurses commit diagnostic errors in the identification of fear and anxiety. Suggestions presented for improving diagnostic accuracy.

Kim MJ: The dilemma of physiological problems: without collaboration, what's left? *Am J Nurs* 85:281, 1985. Discusses the need for the identification and classification of physiological problems nurses use in practice. Stresses the need to represent the diversity in nursing practice by including the collaborative, or interdependent, domain of practice.

Kritek PK: Nursing diagnosis in perspective: response to a critique, *Image* 17:3, 1985. Analyzes and discusses issues raised in a paper published by Shamansky and Yanni (see below).

Leininger AM: Issues, questions, and concerns related to the nursing diagnosis cultural movement from a transcultural nursing perspective, *J Transcult Nurs* 2:23, 1990; and Feild L: Response of Feild to Leininger's nursing diagnosis article, *J Transcult Nurs* 3:25, 1991. Critique and response to the critique of the development of nursing diagnoses from a cultural perspective.

Lindsey AM: Identification and labeling of human responses, *J Prof Nurs* 6:143, 1990. Discusses the need for identifying human responses, risk factors, influencing factors, and interventions. Introduces the concept of life processes that are related in the total functioning human. Relates human responses to life processes, social policy statement, and level of complexity. The need for defining the characteristics and influencing factors is supported.

Loomis ME, Wood DJ: Cure: the potential outcome of nursing care, *Image* 15:4, 1983. Presents a method of classification and proposes that in the diagnosis and treatment of human responses, nurses are capable of curing the actual or potential health problem.

Lunney M: Nursing diagnosis—refining the system, *Am J Nurs* 82:456, 1982. Suggests a naming system for nursing diagnoses that includes (1) the broad pattern or process that is altered or dysfunctional and (2) the specific factors that contribute to the unhealthful response and that are the focus of intervention.

Martens K: Let's diagnose strengths, not just problems, *Am J Nurs* 86:192, 1986. Stresses the importance of identifying positive resources in the client situation and suggests that nursing diagnosis be expanded to include these strengths; gives examples of diagnostic statements of this type.

McKay R, Segall M: Methods and models for the aggregate, *Nurs Outlook* 31:328, 1983. Presents a model for community nursing that incorporates nursing diagnosis as an element to be identified in community research and education.

Mitchell P, Gallucci B, Fought S: Perspectives on human response to health and illness, *Nurs Outlook* 39:154, 1991. Examines the concept of human responses.

Newman MA: Nursing diagnosis: looking at the whole, *Am J Nurs* 84:1496, 1984. Discusses a model that incorporates patterns developed for a taxonomy of nursing diagnoses.

Pridham KE, Schutz ME: Rationale for a language for naming problems, *Image* 17:122, 1985. Suggests that many of the experiences patients have and that nursing addresses defy classification. Views current diagnoses as relevant to other disciplines as well as nursing and thus as not helpful in defining nursing as a distinct discipline. Presents criteria for a nomenclature system.

Rottkamp B, Hurley M: Placement of diagnoses within Taxonomy II: development and process. In Carroll-Johnson R, editor: *Classification of nursing diagnoses: proceedings of the ninth conference,* Philadelphia, 1991, Lippincott, pp 30-34. Major focus of this paper is the conjunction and dysjunction between and among diagnoses and their categorization in Taxonomy II.

Roy C Sr: A diagnostic classification system for nursing, *Nurs Outlook* 23:90, 1975. Explores the rationale for a classification system in nursing. Lists principles of ordering a taxonomy and the deductive approach to its development. Discusses the implications of a diagnostic classification system in nursing practice, education, and research.

Shamansky SL, Yanni CR: In opposition to nursing diagnosis: a minority opinion, *Image* 15:47, 1983. Examines the premises underlying nurses' diagnoses and their impact on clinicians and the health care delivery system.

Shoemaker JK: Essential features of a nursing diagnosis. In Kim MJ, McFarland G, McLean A, editors: *Classification of nursing diagnoses: proceedings of the fifth national conference,* St Louis, 1984, Mosby, pp 104-115. Characteristics of a nursing diagnosis based on a national study.

Simmons DA: *Classification scheme for client problems in community health nursing,* Rockville, MD, 1980, US Government Printing Office. Nomenclature and classification system developed and tested by the Visiting Nurse Service of Omaha to describe nursing problems in community health and to be used in computerized clinical information systems. Many diagnostic categories are similar to the NANDA listing of diagnoses.

Soares CA: Nursing and medical diagnoses: a comparison of essential and variant features. In Chaska N, editor: *The nursing profession: views through the mist,* New York, 1978, McGraw-Hill. Presents a framework for classification of nursing diagnoses.

Stanitis MA, Ryan J: Noncompliance: an unacceptable diagnosis? *Am J Nurs* 82:941, 1982. Discusses the diagnosis of Noncompliance and concludes it is a negative, counterproductive label that may lead to inappropriate nursing behaviors.

Suppe F, Jacox AK: Philosophy of science and the development of nursing theory. In Werley HH, Fitzpatrick JJ, editors: *Annual review of nursing research,* vol 3, New York, 1985, Springer-Verlag. Views taxonomy as a type of conceptual framework and reviews literature on diagnostic taxonomy in the context of philosophy of science and nursing theory development. Includes a review of the evaluation of theories and conceptual frameworks.

Vincent P: Noncompliance may be an appropriate diagnosis, *Nurs Outlook* 33:266, 1985 (letter). Response to the paper by Edel cited above. Suggests the issue to be debated is not *if* Noncompliance is an appropriate nursing diagnosis but *when* it is appropriate. Also see author's response, p. 266.

See References, Chapter 12.

Reports on classification system development (NANDA)

Gebbie KA, Lavin MA, editors: *Classification of nursing diagnoses: proceedings of the first national conference,* St Louis, 1975, Mosby. Reports the first organized effort to classify diagnoses at the First National Conference on Classification of Nursing Diagnoses (1973) and the diagnoses that resulted. Includes papers on various classification systems in medicine; the nature of classification; and its implications for practice, education, and research. Contains diagnoses identified in 1973.

Gebbie KA, editor: *Summary of the second national conference: classification of nursing diagnoses,* St Louis, 1976. National Group for Classification of Nursing Diagnoses. Contains accepted nursing diagnoses, 1975.

Kim MJ, Moritz DA, editors: *Classification of nursing diagnoses: proceedings of the third and fourth national conference,* New York, 1982, McGraw-Hill. Contains accepted nursing diagnoses, 1980. Includes papers on various subjects related to nursing diagnosis, issues in implementation, and research.

Loomis ME, et al: Development of a classification system for psychiatric/mental health nursing: individual response class, *Arch Psychiatr Nurs* 1:16, 1987.

Kim MJ, McFarland G, McLane A, editors: *Classification of nursing diagnoses: proceedings of the fifth conference,* St Louis, 1984, Mosby. Contains new nursing diagnoses accepted in 1982 and papers on classification development and issues, research, implementation, and use in related areas of practice. First bylaws of the newly designated North American Nursing Diagnosis Association (NANDA).

Hurley M, editor: *Classification of nursing diagnoses: proceedings of the sixth conference,* St Louis, 1986, Mosby. Contains accepted nursing diagnoses, 1984. Includes papers on classification, taxonomic structure, quality assurance, DRGs, implementation, and computerization. Includes research papers on specific nursing diagnoses, their use in practice, diagnostic process, and research methodology.

McLane A, editor: *Classification of nursing diagnoses: proceedings of the seventh conference,* St. Louis, 1987, Mosby. Includes major papers presented, developments in diagnosis and taxonomy, research paper abstracts, and current listing of nursing diagnoses, 1986.

Carroll-Johnson R, editor: *Classification of nursing diagnoses: proceedings of the eighth conference,* St Louis, 1990, Mosby. Includes major papers presented, developments in diagnosis and taxonomy, research papers and abstracts, and current listing of nursing diagnoses, 1988.

Carroll-Johnson R, editor: *Classification of nursing diagnoses: proceedings of the ninth conference,* Philadelphia, 1992, Lippincott. Includes major papers presented, developments in diagnosis and taxonomy, research papers and abstracts, and current listing of nursing diagnoses, 1990.

Carroll-Johnson R, editor: *Classification of nursing diagnoses: proceedings of the tenth conference,* Philadelphia, 1993, Lippincott. Includes major papers, developments in diagnosis and taxonomy, research papers and abstracts, and current listing of nursing diagnoses, 1993.

Visiting Nurse Service of Omaha, *Client management information system for community health nursing agencies,* Washington, DC, 1986, US Department of Health and Human Services. Classification of problems in community health nursing. There is an overlap with NANDA diagnostic categories. See References, Chapter 12.

IMPLEMENTATION OF NURSING DIAGNOSIS

Bulechek G, et al: An evaluation guide to assist with implementation of nursing diagnosis, *Nurs Diagn* 1:18, 1990. A guide organized around elements of professional practice is developed to assist with the implementation of nursing diagnosis.

Bryne-Coker et al: Implementing nursing diagnoses within the context of King's conceptual framework, *Nurs Diagn* 1:107, 1990. A tool designed for categorizing NANDA's nursing diagnoses according to the concepts and systems of King's conceptual framework; the utility of the tool was tested.

Maas ML, Specht JP: Implementation of nursing diagnosis: maturation of a professional model of practice. In McCloskey J, Grace H, editors: *Current issues in nursing practice,* ed 2, Boston, 1985, Blackwell Scientific. Discusses the development of a professional model of practice and the implementation of nursing diagnoses.

Rantz M: Implementation of nursing diagnosis: a Symposium, *Nurs Clin North Am* 22:873, 19. Papers describing the process of implementation in various settings.

Thomas N, Newsome G: Factors affecting the use of nursing diagnoses, *Nurs Outlook* 40:182, 1992. Discusses factors affecting nurses and the ability to use diagnoses; cites some data on implementation in practice. The only correlation with self-ratings of ability was the use of diagnoses by the employee setting.

Young MS, Lucas CM: Nursing diagnosis: common problems in implementation, *Top Clin Nurs* 5:68, 1984. Discusses implementing nursing diagnosis in the health care setting, including particular problems of implementation and possible solutions to these problems.

DIAGNOSTIC PROCESS

Agan D: Intuitive knowing as a dimension of nursing, *Adv Nurs Sci* 10:63, 1987. Qualitative study of seven nurses' intuitive knowing.

Aspinall MJ: Development of a patient-completed questionnaire and its comparison with the nursing interview, *Nurs Res* 24:377, 1975. Study that compares the effectiveness of assessment by questionnaire and by interview. More errors were made by unstructured interview, and this method consumed more time. Important limitations of the study are cited.

Aspinall MJ, Tanner CA: *Decision making for patient care: applying the nursing process,* New York, 1981, Appleton-Century-Crofts. Chapter on clinical decision making provides an overview of the subject. Remaining chapters are on specific clinical topics, some of which are nursing diagnoses.

Barrows H, Feltovich P: The clinical reasoning process, *J Med Educ* 21:86, 1987. Describes the badly structured nature of clinical problems and the temporal unfolding of information. Discusses models of the clinical reasoning process.

Benderly B: Everyday intuition, *Psych Today,* 215, September, 1989. Basic description of intuition and current thoughts on its use in everyday and professional thinking.

Benner P: *From novice to expert,* Menlo Park, CA, 1984, Addison-Wesley. Major work on the description of the clinical judgment and expertise of nurses. Defines seven domains of competencies in nursing practice.

Benner P, Tanner C: Clinical judgment: how expert nurses use intuition, *Am J Nurs* 87:23, 1987. Study of intuitive judgments of 21 nurses identified as experts and a description of pattern recognition and its development.

Berner ES: Paradigms and problem solving: a literature review, *J Med Educ* 59:625, 1984. Suggests that Kuhn's ideas help to explain the conflicting research results that have appeared in problem-solving research. Underlying assumptions about the process are explored.

Bieri J, et al: *Clinical and social judgment,* New York, 1966, Wiley. Report of some of the early formulations of information-processing theory as applied in clinical judgment. Reports of methods applicable to nursing studies of judgment.

Billings RS, Marcus SA: Measures of compensatory and noncompensatory models of decision behavior: process tracing versus policy capturing, *Organiz Behav Hum Perform* 31:331, 1983. Presents models for studying decisions that are applicable to the study of clinical judgment in nursing.

Bourbonnais FF, Baumann A: Crisis decision making in coronary care: a replication study, *Nurs Papers (McGill Univ)* 17:4, 1985. Study of the rapid decision making of nurses. Concludes that knowledge and experience are the two most important factors influencing decision making.

Brykczynski K: An interpretive study describing the clinical judgment of nurse practitioners, *Sch Inquiry Nurs Pract* 3:75, 1989. Study of transcripts of 22 nurses' judgments to uncover knowledge embedded in practice using Benner's framework and domains.

Buckhout R: Eyewitness testimony, *Sci Am* 231:23, 1974. Discussion of biases in observation that are applicable to data collection in nursing.

College of Nursing, Texas Women's University: *Monograph, fall 1979: nursing diagnoses,* Denton, TX, 1979, The College of Nursing. An overview of the status of nursing diagnosis. Includes reports of three research studies (concept attainment, relation between logical reasoning and diagnosis, and restlessness).

Corcoran-Perry S, Graves J: Supplemental-information-seeking behavior of cardiovascular nurses, *Res Nurs Health,* 13:119, 1990. This study revealed that patient-specific, institution-specific, and domain knowledge were most frequently sought in decision making.

Dawes R et al: Clinical versus actuarial judgment, *Science* 243:1668, 1989. Discusses the two approaches to decision making. Cites research to support the superiority of the actuarial approach in terms of accuracy and the factors underlying its greater accuracy.

deChesnay M: Problem solving in nursing, *Image* 15:8, 1983. Levels of problems and the nursing process are linked to a change theory to explain the dynamics of labeling clients as difficult patients.

Derdierian A: Etiology: practical relevance. In McLane A, editor: *Classification of nursing diagnoses: proceedings of the seventh conference,* St Louis, 1987, Mosby. Discusses the need for the concept of etiology.

Detmer DE, Fryback DG, Gassner K: Heuristics and biases in medical decision-making, *J Med Educ* 53:682, 1978. Discusses the biases in clinical reasoning. Applicable to nursing diagnosis.

Devine P, Sherman S: Intuitive versus rational judgment and the role of stereotyping in the human condition: Kirk or Spock? *Psychol Inquiry* 3:153, 1992. Examines the potentiality for errors and stereotyping in quick, intuitive, thinking and in the indiscriminate use of social categories.

Doona ME: The judgment process in nursing, *Image* 8:27, 1976. Discusses the importance of clinical judgment in nursing and analyzes phases and types of judgment.

Eckman P, Friesen WV: *Unmasking the face: guide to recognizing emotions from facial expressions,* Englewood Cliffs, NJ, 1975. Prentice-Hall. Assessment guidelines for identifying facial expressions and underlying feelings. Also presents information about emotional states and skill training exercises.

Einhorn HJ, Hogarth RM: Ambiguity and uncertainty in probabilistic inference. *Psychol Rev* 94:433, 1985. A study of how people make decisions under ambiguous and uncertain conditions, such as clinical practice situations.

Elstein AS, et al: Medical decisions in perspective: applied research in cognitive psychology, *Perspect Biol Med* 26:486, 1983. Description of a cognitive model for describing clinical diagnosis in the professions.

Engel J et al: A social judgment perspective on clinical problem solving, *Eval Health Prof* 13:63, 1990. Review of the current status of social judgment theory as applied to reasoning. Describes two problem areas associated with the theory.

Gerrity PL: Perception in nursing: the value of intuition, *Holistic Nurs Pract* 1:63, 1987. Argues for the inclusion of intuition in nursing and that nursing has emphasized sensory perception at the expense of intuitive perception. This, it is argued, leads to seeing the individual in parts but missing the whole person. Sees linear thinking as the mode for clarifying and communicating that which is understood by intuition.

Gordon M: The nurse as thinking practitioner. In Hannah KJ et al, editors: *Clinical judgment and decision making: the future with nursing diagnosis,* New York, 1987, Wiley. Description of the types of clinical judgment used in nursing: diagnostic, therapeutic, and ethical. Describes each and focuses discussion on diagnostic reasoning and judgment.

Gordon M: Predictive strategies in diagnostic tasks, *Nurs Res* 29:39, 1980. Report of a study of nurses' hypothesis testing strategies. Implications for nursing history and diagnosis are discussed.

Gordon M: Nursing diagnosis and the diagnostic process, *Am J Nurs* 76:1276, 1976. Defines nursing diagnosis in terms of concept and structure (PES) and discusses the diagnostic process.

Grier MR: Information processing in nursing practice. In HH Werley, Fitzpatrick, editors: *Annual review of nursing research,* vol 2, New York, 1984, Springer-Verlag. Major review of studies using the information-processing model of judgment and decision making.

Greeno J: A perspective on thinking, *Am Psychol* 44:134, 1989. Outlines the assumptions underlying research on thinking, epistemology, and conceptual competence. Suggests a reformulation.

Hamm R: Moment-by-moment variation in experts' analytic and intuitive cognitive activity, *IEEE Trans Syst Man Cybern* 18:757, 1988. Study analyzing the variations in reasoning in complex engineering tasks.

Hammond KR: Clinical inference in nursing: a psychologist's viewpoint, *Nurs Res* 15:27, 1966. One of a series of articles often quoted as the first studies of clinical judgment in nursing. Presents a 1966 analysis of cognitive tasks encountered by nurses. Views these tasks as complex because the nurse must think "as" the doctor thinks when making judgments.

Hammond K, et al: Direct comparison of the efficacy of intuitive and analytical cognition in expert judgment, *IEEE Trans Syst Man Cybern* 17:753, 1987. Use of a continuum of reasoning in a study of engineers. Accuracy was related to the degree of correspondence of the subjects' reasoning mode with the nature of the task. Emphasizes the need for considering task variables.

Keren G: On the importance of identifying the correct problem space, *Cognition* 16:121, 1984. Discusses the concept of the problem space in the cognitive processing of information.

Kleinmuntz B: Why we still use our heads instead of formulas: toward an integrative approach, *Psychol Bull* 107:296, 1990. Reviews the controversy, biases, and constraints that cause decision errors and proposes correctives.

Knill-Jones RP: Clinical decision making. II. Diagnostic and prognostic inference. *Health Bull* 35:213, 1977. Application of probability and decision theory to clinical inference.

Koran LM: The reliability of clinical methods, data and judgments, *N Engl J Med* 293:695, 1975. Points out the difficulties in the reliability of clinical judgments.

Lanza M, Bantly A: Decision analysis: a method to improve quality of care for nursing practice, *J Nurs Care Quart* 6:60, 1991. Describes decision analysis and indicators of care that can be developed using this method.

Lazare A: The psychiatric examination in the walk-in clinic: hypothesis generation and hypothesis testing, *Arch Gen Psychiatry* 33:96, 1976. Useful in regard to the discussion of hypothesis generation and testing.

Lerners D: Intuition in nursing practice, *J Holistic Nurs* 10:137, 1992. Report of an ethnographic study of intuition that connects findings to caring.

Lindgren C: Diagnostic reasoning in the care of a vocally disruptive, severely demented patient, *Scand J Caring Sci* 6:97, 1992.

Lunney M: Accuracy of nursing diagnoses: concept development, *Nurs Diagn* 1:12, 1990. The concept of accuracy of nursing diagnoses is developed as a first step of theory development related to nursing diagnosis.

Marson D, et al: Psychiatric decision making in the emergency room: a research overview, *Am J Psychiatry* 145:918, 1988. Reviews the methodology and findings of studies in this area and concludes with a synthesis of the findings.

McCarthy MM: The nursing process: application of current thinking in clinical problem solving, *J Adv Nurs* 6:173, 1981. Explores the components of nursing process and diagnosis.

McGuire CH: Medical problem solving: a critique of the literature, *J Med Educ* 60:587, 1985. Review of research findings. Suggests that current research in medical problem solving consists of small samples and microscopic analyses, which have not contributed to the understanding of problem solving.

Mitchell T, Beach L: ". . . Do I love thee: Let me count . . .," Toward an understanding of intuitive and automatic decision making, *Organiz Behav Human Decis Proc* 47:1, 1990. Proposes image theory as a descriptive theory of decision making. Decisions are made to the extent to which alternatives fit with images. Presents research supporting the theory.

Moritz DA: Nursing histories: a guide, yes; a form, no, *Oncol Nurs Forum* 6:18, 1979. The use of a checklist for nursing histories is viewed as a questionable practice. Argues that the way each area in an assessment is pursued and described varies with the concerns and patterns encountered in clients.

Newsome G, Tillman M: Effects of guided design and lecture teaching strategies on knowledge recall and on problem-solving performance of student nurses, *Nurs Diagn* 1:89, 1990. Compares the effect of guided design and lecture teaching strategies on the clinical problem-solving performance of first-quarter student nurses.

Nu NV: Medical problem solving assessment: a review of methods and instruments, *Eval Health Prof* 2:281, 1979. A review of the instruments and methods employed to measure problem solving.

Payne J, Bettman J: Behavioral decision research: a constructive processing perspective, *Ann Rev Psychol* 43:87, 1992. A review of the research in decision making under uncertainty and an overview of the frameworks and aids to decision making.

Phillips LR, Rempusheski VF: Decision-making model for diagnosing and intervening in elder abuse and neglect, *Nurs Res* 34:134, 1985. Presents a model for decision making in suspected elder abuse. The model, which includes variables influencing decision making, is adaptable to nursing diagnosis of other conditions.

Putzier DJ, Padrick KP: Nursing diagnosis: a component of nursing process and decision making, *Top Clin Nurs* 5:21, 1984. Describes the use of nursing diagnosis in each step of nursing process. Views nursing diagnosis as the pivotal factor in decision making. Contrasts this to symptom management and gives some case studies in application.

Radwin L: Research on diagnostic reasoning in nursing, *Nurs Diag* 1:70, 1990. Presents a synthesis of research in diagnostic reasoning to date; identifies common themes and offers suggestions for future work.

Randell B: NANDA versus the Johnson Behavioral Systems Model: is there a diagnostic difference? In Carroll-Johnson R, editor: *Classification of nursing diagnoses: proceedings of the ninth conference,* Philadelphia, 1991, Lippincott, pp 154-160. Examines the most frequently occurring diagnoses generated using the NANDA categories and the Johnson Behavioral Systems Model labels. Defining characteristics and related factors from each set of diagnoses are compared to determine differences in problem identification using the two approaches.

Rew L: Intuition in decision making, *Image* 20:150, 1988. Report of research on intuitive experiences of nurses in critical care and home care settings. Themes were consistent with three characteristics of intuition found in the nursing literature.

Rew L: Intuition: concept analysis of a group phenomenon, *Adv Nurs Sci* 10:49, 1986. Concept analysis using the method of Walker and Avant. Suggestions for application in nursing.

Rew L, Barrow E: Intuition: a neglected hallmark of nursing knowledge, *Adv Nurs Sci* 10:49, 1987. Traces intuition in nursing literature from 1900 to 1985. Concludes that intuition is neglected in the literature.

Rogers JC: Clinical reasoning: ethics, science, art, *Am J Occup Ther* 37:601, 1983. Excellent paper on aspects of clinical reasoning. Discussed in the context of clinical reasoning in occupational therapy.

Rosenhan DL: On being sane in insane places, *Science* 179:250, 1973. Report of a study involving pseudopatients in a psychiatric hospital and the influence of setting on diagnosis. Demonstrates how preconceptions can influence judgment and the labeling of clients.

Shead C, Readance J: An investigation of the inference and mapping processes of the componential theory of analogical reasoning, *J Educ Res* 81:347, 1988. Discusses the theory of analogical reasoning and its five components. Reports a study of the model.

Slater V: Modern physics, synchronicity, and intuition, *Holistic Nurs Pract* 6:20, 1992. Describes Jung's concept of synchronicity. Offers an analysis of this concept and a discussion of intuition.

Smith E, Langston C, Nisbett R: The case for rules in reasoning, *Cogn Sci* 16:1, 1992. Discusses the controversy in the use of abstract rules in reasoning. Proposes guidelines for research to determine if people use rules in reasoning. Suggests a model for combining instance and rule models.

Simon HA: The information-processing explanation of Gestalt phenomena, *Comput Hum Behav* 2:241, 1987. Presents arguments claiming that computer programs in the published literature simulate exactly what Gestalt theorists describe as "insight." This behavior can be explained in terms of recognition processes.

Simon HA: How big is a chunk? *Science* 183:482, 1974. Discusses the concept of chunking information. Applicable to information processing in diagnostic judgment.

Spector R: *Cultural diversity in health and illness,* New York, 1992, Appleton-Century-Crofts. Useful ideas about culture and symptoms and the influence of culture on judgments about other people.

Tanner C et al: Diagnostic reasoning strategies of nurses and nursing students, *Nurs Res* 36:356, 1987. Report of a study of clinical reasoning using high-fidelity simulations.

Young C: Intuition and nursing process, *Holistic Nurs Pract* 1:52, 1987. Reviews the literature on tacit knowing and presents the findings of a study of nurses' judgments and the use of a qualitative knowledge scale.

Zerwekh J: True detectives, *Am J Nurs* 91:30, 1991. Descriptions of public health nurses' critical thinking and reasoning in solving family problems.
See References, chapters 7, 8, and 9.

Functional health patterns

Beyea S, Matzo M: Assessing elders using the functional health pattern assessment model, *Nurse Educ* 14:32, 1989.

Bryant SO, Kopeski LM: Psychiatric nursing assessment of the eating disorder client, *Top Clin Nurs* 8:57, 1986.

Burns C: Development and content validity testing of a comprehensive classification of diagnoses for pediatric nurse practitioners, *Nurs Diagn* 2:93, 1991.

Burns C: *Development and field testing of a classification of diagnoses for use by pediatric nurse practitioners,* Doctoral dissertation, Eugene, OR, 1989, University of Oregon.

Coler MS, Vincent KG: Coded nursing diagnoses on axes: a prioritized, computer-ready diagnostic system for psychiatric-mental health nurses, *Arch Psychiatr Nurs* 1:125, 1987.

Collard A, Jones DA, Fitzmaurice J: The occurrence of nursing diagnosis in ambulatory care. In McLane A, editor: *Classification of nursing diagnoses: proceedings of the seventh conference,* St Louis, 1987, Mosby, pp 283-289.

Corrigan JO: Functional health pattern assessment in the emergency department, *J Emerg Nurs* 12:163, 1986.

Decker SD, Knight L: Functional health pattern assessment: a seasonal farmworker community, *J Comm Health Nurs* 7:141, 1990.

DiBlasi M, Savage J: Revitalizing a documentation system, *Rehabil Nurs* 17:27, 1992.

Dion P, Fitzmaurice J, Baer C: Organization of patient assessment data and nursing diagnosis. In McLane A, editor: *Classification of nursing diagnoses: proceedings of the seventh conference,* St Louis, 1987, Mosby, pp 169-173.

Doyer B, Macker N, Radovich H: Functional health patterns: a post-anesthesia care unit's approach to identification, *J Post-Anesth Nursing* 5:157, 1990.

Gilmartin ME: Patient and family education, *Clin Chest Med* 7:619, 1986.

Gordon M: *Nursing diagnosis: process and application,* New York, 1987, McGraw-Hill, pp 91-161.

Gordon M: Practice-based data set for a nursing information system, *J Med Syst* 9:43, 1985.

Greenlee KK: Effects of implementation of an operational definition and guidelines for the formulation of nursing diagnoses in a critical care setting. In Carroll-Johnson R, editor: *Classification of nursing diagnoses: proceedings of the ninth conference,* Philadelphia, 1991, Lippincott, pp 274-275.

Hanna D, Wyman N: Assessment + diagnosis = care planning: a tool for coordination, *Nurs Manage* 18:106, 1989.

Hartman D, Knudson J: Documentation: a nursing data base for initial patient assessment, *Oncol Nurs Forum* 18:125, 1991.

Henning M: Comparison of nursing diagnostic statements using a functional health pattern and health history/body systems format. In Carroll-Johnson R, editor: *Classification of nursing diagnoses: proceedings of the ninth conference,* Philadelphia, 1991, Lippincott, pp 278-279.

Herberth L, Gosnell DJ: Nursing diagnosis for oncology nursing practice, *Cancer Nurs* 10:41, 1987.

Hirschfield-Bartek J, Dow KH: Decreasing documentation time using a patient self-assessment tool, *Oncol Nurs Forum* 17:251, 1990.

Leahy MK: Using nursing diagnosis as an organizing framework in an integrated curriculum. In *From theory to practice. Abstracts of the second nursing theory congress,* University of Toronto College of Nursing, Toronto, 1988, p 65.

Levin RF, Crosley JM: Focused data collection for the generation of nursing diagnoses, *J Nurs Staff Develop* 4:56, 1986.

McFarland G, Thomas MD: *Psychiatric mental health nursing,* Philadelphia, 1990, Lippincott, pp 499-512.

Mumma CM, editor: *Rehabilitation nursing: concepts and practice: a core curriculum,* ed 2, Evanston, IL, 1987, Rehabilitation Nursing Foundation.

Nettle C, Jones N, Pifer P: Community nursing diagnoses, *Community Health Nurs* 6:135, 1989.

Phelan C, Finnell MD, Mottla KA: A patient self-assessment tool for cardiac rehabilitation, *Rehabil Nurs* 14:81, 84, 1989.

Rantz M, Miller TV: How diagnoses are changing in long term care, *Am J Nurs* 87:360, 1987.

Rossi L: Organizing data for nursing diagnosis using functional health patterns. In McLane A, editor: *Classification of nursing diagnoses: proceedings of the seventh conference,* St Louis, Mosby, pp 97-102.

Tompkins ES: In support of the discipline of nursing: a nursing assessment, *Nurs Connections* 2:21, 1989.

Ward CR: Proportion of specific agreement as a measure of intrarater reliability in the diagnostic process. In McLane A, editor: *Classification of nursing diagnoses: proceedings of the seventh conference,* St Louis, 1987, Mosby, pp 169-173.

Westwell J et al: Health patterns assessment: a form designed to allow psychiatric nurses to practice theoretical pluralism. In *From theory to practice: abstracts of the second nursing theory congress,* Toronto, 1988.

Woodtli MA, Van Ort S: Nursing diagnoses and functional health patterns in patients receiving external radiation therapy: cancer of the head and neck, *Nurs Diagn* 2:171, 1991.

APPLICATION
Specialties and settings

Clark SR: Nursing diagnosis: its application in an ambulatory-care setting, *Top Clin Nurs* 5:57, 1984. Shows, through example, the use of nursing process and nursing diagnosis in the ambulatory care setting.

Davidson SB: Nursing diagnosis: its application in the acute-care setting, *Top Clin Nurs* 5:50, 1984. Attempts to clarify the differences between what nurses diagnose and what physicians diagnose. Uses a conceptual framework and diagnostic process.

Fredette S, Gloriant FS: Nursing diagnosis in cancer chemotherapy, *Am J Nurs* 81:2013, 1981. Discusses the concept of nursing diagnosis and identifies diagnoses in patients undergoing cancer chemotherapy.

Gleit CJ, Tatro S: Nursing diagnoses for healthy individuals, *Nurs Health Care* 2:456, 1981. Suggests more liberal use of diagnosis as a basis for activities related to the promotion of high-level wellness. Also suggests that the use of wellness diagnoses can lead to a more cost-effective health care system.

Guzzetta CE, Dossey BM: Nursing diagnosis: framework, pro-

ANNOTATED BIBLIOGRAPHY **403**

cess and problems, *Heart Lung* 12:281, 1983. Discusses nursing diagnosis, diagnostic process, and issues related to classification.

Hauck MR, Roth D: Application of nursing diagnoses in a pediatric clinic, *Pediatr Nurs* 10:49, 1984. Suggests that nursing diagnoses can help nurses analyze their observations and identify interventions. Views nursing diagnosis as enhancing accountability, responsibility, and pride in nursing care.

Kim MJ: Nursing diagnosis in critical care, *Dimens Crit Care Nurs* 2:5, 1983. Discussion of nursing diagnosis and the issues surrounding diagnosis in critical care.

Lister DW: The nursing diagnosis movement and the Occupational Health Nurse, *Occup Health Nurs* 31:11, 1983. Discusses what nursing diagnosis is and how its implementation is beneficial to nursing care.

McKay R, Segall M: Methods and models for the aggregate, *Nurs Outlook* 31:328, 1983. Discusses how and why graduate programs in public health nursing should clarify the relationship between community and aggregate.

Occup Health Nurs 33: August, 1985. Entire issue is devoted to diagnosis.

Parisi B: Nursing diagnosis: application for renal nurses, *Dial Transplant* 12:362, 1983. The structure of nursing diagnosis and its application to the overall nursing process is defined, and a case report is presented as a learning exercise.

Rantz M, Miller T, Jacobs C: Nursing diagnosis in long term care, *Am J Nurs* 85:916, 926, 1985. Report of the implementation of nursing diagnosis and interdisciplinary care planning in a nursing home. Identifies five common diagnoses in long-term care.

Simmons DA: *Classification scheme for client problems in community health nursing,* Rockville, MD, 1980, HRA-80, US Government Printing Office. Nomenclature and classification system developed and tested by the Visiting Nurse Service of Omaha to describe nursing problems in community health, to be used in computerized clinical information systems. Many diagnostic categories are similar to the NANDA listing of diagnoses.

Symposium on nursing diagnosis, *Heart Lung* 14, 1985. Has four articles related to critical care.

Taylor JW: Nursing management of stroke. I. Acute care, *Cardiovasc Nurs* 21:1, 1985. Identifies nursing diagnoses common in patients in the acute phase after a stroke.

Tilton C, Maloff M: Diagnosing the problems in stroke, *Am J Nurs* 82:597, 1982. Identifies nursing diagnoses common in cerebrovascular accidents.

Care delivery

Delaney C, Mehmert P: Utility of the nursing minimum data set in validation of computerized nursing diagnoses. In Carroll-Johnson R, editor: *Classification of nursing diagnoses: proceedings of the ninth conference,* Philadelphia, 1991, Lippincott, pp 175-179. Assesses the utility of the Nursing Minimum Data Set for validating the defining characteristics of the nursing diagnostic labels associated with alterations in fluid balance.

Gordon M: Practice-based data set for a nursing information system, *J Med Syst* 9:43, 1985. Examines the nursing practice components for a nursing data set within an NIS.

Halloran EJ: Nursing workload, medical diagnosis related

groups, and nursing diagnoses, *Res Nurs Health* 8:421, 1985. Reports a study of these variables and concludes that the best predictors of resources consumed are nursing and medical diagnoses and an acuity factor.

Halloran EJ: RN staffing: more care—less cost, *Nurs Manage* 14:18, 1983. A study on types of staffing and related costs, showing that a more highly qualified staff (and more RNs) can lead to greater attention to total patient needs and decrease the cost of nursing care.

Halloran EJ, Kiley M: Nursing dependency, diagnosis-related groups, and length of hospital stay, *Health Care Financ Rev* 8:27, 1987. Report of a study indicating that nursing diagnoses explain the length of hospital stays.

Halloran E, Halloran DC: Exploring the DRG/nursing equation, *Am J Nurs* 85:1093, 1985. Report of a study demonstrating that predicting total hospital costs may be more accurate using a combination of nursing diagnosis and DRGs, as opposed to using either one alone.

Happ M, Kerr M: Nursing effort and the exchanging human response pattern, *Nurs Diagn* 2:155, 1991. Provides information about how nurses allocate time for the treatment of actual and potential nursing diagnoses from the exchanging human response pattern and outlines areas for further development in diagnosis-based patient classification.

Lancour J: Nursing diagnosis and the effectiveness initiative, *Nurs Diagn* 2:33, 1991. The link between nursing diagnosis, outcomes, and interventions is discussed, and the role of nursing diagnosis in the overall nursing classification scheme is highlighted. Discusses guideline development, dissemination of research findings, data base development, and effectiveness and outcomes research.

Long Island Jewish–Hillside Medical Center: *Computerized nursing care planning: utilizing nursing diagnosis,* Washington, DC, 1985, Oryn Publications. Describes a computer system that incorporates nursing diagnoses. Includes screens for diagnostic categories and information on signs and symptoms, related factors, patient outcomes, nursing care plan, specificities, and evaluations, each validated by a consensus of nurse experts.

McCourt AE: The measurement of functional deficit in quality assurance, *Qual Assur Update* 5:1, 1981. Discusses the diagnoses *Self-Care Deficit* and levels used in formulating the diagnosis.

Rantz M, Miller TV: How diagnoses are changing in long-term care, *Am J Nurs* 87:360, 1987. Compares data on nursing diagnoses in this specialty over a period of years. Changes are related to changes in health care delivery.

Young DE, Ventura MR: Application of nursing diagnosis in quality assessment research, *Qual Assur Update* 4:1, 1980. Discusses the application of nursing diagnosis in the development of diagnostic outcome and the process criteria for three accepted nursing diagnoses. Argues that combining medical and nursing diagnoses more clearly defines the population to be assessed than using medical diagnosis alone.

Werley HH, Grier MR: *Nursing information systems,* New York, 1981, Springer. Report of a research conference on nursing information systems, June 1977. Sections on nursing diagnoses, clinical decision making, standardization of nomenclature, use of diagnosis in client classification–nurse staffing, and other topics related to clinical information processing.

Westfall UE: Nursing diagnosis: its use in quality assurance,

Top Clin Nurs 5:78, 1984. Clarifies the terms *nursing diagnosis* and *quality assurance* by exploring their definitions, the interrelationships of the two, and the operational problems encountered when linking the two.
See References, Chapters 10 and 11.

Education

American Association of Colleges of Nursing: *Essentials of college and university education for nursing,* Washington, DC, 1986, The Association. Describes the essential content of a baccalaureate education. Emphasizes clinical judgment.

Beyerman K: Nursing diagnosis crossword puzzle, *Nurse Educ* 12:45, 1987. Provides a crossword puzzle that can be used as an educational tool.

Fredette S, O'Connor K: Nursing diagnosis in teaching and curriculum planning, *Nurs Clin North Am* 14:541, 1979. Discussion of nursing diagnosis as the focus of theoretical and clinical study in educational programs. Examples are given of increasing competency in diagnosis as the learner progresses in the educational program.

Gaines BC, McFarland MB: Nursing diagnosis: its relationship to and use in nursing education, *Top Clin Nurs* 5:39, 1984. Reviews the concept and presents a study of the use of nursing diagnosis in schools of nursing.

Gebbie KA: Fee-based reimbursement using nursing diagnosis. In McLane A, editor: *Classification of nursing diagnosis: proceedings of the seventh conference,* St Louis, 1987, Mosby, pp 37-52. Raises questions about reimbursement for nursing diagnoses—why it has not occurred, why is it sought, and what are the things to be done before this can happen.

Holden G, Klingner A: Learning from experience: differences in how novice vs expert nurses diagnose why an infant is crying, *J Nurs Educ* 27:23, 1988.

Howe KR, Holmes M, Elstein AS: Teaching clinical decision making, *J Med Philos* 9:215, 1984. Outlines the process and presents teaching methodologies that are applicable to nursing.

Jacoby MK, Adams DJ: Teaching assessment of client functioning, *Nurs Outlook* 29:248, 1981. Discusses the systematic ordering of data in nursing diagnosis and offers guidelines for students.

Kemp VH: Concept analysis as a strategy for promoting critical thinking, *J Nurs Educ* 24:382, 1985. Describes the process of concept analysis and identifies the usefulness of this strategy for the development of critical thinking, which is an essential component of scientific inquiry.

Lee HA, Strong KA: Using nursing diagnosis to describe the clinical competence of baccalaureate and associate degree graduating students: a comparative study, *Image* 17:82, 1985. Report of a study comparing professional and technical nursing students' conceptions of clinical competence with the expectations of their nursing faculty, using a nursing diagnosis framework.

Lunney M: Development of written case studies as simulations of diagnosis in nursing, *Nurs Diagn* 3:23, 1992. Presents guidelines and methods for the systematic development of valid and reliable case studies as simulations of diagnosis in nursing.

Morris JL: Nursing diagnosis: a focus for continuing education, *J Contin Educ Nurs* 13:33, 1982. Report of a continuing education program that uses nursing diagnosis as a focus. Describes implementation of the focus in programming.

Saarmann L, et al: Relationship of education to critical thinking ability and values among nurses: socialization into professional nursing, *J Prof Nurs* 8:26, 1992. A study that compares the critical thinking ability of ADN-prepared, BSN-prepared registered nurses, nursing faculty, and sophomore college students in nursing. Finding: Faculty did not score significantly higher in these abilities when the study was controlled for age, although it is assumed that they are agents of socialization for students.

Thiele J et al: An investigation of decision theory: what are the effects of teaching cue recognition? *J Nurs Educ* 25:319, 1986. An investigation of the effect of teaching cue recognition. Findings: Cue recognition, cue sorting, and cue linking can be taught and can improve the accuracy of clinical decisions.

Watts FN: Clinical judgment and clinical training, *Br J Med Psychol* 53:95, 1980. A detailed exploration of the process of clinical judgment and a review of the research and theory on the teaching of clinical judgment.

Weber J, Smith D: Name that nursing diagnosis: a gaming-simulation, *Nurs Diagn* 2:79, 1991. A gaming-simulation was developed as an alternative strategy for teaching nursing diagnostic skills.

Name and Title Index

SUBJECT INDEX

A

Acquired immune deficiency syndrome (AIDS), 105
  practice guidelines, 220
Activity-exercise pattern, 84-86, 109-112
  activity intolerance, 110
  decreased cardiac output, 112
  developmental delay, 111
  diversional activity deficit, 110-111
  impaired home maintenance management, 110
  ineffective airway clearance, 111-112
  joint contractures, 111
  self-care deficit, 111
  subjective descriptions, 85
Adaptation model, 58-59
  client focus, 58
  nursing goal, 58
  theorist's view of diagnosis, 58-59
Agency for Health Care Policy and Research, 220,
    256, 258, 260, 275
America, 34, 35
American Academy of Nursing Expert Panel, 75
American Association of Colleges of Nursing, 5, 39,
    280, 301
American Association of Critical Care Nurses, 219
American Medical Association, 226
American Nurses Association (ANA), 4-8, 33, 36, 66,
    198, 220, 221, 248, 261, 270, 275, 282, 297,
    304
  Congress of Nursing Practice, 270
  Council on Computer Applications, 8
  Model Practice Act, 33
  Social Policy Statement, 36, 270, 282
  Social Policy Task Force, 7
  Steering Committee on Databases to Support
    Clinical Nursing Practice, 263
  Task Force on Case Management, 268
American Psychiatric Association, 45
Amsterdam, 275
ANA; *see* American Nurses Association
Assessment
  admission documentation, 236
  analytical inference, 143-144

Assessment—cont'd
  categories, 99-100
  clinical information collection, 121-151
  clinical knowledge, 138-140
  critically ill, 97-99
  emergency, 132-133
  format, adapting, 97-99
  formulating diagnostic statement, 197
  functional health patterns, 69-100
  going beyond information given, 143-145
  handling uncertain clues in clinical judgment,
    136-138
  infant and child, 97
  initial, 122-130
    nursing history and examination, 125
    probability of health problems, 124
    psychological set: client, 123-124
    psychological set: nurse, 122-123
    purpose and scope, 122
    structure of information collection, 125
  intuition/analytical thinking, 145-150
  intuitive inference, 144-145
  model, search for unified
    different assessment tool, 66
    diversity in nursing models, 67
    nursing science, 66
    standardization of assessment, 67
    unification of assessment structure, 67
  novice and expert, 146-150
  perceptual recognition, 140-143
  problem-focused, 130-132
    probability of health problems, 131
    purpose and scope, 131
    structure for information collection, 131-132
  professional responsibility, 121
  review of findings, 196-197
  situational context, 122
    cues, 133-136
    nature of clinical information, 133-136
  structure, unification, 67
  systematic approach, 121
  time-lapse reassessment, 133-136

411